The Languages of Psyche

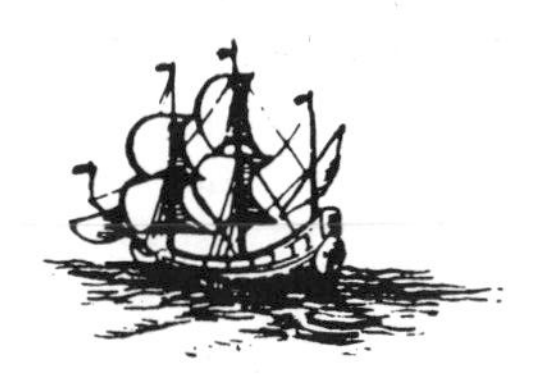

PUBLISHED UNDER THE AUSPICES OF THE
WILLIAM ANDREWS CLARK MEMORIAL LIBRARY
UNIVERSITY OF CALIFORNIA, LOS ANGELES

Publications from the
CLARK LIBRARY PROFESSORSHIP, UCLA

1.
England in the Restoration and Early Eighteenth Century: Essays on Culture and Society
Edited by H. T. Swedenberg, Jr.

2.
Illustrious Evidence: Approaches to English Literature of the Early Seventeenth Century
Edited by Earl Miner

4.
English Literature in the Age of Disguise
Edited by Maximillian E. Novak

5.
Culture and Politics: From Puritanism to the Enlightenment
Edited by Perez Zagorin

6.
The Stage and the Page: London's "Whole Show" in the Eighteenth-Century Theatre
Edited by Geo. Winchester Stone, Jr.

7.
England's Rise to Greatness, 1660–1763
Edited by Stephen B. Baxter

8.
The Uses of Science in the Age of Newton
Edited by John G. Burke

9.
Studies in Eighteenth-Century British Art and Aesthetics
Edited by Ralph Cohen

10.
The Golden & The Brazen World: Papers in Literature and History, 1650–1800
Edited by John M. Wallace

11.
Background to Discovery: Pacific Exploration from Dampier to Cook
Edited by Derek Howse

12.
The Languages of Psyche: Mind and Body in Enlightenment Thought
Edited by G. S. Rousseau

The Languages of Psyche

Mind and Body in Enlightenment Thought

Clark Library Lectures 1985–1986

EDITED BY

G. S. Rousseau

Clark Library Professor, 1985–1986

UNIVERSITY OF CALIFORNIA PRESS

Berkeley Los Angeles Oxford

University of California Press
Berkeley and Los Angeles, California
University of California Press
Oxford, England

Printed in the United States of America

1 2 3 4 5 6 7 8 9

Library of Congress Cataloging-in-Publication Data

The Languages of psyche: mind and body in Enlightenment thought: Clark Library lectures, 1985–1986 / edited by G. S. Rousseau.
p. cm.
ISBN 0–520–07044–5 (alk. paper).—
ISBN 0–520–07119–0 (pbk.: alk. paper)
1. Mind and body—History. 2. Enlightenment. I. Rousseau. G. S. (George Sebastian) II. Title: Clark Library lectures.
BF171.L32 1990
128′.2′09033—dc20 90–34872
CIP

The paper used in this publication meets the minimum requirements of American National Standard for Information Sciences—Permanence of Paper for Printed Library Materials, ANSI Z39.48–1984 ∞

For Norman Thrower,
Director of the Clark Library 1981–1987,
who can read this book,
and
the late Donald G. O'Malley,
who cannot.

CONTENTS

LIST OF PLATES

PREFACE

When Norman Thrower, then the Director of the William Andrews Clark Memorial Library at UCLA, invited me to serve as the Clark Library Professor for 1985–86, I immediately realized that the subject to be privileged should be the mind/body relation viewed within broad cultural and scientific contexts, and against the complexities of Enlightenment theory and practice. Here was a topic that had not been worked over by specialists, or generalists, in the field; a topic, moreover, of terrific contemporary impact, as men and women from diverse walks of life wonder how their minds and bodies—surely parts of one, indivisible, holistic unit—ever came to be separated.

My own research interests in the relations of science and medicine to the imaginative art forms generated during the Enlightenment were so interdisciplinary that I began to envision ways in which these subjects could be transformed into a useful annual series. The mind/body relation inevitably straddles the interstices of the sciences and the humanities: that no-man's-land lying between Scylla and Charybdis—territories still deemed worthy of special study to us today and which we have come to take for granted, yet a relation that was coming into its own during the seventeenth and eighteenth centuries.

More locally in southern California, medicine had been omitted from the Clark Library's programs from the inception of the Clark Professor Series, yet not by design. The late Donald G. O'Malley, a distinguished professor of the history of medicine at UCLA and the author of an important biography of Vesalius, the pioneering Renaissance anatomist, had died in 1969, while in the midst of planning just such a series at the

Clark Library. Dr. O'Malley would have executed his task with the characteristic dedication and thoroughness for which he was known during his lifetime. Had he lived long enough to prepare a volume similar to this one, I know it would have made a significant contribution to the frontiers of knowledge, and although he cannot read this book, I feel certain that he would have encouraged its conception and execution in every possible way. To both these able scholar-administrators—Norman Thrower and D. C. O'Malley—this volume is dedicated.

Yet ultimately the measure of this book's success will be determined by its diverse readership and by the nine contributors, all of whom were willing to take time from their own work and academic-administrative obligations at their home institutions to pursue the common theme of this volume: mind and body during the European Enlightenment. The team itself was vigilantly selected with regard to disciplinary affinity, national origin, geographical location, and even generational point of view, gender, and methodology: all these to provide balance and variety to an area—the complex relations of mind and body in an epoch of intense intellectual ferment—in which new paths prove hard to find. If, then, a common theoretical underpinning is perceived to be missing from the ten essays, or if it is adjudged that here less attention is paid to methodology than some readers would like, this derives, in part, as a direct consequence of the death of the first participant—the late Michel Foucault—and as the result of the liberty given to all the participants ensuring that they could follow their own researches.

Foucault had agreed to provide a theoretical framework of just the type for which he was deservedly renowned—specifically, to illuminate the semiotics and signposts of mind and body during the Enlightenment. Had he lived to participate in this volume, he would no doubt have performed his task with characteristic brilliance and bravura. I was therefore relieved when Roy Porter consented to replace him. Porter had already agreed to participate in the series, but not in the opening slot, and I continue to remain in his debt for assisting me at a time when assistance was direly needed. As if this kindness were insufficient, Porter also collaborated with me in composing the opening essay which, we hope, will tie together the threads of this complex subject.

Chapters 2 through 10 were originally delivered as public lectures in Los Angeles from October 1985 to June 1986, each describing an aspect of the representation of mind and body during the Enlightenment. The introduction was not delivered in the series, but aims to contextualize the topic and introduce the various approaches—not by listing or comparing them in any systematic way but by locating them within a continuum of discourses and critiques suggestive of the immense complexity of the problem. The introduction—"Toward a Natural History of Mind and Body"—also aims to describe the tangled web and vast historiography of the subject.

Even so, our collective approach in the volume remains eclectic, especially with reference to national cultures, and none of the contributors seeks to provide an exhaustive, let alone complete, view of his or her topic in any sense in which completeness can be construed. The approaches, coming from the domains of social history and the history of religions, the history of science and the history of medicine, literary criticism and literary theory, and—of course—philosophy, themselves serve as diversified commentaries on the endurance of the mind/body problem in our time and its resonance over three centuries. That mind and body should continue to serve as vital metaphors for these disciplines—in literary criticism, for example—attests, as well, to the resonance of the concept into our own era. Still, nowhere do the authors (again individually or collectively) suggest that the mind/body split is in any scientific or objective sense *valid*, or endorse it as a philosophically defensible doctrine in any of its dualistic, or neodualistic, versions. Our intention has not been to take sides and decide these matters once and for all, but to trace origins and chart continuities—to tease out the metaphors and tropes that continue to haunt late-twentieth-century civilized discourse. Indeed, the problematization of the notion of *validity* for the mind/body relation is precisely what we have identified as our subject. And we consider it our collective task to assess the status of the split in Europe during the period of the seventeenth and eighteenth centuries (in this book commonly referred to for convenience as the Enlightenment).

Always, our task was eased by the Clark's Librarian, Dr. Thomas Wright, and his deputy, Dr. John Bidwell, and was also facilitated by the staff of the institution, who accord their guests so many acts of kindness. The volume, more specifically its editor, incurred a number of debts during the annual series that must be acknowledged, even if briefly. Susan Green assisted us even before the series opened by meticulous supervision of every aspect of its daily operations; and Carol Briggs, now resident in London but then very much a member of the Clark's staff, proved most useful on those leisurely Friday afternoons when the scholars gathered with the public, delivered their talks, and engaged in lively and sometimes heated debate about these controversial subjects. Dr. Franklin D. Murphy, the former Chancellor of UCLA, supported the series on mind and body with a grant given by the Ahmanson Foundation. Sandra Guideman transformed the long and complex initial manuscript into the final manuscript, which Nicholas Goodhue copyedited for the press. My chair at UCLA, Professor Daniel A. Calder, released me from various duties in the Department of English so that I could focus my attention in 1986–87 on the book, during the year after the series was delivered. Dr. Gerald Kissler, our Vice-Provost at UCLA, supported the series in a number of ways during the actual year, and Provost Raymond Orbach provided us with funding that ensured the publication of this volume. Professor Herbert Morris, our Dean of Humanities in the College of Letters and Science at UCLA, aided us under two hats: in his administrative capacity and, as crucially, as a philosopher who came to some of our meetings and asked hard questions. Most tangibly, Scott Mahler, our editor at the University of California Press, performed a multiplicity of kindnesses and services too numerous to be itemized here.

To all these friends of *The Languages of Psyche,* and to the others whose names do not appear because the Preface would have swelled to Brobdingnagian proportions if the full roll call had been produced, we express our deep gratitude and thanks.

University of California, Los Angeles G. S. Rousseau

CONTRIBUTORS

Carol Houlihan Flynn is Professor of English at Tufts University.

Philippa Foot, regarded by her colleagues as one of the most influential moral philosophers of her generation, holds the Gloria and Paul Griffin Chair in Philosophy at the University of California, Los Angeles, and is Senior Research Fellow at Somerville College, Oxford University, Oxford.

Robert G. Frank, Jr. is Associate Professor of Anatomy and History at the University of California, Los Angeles.

Antonie M. Luyendijk-Elshout is Emeritus Professor of the History of Medicine at the University of Leiden, Holland, and a Trustee of the National Boerhaave Museum.

David B. Morris, formerly Professor of English at the University of Iowa, is a free-lance writer who lives in Kalamazoo, Michigan.

Richard H. Popkin is Adjunct Professor of History and Philosophy at the University of California, Los Angeles, and the doyen of historians of skepticism. He served as Clark Library Professor at UCLA in 1981–82.

Roy Porter is Lecturer in the Social History of Medicine at the Wellcome Institute for the History of Medicine, London, and served as Clark Library Professor at UCLA in 1988–89.

G. S. Rousseau served as Clark Library Professor at UCLA in 1985–86, where he is Professor of English and Eighteenth-Century Studies.

Simon Schaffer is Lecturer in the History and Philosophy of Science at Cambridge University, and a Fellow of Darwin College.

Dora B. Weiner is Professor of Medical Humanities at the University of California, Los Angeles.

EPIGRAPHS

I know that a Triangle is not a Square, and that Body is not Mind, as the *Child knows that Nurse that feeds it is neither the Cat it plays with, nor the Blackmoor it is afraid of,* and the Child and I come by our Knowledge after the same Manner.

—Mary Astell, *The Christian Religion, As Profess'd by a Daughter of the Church of England* (London, 1705), 95.

For mark the Order of things, according to *their* [the metaphysicians'] account of them. First comes that huge Body, *the sensible World.* Then this and its Attributes beget *sensible ideas.* Then out of sensible Ideas, by a kind of lopping and pruning, are made *ideas intelligible, whether specific or general.* Thus, should they admit that MIND was coeval with BODY, yet *till* BODY *gave its Ideas,* and awakened its dormant Powers, it could at best have been nothing more, than *a sort of dead Capacity*: for INNATE IDEAS *it could not possibly have any.*

—James Harris, *Hermes; or, A Philosophical Inquiry concerning Language* (London, 1756), 392–393.

I find my spirits and my health affect each other reciprocally—that is to say, everything that discomposes my mind, produces a correspondent disorder in my body; and my bodily complaints are remarkably mitigated by those considerations that dissipate the clouds of mental chagrin.

—Tobias Smollett, *The Expedition of Humphry Clinker* (London, 1771), Mathew Bramble to Doctor Lewis, June 26.

Descartes appeared to have fallen rather out of love with geometry and physics, and liked to imagine (for this apostle of reason was singularly prone to imagining) the workings of the living organism. Indeed, in spite of his efforts to separate Psyche from the body and from extension, he went to great lengths to find her a cerebral habitation and to demonstrate that this location was indispensable for the purpose of feeling.

—Paul Valéry, *Masters and Friends* (Princeton, 1968), 64–65; originally published in French in 1918.

How is it, that the visual picture proceeds—if that is the right word—from an electrical disturbance in the brain?

—Sir Charles Sherrington, *Man on His Nature* (Cambridge, 1946), 125.

The compulsive urge to cruelty and destruction springs from the organic displacement of the relationship between the mind and body.

—Max Horkheimer and Theodor W. Adorno, *Dialectic of Enlightenment* (New York, 1972), 233; originally published in German in 1944.

Curiously, for a society that believes in a mind superior to the body, we extol behavior in which the mind is said to be absorbed in the body, in contrast to a sexual act in which the mind may be detached from the body. . . . The mind/body dichotomy itself can be seen as an extension of the body, expressing symbolically the separate functions of the left and right hemispheres of the brain.

—John Blacking, *The Anthropology of the Body* (London and New York, 1977), 20.

At one time many people adhered to what the philosopher Gilbert Ryle called the 'official view' of the relationship between mind and body (or brain), which can be traced back at least to Descartes. According to this view, mind (or soul) is a type of substance, a special type of ephemeral, intangible substance, different from, but coupled to, the very tangible sort of stuff of which our bodies are made. Mind, then, is a *thing* which can have states—mental states—that can be altered (by receiving sense data) as a result of its coupling to the brain. But this is not all. The link which couples brain and mind works both ways, enabling us to impress our will upon our brains, hence bodies.

Today, however, these dualistic ideas have fallen out of favor with many scientists, who prefer to regard the brain as a highly complex, but otherwise unmysterious electrochemical machine, subject to the laws of physics in the same way as any other machine.

—P. C. W. Davies et al., *The Ghost in the Atom: A Discussion of the Mysteries of Quantum Physics* (Cambridge, 1986), 32.

Progress lies in the direction of disengagement from the social and medical sciences, and through greater cooperation between historians and literary scholars. The old boundaries between fact and fiction, the real and the imagined, subject and object have been breached. Now comes the task of reconnecting mind and body.

—John R. Gillis, *Annals of Scholarship* 5, 4 (1988): 523.

There is a straight ladder from the atom to the grain of sand, and the only real mystery in physics is the missing rung. Below it, particle physics; above it, classical physics; but in between, metaphysics. All the mystery in life turns out to be this same mystery, the join between things which are distinct and yet continuous, body and mind.

—Tom Stoppard, *Hapgood* (London, 1988), 49–50.

PART ONE

Theories of Mind and Body

ONE

Introduction: Toward a Natural History of Mind and Body

G. S. Rousseau and Roy Porter

I

The mind/body problem has long taxed Western thought. This book is not, however, another contribution to the philosophical argument about mind/body relations per se.[1] Rather, the common endeavor uniting these essays amounts to something different, the desire to explore the *problem* of the mind/body problem. In their different ways, all the authors investigate why it has been the case (and still is) that conceptualizing consciousness, the human body, and the interactions between the two has proved so confusing, contentious, and inconclusive—or, as we might put it, has acted as the grit in the oyster that has produced pearls of thought. Furthermore, the volume as a whole has the wider purpose of taking that mind/body dichotomy which has been such a familiar feature of the great philosophies and locating it within its wider contexts—contexts of rhetoric, fiction, and ideology, of imagination and symbolism, science and religion, contexts of groups and gender, power and politics. To

1. Rigorous study of the mind/body relationship construed in the philosophical sense begins as a subset of the philosophy of mind in the nineteenth century, and a case can be made that there are traces of it evident in eighteenth-century rational thought. By the time the journal *Mind: A Quarterly Review of Psychology and Philosophy* was launched in England in 1876, the mind/body relationship was a widely discussed philosophical topic and a valid field of serious inquiry, as is evident, for example, in books written by diverse types of authors. See, for example, the philosopher George Moore's *The Use of the Body in Relation to the Mind* (London: Longman, 1847), Benjamin Collins Brodie's *Mind and Matter* (New York: G. P. Putnam, 1857), and the famous British psychiatrist Henry Maudsley's medico-philosophical study of *Body and Mind* (London, 1873).

speak of the mind/body problem as if it were a timeless abstraction, a topos for unlimited discussion by countless symposia down the ages, would be to perpetuate mystifications. It must itself be problematized—theorized—in relation to history, language, and culture. And here, the first thing to notice—a bizarre fact—is the paucity of synthetic historical writing upon this profound issue.[2]

By the turn of the twentieth century, discussions of mind/body continued to flourish in the major European and American schools of philosophy, as can be seen in the tradition from Wittgenstein to Gilbert Ryle and A. J. Ayer, and in such works as the well-known philosopher C. D. Broad's *The Mind and Its Place in Nature* (London: Routledge and Kegan Paul, 1925). More recently, see R. W. Rieber, ed., *Body and Mind: Past, Present and Future* (New York: Academic Press, 1980); Neil Bruce Lubow, *The Mind-Body Identity Theory* (Oxford: Clarendon Press, 1974); Michael E. Levin, *Metaphysics and the Mind-Body Problem* (New York: Oxford University Press, 1979); and Norman Malcolm, *Problems of Mind: Descartes to Wittgenstein* (New York: Harper and Row, 1971)—authors writing on the relationship from different perspectives and for different diachronic periods. The literature is vast and continues to produce scholarship, as can be surmised from the entry on "Mind and Body" in the recently published *Oxford Companion to the Mind*, ed. R. L. Gregory (Oxford: Oxford University Press, 1987), 204.

2. The historiography of the mind/body relationship extends, of course, as far back as the Greeks and demonstrates a long tradition of speculation, so abundant that it would be foolish to attempt to provide any sense of its breadth in the space of a note. But we want to comment on the main curves of the heritage of mind and body, especially by noticing the supremacy of mind over body throughout the Christian tradition, and the reinforcement of this hierarchy in the aftermath of Cartesian dualism. Both mind and body received a great deal of attention in the Enlightenment, and it is one of the purposes of this book to annotate this relationship in a variety of discourses, more fully than the matter has been studied before. There is also a large literature, scientific and mystical, secular and religious, in the seventeenth and eighteenth centuries, that treats of the mind's control over the body or the converse: see, for instance, the Paracelsian physician F. M. van Helmont: *The Spirit of Diseases; or, Diseases from the Spirit . . . wherein is shewed how much the Mind Influenceth the Body in Causing and Curing of Diseases* (London, 1694). Other works attempted to demarcate the boundaries of mind and body, such as John Petvin's *Letters concerning Mind* (London: J. and J. Rivington, 1750); John Richardson's (of Newtent) *Thoughts upon Thinking; or, A new theory of the human mind: wherein a physical rationale of the formation of our ideas, the passions, dreaming and every faculty of the soul is attempted upon principles entirely new* (London: J. Dodsley, 1755); and John Rotherham's *On the Distinction between the Soul and the Body* (London: J. Robson, [1760]), a philosophical treatise aiming to differentiate the realm of mind from that of soul. Still other discourses, often medical dissertations written with an eye on Hobbes's *De Corpore* (1655), actually aimed to anatomize the soul as distinct from the brain in strictly mechanical terms; see, for example, Johann Ambrosius Hillig, *Anatomie der Seelen* (Leipzig, 1737). In all these diverse discourses, the dualism of mind and body was so firmly ingrained by the mid eighteenth century that compendiums such as the following continued to be issued: Anonymous, *A View of Human Nature; or, Select Histories, Giving an account of persons who have been most eminently distinguish'd by their virtues or vices, their perfections or defects, either of body or mind . . . the whole collected from the best authors in various languages . . .* (London: S. Birt, 1750).

If we acknowledge a certain plausibility to Alfred North Whitehead's celebrated dictum that all subsequent philosophy is a series of footnotes to Plato, we might be especially disposed to the view that the mind/body

More recently, in the Romantic period, there was realignment of the dualism often in favor of the body, as J. H. Hagstrum has noted in *The Romantic Body: Love and Sexuality in Keats, Wordsworth and Blake* (Knoxville: University of Tennessee Press, 1985). In our century, the discussion has proliferated in a number of directions. On the one hand, there is a vast psychoanalytic and psychohistorical literature that we do not specifically engage in this volume but whose tenets can be grasped, if controversially, in Norman O. Brown's *Life against Death: The Psychoanalytical Meaning of History* (London: Routledge and Kegan Paul, 1957), a classic expression of the Freudian viewpoint; and in Leo Bersani's *The Freudian Body: Psychoanalysis and Art* (New York: Columbia University Press, 1985). On the other, the philosophy of mind within the academic study of philosophy has continued to privilege mind over body. But there is now also a tradition of revaluation that (at least nominally) attempts to view the mind/body relationship neutrally, giving each component allegedly equal treatment no matter which diachronic period is being studied, and still other critiques that view body in relation to society, as, for instance, in A. W. H. Adkins, *From the Many to the One: A Study of Personality and Views of Human Nature in the Context of Ancient Greek Society, Values and Beliefs* (London: Constable, 1970), and in Bryan Turner's *The Body and Society* (Oxford: Basil Blackwell, 1984). Francis Barker's *The Tremulous Private Body: Essays on Subjection* (New York: Methuen, 1984), represents the deconstruction of the body according to the lines of modern literary theory.

Other, more diverse, studies pursuing literary, artistic, political, and even semiotic relationships include: David Armstrong, *Political Anatomy of the Body* (Cambridge: Cambridge University Press, 1983); Leonard Barkan, *Nature's Work of Art: The Human Body as Image of the World* (New Haven: Yale University Press, 1975); *Body, Mind and Death,* readings selected, edited and furnished with an introductory essay by Anthony Flew (New York: Macmillan, 1964); J. D. Bernal, *The World, the Flesh and the Devil: An Inquiry into the Future of the Three Enemies of the Rational Soul* (London: Cape, 1970); Robert E. French, *The Geometry of Vision and the Mind-Body Problem* (New York: P. Lang, 1972); Jonathan Miller, *The Body in Question* (London: Cape, 1978); Gabriel Josipovici, *Writing and the Body* (Brighton: Harvester, 1982); for a literary interpretation, see M. S. Kearns, *Metaphors of Mind in Fiction and Psychology* (Lexington: University Press of Kentucky, 1987). Rebecca Goldstein, the British novelist, has written a novel about the dualism entitled *The Mind-Body Problem* (London, 1985).

During this decade there has been a proliferation of studies of the body in respect of gender, as in: Sandra M. Gilbert and Susan Gubar, *The Madwoman in the Attic: The Woman Writer and the Nineteenth Century Literary Imagination* (New Haven: Yale University Press, 1979); idem, *No Man's Land: The Place of the Woman Writer in the Twentieth Century* (New Haven and London: Yale University Press, 1988); Susan Rubin Suleiman, ed., *The Female Body in Western Culture: Contemporary Perspectives* (Cambridge, Mass.: Harvard University Press, 1985); Catherine Gallagher and Thomas Laqueur, eds., *The Making of the Modern Body* (Berkeley, Los Angeles, London: University of California Press, 1986); Elaine Scarry, *The Body in Pain: The Making and Unmaking of the World* (Cambridge, Mass.: Harvard University Press, 1984). The full range of studies of the body in our time will become apparent when Dr. Ivan Illich's comprehensive bibliography of "The Body in the Twentieth Century" appears.

problem is amongst the most ancient and thorny—yet fundamental and inescapable—in the Western intellectual tradition. For the predication of such differences was one of Plato's prime strategies. In attempting to demonstrate against sophists and skeptics that humans could achieve a true understanding of the world, Plato developed rhetorical ploys that postulated dichotomies between (on the one hand) what are deemed merely fleeting appearances or shadows and (on the other) what are to be discovered as eternal, immutable realities. Such binary opposites are respectively construed in terms of the contrast between the merely mundane and the truly immaterial; and these in turn are shown to find their essential expressions on the one side in corporeality and on the other in consciousness. The construction of such a programmatically dualistic ontology provides the framework for epistemology, since for Plato, the only authentic knowledge—not to be confused with subjective "belief" or "opinion"/is that which transcends the senses, those deceptive windows to the world of appearances. But it is equally the basis for a moral theory, as dozens of philosophers have shown: knowing the good is the necessary and sufficient condition for choosing it, and right conduct constitutes the reign of reason over the tumult of blind bodily appetites.

The Homeric writings are innocent of any such clear-cut abstract division between a unitary incorporeal principle called mind or soul, and the body as such. So too the majority of the pre-Socratic philosophers. But "Enter Plato," as Gouldner put it, and the terms were set for philosophy.[3] And, as Whitehead intimated, the formulations of post-Platonic philosophies can be represented as repeatedly ringing the changes upon such foundational propositions. Admittedly, as early as Aristotle, there was dissent from Plato's postulation of Ideas, or ideal forms, as the eternal verities indexed in the empyrean; yet in practice the Aristotelian corpus affirmed the equally comprehensive sovereignty of mind over matter in the natural order of things, which found expression—ethical, sexual, social, and political—in his images of the good man (the gender is significant) and his superior status within the hierarchies of the family, economy, polity, and cosmos. And in their varied ways, most other influential philosophies of antiquity corroborated the elemental Platonic interpretation of the order of existence as organized through hierarchi-

3. Alvin Gouldner, *Enter Plato: Classical Greece and the Origins of Social Theory* (New York: Basic Books, 1965) emphasizes how Plato makes a break with earlier thought traditions. A good introduction to Plato's strategies is offered by G. M. A. Grube, *Plato's Thought* (Indianapolis: Hackett, 1980). Popper's attack upon Plato is worth remembering in this context: Karl Popper, *The Open Society and Its Enemies* (London, 1945). See also Bennett Simon, *Mind and Madness in Ancient Greece* (Ithaca, N.Y.: Cornell University Press, 1978).

cal dochotomies that dignified the immaterial over the physical, and, specifically, mind over the flesh that was so patently the seedbed of mutability and the harbinger of death. Through its aspirations to "apathy"—and, if necessary, in the final analysis, suicide—Stoicism aimed to reduce the body to its proper insignificance, thereby liberating the mind for its nobler offices. Neoplatonists in the Renaissance and later, with their doctrines of love for higher, celestial beings, likewise envisaged the soul soaring upward, in an affirmation of what we might almost call the incredible lightness of being.

Moreover, the rational expression of the Christian gospel, drawing freely upon Platonic formulas, was to recuperate the radical ontological duality between mind and gross matter in its assertion that "in the beginning was the Word." (Here, of course, are the origins of the logocentrism that proves so problematic to our contemporaries.) Various sects of early Christians, from Gnostics to Manichaeans, took the dualistic disposition to extremes, by mapping the categories of good and evil precisely onto mind and body respectively, and urging modes of living—for example, asceticism or antinomianism—designed to deny the demands of the body in ways yet more drastic than ever the Stoics credited.[4]

II

There is no need in this Introduction to provide a detailed route-map through the history of Western thought, charting the course taken by such dualistic ontologies of mind over matter, mind over body, ever since antiquity gave it its philosophical, and Christianity its theological, expression, and Thomist Scholasticism synthesized the two. Nevertheless, something substantial must be said about the natural history of mind and body. Otherwise, the stunning essays in this volume will appear to be less integrated than they are, and the chapters by Foot and Popkin may appear to fall outside the book's stated scope. In fact, Foot's chapter demonstrates that the accounts of motivation in both Locke and Hume depend upon an antecedent theory of mind and body: as motives belong to the realm of the mind, the emphasis on pleasure and pain in the thought of Locke is not readily understood without taking account of his well-developed mind/body relation. Popkin's claim, in contrast, is

4. F. Bottomley, *Attitudes to the Body in Western Christendom* (London: Lepus Books, 1979); Peter Brown, *The Body and Society: Men, Women and Sexual Renunciation in Early Christianity* (New York: Columbia University Press, 1988).

that racism always depends to a certain extent on the anthropological and biological assumptions of its proponents, and although he assumes rather than adumbrates the point, the biology of an era necessarily reflects a substratum of philosophical ideas concerning empiricism and magic, mechanism and vitalism, materialism and immaterialism, reason and unreason—in short, all those constellations that converged into "mind-body" during the Enlightenment. These ideas, sometimes coherent, sometimes not, fed into the ocean of Enlightenment thought we are calling "mind and body," and although *The Languages of Psyche* does not undertake to compile any proper history or route-map of the conjunction, we (the collective authors) believe that the mind/body relation possesses a rather intricate natural history that must be articulated here if the essays that follow are to be appreciated.

Influential Renaissance teachings on the nature of man and his place in nature—in particular, those of Ficino and Pico—articulated Christian versions of Neoplatonic idealism;[5] Christian Stoicism was soon to have its day. And Descartes's celebrated "proof" of the mind/body polarity—under God, all creation was gross *res extensa* with the sole exception of the human *cogito*—confirmed the priority and superiority of mind with a logical éclat unmatched since Anselm, while providing a vindication of dualism both deriving from, and, simultaneously, legitimating, the "new science" of matter in motion governed by the laws of mechanics. Furthermore—and crucially for the future—Descartes contended that it was upon such championship of the autonomy, independence, immateriality, and freedom of *res cogitans,* the human consciousness, that all other tenets fundamental to the well-being of that thinking subject depended: man's guarantees of the existence and attributes of God, the reality of cosmic order and justice, the regularities and fitnesses of Creation.

Micro- and macrocosmic thinking, ingrained as part of the medieval habit of mind, found itself reinvigorated by the Cartesian dualism. Whether this was owing primarily to religious or secular developments, or again to the challenge given to the "old philosophy" by the "new science," continues to be the subject of fierce controversy among a wide variety of historians on many continents. But the progress of micro-macrocosmic analogies itself is unassailable. For the Malebranchians and Leibnizians, Wolffians and Scottish Common Sense philosophers who

5. Valuable here are Paul Kristeller, *Renaissance Thought* (New York: Harper, 1961); Charles Schmitt and Quentin Skinner, eds., *The Cambridge History of Renaissance Philosophy* (Cambridge: Cambridge University Press, 1988).

manned the arts faculties of eighteenth-century universities, instructing youth in right thinking, the analogy of nature underlined the affinities between the divine mind and the human, each unthinkable except as reflecting the complementary Other. From the latter half of the seventeenth century, it is true, rationalist and positivist currents in the European temper grew increasingly skeptical as to the existence of an array of nonmaterial entities: fairies, goblins, and ghosts; devils and wood demons; the powers of astrology, witchcraft, and magic; the hermetic "world soul," and perhaps even Satan and Hell themselves—all as part of that demystifying tide which Max Weber felicitously dubbed the "disenchantment of the world."[6] Yet subtle arguments were advanced to prove that such a salutary liquidation of false animism and anthropomorphism served but to corroborate nonmaterial reality where it truly existed: in the divine mind and the human. For many eighteenth-century natural philosophers and natural theologians, the more the physical universe was drained by the "mechanicization of the world picture" of any intrinsic will, activity, and teleology, the more patent were the proofs of a mind outside, which had created, sustained, and continued to see that all was good.[7]

It would be a gross mistake, however, to imply that Christian casuistries alone perpetuated canonical restatements of the mastery of mind over body. The very soul of the epistemology and poetics of a Romanticism in revolt against the allegedly materialistic attitudes and aesthetics of the eighteenth century was the championship of mental powers, most commonly finding expression through the idea of the holiness of imagination and the transcendency of genius. Genius and imagination, no matter how designated, had been among the commonest themes of the rational Enlightenment: the basis of its developing discourse of aesthetics; the salt of its political theory, as Locke and Burke showed; even the ideological underpinning of its "scientific manifestoes."[8] Later on,

6. See the argument in R. D. Stock, *The Holy and the Daemonic from Sir Thomas Browne to William Blake* (Princeton: Princeton University Press, 1982).

7. For the relations of God and Nature see Amos Funkenstein, *Theology and the Scientific Imagination from the Middle Ages to the Seventeenth Century* (Princeton: Princeton University Press, 1986).

8. Illuminating on the philosophy of imaginative genius are J. Engell, *The Creative Imagination* (Cambridge, Mass.: Harvard University Press, 1981); P. A. Cantor, *Creature and Creator: Myth-making and English Romanticism* (Cambridge: Cambridge University Press, 1984); and, more generally, G. S. Rousseau, "Science and the Discovery of the Imagination in Enlightenment England," *Eighteenth-Century Studies* 3 (1969): 108–135, and E. Tuveson, *The Imagination as a Means of Grace* (Berkeley and Los Angeles: University of California Press, 1960).

contemporary philosophical Idealism in the form of Hegel-on-horseback likewise interpreted the dynamics of world history as the process whereby *Geist,* or spirit, realized itself in the world, spiraling dialectically upward to achieve ever higher planes of self-consciousness. And we must never minimize the Idealist thrust of the developmental philosophies so popular in the nineteenth-century *fin-de-siècle* era—from Bosanquet and Balfour to Bergson, and influenced by Hegelianism no less than by the *Origin of Species*—which represented the destiny of the cosmos and of its noblest expression, man, as the progressive evolution of higher forms of being out of lower, and in particular the ascent of man from protoplasmic slime to the Victorian mind.[9]

Given this philosophical paean down the millennia affirming the majesty of mind, it is little wonder that so many of the issues which modern philosophy inherited hinged upon mapping out the relationships between thinking and being, mind and brain, will and desire, or (on the one hand) inner motive, intention, and impulse, and (on the other) physical action. In one sense at least, Whitehead was a true child of his time. Twentieth-century philosophers such as G. E. Moore still puzzled over the same sorts of questions Socrates posed, wondering what the shadows flickering on the cave walls really represented, and pondering whether moral truths exist within the realm of the objectively knowable. Not only that, but the kinds of words, categories, and *exempla* in circulation to resolve such issues have continued—for better or worse—to be ones familiarized by Plato, Locke, or Dewey.[10]

To its credit, recent philosophy—as Philippa Foot energetically argues below—has urged the folly of expecting to find solutions to these ancestral problems through honing yet more sophisticated variants upon the formulas traded by post-Cartesian rationalism or Anglo-Saxon empiricism. A few more refinements to utilitarianism or the latest model in associationism will not get us any further than will laboratory experiments in search of the true successor to the pineal gland. And when Richard Rorty pronounces the death of philosophy in his latest tour de force,[11] one wonders to what degree the age-old dualism has conspired to cause it. Rorty, like Foot, suggests that philosophers had just as well throw up their hands—perhaps even do better by denying the dualism

9. See Peter Bowler, *The Eclipse of Darwinism* (Baltimore: Johns Hopkins University Press, 1983).

10. See J. Passmore, *A Hundred Years of Philosophy* (New York: Basic Books, 1966).

11. Richard Rorty, *Philosophy and the Mirror of Nature* (Princeton: Princeton University Press, 1980).

of mind and body altogether. It may be, as Rorty maintains, that, philosophically speaking, "there is no mind-body problem,"[12] and that as a consequence Rorty is entitled, as a professional philosopher, to cast aspersions on, even to crack grammatical jokes about, all those who believe there is. For this reason, Rorty believes that "we are not entitled to begin talking about the mind and body problem, or about the possible identity or necessary non-identity of mental and physical states, without first asking what we mean by 'mental.'"[13] And as a direct consequence of his aim to shatter Cartesian dualism and the philosophies that built on its further dualisms all the way up to Kant, Rorty can announce his own aim in *Philosophy and the Mirror of Nature* as being "to undermine the reader's confidence in the 'mind' as something about which one should have a 'philosophical' view, in 'knowledge' as something about which there ought to be a 'theory' and which has 'foundations,' and in 'philosophy' as it has been conceived since Kant."[14]

Above all, new bearings in philosophy—especially the way Wittgenstein proved a seminal impulse for many, phenomenology for others—have reoriented attention away from the traditional envisaging of emotions, desires, intentions, states of mind, acts of will, and so on, as "things," as inner natural objects with a place within some conceptual

12. Ibid., 7. Rorty's fervor to smash dualism is everywhere apparent. For example, in this same introductory section entitled "Invention of the Mind," Rorty writes: "at this point we might want to say that we have dissolved the mind-body problem" (32), and a few sentences later, on the same page, "the mind-body problem, we can now say, was merely a result of Locke's unfortunate mistake about how words get meaning, combined with his and Plato's muddled attempt to talk about adjectives as if they were nouns."

13. Ibid., 32. Rorty continues this passage by derogating the grand aims of contemporary professional philosophy: "I would hope further to have incited the suspicion that our so-called intuition about what is mental may be merely our readiness to fall in with a specifically philosophical language game." Here Rorty's polemical pronoun ("our") shrewdly hovers between professional philosophers on the one hand and interested amateurs who have thought about the dualism of mind/body on the other.

14. Ibid., 7. The implication would seem to be equally true for the "body." But historically speaking, there have been three species of books about body, all of which have produced a large number of metacritiques in the last century: (1) those written by philosophers of mind with an interest in keeping the dualism (Rorty would say "philosophical language game") alive by diminishing the importance of body when considered in its physiological, or neurophysiological, state; (2) those by scientists (anatomists, physiologists, neurophysiologists, and other empirical laboratory experimenters) often concerned to demonstrate that the dilemmas called linguistic by the philosophers are actually as yet unexplored neurophysiological mysteries related to the workings of the central nervous system; and (3) those by a broad range of historians and other cultural commentators interested in the social dimensions of the mind/body problem when considered with respect to individuals or societies viewed collectively.

geography of the self, the causal connections between which it is our duty to discover by introspection and thought experiments. Such a reified view of being, thinking, and acting—a Marxist critic might say it is no more than is to be expected within commodity capitalism—has sustained devastating attack, and modern crosscurrents in philosophy have been claiming that we should rather attend to the meanings of our moral languages understood as systems of public utterance. Thereby we might escape from the sterilities of a figural mechanics of the mind which, as Alasdair MacIntyre has emphasized, and as Rorty has now demonstrated, threatened to drag moral philosophy down into a morass, and address ourselves afresh to more urgent questions of value and choice.[15]

Comparable processes of revaluation have also transformed literary theory. In England, Victorian criticism (itself sometimes proudly hitched to the wagon of associationist psychophysiology) commonly believed its mission was to judge novelists and playwrights for psychological realism: were their dramatis personae credible doubles of real people? Somewhat later, various schools of criticism, enthused by Freudian dogmas, went one stage further, and took characters out of fiction and set them on the couch, attempting to probe into their psyches (how well was their unconscious motivation grasped?) and into the unconscious of their authors (how were their fictions projections of their neuroses?). Today's criticism has discredited such preoccupations with the physical presence and the psychic potential of characters as banal, as but another form of literal-minded reification. For many theorists today, especially the feminists, the task of dissecting the body of the text is coeval with that of the body of women, while the traditional notion of the authorial mind as creator—a notion reaching its apogee in Romanticism—has yielded to a fascination with genre, rhetoric, and langauge as the informing structures.[16]

15. Alasdair MacIntyre, *After Virtue* (Notre Dame, Ind.: University of Notre Dame Press, 1984).

16. In the process, the human body is abandoned, and discourses consulting the human *form* rather than "the body as text" or "the body as trope" become increasingly rare. Amongst them see John Blacking, *The Anthropology of the Body* (London: Academic Press, 1977); Julia L. Epstein, "Writing the Unspeakable: Fanny Burney's Mastectomy and the Fictive Body," *Representations*, Fall 1986, 131–166; Robert N. Essick, "How Blake's Body Means," in *Unnam'd Forms: Blake and Textuality*, ed. Nelson Hilton and Thomas A. Vogler (Berkeley, Los Angeles, London: University of California Press, 1986). The more usual approach applies the paradigm "read the body—read the text," as if to equate the two through a metonymy, and as discovered in so many (often excellent) works of contemporary feminism (see those mentioned in n. 2 above). But these trends appear to be absent, or at least minimal, in contemporary philosophy; see, for example, Mark Johnson, *The*

We may applaud the transcendence—in philosophy, in criticism, and elsewhere—of crude mechanical models of the operations of thinking and feeling, willing and acting. This is not, however, to imply that the interplay of consciousness and society, of nerves and human nature, has somehow lost its meaning or relevance. Far from it, for it is important, now more than ever, to be able to think decisively about the ramifications of mind and body, their respective resonances, and their intersections, because the practical implications are so critical.

For ours is a material culture that is rapidly replacing the received metaphors that help us understand—or, arguably, mystify—the workings of minds and bodies. Deploying such models is nothing new. To conceptualize the mind, suggested Plato, think of the state; the understanding begins as a blank sheet of paper, argued Locke (for Tristram Shandy, by contrast, its objective correlative was a stick of sealing wax). Above all, during the last few centuries, the proliferation of machinery—watches, steam engines, and the like—has provided models for the functions of corporeal bodies and the processes of the understanding; the image of thinking as a mill, grinding out truths, was especially powerful.

Indeed, as Otto Mayr has remarked, particular forms of technology may even determine—or, at least, shape distinctive ways of viewing the mind itself.[17] Clockwork mechanisms as found in watches yield images of man, individual and social, as uniformly and predictably obeying the pulse of centrally driven systems. Such a behaviorist image of man-the-machine, Mayr suggests, was particularly prominent in the propaganda of ancien régime absolutism (and we may add, in images of factory discipline in the philosophy of manufactures). In Britain, the more complex regulatory equipment of the steam engine, with its flywheels and contrapuntal rhythms, perhaps offered a rather different metaphor of man: that of checks and balances, counterpoised within a more decentralized and self-regulating whole, suggestive perhaps of a kind of individuality in tune with the English ideology. And, more recently, in the aftermath of late-nineteenth-century positivism, neurobiology and neurophysiology have become persuaded that mind is brain, and that

Body in the Mind: The Bodily Basis of Meaning, Imagination and Reason (Chicago: University of Chicago Press, 1987). Further reasons for this recent development, viewed within the context of literary theory, are provided in H. Aram Veeser, ed., *The New Historicism* (London: Routledge, 1989).

17. O. Mayr, *Authority, Liberty and Automatic Machines in Early Modern Europe* (Baltimore: Johns Hopkins University Press, 1986); L. Mumford, *The Condition of Man* (London, 1944); idem, *Technics and Civilization* (New York: Harcourt, Brace and World, 1963).

the brain is an entirely mechanical, machine-like instrument whose operations are barely understood because of the vastness of its complexity.[18] In this sense, the human brain is more complex than the largest computer.[19] This radical mechanism, shunning any traces of vestigial vitalism (of the old Bergsonian or Drieschian varieties), forms the unarticulated basis of practically all laboratory biology and physiology today, yet its roots, vis-à-vis mind and body, extend at least as far back as the eighteenth-century Enlightenment. In a sense, then, mechanism, at least viewed within its mind/body context, has come full circle back to its Cartesian, and somewhat post-Cartesian, model.[20]

Mechanical models—realized in Vaucansonian automata—were obviously integral to Cartesian formulations of man as an intricate piece of

18. For the reciprocity of mind and brain, see Patricia S. Churchland, *Neurophilosophy: Toward a Unified Science of the Mind/Brain* (Cambridge, Mass.: MIT Press, 1986); John Eccles, *The Neurophysiological Basis of Mind* (Oxford: Clarendon Press, 1953); idem, *Brain and Human Behavior* (New York: Springer Verlag, 1972); idem, *The Understanding of the Brain* (New York: McGraw-Hill, 1973); Marc Jeannerod, *The Brain Machine: The Development of Neurophysiological Thought* (Cambridge, Mass.: Harvard University Press, 1985); Morton F. Reiser, *Mind, Brain, Body: Toward a Convergence of Psychoanalysis and Neurobiology* (New York: Basic Books, 1984); Fred A. Wolf, *The Body Quantum: The Physics of the Human Body* (London: Heinemann, 1987). Arguing against the radical mechanism of these positions is Herbert Weiner, M.D., "Some Comments on the Transduction of Experience by the Brain: Implications for Our Understanding of the Relationship of Mind to Body," *Psychiatric Medicine* 34 (1972): 355–380. For the shrewd input of a Nobel laureate in physics on the question of material reciprocity, see E. P. Wigner, Emeritus Professor of Physics at Princeton University, "Remarks on the Mind-Body Question," in *The Scientist Speculates: An Anthology of Partly Baked Ideas*, ed. I. J. Good (New York: Basic Books, 1962), 284–302.

19. Victor Weisskopf, *Knowledge and Wonder: The Natural World as Man Knows It* (Cambridge, Mass.: MIT Press, 1979), 244.

20. The endurance of these Cartesian models, from Descartes to the present, in regard to the mind/body dualism, as well as in such disparate academic territories as linguistics, medicine, and psychology, is discussed in William Barrett, *Death of the Soul: From Descartes to the Computer* (New York: Doubleday, 1986); Richard B. Carter, *Descartes' Medical Philosophy: The Organic Solution to the Mind-Body Problem* (Baltimore: Johns Hopkins University Press, 1983); Harry M. Bracken, ed., *Mind and Language: Essays on Descartes and Chomsky* (Dordrecht and Cinnaminson, N.J.: Foris Publications, 1984); Marjorie Grene, *Interpretations of Life and Mind: Essays around the Problem of Reduction* (London: Routledge and Kegan Paul, 1971); idem, *Descartes* (Brighton: Harvester, 1985); Kenneth Dewhurst and Nigel Reeves, eds. *Friedrich Schiller: Medicine, Psychology and Literature* (Berkeley, Los Angeles, London: University of California Press, 1978); E. H. Lenneberg, *Biological Foundations of Language* (New York: Wiley, 1967); Amélie Oksenburg Rorty, *Essays on Descartes' Meditations* (Berkeley, Los Angeles, London: University of California Press, 1986); Margaret D. Wilson, *Descartes* (London: Routledge and Kegan Paul, 1978); Albert G. A. Balz, *Descartes and the Modern Mind* (New Haven: Yale University Press, 1952). Some of these topics are anticipated in René Descartes, *Lettres de Mr Descartes, où sont traittés les plus belles questions de la morale, physique, médicine, & les mathématiques* (Paris: C. Angot, 1666–1667).

mechanism yoked, however mysteriously, to an undetermined mind—the whole amounting to the notorious "ghost in the machine."[21] Such Cartesian mechanical metaphors—widely condemned by Romantics old and new for their supposedly disembodying and alienating implications[22]—were commonly drawn upon, with rather conservative intent, to reinforce the age-old belief that *homo rationalis* was destined, from above, to govern those below.

But there are also significant differences between these old Romantic views of our world of artificial intelligence and cognition theory. The material analogues in vogue today, by contrast, are arguably far more challenging and less flattering to entrenched human senses of self. Ever since Norbert Wiener and Alan Turing, cybernetics, systems analysis, and the computer revolution have been changing our understanding of the transformative potentialities of machines. If the Babbagian computer was merely a device to be intelligently programmed "from above," the computers of today and tomorrow have intelligence programmed into them, and they possess the capacity to learn, modify their behavior, and "think" creatively—in a sense, to evolve. The more the notion of "machines that think" becomes realized, the more urgent will be the task of clarifying in precisely which ways we believe their feedback circuits differ from ours; or perhaps we will have to say, the ways in which those alien, artificial intelligences believe our calculating operations differ from *theirs*! Human/robot interactions, once the amusing speculations of science fiction, may ironically become the facet of the mind/body problem most critical to that twenty-first century which is but a decade away. What is it, if anything, that gives us a "self," a personality, entitling us to rights and duties in a society denying these to artificial intelligence? Today, as in the seventeenth and eighteenth centuries, the philosophers, especially philosophers of mind, speak out on these vital subjects. John Searle and many others regard "free will"—the traditional predicate of autonomous mind—as an unsatisfactory and obsolete answer.[23] And it is one of the strengths of Philippa Foot's chapter that she demonstrates the eighteenth-century legacy of this continuing problem.

21. For this Cartesian legacy, see Aram Vartanian, *Diderot and Descartes: A Study of Scientific Naturalism in the Enlightenment* (Princeton: Princeton University Press, 1953); and see, of course, Arthur Koestler, *The Ghost in the Machine* (London: Hutchinson, 1976).

22. For modern critics of the supposedly dire consequences of Cartesian dualism, see F. Capra, *The Turning Point: Science, Society and the Rising Culture* (New York, 1982); M. Berman, *The Re-enchantment of the World* (London, 1982).

23. John Searle, *Minds, Brains and Science* (Cambridge, Mass.: Harvard University Press, 1984). Modern neurosurgeons have made useful contributions to this subject, especially within the contexts of the complex ways in which the brain processes language in

III

If airing such issues may still seem frivolous or futuristic, it can hardly be fanciful to focus attention upon the transformations that living bodies and personalities are nowadays undergoing. Spare-part surgery became a *fait accompli* long before philosophers had solved its moral and legal dilemmas. Surgeons have implanted the kidneys, hearts, lungs of other humans, and even other primates. Surely such developments (it might have been thought) must have caused intense anxiety for identity in a culture that still speaks—if metaphorically—of the heart as the hub of passion and integrity, and the brain as the seat of reason and control. But it hardly seems to have proved so. Should we conclude that we are all Cartesians or Platonists—or maybe even Christians—enough to regard the bits and pieces of the body as no more than necessary but contingent appendages to whatever we decide it is that does define our unique essence? One wonders (skeptically) whether we would feel as nonchalant about brain transplants. Are we sufficiently confident in our dualism to believe that acquiring another's brain would not make us another person, or, indeed, a centaur-like monster? Contemporary philosophers such as Thomas Nagel think not,[24] and Professor Foot reminds us to what degree Enlightenment philosophers such as Locke and Hume pondered these matters, albeit in a different key.

And more perplexing perhaps, because more imminent, what of the implantation of fragments of brains, or elements of the central nervous system? Would these involve dislocations of identity?—the equivalent perhaps to the caricaturists' macabre vision of the Day of Judgment when the bodies of those dissected by anatomists and dismembered in war arise, yet with their parts grotesquely muddled and misassembled. Here we seem to be on terrain already laid bare by current practices within psychological medicine. In the psychiatric hospital, advances in neuropsychiatry enable us, through drugs and surgery alike, radically to transform the behavior and moods of the disturbed, so that we colloquially say that they have turned into "another"—indeed, a "new"—person. Can somatic interventions thus make a whole new self? Because the patients involved are "psychopathological" cases, to which regular

relation to a perceived external reality and to the role of the will within this reality, a subject of immense concern to poststructuralist theory, especially Derridean and post-Derridean deconstructionism. Among these Fred Plum, M.D., has been especially eloquent; see, for example, F. Plum, ed., *Language, Communication and the Brain* (New York: Raven Press, 1988); G. Globus, ed., *Consciousness and the Brain* (New York: Plenum, 1976).

24. Thomas Nagel, *Mortal Questions* (Cambridge: Cambridge University Press, 1979); idem, *The View from Nowhere* (New York: Oxford University Press, 1986).

public legal constraints may not apply—or because, to put it crudly, such developments have been largely pioneered in the back wards, out of sight and out of mind—the dystopian implications of such medically induced personality transformations do not always receive full attention.[25]

Yet our dramatically increased capacity to wreak such changes, to make "new men" of old, is obviously a matter of great moment for the natural history of the somatic/psychic interface. The ethical and legal ramifications are obviously epochal—although law courts in their own fashion currently tend to handle such issues on an *ad hoc,* case-by-case basis, often hearing the authority of biology in the distant background. The widening horizons of genetic engineering, reproductive technology, and gender-change operations raise parallel issues as to wherein the unique—and permanent?—human personality should be deemed to reside: is it in genetic material that is essentially somatic, in particular organs, or in an experiential *je ne sais quoi* such as memory? (It may be one thing for the law, another for morality, and something different for the people themselves.)

Finally, though certainly not least, all these issues have been sharpened by our new technologies for managing death. Until quite recently, death was defined by some palpable and natural organic termination: the heart stopped beating, the breath of life expired. Even among the more superstitious and mystical, the "will to live" (Life Force?) was translated into organic dysfunction or disease. Medical technology, however, has marched on, from iron lungs to resuscitators and respirators. The implicit Cartesian in us can happily accept that a person remains alive even after the cessation of spontaneous body activity such as the heartbeat. But does that not leave us without a certain index of death at all?—or, indeed, signs of life? (Are some people simply more dead, or more alive, than others?) Medical attention has, of course, switched to the concept of "brain death"—which itself implicitly trades upon the humanist assumption that what finally defines mortal man is consciousness, while also embodying the more specifically modern faith that, while mind may still be more than brain, the needles registering presence of electrical impulses in the cortex betoken that the mind is still "alive." The paradoxical outcome of this eminently "humane" chain of reasoning is that we nowadays aggresively keep "alive" those in whom none of the indices of consciousness recognizable to the "naked eye" survive.[26]

25. For criticism of invasions of the rights of mental patients, see T. Szasz, *The Myth of Mental Illness* (New York: Paladin, 1961). See also idem, *Pain and Pleasure: A Study of Bodily Feelings* (London: Tavistock Publications, 1957).

26. On the modern medicalization of death see R. Lamerton, *The Care of the Dying* (Harmondsworth: Penguin, 1980).

IV

The argument so far has accentuated two points (the second developed below). First, the question about how we envisage the two-way traffic between mind and body is of fundamental concern for us today as well as for diverse cultural historians concerned with the diachronic past. It determines matters of grave import—ethical, legal, social, political, personal, sexual. The intricacies of exchange between consciousness and its embodiments are not gymnastic exercises designed to tone up mental athletes for the philosophers' Olympics, but are integral to everyone's intimate sense of what being human is and ought to be. Mental and physical interaction is a subject extending far beyond the historian's workshop or the philosopher's purview.[27] Idiomatic expressions—being somebody or nobody, or a nobody, being in or out of one's mind—prove the point beyond a shadow of doubt.

Thus our understanding, private and public, of mind and body has always been deeply important—for the law of slavery no less than for the salvation of souls. Yet it is crucial that we avoid the trap of hypostatizing "the mind/body problem" as if it were timeless and changeless, one of the "perennial questions" of the master philosophers—indeed, itself a veritable Platonic form, immemorially inscribed in the "aether." Toward this goal, amongst others, *The Languages of Psyche: Mind and Body in Enlightenment Thought* is largely dedicated: especially to the contextual dimensions and social implications of the two-way traffic. The terrain is so vast that we (the collective authors) have been able to cover only a few facets of this broad contextualism and historicism, and many volumes would be required to fill in the canvas more adequately. Even in specific terrains, history—social and political, religious and economic—has taken its toll. For one thing, as already suggested, the dilemmas involving disputed readings of psyche/soma relations, and the terms in which discussion has been conducted, have been radically transformed over the centuries.[28]

27. Despite the unassailability of the crucial function they play there. For example, the late American philosopher Susanne Langer devoted her entire professional career to the interaction of mental and physical phenomena in an attempt to generate an aesthetics based on the link. See her *Feeling and Form: A Theory of Art* (New York: Scribner, 1953) and *Mind: An Essay on Human Feeling*, 3 vols. (Baltimore: Johns Hopkins University Press, 1967–1982).

28. Cf. W. I. Matson, "Why Isn't the Mind-Body Problem Ancient?" in *Mind, Matter, and Method*, ed. P. K. Feyerabend and G. Maxwell (Minneapolis: University of Minnesota Press, 1966). This matter of origins viewed within the context of the seventeenth- and eighteenth-century debates is discussed by Douglas Odegard in "Locke and Mind-Body

At one time, to take an example, proof of the existence of a consciousness seemingly independent of this mortal coil counted because it seemed confirmation of a soul destined, as was hoped, for a glorious immortality; nowadays, by contrast, many defend autonomy of the mind against scientistic reductionisms precisely because no such heavenly bliss after death can be expected. Early-eighteenth-century thinkers were not confronted with organ transplants as problems for practical ethics. They did, however, puzzle themselves, at least mock-seriously, about the status of Siamese twins: one body, two heads—but how many souls did such creatures have?[29] Other philosophers and projectors of the time asked what a "soul" was anyway? Did all moving creatures possess one? When was soul acquired? Did it make any sense to ponder a cat's soul or a cow's? Could a black African be said to have the same soul as a white? (Blake's "little black boy" in *Innocence* was born "in the southern wild" and is black: "but oh," he pleads, "my soul is white.") These and other similar questions were asked under as many agendas as there were philosophers. The notion of multiple "personality," of course, came much later, once the techniques of hypnotism and dynamic psychiatry had revealed the disturbing presence of a plurality of apparently hermetically-sealed chambers of the consciousness (*cogito ergo sumus,* as it were).[30] In other words, concepts such as "soul" and "personality" must be handled with care, paying due respect to their resonances in context over time.

Second—and this is the key contention which forms the rationale for this volume—it would be a mistake to speak of the mind/body problem as if it were a conundrum that has always existed. Rather mind/body relations became pressing in the guise of the mind/body *problem* only rather recently, and in response to specific cultural configurations. Above all, it was the eighteenth century (to deploy that diachronic expression somewhat elastically) and the intellectual movement we term the Enlightenment, which problematized this feature of the human condition. How was this so? This is the question—construed in its broadest contexts—which we (the collective authors in this book) aim to address, fully aware that we want to continue dialogue about the matter, rather than to suggest any ultimate explanations or final words.

Dualism," *Philosophy* 45 (1970): 87–105, and Hilary Putnam in "How Old Is the Mind?" in *Exploring the Concept of Mind,* ed. Richard Caplan (Iowa City: University of Iowa Press, 1986).

29. See C. Kerby-Miller, ed., *Memoirs of the Extraordinary Life, Works and Discoveries of Martinus Scriblerus* (New York, 1966), for the sad story of Indamira and Lindamora.

30. See S. P. Fullinwider, *Technologies of the Finite* (Westport, Conn.: Greenwood Press, 1982).

As indicated above, mainline philosophical currents from the Greeks onward adumbrated a mythic conceptual geography which, in its value hierarchy, elevated the ideal above the material, the changeless over the mutable, the perfect over the processual, the mental over the physical, the free over the determined, and superimposed each pair upon the others. Demonstrating such an order of things could not, it is true, be achieved without some ingenuity and acumen. After all, the existence of the eternal form of a table and the survival of the soul beyond the body, are neither of them immediate objects of sense experience.

Nor could such a metaphysic be established without intellectual aplomb. Aristotle's polished conceptualization of nature, for instance, is a far cry from the messy chaos of contrary motions and kaleidoscopic multiplicity of shapes which greets the innocent eye.[31] Christian apologetics in particular had to overcome what prima facie appear to be profound internal tensions, not to say contradictions, in its theology. The Christian faith, zealous in its denigration of the (original) sinfulness of the flesh, set particular value upon the immortal destiny of a unique, personal soul (an element absent, in different ways and for distinct reasons, from both Neoplatonism and Judaism). Yet at the same time, and no less uniquely, the Scriptures revealed that embodied man was made in God's image, that God's own Son was made flesh, and that His incarnation, crucifixion, and resurrection were typologically prophetic of a universal resurrection of the flesh at the impending Last Judgment. Few creeds made too much of the otherworldly, but none so honored the flesh. This particular tension lay at the root of Augustine's ambivalence, forming the substratum of his ethics and epistemology, as well as his troubled view of mind in relation to body.[32] And those Christian exegetes and scholiasts who followed in Augustine's steps commented upon the paradox of flesh and fleshless within a single credo.

Thus the articulation of orthodox Christian theology might well be read as a heroic holding operation, attempting to harmonize the most unlikely partners. Through the Middle Ages and into early modern times, churchmen battled against the flesh, extolling asceticism, mortification, and spirituality, while believers were almost ghoulishly fascinated by the seemingly incorruptible tissues, freshly spurting blood,

31. Michael V. Wedlin, *Mind and the Imagination in Aristotle* (New Haven: Yale University Press, 1989).

32. For Augustine on mind and body see F. Bottomley, *Attitudes to the Body in Western Christendom* (London: Lepus Books, 1979), and Jean H. Hagstrum, *The Romantic Body* (Knoxville: University of Tennessee Press, 1985), chap. 2.

and weeping tears of long-dead saints, yet simultaneously awaiting the resurrection of the body in expectation of a very palpable orgy of bliss in heaven.[33] The endlessly controversial status of the Eucharist—did the sacrament truly mean consuming the blood and body of the Savior? or was it essentially an intellectual *aide-mémoire* of Christ's passion and atonement?—perfectly captures the essential tension between the spirit and incarnation within Christianity.

Nor was the triumph of the "mind over body" metaphysic achieved without opposition. After all, antiquity itself had its atomists and materialists—Democritus, Diogenes, Epicurus, Leucippus, Lucretius—who in their distinct ways discarded the radical dualism of matter and spirit, denied the primacy of spirit, and proposed versions of monistic materialism which reduced the so-called nobler attributes to particles in motion and to the promptings of the flesh under what Bentham much later called the "sovereign masters, of pleasure and pain." The history of orthodox theology from Aquinas onward amounted to a war of words: a logomachy waged on behalf of what Ralph Cudworth, the late-seventeenth-century Platonist, was tellingly to call the *True Intellectual System of the Universe,* against advancing armies of alleged atomists, eternalists, mortalists, materialists, naturalists, atheists, and all their tribe of Machiavellian, Hobbist, and Spinozist fellow travelers, who were all supposedly engaged in hierarchy-collapsing subversion, intellectual, religious, political, and moral.[34]

Many have doubted whether these leveling metaphysical marauders were in fact real (or at least, numerous)—or were rather, as might be said, *ideal,* or ideal types—demonic bogeymen invented to shore up orthodoxy. They have doubted with good reason. Research is uncovering a larger presence of sturdy grass-roots materialism—as exemplified by Menocchio the Friulian Miller, with his cosmology of cheese and worms—than once was suspected.[35]

33. Such paradoxes are brilliantly illuminated in P. Camporesi, *The Incorruptible Flesh: Bodily Mutation and Mortification in Religion and Folklore* (Cambridge: Cambridge University Press, 1988); see also idem, *Bread of Dreams: Food and Fantasy in Early Modern Europe* (Cambridge: Polity Press, 1990); idem, *The Body in the Cosmos: Natural Symbols in Medieval and Early Modern Italy* (Cambridge: Polity Press, 1989).

34. See Amos Funkenstein, *Theology and the Scientific Imagination from the Middle Ages to the Seventeenth Century* (Princeton: Princeton University Press, 1986).

35. E. Le Roy Ladurie, *Montaillou* (New York: Vintage, 1979); Carlo Ginzburg, *The Cheese and the Worms* (New York: Penguin, 1982). For the culture of "plebeian" materialism, see M. Bakhtin, *Rabelais and His World,* trans. H. Iswolsky (Cambridge, Mass., 1968); Peter Stallybrass and Allon White, *The Politics and Poetics of Transgression* (London: Methuen, 1986).

Yet, after every qualification, it is clear that the overarching hierarchical philosophy of the mind/body duo became definitive for official ideologies in a European sociopolitical order which was itself massively and systematically hierarchical.[36] Often articulated through correspondences between the bodies terraqueous, politic, and natural, the mind/body pairing was congruent with, and supported by, comprehensive theories of cosmic order which attributed to every last entity of Creation its own unique niche on that scale of beings stretching from the lowest manifestation of inanimate nature up to nature's God. On this great chain, the material was set beneath the ideal, and man was "the great amphibian," pivotal between the two.[37]

This bonding of mind and body was, moreover, all of a piece—as hinted above—with a divine universe presided over by a numinous celestial wisdom. Were mind not lord over matter—were the relations between man's soul, consciousness, and will on the one side, and his guts and tissues on the other truly baffling and ambiguous, would that not have been a scandal in a cosmos created and ruled by a Transcendent Mind, pure Being? As Simon Schaffer argues below in regard to Joseph Priestley, only what one might call perversely heterodox believers, with theologicopolitical fish of their own to fry, would contend that the doctrines of immaterial minds and souls so cardinal to Christian orthodoxy were downright heresies. Lies, moreover, even inimical to the gospel, and, by contrast, promoting a deterministic philosophical materialism as their pristine faith, were problematical in another way.

There was, of course, abundant scope within Christian belief for heresy, and much of that was radical. Yet most rebel creeds involved attacks upon the banausic "knife-and-fork" materialism of paunchy prelates and the espousal, from Luther through the New Light and the Church of Christ, Scientist, of more intensely spiritual outlooks that established churches with their feet on the ground of Rome or Canterbury allowed. Many of the most exciting, modernizing philosophical movements in the sixteenth and seventeenth centuries aimed to slough off what were seen as the excessively materialist Aristotelian components of Scholasticism, replacing them with the more idealistic doctrinces of Neoplatonism and Neo-Pythagoreanism and dozens of grass-roots varieties of the two. Reijer Hooykaas, the contemporary Dutch historian of

36. L. Barkan, *Nature's Work of Art: The Human Body as Image of the World* (New Haven: Yale University Press, 1975).

37. A. O. Lovejoy, *The Great Chain of Being* (Cambridge, Mass.: Harvard University Press, 1936) remains the classic discussion of the meanings of hierarchical metaphysics.

science, has suggestively drawn attention to the congruence between the Protestant God and the transdendental voluntarism of the "new philosophy."[38] It is a similitude—or at least a convergence—that needs to be weighted in all our discussion of the mind/body relationship in modern times.

Hence the first comprehensive and sustained questioning of mind/body dualism, and the wider cosmology of which it was emblem and authorization, came with the Enlightenment.[39] The relationship was eventually analyzed, explored, questioned, contested, and radically reformulated—a great intellectual wave sweeping over western Europe from the middle of the seventeenth century onward. The terms of the debate were fierce and the stakes (in the cases of scientists and divines) could be high. Indeed, some even rejected root-and-branch its very terms. There was no single line of attack, and certainly no uniform outcome. It was a dialogical undertaking—in Bakhtin's sense—whose grandness could only be gleaned in the architectural magnificence of its details; in the case at hand, in the ramifications and implications of the debate that seemed to touch on every single subject under the sun. But in a multitude of ways, as the contributions to this volume reveal, what hitherto had been taken as a fact of life—albeit not without its difficulties and unrelenting tensions—became deeply problematic to many and repugnant to some.

In certain respects the fabric came apart at the seams not because of ideological animus or ulterior political motives, but because inquiry inevitably uncovered loose threads begging to be pulled. Essentially internal investigations in science and scholarship, new discoveries and technical advances, all served inevitably—though not uncontroversially—to modify the mental map. As Robert Frank shows below, anatomy was one of these fields. Ever since the Renaissance endeavors of Vesalius, Fallopius and others, the forging of more sophisticated techniques of postmortem dissection as part of the rise of anatomy teaching stimulated

38. R. Hooykaas, *Religion and the Rise of Modern Science* (Edinburgh: Scottish Academic Press, 1972). Illuminating also are I. Couliano, *Eros et magie à la Renaissance* (Paris: Flammarion, 1984), and W. Leiss, *The Domination of Nature* (New York, 1972); and, for the long-term retreat of the "animist" worldview, E. B. Tylor's anthropological classic, *Primitive Culture* (1871).

39. Ernst Cassirer, *The Philosophy of the Enlightenment* (Boston: Beacon, 1964) remains the most penetrating account of the metaphysics of the Enlightenment. S. C. Brown, ed., *Philosophers of the Enlightenment* (Brighton: Harvester Press, 1979) contains valuable discussions of *philosophes* from Locke to Kant.

intense curiosity about the relationship between structure and function, normalcy and pathology, the living body and the corpse on the slab.

As well as investigating muscles, bones, and, most celebratedly, the vascular system, seventeenth-century anatomy devoted fertile attention to the nerves. These nerves became the European sport of anatomists and physiologists, whose narrative discourses reveal to what degree the nerves also engaged the imagination, and often, the genius, of these scientists. The pathways between nerve endings, the central nervous system conducted along the spine, and the distinct chambers of the brain were finely traced, above all by the English physician and scientist Thomas Willis, with a precision vastly outstripping Galen's pioneering investigations. Such work invited inferences not merely about the role of the brain both as the receptor of nervous stimuli from the senses and the transmitter of motor signals, but about the localized functions of the distinct brain structures: cerebrum, cerebellum, and so forth. The logic of anatomical investigation was offering every encouragement, not merely to the general intuition that the brain was connected with thinking, but to the more radical prospect that specific pieces of gray matter governed identifiable facets of sensation, ideation, and behavior.[40]

There was of course nothing new in a broad, essentially mechanistic, "medical materialism"—the perception of every doctor (indeed, every patient) that physical states affect consciousness; such views, as Carol Houlihan Flynn emphasizes below, were of a piece with the most orthodox humoralism. What *was* new and challenging about Willis's "neurologia" and "psyche-ologia" was that it pinned down the mind remarkably—even uncomfortably—close to the brain. In making these observations, Willis had no grander ax to grind. Blamelessly orthodox in his Anglicanism and a true-blue royalist in politics, he was no *proto-philosophe.* Even his use of language—a prose style that was closer to Bacon than to the more baroque Sir Thomas Browne and Thomas Burnet of his own time—was remarkably conventional and augured for scientific style the plain prose advocated by Thomas Sprat's *History of the Royal Society.*[41] But his own work and later investigations by others

40. For Willis see also Hansruedi Isler, *Thomas Willis, 1621–1685, Doctor and Scientist* (New York: Hafner, 1968); and on the nerves, J. Spillane, *The Doctrine of the Nerves* (London: Oxford University Press, 1981); G. S. Rousseau, "Nerves, Spirits, and Fibres: Towards Defining the Origins of Sensibility," with a postscript, *The Blue Guitar* (Messina) 2 (1976): 125–153; idem, "Psychology," in *The Ferment of Knowledge,* ed. G. S. Rousseau and Roy Porter (Cambridge: Cambridge University Press, 1980), 143–210.

41. There is no study of Thomas Willis's prose style, certainly no exploration approaching the work that has been completed for Sprat, Thomas Burnet, and other early

such as Albrecht von Haller (the Swiss Enlightenment physiologist) into the nervous system and its functions of irritation and excitability, were easily appropriated by those whose vision of a "science of man" (to complement and complete the "science of nature" which had been so successfully pursued in the seventeenth century) was intended as a weapon of war against the entrenched cosmology, theology, and politics.

V

This is no place to retell the tale of the Enlightenment, or even of the role of scientific materialism within it.[42] As Peter Gay has emphasized, however, we must never forget that the sharpest intellects of the generations from the late seventeenth century forward were primed to be systematically critical of old orthodoxies, and eager to map out new-found worlds, cognitive as well as physical. The voyages of discovery, the philological criticism pioneered by Renaissance humanists, the dazzling techniques of historical inquiry, and the new science accelerating from Galileo to Newton all joined forces to question traditional authorities as graven in the authority of books, including the Book of God's Word and delivered in the ipse dixits of the ancients and the entrenched hand-me-down orthodoxies of metaphysics, Scholasticism, and custom. To set human understanding on a sure footing, searching inquiries had to be initiated into man's nature and his place within the entire living system, into his natural faculties, propensities, and endowments, his history, his social ties, his prospects. And if the proper study of mankind was man, as the great English poet had pronounced, such knowledge (it was claimed) patently could not be plucked down from abstract eternal witnesses or looked up in books, but had to be grounded upon firsthand facts, derived from observation and experiment, subject to the searing

prominent members of the Royal Society. For the debates over rhetoric and science within the Royal Society at this time see Brian Vickers, *In Defence of Rhetoric* (Oxford: Clarendon Press; New York: Oxford University Press, 1988); idem, ed., *Occult and Scientific Mentalities in the Renaissance* (Cambridge: Cambridge University Press, 1984); also useful for the linguistic milieu of all those post-Cartesian figures is *Rhetoric and the Pursuit of Truth: Language Change in the Seventeenth and Eighteenth Centuries: Papers Read at a Clark Library Seminar, 8 March 1980,* by Brian Vickers and Nancy S. Struever (Los Angeles: William Andrews Clark Memorial Library, University of California, Los Angeles, 1985); and Hans Arsleff, *From Locke to Saussure: Essays on the Study of Language and Intellectual History* (Minneapolis: University of Minnesota Press, 1982).

42. For admirable introductions, see Peter Gay, *The Enlightenment: An Interpretation,* 2 vols. (New York: Vintage, 1966–1969); Norman Hampson, *The Enlightenment* (Harmondsworth: Penguin Books, 1968).

sunlight of criticism.[43] Yet few pursuits in the history of science in the modern age invigorated empiricism more than the dilemma of mind and body. It was a dualism almost guaranteed to elicit the latest strain in every man and woman.

The mobilization of such programs—Hume spoke for his age in expressing his aspiration to become the Newton of the moral sciences—broke down, or at least left uncertain and indeterminate, that overarching structure of analogies and correlations between the microcosm of man and the macrocosm of the universe which had been the guarantor of traditional epistemologies. This was the larger "breaking of the circle" about which the late Marjorie Hope Nicolson has written so eloquently,[44] but the collapse was felt as much in the domain of mind and body as in the organic and inorganic sciences. Indeed, Hume's skeptical *Dialogues of Natural Religion* questioned the very possibility that man could attain to any determinate understanding of his (teleological) station within the cosmos, or any grasp of the meaning of the universe, just as his radical moral philosophy appeared to deny that the order of the natural world could provide the basis for an ethical code by which to live.[45]

Hence in a multitude of ways, Enlightenment inquirers convinced themselves that the highest priority for a true understanding of man—to serve as the basis for the critique and reform of society—must be (to use Hume's terms) an *Inquiry into Human Nature.* This was an endeavor conducted in a variety of fields or disciplines—we may anachronistically call them politics, religion, aesthetics, psychology, anthropology, history, and so forth—by the distinguished succession of thinkers from Bayle and Locke, through Montesquieu, Voltaire, Hume, and La Mettrie, and on to Helvetius, Diderot, d'Holbach, Rousseau, Lessing, and Herder, to say nothing of innumerable lesser figures. Their outlooks were often remarkably diverse, as they debated and disagreed on levels extending beyond methodological and clerical ones. Also, their vantages differed in accordance with national and regional cultures and changed over

43. Paul Hazard, *The European Mind, 1680–1715* (Cleveland: Meridian, 1963), and idem, *European Thought in the Eighteenth Century: From Montesquieu to Lessing* (Cleveland: Meridian, 1963) capture, in vivid language, the effervescence of intellectual transformation produced by the new science, scholarship, and geographical discoveries. See also R. F. Jones, *Ancients and Moderns: A Study of the Background of the Battle of the Books* (St. Louis: Washington University Press, 1936).

44. See M. H. Nicolson, *The Breaking of the Circle: Studies in the Effect of the "New Science" upon Seventeenth-Century Poetry,* rev. ed. (New York: Columbia University Press, 1960).

45. See David Hume, *Dialogues concerning Natural Religion,* ed. N. Kemp Smith (New York: Social Science Publishers, 1948).

time.[46] Yet when viewed as a whole, the movement served to destroy the traditional notion—the creed of Milton, Pascal, Racine, and Bossuet—that man had been placed in a divinely ordered universe as a unique compound of immaterial and immortal soul and mundane, mortal body, as Sir Thomas Browne's "great amphibian":

> to call ourselves a Microcosm, or little World, I thought it onely a pleasant trope of Rhetorick, till my neer judgement and second thoughts told me there was a real truth therein. For first we are a rude mass, and in the rank of creatures which onely are, and have a dull kind of being, not yet priviledged with life, or preferred to sense or reason; next we live the life of Plants, the life of Animals, the life of Men, and at last the life of Spirits, running on in one mysterious nature those five kinds of existences, which comprehend the creatures, not onely of the World, but of the Universe. Thus is Man that great and true *Amphibium,* whose nature is desposed to live, not onely like other creatures in divers elements, but in divided and distinguished worlds; for though there be but one to sense, there are two to reason, the one visible, the other invisible.[47]

Many *philosophes,* sketching in what was often called a "natural history" of man, believed it was imperative to treat man less as a fixed and final object of creation, an "Adam," than as the product of time, circumstances, and milieu—the creature of education (as Locke, Condillac, and Helvetius especially stressed),[48] of climate and physical environment (Montesquieu), of physical evolution (Buffon, Erasmus Darwin, and Lamarck),[49] or of history (Vico, Boulanger, Ferguson, Miller, Herder).[50] Man's physique and consciousness were both the result of processes of

46. A point argued in Roy Porter and Mikulas Teich, eds., *The Enlightenment in National Context* (Cambridge: Cambridge University Press, 1981).

47. *The Works of Sir Thomas Browne,* ed. Geoffrey Keynes, 6 vols. (London: Faber and Gwyer, 1928–1931), 1:47 (sec. 34). Browne, like Willis, conducted a thriving medical practice all his life, but the intersection of his literature and medicine, especially viewed within the medicolinguistic realm, or in relation to mind/body dualism, has not been explored. Such fine books as Thomas N. Corns's *The Development of Milton's Prose Style* (Oxford: Clarendon Press, 1982) discuss baroque English style in the age of Browne but omit these seminal scientific figures.

48. See, for instance, D. W. Smith, *Helvetius: A Study in Persecution* (Oxford: Clarendon Press, 1965), a fine account of the pioneering utilitarian.

49. For the history of man set in the context of vibrant ideas of life see Jacques Roger, *Les sciences de la vie dans la pensée française au XVIII siècle* (Paris: Colin, 1963).

50. For Enlightenment conjectural histories of man see Gladys Bryson, *Man and Society: The Scottish Inquiry of the Eighteenth Century* (Princeton: Princeton University Press, 1945); J. H. Brumfitt, *Voltaire, Historian* (Oxford: Oxford University Press, 1958); P. Rossi, *The Dark Abyss of Time: The History of the Earth and the History of Nations from Hooke to Vico* (Chicago: University of Chicago Press, 1984).

natural and social advancement from savagery to civilization, from rudeness to refinement. Or, as some saw it—a point emphasized below in Richard Popkin's essay on the Jewish question—possibly the result of a deterioration from some pristine golden age through to latter-day decadence. In the process of such dynamic interaction with the environment, of learning and adaptation, body and awareness had endlessly, indefinitely interacted. Consciousness (both individual and collective) developed out of the senses, and the senses themselves—whether considered in terms of the individual adult maturing from infancy or in terms of the collective psychohistory of the species—had equally been the product of dynamic processes of refinement, atunement, or, possibly, enfeeblement.[51]

Nevertheless, it would be grossly misleading to imply that Enlightenment thought was programmatically atheistic or revolutionary, or even optimistic about the prospects of radical praxis.[52] Diderot's dialogues hardly share the practical confidence of Lenin's tone: *What Is to Be Done?*; the conclusions of *Candide* and *Rasselas* are conclusive within an intentional inconclusiveness; and so self-conscious a work of advanced thought as *Tristram Shandy* is ultimately an elegy—an *English* elegy—to inaction. Yet the Enlightenment advanced visions of man's life that saw his essence lying in change, process, transformation, becoming—anything but a fixed point on an inflexible scale. Man had less of a nature than of a history, or rather his history was his nature. He was made by the sum of all the determining forces; but out of the resources of his milieu man also made himself—and, through the dynamic dialectic of habit and education, constantly remade himself over and again. And this was a process, as Diderot emphasized so clearly, long before Marx, in which material circumstances shaped consciousness even as consciousness itself changed material circumstances. Thinking was thus an expression of being, and self was a creature of experience. A radical prospect—indeed, a daunting one, when a Laurence Sterne (whose hero tells us, deferring to Locke, that a man's mind is a veritable history book) goes on to have his hero asked "Who are you?," to which his only response is, "Don't puzzle me."[53]

51. For ideas about the malleability of man see J. Passmore, *The Perfectibility of Man* (London: Duckworth, 1972).

52. See Henry Vyverberg, *Historical Pessimism in the French Enlightenment* (Cambridge, Mass.: Harvard University Press, 1958).

53. Laurence Sterne, *The Life and Opinions of Tristram Shandy*, ed. C. Ricks (Harmondsworth: Penguin, 1967).

Man was thus a creature less of fixed being than of becoming. Lockeans denied he was born naturally endowed with a full complement of innate ideas and moral understanding. Experience was all, and experience was derived from the senses and was mediated by the highly somatic mechanisms of pleasure and pain. Thus, a tacit materialism was seeping in through the cracks, as is illustrated by Locke's canny acknowledgment that there was nothing incompatible with the divine creation in the possibility of "thinking matter"—though it was not a notion he expressly espoused.[54] Yet the radical transformation of mind/body concepts had less to do with doctrinaire materialism than with the softening-up process whereby man's faculties, traditionally taken as "given," such as the will, or the understanding conceived as the "candle of the Lord,"[55] as a divinely endowed "ratio recta," were subjected to intense scrutiny, one might almost say "deconstructed." It is as if their operations were itemized, part by part and one by one, and the contingencies and vagaries of consciousness thereby accentuated.

Thus, in moves whose inadequacy Philippa Foot criticizes below, the various forms of utilitarianism attempted, in the name of scientificity, to reduce the exercise of moral judgment to sets of component decisions taken in a lawlike way on the basis of the operation of the mechanisms of desire and aversion. Likewise, epistemological associationism pictorialized the processes whereby edifices of knowledge were built up out of the primitive building bricks of sense impressions.[56] As Locke's revolutionary *Essay concerning Human Understanding* shows, associationism was not necessarily committed to a materialist physiology; yet, as in Hartley's subsequent system, it often was. As Foucault (in such well-known books as *Madness and Civilization* and *Discipline and Punish*) and other scholars have noted, theory and practice in such eighteenth-century endeavors as child rearing, pedagogy—not least instruction for the deaf and blind—and penology was the radical new model of a will which was neither free nor instinctually wicked but malleable and available for conditioning in a controlling environment. These developments assumed an understanding for simpler concepts—attention, learning languages ver-

54. John Yolton, *John Locke and the Way of Ideas* (New York: Oxford University Press, 1956); idem, *Thinking Matter: Materialism in Eighteenth-Century Britain* (Minneapolis: University of Minnesota Press, 1983); idem, *Perceptual Acquaintance from Descartes to Reid* (Minneapolis: University of Minnesota Press, 1984).

55. The favorite Cambridge Platonist image; see Rosalie Colie, *Light and Enlightenment* (Cambridge: Cambridge University Press, 1957).

56. Perhaps the finest discussion of the rise of such mechanistic imagery of thinking remains Elie Halevy, *The Growth of Philosophic Radicalism* (London: Faber and Faber, 1928).

bal and symbolic, reading—which have yet to be fully studied.[57] Even so, by the middle of the eighteenth century it was perfectly clear to those who entered into such physiological and psychological discussion that consciousness, like memory and desire, was not an activity that could profitably be discussed without full recourse to both mind and body.

Such developments had many faces. Reflecting widespread contemporary excitement, many of our historians have been enthusiastic about the Enlightenment "discovery" of man and its formulation of new, scientific, secular concepts of the personality and identity; about the birth of self-awareness and the exhilarating odyssey of individualism that occurred during that period; and about the growing importance of the notion of *Bildung,* with its proclamation, paralleling the Kantian *sapere aude,* dare to be wise, of *esse aude,* dare to be, or to become, asserting the true emancipation of mankind from ancient, self-imposed, fetters. At the end of this avenue lies the declaration of the rights of man: startlingly secular, individualist, utilitarian.[58] And from these natural rights—natural because they derive from man's anatomy and physiology, his or her body as much as any other consideration—follows the modern state with its peculiar blend of democratic liberty and social control.

Or one could speak in more pessimistic tones of the dissolution of traditional stable senses of self, soul, and of social obligation in that welter of indulgent narcissism and moral solipsism encouraged by the fashion-

57. Attention, learning to read, and language theory as it reflected the relation of words to things were subjects of supreme significance throughout the Enlightenment, and those who wrote on these subjects—from whatever vantage point—inevitably found themselves commenting upon mind and body. Among these, for example, were such diverse thinkers as the Swiss classicist Samuel Werenfels, the opponent of false sublimity and author of *A Discourse of Logomachys, or controversys about words, so common among learned men. To which is added, A Dissertation concerning Meteors of Stile, or false sublimity* (London: W. Taylor and E. Sanger, 1711); the English philologist James Harris, the author of the 1756 *Hermes* (reprint, Menston, Yorks.: Scolar Press, 1968), from whose work the passage in our epigraph is taken; the illustrious French philosopher–social commentator Condorcet, in his *Progress of the Human Mind* (see the edition by Stuart Hampshire et al. [London: Weidenfeld and Nicolson, 1955]); and Charles Bonnet, the Swiss naturalist whose psychology of mind and body formed the basis of his very interesting theories of attention and learning. For Bonnet, see *Considérations sur les corps organisés, où l'on traite d leur origine, de leur dévelopment, de leur réproduction, &c. & où l'on a rassemblé en abrégé tout ce que l'histoire naturelle offre de plus certain & de plus intéressant sur ce sujet,* 2d ed. (Amsterdam: Marc Michel Rey, 1768); idem, *Essai analytique sur les facultés de l'âme* (reprint, New York: Olms, 1973); idem, *Essai de psychologie* (reprint, New York: Olms, 1978); as well as Lorin Anderson, *Charles Bonnet and the Order of the Known* (Dordrecht: D. Reidel, 1982). G. Murphy, in *Psychological Thought from Pythagoras to Freud* (New York: Harcourt, Brace, 1968), does not identify "attention" as a valid category until the nineteenth century, but it was surely a crucial category in the eighteenth-century Enlightenment.

able new sensibility and the utilitarian hedonic calculus. The erosion of that value hierarchy which the mind/body template had inexorably underwritten was (in ths reading) that highroad to nihilism trodden (in the eyes of many scholars, as David Morris underlines below) by none other than that hero of the late Enlightenment, the Marquis de Sade.[59]

Or, as a third possibility, one might eschew premature judgments beteen optimistic and pessimistic readings, the visions of self-emancipation and self-imprisonment, and rather preserve a studied ambivalence, echoing the open question of Diderot's final drama, *Est-il bon? Est-il mechant?* Which ever line is taken, what seems beyond dispute is the Enlightenment conviction that to know the world it was vital first to know the knower; to look within man was to grasp his faculties, dispositions, and potentialities; but the latter could not be accomplished without first inquiring into the boundaries of the body, the status of consciousness, and the interplay between the two. Whether viewed dialectically, as Kant and Blake would, or more simply as contrary states of body and mind, interplay required consultation of *both*. One without the other—say mind without body, or body without consciousness—entailed an epistemological, even ontological, impossibility—a constituted anomaly whose just proportions could only be set straight by consultation of the Other. In this radical inclusiveness lay much of the elusive originality of Enlightenment thinking on mind and body, whether viewed along English, French, German, or any other national lines.[60]

VI

Above all, the Enlightenment did actually generate, almost for the first time in Western culture, a thoroughgoing materialist strand, which was

58. For the eighteenth century as an era of the achievement of self-identity see S. D. Cox, *"The Stranger within Thee": Concepts of the Self in Late-Eighteenth-Century Literature* (Pittsburgh, 1980); J. O. Lyons, *The Invention of the Self* (Carbondale: Southern Illinois University Press, 1978); P. M. Spacks *Imagining a Self* (Cambridge, Mass.: Harvard University Press, 1976); J. N. Morris, *Versions of the Self* (New York, 1966); for philosophical background see H. E. Allison, "Locke's Theory of Personal Identity: A Re-examination," in *Locke on Human Understanding: Selected Essays*, ed. I. C. Tifton (Oxford, 1977), 105–122.

59. Lester G. Crocker, *An Age of Crisis: Man and World in Eighteenth-Century France* (Baltimore: Johns Hopkins University Press, 1959); idem, *Nature and Culture: Ethical Thought in the French Enlightenment* (Baltimore: Johns Hopkins University Press, 1963). Crocker highlights the dilemmas produced by Enlightenment naturalism, subjectivism, and relativism.

60. See Peter Gay, *The Enlightenment: An Interpretation*, 2 vols. (New York: Vintage, 1966–1968); and Roy Porter and Mikulas Teich, eds., *The Enlightenment in National Context* (Cambridge: Cambridge University Press, 1981).

generally—though not necessarily, as the cases of Hartley and Priestley amply testify—associated with a strident religious freethinking verging on atheism: true materialism would expose theistic idealism as false consciousness. This was an agenda whose vitality remains to be explored and measured for the latter part of the eighteenth century. Taking up suggestions such as Locke's hints of the possibility of "thinking matter," the suggestion was widely investigated and disseminated—it is bandied about as a shocking commonplace by Diderot—that mind might be fully and entirely comprehended by the activities of the brain, nerves, and juices, and that thought was nothing but the secretion of the brain just as bile was the secretion of the stomach. From the middle of the eighteenth century, this materialist agenda became privileged. La Mettrie first comprehensively spelt out a materialism applied to man in *L'homme machine,* d'Holbach expounded a totally materialistic vision of the cosmos in his *Système de la nature,* and the Ideologues later systematized a functionalist philosophy of thinking, in which they emphasized that the phenomena of consciousness were purely the products of the fine-tuned organization of matter.[61] It may appear an odd position—this radical materialist notion of consciousness and ideation. Yet it was widely explored and—what is more—continues to find staunch champions among the elite of our contemporary neurobiological and neurophysiological establishment who continue to insist that brain is matter, thought brain, and (as John Keats, the young doctor-poet, might have remarked) that this is all we need to know. To be sure, the sociobiologists and environmentalists have countered this extreme materialist position, but the results are still out, and it would be imprudent and premature to believe that one or another position lies close to any agreed-upon truth. This fierce ambiguity underlies some of (but not all) the eternal fascination of mind and body.

In the eighteenth century, materialist outlooks appeared in many other guises too, such as Erasmus Darwin's pioneering version of biolog-

61. For Enlightenment historical and critical exposés of religion as false consciousness, see Frank E. Manuel, *The Eighteenth Century Confronts the Gods* (New York: Atheneum, 1967); R. Knox, *Enthusiasm* (London, 1950); B. R. Kreiser, *Miracles, Convulsions and Ecclesiastical Politics in Early Eighteenth-Century Paris* (Princeton: Princeton University Press, 1978); G. Rosen, "Enthusiasm: 'A Dark Lanthorn of the Spirit,'" *Bulletin of the History of Medicine* 42 (1958): 393–421; H. Schwartz, *Knaves, Fools, Madmen, and That Subtile Effluvium: A Study of the Opposition to the French Prophets in England, 1706–1710* (Gainesville: University Presses of Florida, 1978). For materialism, see in particular Margaret C. Jacob, *The Radical Enlightenment: Pantheists, Freemasons and Republicans* (London: George Allen and Unwin, 1981); A. C. Kors, *D'Holbach's Circle: An Enlightenment in Paris* (Princeton: Princeton University Press, 1977).

ical evolutionism. This version envisaged the evolution of all forms of organic activity out of the first living filament, driven by an urge to aspire to higher levels of sensory enjoyment. The inherent drives of wriggling matter eventually blossomed forth in the human consciousness.[62] This Darwinian position greatly influenced early Romantic thinkers, in England and on the Continent, who derived much of their sense of mind and body form Darwin's materialist biology, perhaps even more so than from the great philosophical tradition extending from Hobbes and Locke to Kant and the Germans.

It is no accident that Darwin—like La Mettrie, Hartley, Cabanis, and literally dozens of others who would figure into a detailed study of mind and body—was a physician. For, as Dora Weiner emphasizes in her essay below, the most powerful, yet profoundly ambiguous, toehold for a mode of materialism within traditional European thought had been the discourse of medicine—a discourse as vast as it was diverse. Doctors had long enjoyed a notoriety for what we might call their professional materialism, alongside their proverbial (if probably unjustified) reputation for atheism. Traditional humoral medicine was materialist through and through, if we mean by that that it acknowledged—as must any medicine worth its salt—the central role of psychosomatic and somatopsychic activities in determing health and disease. No doctor or patient earnestly examining the parameters of sickness could question that physical disorders—or indeed medical drugs—affected mental states, or, vice versa, that physical health depended to no mean degree upon emotional disposition, states of mind, and so forth. The placebo effect was highly familiar to doctors attuned to the magic of sympathy and the strength of imagination in governing matters of health.[63] Medicine was permitted this potentially threatening perspective, in part because the needs of practice required it, and, far more so, because, dealing definitionally with pathological states, with the diseased individual, the ground rules governing normal human values were obviously suspended. One

62. Maureen MacNeil, *Under the Banner of Science: Erasmus Darwin and His Age* (Manchester: Manchester University Press, 1987); see D. King-Hele, *Erasmus Darwin and the Romantic Poets* (New York: St. Martin's Press, 1986), for this theory of consciousness amongst Romantic *literati.*

63. For explication see L. S. King, "The Power of the Imagination," in *The Philosophy of Medicine: The Early Eighteenth Century* (Cambridge, Mass.: Harvard University Press, 1978), chap. 7; Owsei Temkin, *Galenism: The Rise and Decline of a Medical Philosophy* (Ithaca, N.Y.: Cornell University Press, 1973); and more broadly, idem, "Health and Disease," in *Dictionary of the History of Ideas,* ed. P. P. Wiener et al., vol. 2 (New York: Scribner's, 1973), 395–407.

might incidentally compare the license granted the satirist or caricaturist to imply that his target was none other than an insect, a wild beast, or a machine. Such "medicinal" satire did not derogate from the dignity of human nature precisely because it exposed the sickness of those who truly threatened it.[64]

Furthermore, despite an older and erroneous historiography, Cartesian philosophy no more undermined the traditional psychosomatic medical perspective than the "scientific revolution" of the seventeenth century destroyed humoral medicine (although, as we have seen a new emphasis upon the key role played by the nervous system is everywhere evident).[65] It is hardly surprising in such circumstances that medicine (broadly understood) proved one of the key sites for the further elucidation of the seemingly infinitely complex and shifting relations between consciousness and corporeality.

This development is highly evident in Antonie Luyendijk-Elshout's paper. It is widely argued these days, in part following Foucault, that the age of reason could not tolerate "unreason" and had to sequestrate and silence it in the "great confinement"; and that, by consequence, eighteenth-century therapeutics for the mad fell back more heavily

64. But it did not call in question the semiology of disease and the role of imagination within this semiotic system of medical diagnosis. Also, satires on the imagination in the period reflected the intersection of these two realms: medical and literary—in such works, for example, as (in England) Dr. Malcolm Flemyng's *Neuropathia* (London, 1747) and (in Italy) the polymathic Lodovico Antonio Muratori's book on imagination, human health, and dreams (1747). For medical satire, see M. H. Nicolson and G. S. Rousseau, *This Long Disease My Life: Alexander Pope and the Sciences* (Princeton: Princeton University Press, 1968), but there remains no in-depth study of the medicalization of the imagination in the Enlightenment, as G. S. Rousseau noted two decades ago in "Science and the Discovery of the Imagination in Enlightened England," *Eighteenth-Century Studies* 3 (1969): 108–135.

65. Modern critiques of Cartesian dualism stress the continuing degree of psychosomatic interplay, even in the discussion of brutes, for the latter of which see L. Cohen Rosenfeld, *From Beast-Machine to Man-Machine: The Theme of Animal Soul in French Letters from Descartes to La Mettrie* (New York: Oxford University Press, 1940). See also T. Brown, "Descartes, Dualism and Psychosomatic Medicine," in *The Anatomy of Madness,* ed. W. F. Bynum, Roy Porter, and Michael Shepherd, 2 vols. (London, 1985), 2: 40–62; Sylvana Tomaselli, "Descartes, Locke and the Mind/Body Dualism," *History of Science* 22 (1984): 185–205; R. B. Carter, *Descartes' Medical Philosophy* (Baltimore: Johns Hopkins University Press, 1983); L. J. Rather, *Mind and Body in Eighteenth-Century Medicine* (Berkeley and Los Angeles: University of California Press, 1965); idem, "Old and New Views of the Emotions and Bodily Changes," *Clio Medica* 1 (1965): 1–25. A contrary interpretation is to be found in P. Lain Entralgo, *Mind and Body: Psychosomatic Pathology: A Short History of the Evolution of Medical Thought* (London: Harvill, 1955).

upon mechanical and medical means to restrain the body.[66] This marginalization of the Enlightenment doctors was almost unprecedented—it is said—in Western civilization. But Dr. Luyendijk-Elshout's paper shows that this interpretation is far too simplistic a reading, and demonstrates the point by using students' medical dissertations, which have rarely been consulted. The "mad-doctors" assessed by our Dutch historian of medicine fully understood the importance of mental and emotional precipitants of the sicknesses of their charges, just as they intertwined medical and moral treatments in their often highly original therapeutics. Medical concepts, centered upon the mediating role of the nerves, and psychophysiological categories, such as the idea of the passions of the soul and their pathology, effectively established the interlinkage. The result was a more elaborate and psychopathological medical theory than we (collectively, that is) have recognized: one taking account of dreams and visions, nightmares and hallucinations, fantasies and phantasmagorias—an entire underworld of dark subconscious passions often sinking the patient in a sea of mental conflict. The nerves could not be forgotten, of course, prime movers that they were. Yet even they were only a part of the evidence heard by the Enlightenment physician, who also listened to the cries and whispers of the spectral, nighttime world of his patients.[67]

A similar conclusion emerges from Carol Flynn's discussion of key concepts of health and disease as they figured in medical tracts, practical medical advice, therapeutics, and fiction in the eighteenth century. Doctors and laymen were equally aware that the organism possessed a rather mysterious and often mocking wisdom of its own. Both the clergyman-novelist Laurence Sterne and the physician-novelist Tobias Smollett—each suffering from a consumption he clearly knew would prove fatal and cause early death—expressed in their writings the perception that states of health and disease were not gross matters of mechanism, nor entirely under the control of imperious reason. Each recognized that his

66. See classically M. Foucault, *Madness and Civilization*. Similar views are to be found in the Frankfurt School interpretation of the Enlightenment, as in, for example, Max Horkheimer and Theodor W. Adorno, *Dialectic of Enlightenment* (New York: Herder and Herder, 1972).

67. This spectral, nighttime world is just beginning to receive attention, although no one has written so lucidly about it as Luyendijk-Elshout below; see Terry Castle, "Phantasmagoria," *Critical Inquiry* 15 (1988): 32–49. N. Kiessling's valuable study *The Incubus in English Literature: Provenance and Progeny* ([Pullman]: Washington State University Press, 1977) treats the literary dimension without consulting its medical underbelly.

best hope for health depended deeply upon the animated expression of his own personality in action,[68] in motion, in the velocity of change. *Au fond,* it was a recipe for health lying proximate to our twentieth-century holistic views that celebrate the unity of mind and body, the constant occupation of the imagination, and motion, or exercise, elevated to new degrees of sophistication.

Medicine, with, as we have seen, its materialist undertow, diagnoses sickness and proffers remedy. As Peter Gay has pointed out, the *philosophes* adored the picturing of themselves as physicians to a priest-ridden, poverty-stricken ancien régime they regarded as sick, materially, intellectually, and spiritually.[69] Indeed, they diagnosed such traditional theological and metaphysical conceptions as the absolute mind/matter, or mind/body dualisms, or the disembodied soul, or the dogmatic espousal of free will, and its correlate, sinfulness, as themselves symptoms of mental folly or even derangement. Such "fictions" became the targets of those unmasking campaigns for disillusionment and demystification that animated much of the best Enlightenment criticism.

Thus *philosophes* made free with attacking forms of consciousness as diseased, as the expressions of psychopathology. Metaphysical dogmatizing, system-building, religious ravings, and speaking in tongues—these (critics argued) were not rational minds at work but the shriekings of the sick and suffering. "The corruption of the senses is the generation of the spirit," Swift sardonically remarked, in a materializing formulation that any competent *philosophe* might have appropriated.[70] Likewise, Enlightenment pundits enjoyed representing supposed proofs of "free consciousness" as quintessential expresions of *false* consciousness, analogous to nightmares, ghosts, specters, incubi, and succubi; the entire range of somnambulism or mesmeric phenomena thus offered manna to satirists. "The sleep of reason produces monsters," judged Goya, for whom so much official culture betrayed an ingrained psychopathology.[71]

68. See D. Furst, "Sterne and Physick: Images of Health and Disease in *Tristram Shandy*" (Ph.D. diss., Columbia University, 1974); J. Rodgers, "Ideas of Life in *Tristram Shandy*: Contemporary Medicine" (Ph.D. diss., University of East Anglia, 1978); A. Cash, *Laurence Sterne: The Early and Middle Years* (London: Methuen, 1975); and for Smollett, G. S. Rousseau, *Tobias Smollett: Essays of Two Decades* (Edinburgh, 1982).

69. See P. Gay, "The Enlightenment as Medicine and as Cure," in *The Age of the Enlightenment: Studies Presented to Theodore Besterman*, ed. W. H. Barber (Edinburgh: St. Andrews University Publications, 1967), 375–386.

70. J. Swift, *A Tale of a Tub and Other Satires*, ed. K. Williams (London: Everyman, 1975), 191–194.

71. Ronald Paulson, *Representations of Revolution, 1789–1820* (New Haven: Yale University Press, 1983).

It is one of the goals of this book that we should see to what degree this was a psychopathology widely disseminated throughout the various layers and segments of Enlightenment culture—medically generated, perhaps, but also widespread elsewhere, having filtered down to many parts of society through its popular theologies and mythologies of the flesh.

In Enlightenment knockabout histories, entire disciplines such as Scholastic metaphysics or dogmatic theology were relegated to the status of mere delusion, mental aberrations, or, at best, products of a species in its immaturity, a stage in the progress from mental infancy up to modern maturity. Thus Idealism was exposed to the whiplash of criticism as the archetype of false consciousness. As Simon Schaffer emphasizes below, formulating theories of "fictions" was integral to the endeavors of reformers such as Bentham. He represented the very idea of the immortal soul as the fabrication of vested interests, above all the clergy, eager to indoctrinate the masses with beliefs that magnified their own authority, and, more broadly, systematically promoting a self-serving "fiction" of the superiority of the spiritual over the physical, head over hand, priesthood over people. For radical *philosophes,* the very notions of God, Satan, and all other nonmaterial powers were phantoms of priestcraft, fabricated to keep the people in their place. Yet the line from Hartley (who was also a physician) to Priestley, and then Priestley to Bentham, has not been studied in this light: as a discourse of radical will, part mind, part body, and thoroughly soaked in the elaborate medico-philosophical labyrinth of the time. *The Languages of Psyche* aims to open up this avenue for further exploration.

More comprehensively, and even constructively, such diagnoses of the psychopathology of the ancien régime were incorporated into a systematic sociohistorical critique through the program of the Idéologues, notably Cabanis.[72] For these intellectuals living in times of revolutionary social change, expressions of thought were to be treated as one of many products of the integrated, unified human organism. Such unity may have been more imagined than scientifically demonstrable, and it also happened to follow in the footsteps of the giant waves of vitalism sweeping over late Enlightenment thought.[73] But the idea of a complex or-

72. Sergio Moravia, *Il pensiero degli Idéologues* (Florence: La Nuova Italia, 1974); M. Staum, *Cabanis: Enlightenment and Medical Philosophy in the French Revolution* (Princeton: Princeton University Press, 1980).

73. The classic statement is, of course, by Jacques Roger, *Les sciences de la vie* (Paris: Colin, 1963), but Bakhtin has added to the discussion in his 1926 statement about the "dialogism of vitalism" in which both Enlightenment mechanists and vitalists are seen as more entrenched in "the Other" than has been acknowledged; see Michael Bakhtin,

ganic form as the basis of a unified human organism was so strong that it invigorated this research program continuously, especially in France and in centers of learning where French influence held sway. It was thus axiomatic for them—within the mind/body context—that consciousness could not be regarded on its own terms but had to be understood as complementing the thinker, whose ideas were to be read as functional to his interests. In thus developing the notion of "ideology" into an analytic weapon—the weapon that was eventually transformed through the breakdown of other vital connections into nineteenth-century sociology and twentieth-century sociology of knowledge—the Idéologues proved astute commentators upon their own times.

For they—and others besides them—were perceiving that traditional doctrines of consciousness were obsolete; in this sense, traditional concepts of the old mind/body dualism being just as out of date. It was no longer plausible to maintain that the order of things, natural and social, was to correspond to Truths, revealed in Scripture, enshrined by the Church, and expounded by right reason. Such prescriptive visions had to yield to analytic accounts that acknowledged and explained the sociohistorical fact that information, ideas, images, public opinion, and propaganda—in short, ideology—were increasingly playing a crucial, indeed, a dominant, role in ordering and managing society.[74] So magisterial was the authority of knowledge in the high Enlightenment. The very power of the *philosophes,* the spread of books and the press (the fourth estate), was making Swift's dictum that "the pen is mightier than the

"Sovremennyi Vitalizm" (Contemporary vitalism), *Chelovek i Priroda* 1 (1926): 9–23, 33–42, and G. S. Rousseau's analysis of this work in relation to the traditions of Enlightenment vitalism: "Bakhtin and Enlightenment: An Essay on Vitalism for Our Times," in *The Crisis of Modernism: Bergson and the Vitalist Tradition,* ed. Frederick Burwick and Paul Douglass (Cambridge: Cambridge University Press, 1990). For vitalism as it impinges on the mind/body question, see the now classic early-twentieth-century statement by Hans Driesch, *The History and Theory of Vitalism* (London: Macmillan, 1914); and idem, *Mind and Body,* trans. Theodore Besterman (New York: L. MacVeagh, the Dial Press, 1927). The role of vitalism in relation to mind and body was widely studied in the eighteenth century in medical dissertations, especially in middle European universities, and in relation to Stahl's animism and Barthez's medical theory (discussed in Rousseau above). Vitalism in general was fully considered by the German psychologist Ferdinand Carus in his *Geschichte der Psychologie* (Halle, 1795).

74. See Raymond Williams, *The Long Revolution* (London: Chatto and Windus, 1961); Elizabeth Eisenstein, "On Revolution and the Printed Word," in *Revolution in History,* ed. Roy Porter and Mikulas Teich (Cambridge: Cambridge University Press, 1986) 186–205; Robert Darnton, *The Business of Enlightenment: A Publishing History of the Encyclopédie, 1775–1800* (Cambridge, Mass.: Harvard University Press, 1979); idem, *The Literary Underground of the Old Regime* (Cambridge, Mass.: Harvard University Press, 1982).

sword" prove prophetic, and confirming Hume's view that mankind is governed, *au fond,* by "opinion." Wishful thinking aside, it was hardly fortuitous that it was the *philosophes* who made such observations, because in their war to displace priests and official propagandists as the mouthpieces of society, they became masters of the media in an increasingly opinion-conscious society.

Yet here lies a profound paradox that may stand as the summation of that multitude of ironies that sprang out of the mind/body dialectic. Enlightenment thinking, as we have suggested, was profoundly critical of the theological-metaphysical myth of the autonomy of mind and its correlate, free will. Such fictions sanctioned priestcraft, superstition, and hellfire. *Philosophes* anatomized such absurdities and their wider practical manifestations—the irrationalities of credulity, faith, devotion, magic, spells, folklore, and faith healing.[75] Yet the whole body of such beliefs and practices proved amazingly resilient. Explaining the acceptance and continuing purchase of such nonsense presented no small problem, especially for reformers desperately trying to convince themselves and the world that mankind was growing ever wiser in what Paine called the *Age of Reason.* Worse still, progressives had to face the embarrassing fact that many such absurd beliefs and practices appeared to be efficacious. Old charms and new mesmerism might be stuff and nonsense, silly mumbo jumbo from the viewpoint of Newtonian science; yet both seemed to possess curative properties and to exercise strange "occult" powers, if only because of the deviousness of the human imagination.[76] Might not human nature and the human mind then also harbor dark mysteries? Mysteries impenetrable to any science, Newtonian or even more advanced? Impenetrable forever?

VII

An ominous cloud hovered over the Enlightenment: the fear that, for all their faith in the progress of humanity, all their secular evangelizing,

75. See K. V. Thomas, *Religion and the Decline of Magic* (Harmondsworth; Penguin, 1973); and also H. Leventhal, *In the Shadow of the Enlightenment: Occultism and Renaissance Science in Eighteenth-Century America* (New York: New York University Press, 1976).

76. On mesmerism and similar sympathetic powers see W. Falconer, *A Dissertation on the Influence of the Passions upon Disorders of the Body* (London: C. Dilly, 1788); John Haygarth, *Of the Imagination, as a Cause and as a Cure of Disorders of the Body* (Bath: Cadell and Davies, 1800); and, amongst modern scholarship, R. Darnton, *Mesmerism and the End of the Enlightenment in France* (Cambridge, Mass., 1968); Jonathan Miller, "Mesmerism," *The Listener,* 22 Nov. 1973, 685–690; Roy Porter, "Under the Influence: Mesmerism in England," *History Today,* September 1985, 22–29.

all their optimistic demythologizing crusades, the human animal himself might not prove fit for the programs of education, organization, and consciousness-raising that the *philosophes* were mobilizing. Might there be some secret soul within? Some metaphysical *je ne sais quoi* no microscope could ever detect? For the Voltaire of *Candide,* as well as the Johnson of *Rasselas,* man seemed only to have the definitive capacity for making himself miserable. For the Diderot of *Rameau's Nephew,* man was all antitheses (perhaps like Pope's vile Sporus), a chameleon, a monster even. And the Shandy males (in what remains one of the most highly genderized "cock and bull" stories in any language) argued themselves into incapacity. The culture of sensibility thus seemed to entrap itself in a maze of contradictions, and not least, as that famous if corpulent "nerve doctor" George Cheyne contended long before Freud, the pursuit of civilization brought only the discontents of the "English Malady."[77] All these ironies were encapsulated in that archetypal Enlightenment disorder variously called hypochondria,[78] melancholy, hysteria, low spirits, depression. Call it by any other name, wax skeptical even, it remained psychological misery nonetheless.

Stated otherwise, the eighteenth century that aimed to erect a Newtonian moral science, discover the laws of thinking and action, and generate social technologies to pave the way for progress, increasingly stumbled upon hidden depths within the human animal that hindered organized improvement. The boundless and willful anarch, the imagination, was one such sphere. Enlightenment writers continually expressed their anxieties at what Samuel Johnson brilliantly called "the

77. On sensibility see Erik Erametsa, *A Study of the Word "Sentimental" and of Other Linguistic Characteristics of Eighteenth-Century Sentimentalism in England* (Helsinki, 1951); Janet Todd, *Sensibility: An Introduction* (London: Methuen, 1986); L. Bredvold, *The Natural History of Sensibility* (Detroit, 1962); more broadly cultural are S. Moravia, "The Enlightenment and the Sciences of Man," *History of Science* 18 (1980): 247–268; idem, "From 'Homme machine' to 'Homme sensible': Changing Eighteenth-Century Models of Man's Image," *Journal of the History of Ideas* 39 (1978): 45–60; K. Figlio, "Theories of Perception and the Physiology of Mind in the Late Eighteenth Century," *History of Science* 13 (1975): 177–212; and on the positioning of the "English Malady," as Cheyne christened the peculiar nature of English melancholy within the wider history of mental illness, see Stanley W. Jackson, *Melancholia and Depression from Hippocratic Times to Modern Times* (New Haven: Yale University Press, 1986).

78. See E. Fischer-Homberger, "Hypochondriasis of the Eighteenth Century, Neurosis of the Present Century," *Bulletin of the History of Medicine* 46 (1972): 391–401. For the politics of hypochondria in Britain see Roy Porter, "The Rage of Party: A Glorious Revolution in English Psychiatry?" *Medical History* 29 (1983): 35–50; and much other recent scholarship devoted to the medical career of Dr. George Cheyne.

hunger of imagination," that power of wishing or fantasizing which captivated the consciousness and paralyzed the will, driving individuals into dreamworlds of delusion and flights of phantasmagoria. Imaginaton—and worse still, fancy—had disturbingly ambiguous resonances.[79]

Not least, growing fears were expressed that exercise of imagination entailed the direst practical consequences for both genders. A growing literature laid bare the dangers of fantasy-induced nymphomania in young women, and, above all, masturbation in both sexes.[80] Earlier ages had construed masturbation as a relatively harmless physical abuse, in response to ordinary genital irritation. Enlightenment doctors such as Samuel Tissot, however, reconceptualized onanism not as physically stimulated but as the product of a warping of the mind, overheated by diseased imagination. As such, it was more perilous. Indeed, because imagination was so central, onanism was far more dangerous than mere fornication, more habit-forming, more corrupting of the fabric of character, and ultimately more deleterious in its long term effects.

In other fields too, as Roy Porter's chapter suggests, Enlightenment writers grew preoccupied with the evil consequences of vices which they saw as stemming from mental habits. Excessive drinking paradoxically ceased to be regarded as a vice of excess, with essentially physical sequelae, and increasingly was diagnosed as the expression of mental disorder. Narcotic-taking was also seen in a similar light to drunkenness. Coleridge presents the paradox of a thinker whose Romantic commitments made him unfold a heroic vision of the transcendental indepen-

79. For the ambushes of imagination, see S. Cunningham, "Bedlam and Parnassus: Eighteenth-Century Reflections," *Eighteenth-Century Studies* 24 (1971): 36–55; Roy Porter, "The Hunger of Imagination: Approaching Samuel Johnson's Melancholy," in *The Anatomy of Madness*, ed. W. F. Bynum, Roy Porter, and Michael Shepherd (London, 1985), 1:63–88.

80. G. S. Rousseau, "Nymphomania, Bienville and the Rise of Erotic Sensibility," in *Sexuality in Eighteenth-Century Britain*, ed. P. -G. Boucé (Manchester: Manchester University Press, 1982), 95–120; Roy Porter, "Love, Sex and Madness in Eighteenth Century England," *Social Research* 53 (1986): 211–242. And for masturbation, see P. -G. Boucé, "Les jeux interdits de l'imaginaire: Onanism et culpabilisation sexuelle au XVIIIe siècle," in *La folie et le corps*, ed. J. Ceard (Paris: Presses de l'Ecole Normale Supérieure, 1985), 223–243; E. H. Hare, "Masturbatory Insanity: The History of an Idea," *Journal of Mental Science* 108 (1962): 1–25; R. H. MacDonald, "The Frightful Consequences of Onanism," *Journal of the History of Ideas* 28 (1967): 323–341; J. Stengers and A. Van Neck, *Histoire d'une grande peu . La masturbation* (Brussels: University of Brussels Press, 1984); L. J. Jordanova, "The Popularisation of Medicine: Tissot on Onanism," *Textual Practice* 1 (1987): 68–80; and for a wider vision of bourgeois culture as leading to a masturbatory privatization of the body, F. Barker, *The Tremulous Private Body* (New York: Methuen, 1984).

dent mental faculties of reason and imagination, but whose everyday addition to opium—he called it a "*free-agency-annihilating* Poison"—illustrates both the practical reality of growing addiction to narcotics and its recognition as a disease of the mind. Yet Coleridge was the prophet of mental autonomy who enslaved himself. In his *View of the Nervous Temperament,* delivered almost at the graveside of the Enlightenment, the British physician Thomas Trotter exposed the modern philosophy of desire—classically expressed in the terms of utilitarianism—as the pathogenic agent perverting civilization into a drug culture, a mocking materialization of that scientific vision of mechanical man, subject to the laws of cause and effect, so dear to the Enlightenment.[81]

Thus, in one of the great ironies of history, that "mind" which the Enlightenment set out to expose as a "fiction" fought back and reasserted itself, in surprising and troublesome fashions. For one thing, its pathological face was revealing itself. For late-eighteenth-century medicine was, as Dora Weiner demonstrates below, coming to recognize that lunacy was not just seated in the blood, nerves, or brain, but was an authentically *mental* disorder, requiring to be treated with "moral" means (the limitations of such methods would not become apparent until rather later).[82] For another, mind went underground. As Ellenberger and Whyte have shown, the notion of the "unconscious" was taking on an at least inchoate existence in the age of sensibility, coming out in the culture of Romanticism. The Age of Reason closed, so to speak, with increasing, if grudging, homage to its opposite.[83]

Profound currents of Enlightenment thought, we have argued, set about challenging the sovereignty of Mind, because it regarded that

81. See Roy Porter, ed., Introduction to Thomas Trotter, *An Essay, Medical, Philosophical, and Chemical, on Drunkenness* (London: Routledge, 1988; 1st ed., 1804). See also idem, "The Drinking Man's Disease: The Prehistory of Alcoholism in Georgian Britain," *British Journal of Addiction* 80 (1985): 384–396. For other paradoxes arising out of the mind/body problem and the emergence of ideology, see idem, *Mind-forg'd Manacles: A History of Madness in England from the Restoration to the Regency* (London: Athlone, 1987); idem, "Body Politics: Aproaches to the Cultural History of the Body," in *Historiography Today,* ed. P. Burke (London: Polity Press, forthcoming).

82. On moral therapy see A. Digby, *Madness, Morality and Medicine* (Cambridge: Cambridge University Press, 1985); idem, "Moral Treatment at the York Retreat," in *The Anatomy of Madness,* ed. W. F. Bynum, Roy Porter, and Michael Shepherd, 2 vols. (London, 1985), 2: 52–72; W. F. Bynum, "Rationales for Therapy in British Psychiatry 1780–1835," *Medical History* 18 (1974): 817–834.

83. L. L. Whyte, *The Unconscious before Freud* (New York: Doubleday, 1962); H. P. Ellenberger, *The Discovery of the Unconscious: The History and Evolution of Dynamic Psychiatry* (New York, 1971).

sovereignty, in its traditional hierarchico-theological forms, as objectively reactionary and ideologically subservient to tyrannies, personal, social, and political. Mind/body dualism was an instrument of power. Progressives such as Condorcet aimed to undermine such traditions by insisting that consciousness was merely an expression of body-based impressions and sensations.[84] Yet across the spectrum of experience the result was not as expected. For one thing, Romanticism emerged—eventually throughout Europe—as a triumphant vindication of mental individuality, an irreducible integrity, a celebration of uniqueness. And at the same time a mocking deviousness of the will asserted its resistance, manifest in its extreme form as mental morbidity, or what Freud honored as the psychoneuroses. These twin developments might respectively be represented as, on the one hand, the naturalization of theism, and, on the other, the survival of satanic possession.

Together they paradoxically combined to ensure the endurance of the age-old dualism. Throughout the nineteenth century—long after one can validly conjure up Enlightenment debates of any type—fierce challenges to mind were made. These came not only from expected quarters—in the name of credos and cults, the church at large, all the arts—but also from such newly developing academic subjects as anthropology, sociology, psychology, and, in some ways most crucially, from the newly privileged discourse of psychiatry. Body and consciousness played elusive roles in this nineteenth-century evolution of an old relationship: by now a worn-out dialectic, even a reciprocity. Too amorphous to be pinned down or pegged to anything concrete in an age of incremental positivism, consciousness was still viewed either in its mental or physical states, but rarely as the expression of a holistic unit called man or woman. Those who persistently pleaded for body tended to enforce the dualism, in its rhetorical antithesis more forcefully than anywhere else.

Thus minds and bodies were assured a legacy as individual entities, even by those whose unequivocal aim in the nineteenth century, and afterward, was to quash its durability. As the nineteenth century wore on, ever persuaded that its scientific discoveries were new and complacent in the belief that its predecessor (the century of Enlightenment)

84. K. M. Baker, *Condorcet: From Natural Philosophy to Social Mathematics* (Chicago: University of Chicago Press, 1975) is a fine study of the late Enlightenment's most important social scientist-cum-prophet. Also relevant are R. V. Sampson, *Progress in the Age of Reason* (London: Heinemann, 1956), and C. Vereker, *Eighteenth-Century Optimism* (Liverpool: Liverpool University Press, 1967).

had uncovered nothing worthy of preservation, its discourses of mind and body became politically more explosive than they had been. Pardoxically again, the dialogue acquired a type of collective authority that enfranchised, even guaranteed, the survival of the already age-old dualism.

Looking back from the vantage point of our century, one can predict that such a sensitized view of mind and body will result in impasse. Indeed, as the nineteenth century wore out, it became practically impossible to become dialogical about mind and body in any open-ended sense (here Bakhtin was the great exception). If mind was construed as Self, and body as Other—a fair construction considering the degree to which man's rationality was celebrated in the long nineteenth century—one sees why neutral debates could not be held about the mind/body relationship which were incorporative, recuperative, or homogenizing of the Other. By the turn of the twentieth century, the desire to understand otherness—whether mind *or* body—was no longer ideologically or even politically acceptable, except as small waves and insignificant currents in an ocean of selfhood. The mainstream remained divided, as laboratory dualists and philosophical monists, for example, worked independently of the Other. Our dominant late-twentieth-century attitude to mind and body, in contrast, has entailed something of a denouement: less polarized, less dialogical, a topic less urgent among those who plead for integration, as entire segments of civilized society concede that they are entrapped in the dualism while hoping to escape from it, or dismiss its existence, altogether.

TWO

Barely Touching: A Social Perspective on Mind and Body

Roy Porter

It is a mark of the perduring Idealism of our culture that the "body" side of the mind/body relationship has been neglected, or, to put the same point another way, that the major studies of the mind/body problem have been philosophical rather than material-social. Even the direct physical anguish of the flesh, as in the experience of disease, fails to challenge our preferences. The nineteenth-century tuberculosis victim, his or her body wasting away, was somehow "spiritualized" by the process, just as in an analogous way, twentieth-century Freudianism represents a final if backhanded vindication of the ultimate sovereignty of consciousness.

Perhaps this is changing. Perhaps today's newly heightened sense of the ultimate fragility of the body, seemingly threatened with extinction from one quarter by neutron bombs, from another by AIDS, will at last engender a fundamental cultural reversal. The odds are probably against it. History suggests rather the enormous capacity of Idealism in its various forms to rise above the threats. The history of the cursed body and of mind triumphant over matter is long and involved, but ultimately clearly defined.

Back in mid-eighteenth-century Yorkshire, Dr. Slop anathematizes Obadiah:

> "May he . . . be damn'd," (for tying these knots). "May he be cursed in eating and drinking, in being hungry, in being thirsty, in fasting, in sleeping, in slumbering, in walking, in standing, in sitting, in lying, in working, in resting, in pissing, in shitting, and in bloodletting.

> "May he (Obadiah) be cursed in all the faculties of his body.
>
> "May he be cursed inwardly and outwardly. – May he be cursed in the hair of his head. – May he be cursed in his brains, and in the vertex," (that is a sad curse, quoth my father) "in his temples, in his forehead, in his ears, in his eye brows, in his cheeks, in his lips, in his throat, in his shoulders, in his wrists, in his arms, in his hands, in his fingers.
>
> "May be damn'd in his mouth, in his breast, in his heart and purtenance down to the very stomach. . . . may there be no soundness in him."[1]

Thus the fate of Obadiah, cursed in his body. Yet the same malediction seems to have hung over all the males in the Shandy household. Tistram's own complaint—the loss of his animal spirits, of his nose, of his name, of his foreskin, and almost of his life—

> *I can now scarce draw [breath] at all, for an asthma I got in skating against the wind in Flanders*[2]

merely echoes the evils heaped on the bodies of his father (a man "phthisical" and racked with a sciatica),[3] his brother Bobby ("a lad of wonderful slow parts" who expired in his youth),[4] his uncle Toby, wounded in the groin at the seige of Namur, alongside his faithful servant Trim (likewise "disabled for the service"),[5] and not least Parson Yorick, victim like Sterne himself of consumption, whose death is commemorated by a double page of black humor ("Alas, poor Yorick!").[6] It is in short a "dirty planet,"[7] whose "strange fatalities"[8] curse Everyman

1. L. Sterne, *The Life and Opinions of Tristram Shandy,* ed. C. Ricks (Harmondsworth: Penguin, 1967), 185–187. For recent work on the body in Sterne see M. New, "At the Backside of the Door of Purgatory," in *Laurence Sterne: Riddles and Mysteries,* ed. V. Grosvenor-Myer (London: Vision, 1984), 15–23; J. Berthoud, "Shandeism and Sexuality," ibid., 21–88; E. A. Bloom and L. D. Bloom, "'This Fragment of Life': From Process to Mortality," ibid., 57–74; Roy Porter, "Against the Spleen," ibid., 84–98; D. Furst, "Sterne and Physick: Images of Health and Disease in *Tristram Shandy*" (Ph.D. Diss., Columbia University, 1974); L. S. King, *The Medical World of the Eighteenth Century* (Chicago: University of Chicago Press, 1958); J. Rodgers, "Ideas of Life in *Tristram Shandy*: Contemporary Medicine" (Ph.D. diss., University of East Anglia, 1978).
2. Sterne, *Tristram Shandy,* 40.
3. Ibid., 219.
4. Ibid., 67.
5. Ibid., 114.
6. Ibid., 233–234.
7. Ibid., 40.
8. Ibid., 136.

the homunculus—"skin, hair, fat, flesh, veins, arteries ligaments, nerves, cartilage, bones" and all.[9]

So the bodies of the Shandy family are cursed to a man. Yet a similar blight seems to infect the study of the history of the body.[10] Of course, the mind/body problem as such has attracted great minds, historians of philosophy have minutely scrutinized theories of consciousness—John Yolton's brace of books, *Thinking Matter* and *Perceptual Acquaintance,* are admirable recent examples—and we have glorious studies of ideologies and mentalities from *The Savage Mind* and *The Greek Mind* to *The Victorian Frame of Mind.*[11] Yet with a handful of honorable exceptions—Mikhail Bakhtin is one, Norbert Elias another—the body side of the mind/body relation remains curiously neglected, perhaps echoing that late-Victorian moment when the journals *Mind* and *Brain* were founded in quick succession, but no *Body.*[12] Even Marxism, heeding Marx's lofty contempt for vulgar biologism—man is what he eats—has failed to generate a historical materialism of the body.[13]

In fact, for services rendered in concentrating our minds upon the body one scholar stands out head and shoulders above the rest, Michel Foucault, who but for his desperately premature death in 1985 would surely have contributed to this series.[14] Foucault dislodged the Cartesian

9. Ibid., 36.

10. There is a lively discussion on the inadequacies of histories and sociologies of the body in B. S. Turner, *The Body and Society: Explorations in Social Theory* (Oxford: B. Blackwell, 1984). It is less clear whether Turner's own formulations offer a way forward. There is a stimulating discussion of the neglect of the body in literature in Virginia Woolf's essay, "On Being Ill," in *Collected Essays,* vol. 4 (London: Hogarth Press, 1967), 193–203. For Woolf's own problems with "embodiment" see S. Trombley, *"All That Summer She Was Mad": Virginia Woolf and Her Doctors* (London: Junction Books, 1981). And more generally see the discussion in G. S. Rousseau, "Science and Literature: The State of the Field," *Isis* 69 (1978): 583–591; idem, "Literature and Medicine: The State of the Field," *Isis* 72 (1981): 406–424.

11. J. Yolton, *Thinking Matter: Materialism in Eighteenth-Century Britain* (Minneapolis: University of Minnesota Press, 1983); idem, *Perceptual Acquaintance from Descartes to Reid* (Minneapolis: University of Minnesota Press, 1984); C. Levi-Strauss, *La pensée sauvage,* trans. as *The Savage Mind* (London: Weidenfeld and Nicolson, 1965); W. E. Houghton, Jr., *The Victorian Frame of Mind, 1830–1870* (New Haven: Yale University Press, 1957).

12. M. Bakhtin, *Rabelais and His World,* trans. H. Iswolsky (Cambridge, Mass.: MIT Press, 1968); N. Elias, *The Civilizing Process* (Oxford: B. Blackwell, 1983).

13. See the discussion in Turner, *The Body and Society,* 5–6, 99–101.

14. Foucault's main relevant works are *Madness and Civilization: A History of Insanity in the Age of Reason* (London: Tavistock, 1967); *The Order of Things: An Archaeology of the Human Sciences* (London: Tavistock, 1970); *The Archaeology of Knowledge* (London: Tavistock, 1972); *The Birth of the Clinic: An Archaeology of Medical Perception* (London:

privileging of the subject, of the *cogito,* in arguing that the true object of the disciplines, of the exercise of *savoir-pouvoir,* has been the body, focal point of the clinic, asylum, school, reformatory, prison, parade ground, bed. Foucault exposed the folly of taking the bourgeois disparagement of the flesh at face value. Sexual repression was sexual expression; every technique for subduing the flesh was but another mode of empowering it.[15]

The scale of our loss in Foucault's death is only underlined by the crass extravagance of his epigoni. Take for example Francis Barker's *The Tremulous Private Body,* subtitled *An Essay on Subjection,* issued in 1985. Here is his verdict on Pepys, or rather, as he insists, "the Pepysian text":

> the body in the Pepysian text is no more than a monstrous discourse at least in so far as the subject experiences itself as initiator of its own speech. . . . Disinherited and separate, the body is traduced as a rootless thing of madness and scandal and then finally, in its object-aspect, it is pressed into service.[16]

Is this Pepys? The phrase "monstrous discourse" invites the riposte: if the cap fits. The willfulness of Barker's thesis that the triumph of the bourgeoisie involved the disappearance of the body and its replacement by the book simply brings home the need for investigation rather than sloganizing.

Indeed, study of the mind/body problem has been bedeviled all along by ax-grinders. How often have philosophers, insensitive to anachronism, invoked a Cartesian dualism—tailored after whatever mode of rationalism or dualism happened currently to be in vogue—to explain all manner of twists and turns of ideas, with scant regard for the historical Descartes or for his actual reception or reputation?[17] But more distorting still are those moralists who would use the mind/body relation to redress the human condition or peddle new metaphysics.[18] Writes Fritjof Capra in *The Turning Point:*

Pantheon, 1973); *Discipline and Punish: The Birth of the Prison* (Harmondsworth, Penguin, 1979); *The History of Sexuality,* vol. 1, *An Introduction* (London: Penguin, 1978). See also M. Foucault, *Power/Knowledge,* ed. C. Gordon (Brighton: Harvester, 1980), especially the essay "Body/Power," 55–62.

15. See especially Foucault, *History of Sexuality,* 3–14.

16. F. Barker, *The Tremulous Private Body* (London: Methuen, 1984).

17. An instance of this can be found, for example, in M. D. Wilson, "Body and Mind from the Cartesian Point of View," in *Body and Mind: Past, Present and Future,* ed. R. W. Rieber (New York: Academic Press, 1980).

18. E.g., M. Berman, *The Re-enchantment of the World* (Ithaca, N.Y.: Cornell University Press, 1982); F. Capra, *The Turning Point: Science, Society and the Rising Culture* (New York: Wildwood, 1982).

> The Cartesian division between mind and matter has had a profound effect on Western thought. It has enabled huge industries to sell products—especially to women that would make us owners of the "ideal body"; it has kept doctors from seriously considering the psychological dimensions of illness, and psychotherapists from dealing with their patients' bodies.[19]

Yet this is, of course, baloney. Descartes himself never denied the utter interdependence of mind and body. As he put it:

> The mind depends so much on the temperament and disposition of the bodily organs that, if it is possible to find a means of rendering men wiser and cleverer than they have hitherto been, I believe that it is in medicine that it must be sought.[20]

Furthermore, as L. J. Rather's admirable study of Jerome Gaub has shown, post-Cartesian medicine indeed remained thoroughly psychosomatic and somato-psychic.[21] To father Descartes with praise or blame for the "ghost in the machine" is no substitute for accurately probing what happened.

To be precise, we need thick-textured study of the body, unprejudiced by timeless philosophical dualisms or Lovejoyan unit-ideas—remember that Homer had no general term for "mind" or "body"—[22] research which contextualizes the human frame within specific sociocultural frames of reference, sensitive to experience, representations and meaning. And in undertaking this, it will be as well to go back to banausics, and remember that in medieval and early modern Europe—that civilization of faith—the human body had a power and prominence

19. Capra, *Turning Point,* 23, 44.

20. Quoted in T. Brown, "Descartes, Dualism and Psychosomatic Medicine," in *The Anatomy of Madness,* ed. W. F. Bynum, Roy Porter, and Michael Shepherd, 2 vols. (London: Tavistock, 1985), 2: 40–62. See also R. B. Carter, *Descartes' Medical Philosophy* (Baltimore: Johns Hopkins University Press, 1983), who demonstrates the extent of Descartes's own explorations of psychosomatic interplay; see, e.g., pp. 113–114.

21. L. J. Rather, *Mind and Body in Eighteenth-Century Medicine* (London: Wellcome, 1965). For discussions of medical continuity, the irrelevance of the "Cartesian" dualism, and the continuation of psychosomatic approaches to health and personality see W. F. Bynum, "Health, Disease and Medical Care," in *The Ferment of Knowledge,* ed. G. S. Rousseau and Roy Porter (Cambridge: Cambridge University Press, 1980), 211–255; G. S. Rousseau, "Psychology," ibid., 143–210; L. S. King, *The Medical World of the Eighteenth Century* (Chicago: University of Chicago Press, 1958).

22. Bennett Simon, *Mind and Madness in Ancient Greece* (Ithaca, N.Y.: Cornell University Press, 1978); W. I. Matson, "Why Isn't the Mind-Body Problem Ancient?" in *Mind, Matter, and Method,* ed., P. K. Feyerabend and G. Maxwell (Minneapolis: University of Minnesota Press, 1966).

never again to be matched: it was the measure of all things. It was muscle power that tamed the animals, tilled the fields, and made what were—literally—the manufactures. It was man power that built the cathedrals and won the battles—still, in the Renaissance, spectacles of hand-to-hand combat. In what Laslett has called the face-to-face society,[23] it was the personal stature, strength, physique, and stamina of rulers that held the balance between government and anarchy. From trial by ordeal to judicial torture, courtroom procedures put the body to the test; and justice was meted out against the flesh from whippings to the faggot and the gallows.[24] Even after death, the corpse was not spared, often being left to hang in chains as a lesson to the living (yet felons' corpses were touched for their supposed miraculous healing properties).[25] The elementary functions of keeping body and soul together really mattered. Here is a late-seventeenth-century child, Mary Nelthorpe, writing to her mother about the state of her health:

> This is to lett my Mother know
> Her Worme is well from top to toe,
> Except my Bumps, they so exceed
> They make me scratch untill I Bleed;
> But now I think ont, It is fitt,
> To lett you know how oft I shitt,
> Two stooles a day, but sometimes none
> Take one time with another one;
> And that I may not one thing miss;
> Bout twice as oft I goe to piss.[26]

Standard histories tell us that Christianity was a religion of the spirit, the soul's quest for Heaven. But, as Piero Camporesi has brilliantly demonstrated, for the common flock what commanded belief was Christ's body nailed to the Cross, the mortifications of holy men, the marvels of saints' corpses that gushed blood or remained incorruptible, healing miracles, the promise of the resurrection of the body.[27]

Bodies were pregnant with meaning. There were the symbols of the Body Politic, of the King's Two Bodies, and of the Corpus Christi, that *corpus mysticum* which was the Church. The Royal Touch cured scrofula,

23. P. Laslett, *The World We Have Lost* (London: Methuen, 1978).

24. See Foucault, *Discipline and Punish.*

25. P. Linebaugh, "The Tyburn Riot against the Surgeons," in *Albion's Fatal Tree*, ed. D. Hay, P. Linebaugh, and E. P. Thompson (London: A. Lane, 1975), 65–118.

26. Hertford Record Office. I owe this quotation to the kindness of Dr. Linda Pollock of Churchill College, Cambridge.

27. P. Camporesi, *La carne impassibile* (Milan: Saggiatore, 1983).

and aristocratic lineage spelt out the mystique of blood.[28] And the ritual theater of the body was played out not least on the stage itself littered in Shakespeare's age with corpses, just as from Petrarch to Donne, poetry both sacred and profane pursued the paradoxes of the human clay.

Of course, to say the body was prominent is not to say it was held in good odor. In a biological ancien régime where life expectations were low and whose creed blamed original sin for bringing death and disease into the world, vile bodies drew deep disgust. "Inter urinas et faeces nascimur," pronounced St. Augustine, developing a dualism of the body seen as the prison house of the soul, echoed later by the Puritan Oliver Hayward's "Alas, the best man is two men."[29] In his *Second Anniversary*, John Donne addressed his own soul:

> Think further on thyself, my soul, and think
> How thou at first wast made but in a sink
> This curded milk, this poor unlittered whelp,
> My body, could, beyond escape or help,
> Infect thee with original sin and thou
> Couldn't neither then refuse, nor leave it now.[30]

Small wonder the term "body" itself became a synonym for corpse, that Swift might surmise "surely mortal man is a broomstick,"[31] or that on his return to England, Lemuel Gulliver, his hero, "could not endure my wife or children in my presence, the very smell of them was intolerable";[32] or, more generally, that when satirists wished to deflate the pretensions of poets, kings, or philosophers, they showed that their inflated status arose at bottom only from diseases of the guts.[33] In Swift's classic

28. M. Bloch, *The Royal Touch* (London: Routledge and Kegal Paul, 1978); R. Crawfurd, *The King's Evil* (Oxford: Clarendon Press, 1911).

29. *The Diaries of Oliver Heywood,* ed. J. H. Turner, vol. 3 (London, 1882), 304.

30. See the discussion in J. Broadbent, "The Image of God, or Two Yards of Skin," in *The Body as a Medium of Expression,* ed. J. Benthall and T. Polhemus (London: A. Lane, 1975), 305–326; and J. Carey, *John Donne: Life, Mind and Art* (London: Faber and Faber, 1981), chap. 5, "Bodies."

31. J. Swift, "A Meditation upon a Broomstick," in J. Swift, *A Tale of a Tub and Other Satires,* ed. K. Williams (London: Everyman, 1975), 191–194.

32. See the illuminating discussion in N. O. Brown, *Life against Death* (London: Routledge and Kegan Paul, 1968), 171 f.

33. See, for instance, C. Kerby-Miller, ed., *Memoirs of the Extraordinary Life, Works and Discoveries of Martinus Scriblerus* (New York: Russell and Russell, 1966), 107 ff.; and the descriptions in M. V. Deporte, "Digressions and Madness in *A Tale of a Tub* and *Tristram Shandy,*" *Huntington Library Quarterly* 34 (1970): 43–57; R. Paulson, *Theme and Structure in Swift's Tale of a Tub* (New Haven: Yale University Press, 1960); J. R. Clark, *Form and Frenzy*

formula, "the Corruption of the Senses is the generation of the Spirit"; "the same Spirits which in their superior Progress would conquer a Kingdom, descending upon the Anus, conclude in a Fistula."[34]

Yet Christianity also held the body in an esteem other sects—for example, the Gnostics—or philosophies such as the Stoic found contemptible. After all, Scripture taught man was made in God's image, God's only son became flesh, and then rose from the dead, so presaging the general resurrection of the body at the Last Judgment.[35] How could the body be more highly honored than by the Catholic sacrament of the Eucharist, which brought Christ's very blood and body to the lips of the faithful?

If man were made in God's image, his body must be almost holy. A Puritan drew the natural inference:

> Whereas our bodies are God's workmanship, we must glorify him in our bodies. . . . yea, we must not hurt or abuse our body, but present them as holy and loving sacrifices unto God.[36]

In the Renaissance nude, the body became a veritable emblem of the soul, just as human anatomy became incorporated in a natural theology of design. Man's body was a microcosm epitomizing the order and meaning of the cosmos; and so, too, according to the physiognomy, the outer case itself was an index of the soul.

Bodies thus carried complex and contradictory messages, and minds felt confused about embodiment. Tristram Shandy expressed his admiration for

> the Pythagoreans (much more than ever I dare tell my Jenny) for their "*getting out of the body, in order to think well.*" No man thinks right, whilst he is in it.[37]

in Swift's Tale of a Tub (Ithaca, N.Y.: Cornell University Press, 1970); D. B. Morris, "The Kinship of Madness in Pope's *Dunciad*," *Philological Quarterly* 51 (1972): 813–831; G. Rosen, "Form of Irrationality in the Eighteenth Century," *Studies in Eighteenth-Century Culture* 2 (1972): 255–288.

34. J. Swift, "A Tale of a Tub," in *A Tale of a Tub and Other Satires*, K. Williams (London: Everyman, 1975), 1–136; "A Discourse concerning the Mechanical Operations of the Spirit," ibid., 167–190.

35. A point justly emphasized in F. Bottomley, *Attitudes to the Body in Western Christendom* (London: Lepus, 1979).

36. William Perkins, quoted in A. Wear, "Puritan Perceptions of Illness in Seventeenth Century England," in *Patients and Practitioners: Lay Perceptions of Medicine in Pre-Industrial Society*, ed. Roy Porter (Cambridge: Cambridge University Press, 1985), 55–100, at 63.

37. Sterne, *Tristram Shandy*, 472.

Events of course prove him right, no one does think right in his body (and yet they don't think right out of them either). But, as Tristram admits, mind cannot declare unilateral independence from the body, they are but two faces of the same coin; or rather

> A man's body and his mind, with the utmost reference to both I speak it, are exactly like a jerkin, and a jerkin's lining; rumple the one—you rumple the other.[38]

So for man, Sir Thomas Browne's great "amphibian," the coexistence of body and soul was a fact of life; or rather its great mystery. For

> How mind acts upon matter, will, in all probability, ever remain a secret [as Dr. William Buchan admitted]. It is sufficient for us to know that there is established a reciprocal influence betwixt the mental and corporeal parts, and that whatever disorders the one likewise hurts the other.[39]

Theories proliferated through the Scientific Revolution and the Enlightenment unraveling the knot of mind and body, what Tristram Shandy termed this "junketting piece of work betwixt [our bodies] and our seven senses"—[40] so many, in fact, that one of the choicer jokes of the *Anti-Jacobin Review* was to carry a mock advertisement of a forthcoming publication:

38. Ibid., 174. Compare p. 356: "I said, 'we were not stocks and stones'—'tis very well. I should have added, nor are we angels, I wish we were,—but men cloathed with bodies, and governed by our imaginations."

39. William Buchan, *Domestic Medicine* (London, 1776). Cf. this discussion in the correspondence of two young men in the eighteenth century:

> In our conversations about matter and spirit, you expressed some doubts whether although matter operates on spirit, spirit can act upon matter, and asked whether a man had ever been known to think himself into a fit of the gout. It did not immediately strike me that there were cases where actual diseases of the body were evidently occasioned by perturbations of the mind. Instances of the force of imagination in pregnant women are notorious. Convulsions and fainting are common effects of fear, an extreme degree of which has been said to turn the hair white. And I have heard an odd story of a man at Edinburgh that was persuaded, by the stratagem of some physician, into a fever. But these kinds of cases, however authentic, are of no weight in the controversy concerning the nature of the soul, as they require that the soul should be previously shewn to be spirit.

J. James to J. Boucher, *The Letters of Richard Radcliffe and John James*, ed. M. Evans (Oxford: Clarendon Press, 1888), 155. Or as a late-eighteenth-century madhouse-keeper put it, "The action of the mind on the body, and of the body on the mind, after all that has been written, is as little understood, as it is universally felt; and has given birth to endless conjecture, and perpetual error" (B. Faulkner, *Observations on the Cruel and Improper Treatment of Insanity* [London, 1789]).

40. Sterne, *Tristram Shandy*, 356.

> The influence of Mind upon Matter, comprehending the whole question of the Existence of Mind as Independent of Matter, or as co-existent with it, and of Matter considered as an intelligent and self-dependent Essense, will make the subject of a larger poem in 127 Books, now preparing.[41]

Such theories form the subject of John Yolton's recent *Thinking Matter,* and it would be illuminating to give Yolton's strictly history-of-ideas analysis an added dimension by exploring the possible social roots and ramifications of the various resolutions. Were materialists radicals? Did dualism support the social hierarchy?[42] Yet my aim here is somewhat different. For I examine actual perceptions, experiences, and modes of mind and body, their bonds and boundaries in specific contexts of use, in order to sound their resonances—scientific, experiential, symbolic—and why these were to modulate.

I shall explore one instance in some detail, the problem of madness, melancholy, and similar forms of disturbance. Today's parlance—mental illness being wrong in the head, psychiatric disorder—instantly reveals our own cognitive map: madness is in the mind. But that was not the common perception three centuries ago. Then insanity was, or at least sprang from, a disease of the body. Insanity was not typically regarded as a condition of an "occult" faculty, such as the psyche, mind, soul, or personality, even though it was a distemper involving disordered thoughts and feelings.[43] "Madness is as much a corporal distemper as the gout or asthma." Today we readily associate such sentiments with the aggressively "medically materialist" wing of the psychiatric profession. But these were actually the words of Lady Mary Wortley Montagu, giving voice to a commonplace of Georgian culture.[44]

Lady Mary's lay view was endorsed by physicians of every school. For their part, the medical old guard identified insanity as typically an imbalance of the humors produced in the digestive system, mania being

41. *Poetry of the Anti-Jacobin* (London, 1851), 84.

42. The anthropological speculations of Mary Douglas are intriguing here. See *Natural Symbols* (London: Pantheon, 1970).

43. Michel Foucault, *Madness and Civilization: A History of Insanity in the Age of Reason,* trans. Richard Howard (New York: Random House, 1965) has an important discussion: see chap. 3; and Michael MacDonald, *Mystical Bedlam: Madness, Anxiety and Healing in Seventeenth-Century England* (Cambridge: Cambridge University Press, 1981); M. G. Hay, "Understanding Madness: Some Approaches to Mental Illness" (Ph.D. thesis, University of York, 1979).

44. *Letters from Lady Mary Wortley Montagu,* ed. R. Brimley Johnson (London: Everyman edition, 1925), 465. G. S. Rousseau has drawn attention to this passage in "Psychology," in *The Ferment of Knowledge,* ed. G. S. Rousseau and Roy Porter (Cambridge: Cambridge University Press, 1980), 143–210, 206.

a superfluity of choler, melancholy too much black bile.[45] Newer iatrochemists, by contrast, attributed craziness to acid and sour chemical ferments, whose sharp particles scoured and inflamed the fibers. Or, more fashionably still, as George Rousseau has emphasized, physicians built on Thomas Willis's pioneer neurology to contend that disturbance lay in defective nerves: their lack of tone or elasticity due to clogging checked the flow of animal spirits, thus depressing the mood.[46]

Rivalries between particular schools of anatomy and physiology, however, were about details. All shared a common conviction that the source was organic. As the Newtonian physician, Dr. Nicholas Robinson, put it in the 1720s:

> Every change of the Mind, therefore, indicates a Change in the Bodily Organs;[47]

His contemporary, George Cheyne, the king of the "hyp doctors," concurred:

> I never saw a person labour under severe obstinate, and strong nervous complaints, but I always found at last, the stomach, guts, liver, spleen, mesentery, or some of the great and necessary organs or glands of the belly were obstructed, knotted, schirrous, spoiled or perhaps all these together.[48]

The etiology is particularly striking for those diseases, such as hysteria or hypochondria, which later generations would come to regard primarily as psychic, as functional disorders, whose physical symptoms were but secondary somatizations. Traditional medical theory, however, regarded these as regular somatic diseases. Of course, as Sydenham and Willis were at pains to prove, medicine no longer accepted antiquity's attribu-

45. For explication of the complexities of black bile and choler see L. Babb, *The Elizabethan Malady: A Study of Melancholia in English Literature from 1580 to 1640* (East Lansing: Michigan State University Press, 1951); idem, *Sanity in Bedlam: A Study of Robert Burton's Anatomy of Melancholy* (East Lansing: Michigan State University Press, 1955).

46. Fundamental here is G. S. Rousseau, "Nerves, Spirits, and Fibres: Towards Defining the Origins of Sensibility," with a postscript, *The Blue Guitar* (Messina) 2 (1976): 125–153; idem, "Psychology," in *The Ferment of Knowledge*, ed. G. S. Rousseau and Roy Porter (Cambridge: Cambridge University Press, 1980).

47. N. Robinson, *A New System of the Spleen* (London: Bettesworth, 1729), quoted in Richard Hunter and Ida Macalpine, *Three Hundred Years of Psychiatry, 1535–1860* (London: Oxford University Press, 1963), 344.

48. George Cheyne, *The English Malady; or, A Treatise of Nervous Diseases of all Kinds* (London: Strahan and Leake, 1733), quoted in Richard Hunter and Ida Macalpine, *Three Hundred Years of Psychiatry, 1535–1860* (London: Oxford University Press, 1963), 184.

tion of hysteria to the wandering womb.[49] Yet that did not make it any the less organic, for (as Willis argued) hysteria was

> chiefly and primarily convulsive, and chiefly depends on the brain, and the nervous stock being affected.[50]

No wonder it struck women worse than men: their nervous systems were weaker.

Paralleling hysteria was hypochondria, which likewise was not classed as a disorder of the understanding (the morbid obsessions of mere *malades imaginaires*) but rather as an organic distemper. There had of course been a traditional humoral etiology for it.

> The primitive Doctors [Richard Blackmore stated] imagined that all Hypochondriacal Symptoms were derived from a Collection of black Dregs and Lees separated from the Blood and lodged in the Spleen, whence, as they supposed, noxious Reeks and cloudy Evaporations were always ascending to the superior Regions (the Chest, the Heart, and Head).[51]

Yet this was ignorance, concluded Blackmore; the new anatomy could account for it much better as a defect of nervous organization.

Or take the vapors, that complaint involving fainting and fits traditionally blamed on the fumes given off by a distempered womb, rising up through the internal organs.[52] But falsely, argued Dr. John Purcell. For in reality vapors were an organic obstruction located

49. I. Veith, *Hysteria: The History of a Disease* (Chicago: University of Chicago Press, 1965); J. Boss, "The Seventeenth-Century Transformation of the Hysteric Affection," *Psychological Medicine* 9 (1979): 221–234.

50. Quoted in Richard Hunter and Ida Macalpine, *Three Hundred Years of Psychiatry, 1535–1800* (London: Oxford University Press, 1963), 190. See Jeffrey M. N. Boss, "The Seventeenth-Century Transformation of the Hysteric Affection," *Psychological Medicine* 9 (1979): 221–234. See also Hansruedi Isler, *Thomas Willis, 1621–1685, Doctor and Scientist* (New York: Hafner, 1968); J. Spillane, *The Doctrine of the Nerves* (London: Oxford University Press, 1981). For important background see J. Wright, "Hysteria and Mechanical Man," *Journal of the History of Ideas* 41 (1980): 233–247.

51. Sir R. Blackmore, *A Treatise of the Spleen and Vapours* (London, 1725), quoted in Richard Hunter and Ida Macalpine, *Three Hundred Years of Psychiatry, 1535–1860* (London: Oxford University Press, 1963), 320.

52. For the spleen—both an abdominal organ and a fashionable term for melancholy—see C. Moore, *Backgrounds of English Literature 1700–1760* (Minneapolis: University of Minnesota Press, 1963); O. Doughty, "The English Malady of the Eighteenth Century," *Review of English Studies* 2 (1926): 257–269; E. Fischer-Homberger, "Hypochondriasis of the Eighteenth Century—Neurosis of the Present Century," *Bulletin of the History of Medicine* 46 (1972): 391–401; Roy Porter, "The Rage of Party: A Glorious Revolution in English Psychiatry?" *Medical History* 27 (1983): 35–50.

> in the Stomach and Guts; whereof the Grumbling of the one and the Heaviness and uneasiness of the other generally preceding the Paroxysm, are no small Proofs.[53]

Noting that one of Hippocrates' greatest contributions to medicine was his recognition that epilepsy was not a divine affliction ("the sacred disease") but natural, Purcell insisted the vapors were akin to epilepsy, indeed that "an epilepsie, is Vapours arriv'd to a more violent degree."[54]

And—the exemplary case—melancholy too was similarly located on the etiological map. The waning of humoralism left early Georgian physicians disinclined to see it literally as the product of black bile.[55] Rather, Willis had insisted, "Melancholy . . . is a complicated Distemper of the Brain and Heart."[56]

Yet, in discarding humoralism, such physicians had no intention of setting mentalist theories in their place. Far from it. Humoralism had proved merely semantic, a will-o'-the-wisp. It was to make way for explanations grounded securely in mechanical operations. For, Dr. Nicholas Robinson insisted, insanity was not a mere matter of "imaginary Whims and Fancies, but real Affections of the Mind, arising from the real, mechanical Affections of Matter and Motion."[57] If craziness was

53. John Purcell, *A Treatise of Vapours, or, Hysterick Fits* (London: E. Place, 1707), quoted in Richard Hunter and Ida Macalpine, *Three Hundred Years of Psychiatry, 1535–1860* (London: Oxford University Press: 1963), 291; O. Temkin, *The Falling Sickness* (Baltimore: Johns Hopkins University Press, 1974).

54. Purcell, *Treatise of Vapours,* quoted in Richard Hunter and Ida Macalpine, *Three Hundred Years of Psychiatry, 1535–1860* (London: Oxford University Press, 1963), 291. See also E. Fischer-Homberger, "Hypochondriasis of the Eighteenth Century—Neurosis of the Present Century," *Bulletin of the History of Medicine* 46 (1972): 391–401.

55. R. Klibansky, *Saturn and Melancholy* (London: Nelson, 1964); Stanley W. Jackson, "Melancholia and the Waning of the Humoral Theory," *Journal of the History of Medicine and Allied Sciences* 33 (1978): 367–376; T. H. Jobe, "Medical Theories of Melancholia in the Seventeenth and Early Eighteenth Centuries," *Clio Medica* 19 (1976): 217–231.

56. T. Willis, quoted in Richard Hunter and Ida Macalpine, *Three Hundred Years of Psychiatry, 1535–1860* (London: Oxford University Press, 1863), 190. See also E. S. Clarke and C. D. O'Malley, *The Human Brain and Spinal Cord* (Berkeley and Los Angeles: University of California Press, 1968); E. S. Clarke and Kenneth Dewhurst, *An Illustrated History of Brain Function* (Oxford: Sandford Publications, 1972).

57. N. Robinson, *A New System of the Spleen* (London, 1729), quoted in Richard Hunter and Ida Macalpine, *Three Hundred Years of Psychiatry, 1535–1860* (London: Oxford University Press, 1983), 344. Robinson continued (345):

> Upon these Grounds, then it clearly appears, that neither the Fancy, nor Imagination, nor even Reason itself, the highest Faculty of the Understanding, can feign a perception, or a Disease that has no Foundation in Nature; cannot conceive the Idea of an Indisposition, that has no Existence in the Body; cannot feel pain or Uneas-

thus fundamentally organic,[58] physical remedies were clearly called for. That is what we find. Thomas Willis himself advocated a regime of close confinement and whippings, which probably reflected contemporary practice at Bethlehem (Bedlam), and drugs formed the staple of medication for the mad in the seventeenth and eighteenth centuries. Drawing on old humoral medicine, Robert Burton had listed hundreds of purges, vomits, and simples for melancholy, including laurel, white hellebore, and tobacco ("divine, rare, super-excellent tobacco . . . a sovereign remedy to all disease")[59] and some more exotic drug cocktails as well. Suffering from "head melancholy"?

> iness in any part, unless there be pain or Uneasiness in that part; The affected Nerves of that Part must strike the Imagination with the Sense of Pain, before the Mind can conceive the Idea of Pain in that part; and therefore, it is in vain to go about to persuade any Man, that he is perfectly at Ease, while he, at the same Time, perceives himself in great pain and Anguish from divers Affections of the Body. . . . While the Nerves, therefore, are in good plight, the Ideas they convey through any of the Senses will be regular, just, and clear; upon which the Understanding will judge and determine of Objects, as they are, by the Laws of Nature, made to exist to a Mind fitly dispos'd, with proper Organs to receive their Impression: But if the Structure or Mechanism of these Organs happen to be disorder'd, and the Springs of the Machine out of Tune; no Wonder the Mind perceives the Alteration, and is affected with the Change.

More generally see, for this mechanical "physiological psychology," M. V. Deporte, *Nightmares and Hobbyhorses* (San Marino, Calif.: Huntington Library, 1974), 125 f.; L. J. Rather, "Old and New Views of the Emotions and Bodily Changes," *Clio Medica* 1 (1965): 1–25; T. H. Jobe, "Medical Theories of Melancholia in the Seventeenth and Early Eighteenth Centuries," *Clio Medica* 11 (1976): 217–231; Esther Fischer-Homberger, *Hypochondrie, Melancholie bis Neurose: Krankheiten und Zustandbilden* (Bern: Huber, 1970).

58. And physical causes were often held responsible. See *The Private Letters of Dorothea Lieven* ed. P. Quennell (London: J. Murray, 1937), 86:

> *The 27th*
> I was upset yesterday at the death of a man whom I knew very well, for he was attached to the Court of the late Princess Charlotte of Wales, a man called Hardenbrot, remarkable for his enormous nose. It is less than three weeks since he came to call on me. I was alone with him. He told me that he was sometimes seized by fits of madness, during which he was not responsible for his actions. At this alarming information, I went up to the bell-cord and stood sentinel until the Duke of York came in and rescued me from our tête-à-tête. Afterwards, I told my husband that I thought Hardenbrot was talking very incoherently. He made enquiries and was told that he was in excellent health and had never shown any sign of madness. Two days later, he went off his head. He was put in charge of two doctors from Bedlam and died yesterday in a violent fit of madness. Don't ever think of eating lobster after dinner: that is what the poor lunatic used to do.

59. Robert Burton, *The Anatomy of Melancholy* (1621), ed. A. R. Shilleto (London: George Bell and Sons, 1898). Second partition, "The Cure of Melancholy."

> Take a Ram's head that never meddled with an Ewe, cut off at a blow, and, the horns Only taken away, boil it well skin and wool together, after it is well sod, take out the brains, and put these spices to it, Cinnamon, Ginger, Nutmeg, Mace, Cloves, in equal parts of half an ounce, mingle the powder of these spices with it, and heat them in a platter upon a chafing-dish of coals together, stirring them well, that they do not burn; take heed it be not overmuch dried, or dryer than a Calves brains ready to be eaten. Keep it so prepared, and for three days give it the patient fasting, so that he fast two hours after it. It may be eaten with bread in an egg, or broth, or any way, so it be taken.[60]

The coming of the new mechanical philosophy changed the drugs but not the drugging.

> No Man can have a tenderer, or more compassionate Concern for the Misery of Mankind than myself [argued Dr. Robinson]: yet it is Cruelty in the highest degree, not to be bold in the Administration of Medicines. . . . It is owing to these safe Men, that do but little good, and a great deal of real Mischief, that chronick Diseases are so rife now-a-days, and so generally incurable. . . . In this Case, therefore, the most violent Vomits, the strongest purging Medicines, and large Bleedings, are to be often repeated.[61]

Nor was faith in organic remedies just a quirk of the doctors, for laymen and patients had equal faith in medicine. The nonconformist divine, Richard Baxter, advised: "neglect not physick."[62] Despairing patients might bewail

> that physick cannot Cure Souls, yet they must be perswaded or forced to it. I have known a Lady deep in Melancholy, who a long time would neither speak, nor take Physick; nor endure her Husband to go out of the Room, and with the Restraint and Grief he died, and she was cured by Physick put down her Throat, with a Pipe by Force.[63]

Even John Wesley—a man who often challenged the organic diagnoses of madness, regarding many cases as instances of demoniacal possession—was free in recommending medical cures:

60. Ibid.

61. N. Robinson, *A New System of the Spleen* (London, 1729), quoted in Richard Hunter and Ida Macalpine, *Three Hundred Years of Psychiatry, 1535–1800* (London: Oxford University Press, 1963), 340.

62. R. Baxter, *The Signs and Causes of Melancholy,* quoted in Robert Hunter and Ida Macalpine, *Three Hundred Years of Psychiatry, 1535–1860* (London: Oxford University Press, 1963), 340.

63. Ibid.

> Boil the Juice of ground ivy with sweet oil and white wine into an ointment. Shave the head, anoint it therewith, and chafe it every other day for three weeks. Bruise also the leaves and bind them on the head and give three spoonsful of the juice, warm, every morning. Or, be electrified. (tried). Or, set the patient with his head under a great water-fall as long as his strength will bear, or pour cold water on his head out of a tea-kettle. Or, let him eat nothing but apples for a month.[64]

So the spectrum of troubles ranging from raving insanity to what we should today label neurosis was typically regarded as seated in the body. Indeed, the very term "neurosis"—a coining of the great Edinburgh professor William Cullen—was originally used not, as today, to signal the perplexing no-man's-land of functional disorders, but neuropathologically, to classify physical lesions. As Cullen put it, the neuroses were

> all those preternatural affections of sense and motion, which are without pyrexia as a part of the primary disease, and all those which do not depend upon a topical affection of the organs, but more upon general effection of the nervous system, and of those powers of the system upon which sense and motion more especially depend.[65]

The conceptual geography I have been mapping may seem strange to our psychiatrically primed minds. We are familiar of course with the kind of medical imperialism today found particularly amongst neurophysiologists, which aims to incorporate all personality disturbance within somatic medicine—for how else can research and therapy be scientific? And Lain Entralgo has demonstrated how rigid was the organicism that became the trademark of regular medicine from Galen onward[66]—witness Coleridge's caustic verdict on the physicians:

> They are *shallow* animals; having always employed their minds about Body and Gut, they imagine that in the whole system of things there is nothing but Gut and Body.[67]

64. J. Wesley, *Primitive Physick* (reprint, Santa Barbara, Calif., n.d.), 87; G. S. Rousseau, "John Wesley's *Primitive Physick* (1747)," *Harvard Library Bulletin* 16 (1968): 242–256; A. W. Hill, *John Wesley among the Physicians* (London: Epworth, 1958).

65. W. Cullen, *First Lines in the Practice of Physic* (Edinburgh, 1784), quoted in Richard Hunter and Ida Macalpine, *Three Hundred Years of Psychiatry, 1535–1860* (London: Oxford University Press, 1963), 473. See J. M. López Piñero, *Historical Origins of the Concept of Neurosis*, trans. D. Berrios (Cambridge: Cambridge University Press, 1983).

66. P. Lain Entralgo, *Mind and Body* (London: Harvill, 1955).

67. Coleridge to Charles Lloyd, Sr., 14 Nov. 1796, *Collected Letters of Samuel Taylor Coleridge* ed. E. L. Griggs, vol. 1 (Oxford: Clarendon Press, 1956), 256.

And yet it would be a great mistake to interpret the prevalent somaticism as a sort of doctors' conspiracy. Nicholas Jewson has suggested how far the traditional physician had to defer to patients' expectations—the clinical encounter was a delicate process of negotiation;[68] and in what we would call psychiatric disorders abundant evidence suggests it was sufferers at least as much as physicians who opted for organic interpretations. As George Cheyne explained, he was often put on the spot when confronted with cases of depression because such conditions were easily jeered at by the vulgar as marks of "peevishness," "whim," "ill humour," or, amongst women, of "fantasticalness" or "coquetry."[69] Or, more seriously, troubled spirits were all too readily taken as but a hairsbreadth away from outright insanity. Hence care was needed before advancing terms like "nervous" in consultations, and patients would expect a real disease diagnosis. Indeed, the dictates of humanity required it. For though the herd might suppose that these maladies were "nothing but the effect of Fancy, and a delusive Imagination, yet . . . the consequent Sufferings are without doubt real and unfeigned."[70] Cheyne's solution was to emphasize organic origins:

> Often when I have been consulted in a Case . . . and found it to be what is commonly call'd Nervous, I have been in the utmost Difficulty, when desir'd to define or name the Distemper, for fear of affronting them or fixing a Reproach on a Family or Person. If I call'd the Case Glandular with nervous Symptoms, they concluded I thought them pox'd, or had the King's Evil. If I said it was Vapours, Hysterick or Hypochondriacal Disorders, they thought I call'd them Mad or Fantastical.[71]

Dr. Richard Blackmore faced the same doctor's dilemma:

> This Disease, called Vapours in Women, and the Spleen in Men, is what neither Sex are pleased to own. A Man cannot ordinarily make his Court worse, than by suggesting to such patients the true Nature and Name of

68. N. Jewson, "The Disappearance of the Sick Man from Medical Cosmology 1770–1870," *Sociology* 10 (1976): 225–244; idem, "Medical Knowledge and the Patronage System in Eighteenth-Century England," *Sociology* 8 (1974): 369–385; Roy Porter, ed., *Patients and Practitioners: Lay Perceptions of Medicine in Pre-Industrial Society* (Cambridge: Cambridge University Press, 1985).

69. G. Cheyne, quoted in L. Feder, *Madness in Literature* (Princeton: Princeton University Press, 1980), 170.

70. Ibid.

71. George Cheyne, *The English Malady; or, A Treatise of Nervous Diseases of All Kinds* (London: Strahan and Leake, 1733), quoted in Richard Hunter and Ida Macalpine, *Three Hundred Years of Psychiatry, 1535–1860* (London: Oxford University Press, 1963), 353.

> their Distemper. . . . One great Reason why these patients are unwilling their Disease should go by its right Name, is, I imagine, this, that the Spleen and Vapours are, by those that never felt their Symptoms, looked upon as an imaginary and fantastick Sickness of the Brain, filled with odd and irregular Ideas. . . . This Distemper, by a great Mistake, becoming thus an Object of Derision and Contempt: the persons who feel it are unwilling to own a Disease that will expose them to Dishonour and Reproach.[72]

In other words it reassured patients to root their troubles in the body, for that made them real while reducing responsibility. Take for example the case of the nonconformist minister Richard Baxter.[73] Baxter experienced a Pandora's box of internal maladies, occasioning excruciating pain and still greater fears, associated with what he intuited to be large kidney stones. He tried many remedies, some from the doctors, some home brews; and consulted up to thirty-six physicians all at once, without relief or remedy. The real blow came when "divers eminent physicians agreed that my disease was the hypochondriack melancholy." What exactly the doctors meant by that we cannot be sure. For Baxter, however, the term carried unwelcome overtones of malingering, delusion, and real madness. His amour-propre had to deny it.

> My distemper never went to so far as to possess me with any inordinate fancies, or damp me with sinking sadness, although the physicians call'd it the hypochondriack melancholy.

Feeling threatened by the doctors, Baxter needed to legitimate his disease and his sick role—by tracing its true body site:

> I thought myself, that my disease was almost all from debility of the stomach, and extream acrimony of blood by some fault of the liver.

Baxter's autobiography makes it quite clear that the mere *malade imaginaire* could expect no pity from ordinary people—any more than did Molière's hero. Indeed, he would be a figure of fun. On being rumored to be hypochondriacal, Baxter reports, "I became the common talk of the city, especially the women."

72. Sir R. Blackmore, *A Treatise of the Spleen and Vapours* (London, 1725), quoted in Richard Hunter and Ida Macalpine, *Three Hundred Years of Psychiatry, 1535–1860* (London: Oxford University Press, 1963), 320.

73. For my discussion of Baxter, I rely on Andrew Wear, "Puritan Perceptions of Illness in Seventeenth-Century England," in *Patients and Practitioners: Lay Perceptions of Medicine in Pre-Industrial Society,* ed. Roy Porter (Cambridge: Cambridge University Press, 1985), 55–99. The extracts that Wear cites are from Baxter's *Reliquiae Baxterianae* (London: Parkhurst, 1898), 9–10, 173.

Hence sympathetic doctors and their patients would collude in diagnoses that realized such conditions by rooting them in the body. As even Bishop John Moore in a sermon in 1692 on Religious Melancholy stated, such troubles were truly "Distempers of the Body, rather than Faults of the Mind."[74] Still, however, the ambiguities ran deep. When Dr. John Radcliffe told Queen Anne she was suffering from the vapors, she sacked him; it was too ambivalent a term to be applied to royalty.[75]

There was another, even stronger reason why sufferers did not want depression to be judged "in the mind" rather than "in the body": the imputation of serious disturbance of the Reason or imagination. Renaissance minds were in no doubt as to the extraordinary cosmic powers exercised by imagination: it was the sustaining force of sympathy, astrology, magic; it engendered fascination.[76] Physicians were of course rather ambivalently aware that imagination had great powers for *curing* diseases, as the successes of "faith" healers and quacks from Valentine Greatrakes through to Mesmer testified, though the faculty considered it scandalous that maladies unresponsive to the best medicines proved susceptible to mumbo jumbo and suggestion. But doctors chiefly warned of the power of imagination to do harm.[77] As Nehemiah Grew put it:

> Phancy . . . also operates . . . in the production of Diseases. Consumptions often come with Grief. From Venereal Love, Madness, and Hysterick Fits.[78]

Typical was the reputed capacity of the imagination in women, at conception or during pregnancy, to impress whatever preoccupied their imaginations upon their unborn child. A woman whose imagination was seized by a strange sight would indeed give birth to a monster.[79]

74. J. Moore, "Of Religious Melancholy," quoted in Richard Hunter and Ida Macalpine, *Three Hundred Years of Psychiatry, 1535–1860* (London: Oxford University Press, 1963), 252.

75. J. B. Nias, *Dr. John Radcliffe: A Sketch of His Life* (Oxford: Clarendon Press, 1918), 16, 18.

76. See D. F. Bond, "'Distrust' of Imagination in English Neoclassicism," *Philological Quarterly* 14 (1937): 54–69, and idem, "The Neoclassical Psychology of the Imagination," *ELH* 1 (1937): 245–264; C. E. McMahon, "The Role of Imagination in the Disease Process: Pre-Cartesian History," *Psychological Medicine* 6 (1976): 179–184; I. Couliano, *Eros et magie à la Renaissance* (Paris: Flammarion, 1984).

77. John Haygarth, *Of the Imagination, as a Cause and as a Cure of Disorders of the Body* (Bath: Cadell and Davies, 1800).

78. Nehemiah Grew, *Cosmologia Sacra* (London: Rogers et al., 1701), quoted in Richard Hunter and Ida Macalpine, *Three Hundred Years of Psychiatry, 1535–1860* (London: Oxford University Press, 1963), 285.

79. It was still part of popular medicine to believe that the mother had the power to

Within classical humanism, imagination was thus a very mixed blessing. Slipping the reins of reason, it ran riot and became dangerous, as appears in the distrust of dreaming so frequently expressed in the Stuart and Georgian ages. If (as Goya was later to put it) the sleep of reason produces monsters, there was every reason for medical theorists to promote bodily explanations for dreams and nightmares, commonly regarded as a form of demonical possession. Nightmare, physicians typically argued, was not literally a matter of being hagridden but was due to heavy suppers or bad sleeping posture.[80]

Thus one popular association was the slippery slope from the anarchy of imagination to out-and-out insanity. "Madness," Samuel Johnson told Fanny Burney, "is occasioned by too much indulgence of imagination." No wonder the idea that pains, perturbations, and quirks of behavior stemmed from rebellious imagination was so distressing. When Johnson confessed that his fidgets, tics, and convulsions were not organic but bad habits, or admitted he was in the grip of religious scruples, it was with the direct awareness of "the dangerous prevalence of imagination." Samuel Johnson dreaded encroaching insanity.[81]

imprint onto her conceptus whatever was in her imagination at the moment of conception. For this vision of the malign power of the imagination, see Bond, "'Distrust' of Imagination" idem, "Neoclassical Psychology"; S. Cunningham, "Bedlam and Parnassus: Eighteenth-Century Reflections," *Eighteenth-Century Studies* 24 (1971): 35–55; and G. S. Rousseau, "Smollett, Wit and Tradition of Learning in Medicine," in *Tobias Smollett: Essays of Two Decades* (Edinburgh: T. and T. Clark, 1982), 160–183.

80. M. Weidhorn, *Dreams in Seventeenth-Century English Literature* (The Hague: Mouton, 1970); John Bond, *An Essay on the Incubus, or Night-Mare* (London: Wilson and Durham, 1753); Thomas Tryon, *A Treatise of Dreams and Visions* (London, 1689), quoted in Richard Hunter and Ida Macalpine, *Three Hundred Years of Psychiatry, 1535–1860* (London: Oxford University Press, 1963), 233.

81. Roy Porter, "The Hunger of Imagination: Approaching Samuel Johnson's Melancholy," in *The Anatomy of Madness,* ed. W. F. Bynum, Roy Porter, and Michael Shepherd, 2 vols. (London: Tavistock, 1985), 1:63–88. For Johnson's mental maladies see R. Macdonald Ladell, "The Neurosis of Dr. Samuel Johnson," *The British Journal of Medical Psychology* 9 (1929): 314–323; R. Brain, "The Great Convulsionary" and "A Post Mortem on Dr. Johnson," in *Some Reflections on Genius and Other Essays* (London: Pitman Medical, 1960), 92–100; K. Grange, "Dr. Samuel Johnson's Account of a Schizophrenic Illness in *Rasselas* (1759)." *Medical History* 6 (1962): 160–169; R. B. Hovey, "Dr. Samuel Johnson, Psychiatrist," *Modern Language Quarterly* 15 (1954): 321–355; K. T. Read, "This Tasteless Tranquillity: A Freudian Note on Johnson's *Rasselas,*" *Literature and Psychology* 19 (1969): 61–62; K. Balderston, "Johnson's Vile Melancholy," in *The Age of Johnson,* ed. F. W. Hilles and W. S. Lewis (New Haven: Yale University Press, 1964), 3–14. For the wider context of Johnson's view of the interconnectedness of idleness, imagination, and madness see R. Voitle, *Samuel Johnson the Moralist* (Cambridge, Mass.: Harvard University Press, 1961); W. B. C. Watkins, *Perilous Balance* (Princeton: Princeton University Press, 1939); A. Sachs,

Even worse, however, might be the prospect of being "possessed" not by one's own imagination but by forces from Beyond, unearthly powers. Scriptural Protestantism envisaged the drama of salvation as a literal psychomachy. If God and the Devil battled for every soul, the likelihood of being personally invaded by Satan, perhaps in disguise, may never have seemed very remote to the pious. Seventeenth- and eighteenth-century spiritual autobiographies—by definition, of course, the memoirs of survivors—commonly tell of infiltration by emissaries of the Devil, invasion being particularly dangerous at times of physical weakness, anxiety, and sickness, when resistance would be low (illness was the Devil's bath, commented Burton).[82] Such struggles were every Christian's cross. And yet the prospects of sin, damnation, and hell must have loomed terrifyingly. Wasn't there every reason then for sufferers to blot out the fear that such were the symptoms of diabolical invasion, taking refuge instead in a comforting physical explanation, located in the diaphragm not in devils, in the spleen not in Satan?

Of course, there was also a tradition of divine madness—hearing voices, seeing visions, receiving prophecy, speaking in tongues. Once part of the Christian mainstream, by the second half of the seventeenth century it had shrunk to being the shibboleth of the sectaries.[83] Yet their claims to be in possession of higher truth and under the direction of higher powers threatened ecclesiastical authority and scandalized Enlightenment reasonableness. Enthusiasm's sting could however be drawn by "medicalization." "Divine madness" did indeed exist, but it was not, after all, a matter of literal inspiration by otherworldly powers, higher or lower, but a species of organic madness.[84] As Nicholas Robinson in-

Passionate Intelligence (Baltimore: Johns Hopkins University Press, 1967); P. K. Alkon, *Samuel Johnson and Moral Discipline* (Evanston, Ill.: Northwestern University Press, 1967).

82. D. P. Walker, *Spiritual and Demonic Magic from Ficino to Campanella* (London: Warburg Institute, 1958); idem, *Unclean Spirits: Possession and Exorcism in France and England in the Late Sixteenth and Early Seventeenth Centuries* (London: Scolar Press, 1981); Keith Thomas, *Religion and the Decline of Magic* (Harmondsworth: Penguin, 1973); Don Cameron Allen, "The Degeneration of Man and Renaissance Pessimism," *Studies in Philology* 35 (1938).

83. M. MacDonald, *Mystical Bedlam* (Cambridge: Cambridge University Press, 1981).

84. R. A. Knox, *Enthusiasm* (Oxford: Clarendon Press, 1950); B. R. Kreiser, *Miracles, Convulsions and Ecclesiastical Politics in Early Eighteenth-Century Paris* (Princeton: Princeton University Press, 1978); G. Rosen, "Enthusiasm: 'A Dark Lanthorn of the Spirit,'" *Bulletin of the History of Medicine* 42 (1958): 393–421; G. Williamson, "The Restoration Revolt against Enthusiasm," *Studies in Philology* 30 (1933): 571–603; S. I. Tucker, *Enthusiasm: A Study in Semantic Change* (Cambridge: Cambridge University Press, 1972); H. Schwartz, *Knaves, Fools, Madmen, and That Subtile Effluvium: A Study of the Opposition to the French Prophets in England, 1706–1710* (Gainesville: University Presses of Florida, 1978).

sisted, the transports of a George Fox or of the French Prophets were nothing more than "mere madness" arising from "the stronger impulses of a warm brain."[85]

Overall then, attributing disordered spirits to the body proved highly serviceable. It protected the sufferer from ridicule. It convinced him that his reason or soul wasn't at risk from rampant imagination or Satanic possession—but that low sectaries' religious inspirations were nothing more than hot air. Of course, the lowly origin of such disorders, seated in the bowels, might be shameful, but that was increasingly remedied by the new anatomy that rerouted the site of the lesion away from the guts and up toward the head, through those superfine, light, delicate fibers, the nerves.

Moreover, identifying melancholy as a disease of the body opened the way to a sociology of illness highly attractive to the polished elite of Georgian England. For, under George Cheyne's designation of "the English malady," depression became a life-style disorder.[86] The pressures of hard, high, and fast living, the demands of the *ton* or the town, the constraints of fashion, hot rooms, rich food, fine wines, late nights, excitement, etiquette—all subjected the physical constitution to intense strain. Becoming low-spirited under such pressures was the cross of High Society, the distinguishing stigmata of those fine spirits, those sensitive souls singled out for excellence. Above all, such low-spirited ladies and gentlemen were patently not fundamentally warped in the will but deserved sympathy. As Cheyne said flatteringly:

> [the English Malady] is as much a bodily Distemper as the Small-Pox or a Fever; and the Truth is, it seldom, and I think never happens or can happen, to any but those of the liveliest and quickest natural parts, whose Faculties are the brightest and most spiritual, and whose Genius is most keen and penetrating, and particularly where there is the most delicate Sensation and Taste, both of Pleasure and pain. So equally are the good and bad Things of this mortal State distributed! For I seldom ever observ'd a heavy, dull, earthy, clod-pated Clown, much troubled with nervous Disorders.[87]

85. N. Robinson, *A New System of the Spleen* (London, 1729).

86. Roy Porter, "The Rage of Party: A Glorious Revolution in English Psychiatry?" *Medical History* 27 (1983): 35–50; O. Doughty, "The English Malady of the Eighteenth Century," *The Review of English Studies* 2 (1926): 257–269.

87. G. Cheyne, *The English Malady* (London, 1733), ii. Similar characterizations of the English malady continue throughout the century. Compare T. Beddoes, *Hygeia*, 3 vols. (Bristol, 1802–1803), 3:4.

I have so far been exploring a pseudoparadox, the diagnostic prominence given to the body in what we now call "mental disorder." Within the larger priorities of the mind/body hierarchy, it is, of course, no paradox at all, in that the body could be safely blamed for such distempers precisely because it was so gross. But that does require us next to face a more taxing question: how, when, and why did mental disorder itself emerge? To explain this, a changing set of strategies will need to be scrutinized. But first the shift itself must be pinned down. If we examine English writings on madness after about the mid-eighteenth century, very different messages ring out. Now it is claimed that insanity and its brood are indeed of the psyche. Take in 1789 the view of Andrew Harper (who, as a surgeon, was hardly likely to be biased against somatic views):

> [insanity] must depend upon some specific alteration in the essential operations and movements of the mind, independent and exclusive of every corporal, sympathetic, direct, or indirect excitement, or irritation whatever.[88]

A few years later, William Halloran, the Irish mad-doctor, took a similar line. There was indeed a delirium that was organic; but there was also a madness genuinely seated in the mind, manifest in delusion. It was vital to attend to that distinction, since quite separate therapies were indicated. Above all, as he put it, "the malady of the mind . . . is, for the most part, to be treated on moral principles."[89]

88. Andrew Harper, *A Treatise on the Real Cause and Cure of Insanity* (London: Stalker and Waltes, 1789). quoted in Richard Hunter and Ida Macalpine, *Three Hundred Years of Psychiatry, 1535–1860* (London: Oxford University Press, 1963), 522.

89. W. S. Hallaran, *An Enquiry into the Causes Producing the Extraordinary Addition to the Number of Insane* (Cork: Edwards and Savage, 1810), quoted in Richard Hunter and Ida Macalpine, *Three Hundred Years of Psychiatry, 1585–1860* (London: Oxford University Press, 1963), 653. Hallaran argued:

> To illustrate this seemingly paradoxical position, I would advert to the many well authenticated instances of insanity, as they have occurred within the last twenty five years especially, and are noted on the records of our Lunatic Asylum. Amongst those are several which have owed their origin to mental causes, strictly speaking: such as dread of punishment, loss of friends, shame, sudden terror, remorse, etc. Having marked their progress, it was not difficult to contrast them with others of an opposite class, which had been occasioned by violent excesses of various kinds, and by which, the free action of the brain in particular, and of the lungs, together with the abdominal viscera in general, had been principally and individually engaged. . . . Here I am aware of exposing myself to animadversion, by seeming to admit the existence of insanity, independently of that intimate connexion which has been so generally supposed to prevail between it and the brain.

Indeed, this new perception of the autonomy of mental disorder spurred an epochal transformation in therapy. Back in the 1720s, Nicholas Robinson had concluded that druggings were the only answer:

> It is not long ago since a very learned and ingenious Gentleman, so far started from his Reason, as to believe, that his Body was metamorphos'd into a Hobby-Horse, and nothing would serve his Turn, but that his Friend, who came to see him, must mount his Back and ride. I must confess, that all the philosophy I was Master of, could not dispossess him of this Conceit: till, by the Application of generous Medicines, I restor'd the disconcerted Nerves to their regular Motions, and, by that Means, gave him a Sight of his Error.[90]

But by the 1750s, William Battie, who adopted a highly Lockean theory of madness viewed as deluded imagination stemming from misassociation of ideas, publicly scorned the time-honored Bethlem ancien régime of vomits and venesection, pronouncing that management could do far more than medicine.[91]

Indeed, "management" became the therapeutic watchword of the last decades of the century. What was meant was a new intensity of person-to-person contact between physician and patient.[92] The precise inflections of the disposition and behavior of the lunatic had to be grasped, addressed, and attacked. Deploying a rich array of tactics, the physician had to take charge, substituting his command for that of the delusional system. At its most theatrical, this might mean fixing the patient with the eye, a technique perfected by the Rev. Dr. Francis Willis, the mad-doctor brought in to treat George III.[93] Questioned by Members of Parliament about what John Haslam was later to call "this fascinating power,"[94] Willis offered a demonstration:

> "Place the candles between us, Mr. Burke," replied the Doctor, in an equally authoritative tone—" and I'll give you an answer. There, sir! by the EYE! I should have looked at him *thus*, Sir—*thus*!" Burke instantaneously averted his head, and, making no reply, evidently acknowledged this *basiliskan* authority.[95]

90. N. Robinson, *A New System of the Spleen* (London, 1729).

91. W. Battie, *A Treatise on Madness* (London: Brunner/Mazel, 1958), 59–81.

92. R. Porter, "Was There a Moral Therapy in Eighteenth-Century Psychiatry?" *Lychnos*, 1981/2: 12–16.

93. See I. Macalpine and R. Hunter, *George III and the Mad Business* (London: Allen Lane, 1969).

94. John Haslam, *Observations on Madness and Melancholy*, 2d ed. (London, 1809), 271.

95. Quoted in Ida Macalpine and Richard Hunter, *George III and the Mad Business* (London: Allen Lane, 1969), 271–272.

Paralleling Willis in management by spectacle was William Pargeter. Case histories show how crucial for him was the idea of gaining mental superiority over his patient:

> When I was a pupil at St. Bartholomew's Hospital, as my attention was much employed on the subject of insanity, I was requested . . . to visit a poor man . . . disordered in his mind. I went immediately to the house, and found the neighbourhood in an uproar. The maniac was locked in a room, raving and exceedingly turbulent. I took two men with me, and learning that he had no offensive weapons, I planted them at the door, with directions to be silent, and to keep out of sight, unless I should want their assistance. I then suddenly unlocked the door—rushed into the room and caught his *eye* in an instant. *The business was then done*—he became peaceable in a moment—trembled with fear, and was as governable as it was possible for a furious madman to be.[96]

One facet of this move from medicines to management was the expectation of greater therapeutic humanity. As Dr. John Ferriar put it:

> It was formerly supposed that lunatics could only be worked upon by terror. Shackles and whips, therefore, became part of the medical apparatus. A system of mildness and conciliation is now generally adopted, which, if it does not always facilitate the cure, at least tends to soften the destiny of the sufferer.[97]

Yet management therapy certainly never advocated kindness for kindness' sake. Far from it, for the model of madness infecting the mind and not the body involved the assumption that the madman's mind was peculiarly devious, warped, intractable. Hence, William Pargeter stressed,

> The *government* of maniacs is an art, not to be acquired without long experience, and frequent and attentive observation. As maniacs are extremely subdolous, the physician's first visit should be by *surprize*. He must employ every moment of his time by mildness or menaces, as circumstances direct, to gain an ascendancy over them, and to obtain their favour and prepossession. If this opportunity be lost, it will be difficult, if not impossible to effect it afterwards; and more especially, if he should betray any signs of timidity. He may be obliged at one moment, according

96. W. Pargeter, *Observations on Maniacal Disorders* (Reading: for the author, 1972), quoted in Richard Hunter and Ida Macalpine, *Three Hundred Years of Psychiatry, 1535–1810* (London: Oxford University Press, 1963), 510.

97. John Ferriar, *Medical Histories and Reflections*, 3 vols. (London: Cadell and Davies, 1795), quoted in Richard Hunter and Ida Macalpine, *Three Hundred Years of Psychiatry, 1535–1860* (London: Oxford University Press, 1963), 545.

to the exigency of the case, to be placid and accommodating in his manners, and the next, angry and absolute.[98]

Joseph Mason Cox, proprietor of the famous Fishponds Asylum, agreed:[99]

> The essence of management results from experience, address, and the natural endowments of the practitioners, and turns principally on making impressions on the senses. Since lunatics are artful, and their minds intensely fixed on the accomplishments of any wild purpose conjured up by the disease, physicians should be constantly on their guard: their grand object is to procure the confidence of the patient or to excite fear. . . . Whatever methods are adopted in order to secure either fear or confidence, deception is seldom admissible, no promise should remain unfulfilled, nor threat unexecuted.[100]

This was because the madman's will had to be won over. Public opinion was scandalized that Francis Willis allowed George III a razor to shave himself with. Willis was firm in his own defense before the Parliamentary Committee:

> It is necessary for a physician . . . to be able to judge, at the Moment, whether he can confide in the Professions of his Patient, and I never was disappointed in my Opinion.[101]

Transferred to a more institutional setting, moral management mutated into moral therapy, most notably at the York Retreat, opened in 1796, run by the Quaker Tuke family.[102] The Tukes likewise elevated mind above body, stating,

98. W. Pargeter, *Observations on Maniacal Disorders* (Reading: for the author, 1792), quoted in Richard Hunter and Ida Macalpine, *Three Hundred Years of Psychiatry, 1535–1860* (London: Oxford University Press, 1963), 539.

99. J. M. Cox, *Practical Observations on Insanity* (London, 1806), 42–43. See also M. Donnelly, *Managing the Mind* (London: Tavistock, 1983).

100. J. M. Cox, *Practical Observations on Insanity* (London, 1806), quoted in Richard Hunter and Ida Macalpine, *Three Hundred Years of Psychiatry, 1535–1860* (London: Oxford University Press, 1963), 596.

101. Quoted in Ida Macalpine and Richard Hunter, *George III and the Mad Business* (London: Allen Lane, 1969), 275.

102. A. Digby, *Madness, Morality and Medicine* (Cambridge: Cambridge University Press, 1985); "Moral Treatment at the York Retreat," in *The Anatomy of Madness,* ed. W. F. Bynum, Roy Porter, and Michael Shepherd, 2 vols. (London: Tavistock, 1985), 2: 52–72; F. Godlee, "The Retreat and Quakerism," ibid. 2: 73–85; A. Scull, *Museums of Madness* (London: Allen Lane, 1979), 68; W. F. Bynum, "Rationales for Therapy in British Psychiatry 1780–1825," *Medical History* 18 (1974): 817–834.

> The physician plainly perceived how much was to be done by moral and how little by medical means.[103]

But management had special connotations at the Retreat. For little value was placed on the virtuosity of the doctor. Instead the emphasis was on community. Its atmosphere was that of the family, its aim through example and the distribution of praise and disapproval to rekindle healthy rational and moral responses in the insane. As Charles Gaspard de La Rive rightly perceived:

> You see, that in the moral treatment, they do not consider the patients as absolutely deprived of reason, that is to say, as inaccessible to the emotions of fear, hope, sentiment and honour. They consider them . . . as children who have a superfluity of strength, and who would make a dangerous use of it; their punishment and rewards must be immediate, because anything at a distance has no effect upon them. A new system of education must be adopted.[104]

Foucault interpreted moral therapy as the imposition of radical chains. The Retreat could dispense with manacles of iron, because it caged the patients in manacles of mind; psychiatric control was so much more thorough, silent, and less scandalous.[105] Yet Foucault's seems a peculiarly paranoid judgment, given that the Retreat did indeed succeed in restoring such a high percentage of its patients to the outside world, and (as Ann Digby's new study has shown) so many ex-patients were deeply grateful for the care they received.[106] Yet Foucault's comment rightly draws attention to one point: the concern of the Retreat with the reform of mind. The Retreat formed part of the new psychiatric space.[107]

It made sense to early Georgian minds to treat behavioral disorders as a matter of the body. By 1800, they had largely become affairs of the mind.

103. S. Tuke, *A Description of the Retreat at York* (York, 1813), 151.

104. Quoted in Alexander Walk, "Some Aspects of the 'Moral Treatment' of the Insane up to 1845," *Journal of Mental Science* 100 (1954): 817.

105. Michel Foucault, *Madness and Civilization: A History of Insanity in the Age of Reason,* trans. Richard Howard (New York: Random House, 1965).

106. A. Digby, *Madness, Morality and Medicine* (Cambridge: Cambridge University Press, 1985); "Moral Treatment at the York Retreat," in *The Anatomy of Madness,* ed. W. F. Bynum, Roy Porter, and Michael Shepherd, 2 vols. (London: Tavistock, 1985), 2: 52–72.

107. M. Fears, "Therapeutic Optimism and the Treatment of the Insane," in *Health Care and Health Knowledge,* ed. R. Dingwall (London: Croom Helm, 1977), 66–81; "The 'Moral Treatment' of Insanity: A Study in the Social Construction of Human Nature" (Ph.D. thesis, University of Edinburgh, 1978).

Why? How did the idea of mental disorder become acceptable? How did terms like "hysteria," "hypochondria," and "neurosis" mutate into having the psychiatric meanings with which we are familiar? Indeed, how did the disciplines now known as psychiatry and psychology acquire independent existence from the early nineteenth century (the term "psychiatry" was an import from Feuchtersleben's German)?[108] I shall hint at some developments which worked together in this direction.

For one thing, treating the mad was developing into a more specialist occupation. Mad-doctors wanted to distinguish themselves over and against general medicine. To be able to claim an expertise of the mind was a mark of independence.

Moreover, mad-doctors were increasingly operating in their own distinctive site, the asylum. From Battie through to the Tukes and Edward Long Fox, many headed small private asylums for respectable clients.[109] The physician was entrepreneur, and personal contact was maximized. Treating the mad face-to-face, in the quasi-domestic intimacy of the small asylum, the energetic and human physician developed an unprecedented familiarity with the complex, ambivalent, defensive, self-protective preoccupations of the lunatic confined within the hothouse environment of the madhouse. They could see method in madness, and gain experience of behavior patterns that demanded explanation in terms more individual than the categories of gross pathological anatomy. The mentalization of lunacy was in large part a consequence of the institutionalization of the mad and their protracted clinical observation.

Yet it was not only the proto-psychiatrists who came to formulate the idea of mental disorder. Thus Coleridge was to insist:

> Madness is not simply a bodily disease. It is the sleep of the spirit with certain conditions of wakefulness; that is to say, lucid intervals.[110]

And this layman's opinion indicates we need to cast our explanatory net wider, exploring shifts in general social perceptions of self and society, danger and prestige, personality and propriety. So great had been the disorder of the Stuart century—that century of revolution—that the risk

108. For some of these mutations see Roy Porter, "The Doctor and the Word," *Medical Sociology News* 9 (1983): 21–28; see also G. S. Rousseau, "Psychology," in *The Ferment of Knowledge*, ed. G. S. Rousseau and Roy Porter (Cambridge: Cambridge University Press, 1980), 143–210.

109. W. Parry-Jones, *The Trade in Lunacy* (London: Routledge and Kegan Paul, 1972), 74 f.; Andrew Scull, "From Madness to Mental Illness: Medical Men as Moral Entrepreneurs," *European Journal of Sociology* 16 (1975): 219–261.

110. Quoted in V. Skultans, *Madness and Morals* (London: Routledge and Kegan Paul, 1975), 16.

of disorder to the soul or self was intolerable, and deviations from Right Reason were abominated as culpable lunacy. By contrast, the peace, prosperity, and civility of Georgian society relaxed the old stringent social and self controls. Waning religious zeal, secularization even, meant that for polite society the threat of diabolical possession was reduced to a ghost from the past, a gothic survival. In the consumer society—whose atmosphere was one of increasing cultural pluralism and artistic tolerance—self-expression and the cultivation of sensibilities by people of feeling found new acceptance.

Rationalized by the Lockean philosophy of liberty, individuality, and the subjective understanding, the inner world of feelings could count for more.[111] Suspicions about imagination were disarmed, and the search for self-identity could become an engrossing activity, the avocation of the finer, nobler soul. Such quests for New Found Lands of inner space—what Thomas Gray called "the stranger within thee"—are perhaps signaled by a remark of Boswell's in his *Hypochondriack* column: "There is too general a propensity to consider Hypochondria as altogether a bodily disorder: mens *sana*—a healthful mind—quite distinct from corpore *sano*—a sound body."[112]

In Boswell, whom Johnson rebuked for flirting with melancholy,[113] and many of his refined contemporaries we detect a willingness to risk the equivocations of a free-floating mental and imaginative condition, paving the way for the Romantic credo that if Consciousness or Imagination were the supreme faculty, it must be sovereign in Madness no less than in Reason, or, more scurrilously, in Byron's vignette of Keats at work on his poetry, "f--gg--g his imagination."[114]

Attributing madness to the body had been a resource for coping with

111. For the eighteenth-century quest for self-identity see P. M. Spacks, *Imagining a Self* (Cambridge, Mass.: Harvard University Press, 1976), especially chap. 5; J. N. Morris, *Versions of the Self* (New York: Basic Books, 1966); for the Lockean philosophical background to this see H. E. Allison, "Locke's Theory of Personal Identity: A Reexamination," in *Locke on Human Understanding: Selected Essays*, ed. I. C. Tipton (Oxford: Oxford University Press, 1977), 105–122; S. D. Cox, *"The Stranger within Thee": Concepts of the Self in Late-Eighteenth-Century Literature* (Pittsburgh: University of Pittsburgh Press, 1980); J. O. Lyons, *The Invention of the Self* (Carbondale: Southern Illinois University Press, 1978).

112. James Boswell, *Boswell's Column*, introduction and notes by Margery Bailey (London: Kimber, 1951), 319.

113. A. Ingram, *Boswell's Creative Gloom* (London: Macmillan, 1982).

114. Thus Byron:

> Mr. Keats, whose poetry you enquire after, appears to me that I have already said: such writing is a sort of mental masturbation f--gg--g his Imagination. I don't mean he is indecent, but viciously soliciting his own ideas into a state, which is neither poetry nor any thing else but a Bedlam vision produced by raw pork and opium.

chaos. After all, through the claims of the sectaries to direction by powers from Beyond, the real threats to order had come not from the body but from the spirit.[115] But by the close of the eighteenth century all had changed. Enlightenment materialism had become incorporated in the French Revolution and in radical materialist sciences such as phrenology. Now it was medical materialism that jeopardized hierarchy. The mind that would now accept mental illness was the one that identified civilization's future with the supremacy of mind, indeed with the march of mind.[116]

I have concentrated upon lunacy. Given time, intriguing parallels and contrasts could be traced in other areas of the mind/body interface. Here I can do no more than hint at a few. Take sex. The sex advice books of the late seventeenth century such as Nicolas Venette's *Tableau de l'amour conjugal* and *Aristotle's Masterpiece* present an extremely organic view of sex: it is essentially seen as a body urge, indeed a body purge, a physiological mechanism for discharging surplus passion or fluid, Nature's provision for the preservation of the race. Failures such as impotence or sterility are put down to organic causes to be set to rights by organic remedies—drugs, diet, surgery, and so forth.[117]

Sexual discourse had changed quite remarkably however by the end of the eighteenth century.[118] By then the dominant assumption was that

In *Byron: Selected Prose,* ed. P. Gunn (Harmondsworth: Penguin, 1972), 357. More generally see G. S. Rousseau, "Science and the Discovery of the Imagination in Enlightenment England," *Eighteenth-Century Studies* 3 (1969–70): 108–135; E. Tuveson, "Locke and Sterne," in *Reason and Imagination: Studies in the History of Ideas 1600–1800* ed. J. A. Mazzeo (New York: Columbia University Press, 1962); idem, *The Imagination as a Means of Grace* (Berkeley and Los Angeles: University of California Press, 1960); idem, "Locke and the Dissolution of the Ego," *Modern Philology* 52 (1955): 159–174; K. MacLean, *John Locke and English Literature of the Eighteenth Century* (New Haven: Yale University Press, 1936).

115. See P. Fussell, *The Rhetorical World of Augustan Humanism* (Oxford: Oxford University Press, 1965).

116. J. Engell, *The Creative Imagination* (Cambridge, Mass.: Harvard University Press, 1981).

117. Roy Porter, "Spreading Carnal Knowledge or Selling Dirt Cheap? Nicolas Venette's *Tableau de L'amour conjugal* in Eighteenth-Century England," *Journal of European Studies* 14 (1984): 235–255.

118. For the shifts see Roy Porter, "The Sexual Politics of James Graham," *British Journal for Eighteenth-Century Studies* 5 (1982): 109–206; P. Wagner, *Eros Revived* (London: Secker and Warburg, 1988); idem, "Research the Taboo: Sexuality and Eighteenth-Century English Erotica," *Eighteenth-Century Life* 3 (1983): 108–115; P. -G. Boucé, "Aspects of Sexual Tolerance and Intolerance in Eighteenth-Century England," *British Journal for Eighteenth-Century Studies* 3 (1980): 180; Vern L. Bullough, *Sexual Variance in Society and History* (Chicago: University of Chicago Press, 1976); Alex Comfort, *The Anxiety Makers* (London: Nelson, 1967).

sex was all in the head. On the one hand, writers on what were becoming singled out as sexual diseases, soon to be the perversions—Tissot on masturbation, Bienville on nymphomania—were increasingly arguing that the blame for sexual vices lay not with some organic lesion but in the diseased mind.[119] For Bienville, "the imagination is the *sole* contriver" of self-abuse.[120] On the other hand, a noted physician such as John Hunter had demonstrated in a famous case-study how impotence could be overcome by acknowledging that the defect lay in the mind, and so proceeding psychologically rather than physiologically.[121] Not least, James Graham, in his notorious *Lecture on Generation*, urged that the key to sexual performance lay in stimulating the imagination:

> How astonishing is the force of the imagination of the bodily faculties! Some of you, gentlemen, may perhaps have experienced that the imagination being intensely rivited, at certain times, on a very beautiful or much loved woman, it will make a man enjoy a plain one with almost equal ardour.[122]

How do we explain the shifts in *this* field? The forces are complex and confused. As part of the movement toward heightened sensibility, sex itself was being elevated, sublimated into the ideal realm of the mental pleasures.[123] But at the same time, as sexual abuses such as masturbation became recognized as resistant to eradication, that sad conclusion suggested that their source must be deeply hidden, in the convoluted, deviant labyrinth of the imagination.

119. See Foucault, *The History of Sexuality*; F. J. Barker-Benfield, *The Horrors of the Half-Known Life* (New York: Harper and Row, 1976).

120. See Peter Wagner, "The Veil of Science and Morality: Some Pornographic Aspects of the ONANIA," *British Journal for Eighteenth-Century Studies* 4 (1983): 179–184; G. S. Rousseau, "Nymphomania, Bienville and the Rise of Erotic Sensibility," in *Sexuality in Eighteenth-Century Britain*, ed. P. -G. Boucé (Manchester: Manchester University Press, 1982), 95–120.

121. Quoted in R. Hunter and I. Macalpine, *Three Hundred Years of Psychiatry, 1535–1860* (London: Oxford University Press, 1963), 494.

122. J. Graham, *A Lecture on the Generation, Increase, and Improvement of the Human Species* (London, 1780?), 50.

123. For the Enlightenment's libido-liberating claim that the erotic is the healthy see J. Hagstrum, *Sex and Sensibility: Erotic Ideal and Erotic Love from Milton to Mozart* (Chicago: University of Chicago Press, 1980); Roy Porter, "Mixed Feelings: The Enlightenment and Sexuality in Britain," in *Sexuality in Eighteenth-Century Britain*, ed. P. -G. Boucé (Manchester: Manchester University Press, 1982), 1–27; idem, "The Sexual Politics of James Graham," *British Journal of Eighteenth-Century Studies* 5 (1982): 199–205; P. -G. Boucé, "Some Sexual Beliefs and Myths in Eighteenth-Century Britain," in *Sexuality in Eighteenth-Century Britain*, 28–47.

A parallel story can surely be told of drunkenness.[124] Doctors traditionally deplored drunkenness as a constitutional malaise. Within humoral medicine, the drunken fever was a mark of a lack of moderation; the consequence of habitual intoxication was the ruin of the stomach and the inflammation of the brain, even to insanity. But in the Gin Age, as a succession of physicians gave more critical attention to hard drinking—Cheyne and Lettsom stand out—attention switched to the disposition to drunkenness—they sometimes spoke of "addiction"—taken as a malady of the will, culminating in Thomas Trotter's express statement of 1804 that habitual drunkenness was not just a disease but "a disease of the mind" (the concept of alcoholism was to follow a generation later).[125] Here, I suggest, as in the case of sexual perversions, a growing recognition of the intractability of the habit, and its unresponsiveness to medication, helped direct the medical gaze within, into the inner space of the delinquent, recalcitrant will.

Mesmerism offers a parallel change and a similar challenge. As is well known, Franz Anton Mesmer himself was adamant that he performed his cures through the agency of a natural superfine medium, the animal magnetic fluid. That guaranteed that his technique was truly scientific. By contrast, it was his critics, especially the devastating French Commission of 1784, who insisted that Mesmer's cures were mere suggestion, were all due to transference from mind to mind. Mesmer could never come to terms with the idea of purely psychic efficacy, yet his follower Puysegur happily discarded the animal magnetic fluid and accepted a psychological explanation. He thus paved the way for hypnotism, Victorian spiritualism, and dynamic psychiatry, anticipating the course taken by the young Freud in shifting away from neurophysiology toward therapies that steadily grew less somatic: from cocaine, to hypnosis by pressure, to free associations and the talking cure.[126]

124. For a recent discussion of this issue see Roy Porter, "The Drinking Man's Disease: The Prehistory of Alcoholism in Georgian Britain," *British Journal of Addiction* 80 (1984).

125. T. Trotter, *An Essay, Medical, Philosophical and Chemical, on Drunkenness* (London, 1804).

126. For mesmerism in France see R. Darnton, *Mesmerism and the End of the Enlightenment in France* (Cambridge, Mass.: Harvard University Press, 1968); G. Sutton, "Electric Medicine and Mesmerism," *Isis* 72 (1981): 375–392; V. Buranelli, *The Wizard from Vienna: Franz Mesmer and the Origins of Hypnotism* (London: P. Owen, 1976); F. A. Mesmer, *Mesmerism: A Translation of the Original Scientific and Medical Writings of F. A. Mesmer, M.D.*, trans. George Bloch (Los Altos, Calif.: Kaufman, 1980); F. Rausky, *Mesmer, ou la révolution thérapeutique* (Paris: Payot, 1977). The early history of English mesmerism awaits its author. For contemporary accounts and attacks see J. Martin, *Animal Magnetism Examined* (London, 1790), and [anon.], *The Wonders and Mysteries of Animal Magnetism Displayed* (London, 1791).

Physiognomy underwent a similar psychological sublimation. Traditional physiognomy had been somatic through and through, postulating that character embossed itself directly upon the face or body. This came to seem hideously crude to eighteenth-century savants aware of hypocrisy and the mask, and subscribing to the New Philosophy's view that Nature's essence lay not in surface qualities but underneath. But Lavater was to develop a new physiognomical gaze—using what he called "an additional eye," his mind's eye, to peer behind transient, fleeting expressions and catch the hidden, secret soul.[127]

Foucault's work is highly suggestive for grasping the meaning of shifts from attention to the body to attention to the mind. In *Discipline and Punish,* for example, he showed how physical torture and corporal punishment gave way to the systematic penalization of the mind ("punishment should strike the soul rather than the body," wrote Mably)—and, more importantly, in the new penology, to the goal of the reform of the criminal mind.[128] Foucault's signal contribution was to deny that this switch should automatically be seen as liberal and humane. The emergence of disciplines such as psychiatry did not constitute "progress" but simply registered new configurations of *savoir-pouvoir,* inscribed in particular institutional structures—the asylum, the prison. But Foucault never ventured a more comprehensive social viewpoint, presumably fearing that the rigor of textual analysis would be sapped by the reentry of flabby social history, with all its people.

Yet surely we need that wider framework—of people, not just prison manuals and penitentials—as if we are to avoid the impression Foucault's books all too readily give that history has been one relentless encroachment of disciplines, controls, and their accompanying discourses. Indeed, his unfinished history of sexuality seems to hint that he himself was willing to broaden his approach. For there he hypothesizes in the first volume how growing bourgeois attention to health in the eighteenth

See also Jonathan Miller, "Mesmerism," *The Listener,* 22 Nov. 1973, 685–690; Roy Porter, "Under the Influence: Mesmerism in England," *History Today,* September 1985, 22–29. For the later legacy, see H. Ellenberger, *The Discovery of the Unconscious* (New York: Basic Books, 1971).

127. See G. Tytler, *Physiognomy in the European Novel* (Princeton: Princeton University Press, 1982); M. Shortland, "Barthes, Lavater and the Visible Body," *Economy and Society* 14 (1985): 273–312; M. Shortland, "The Body in Question: Some Perceptions, Problems and Perspectives of the Body in Relation to Character, c. 1750–1850" (Ph.D. thesis, Leeds University, 1985); Roy Porter, "Making Faces: Physiognomy and Fashion in Eighteenth-Century England," *Etudes anglaises* 38 (1985): 385–396.

128. Foucault, *Discipline and Punish,* 95.

century might be seen as a counterweight to the aristocratic concentration on blood.[129] But he did not proceed to examine the wider class dynamics of such developments, did not explore how the growing bourgeois stress upon the mind, upon body purification, delicacy, and social distance, formed tactics for dematerialization, designed to segregate the propertied and the polite from the *hoi polloi,* as part of that separation of high and low life which formed such a key feature of the eighteenth century.[130]

Mind was to be cordoned off from body, just as the polite were not to be touched by the great unwashed. As that quintessential bourgeois, Mary Anne Schimmelpenninck, was to put it:

> every class of society has its own glory. The poor, his physical strength; the middle, the power of mental research; the elevated, the charm of manner, the amalgam which fits them as keystones to solidify the arch of society. Then let us each rejoice in our own, and rejoice in our neighbours' gifts, but not expect to find all united in one.[131]

Let us nudge these speculations about mind, muscles, and manners one stage further. For in other important ways, broad social changes were to bring mind to the fore. The century from the Scientific Revolution to the Industrial Revolution saw a staggering expansion of human productive powers for the mastery of Nature and the management of matter. The consequence of these scientific and material transformations had been to empty Nature of mind—what Weber called the disenchantment of the world, or Couliano has more recently termed the de-eroticization of Nature.[132]

129. Foucault, *The History of Sexuality.*

130. For the rise of sensibility see Erik Erametsa, "A Study of the Word 'Sentimental' and of Other Linguistic Characteristics of Eighteenth-Century Sentimentalism in England" (Thesis, Helsinki, 1951); R. S. Crane, "Suggestions towards a Genealogy of the Man of Feeling," *ELH* 1 (1934): 205–230; G. S. Rousseau, "Nerves, Spirits, and Fibres: Towards Defining the Origins of Sensibility," with a postscript, *The Blue Guitar* (Messina) 2 (1976): 125–153; L. Bredvold, *The Natural History of Sensibility* (Detroit: Wayne State University Press, 1962); S. Moravia, "The Enlightenment and the Sciences of Man," *History of Science* 18 (1980): 247–268; K. Figlio, "Theories of Perception and the Physiology of Mind in the Late Eighteenth Century," *History of Science* 13 (1975): 177–212. For the opening up of cultural divides see P. Burke, *Popular Culture in Early Modern Europe* (London: Temple Smith, 1978); for the changing role of the public see R. Sennett, *The Fall of Public Man* (Cambridge: Cambridge University Press, 1974).

131. C. C. Hankin, ed., *Life of Mary Anne Schimmelpenninck,* 2 vols. (London, 1858), 2: 127.

132. I. Couliano, *Eros et magie à la Renaissance* (Paris: Flammarion, 1984); W. Leiss, *The Domination of Nature* (New York: Brazillier, 1972).

The world soul vanished, Nature was reduced to matter, or what natural philosophers commonly called body. But while consciousness and sympathy were thus being drained from Nature, they were being concentrated in man's mind. As E. B. Tylor was later to argue:

> Animism, indeed, seems to be drawing in its outposts, and concentrating itself on the first and main position, the doctrine of the human soul.[133]

Crucially, this rise of dominion in science, discovery, and industry afforded man new experience of Mind over Matter, reinforcing that sense of the human mind as the source of power and creation so prominent in late-eighteenth-century sources from German Idealism to English Romanticism.[134] It was but a short step to the Victorian identification of destiny with the March of Mind.

If one embodiment of this new sense of will was the entrepreneur, he was closely paralleled by the emergent intellectual. When the history of the intelligentsia is properly written, we will at last have a better appreciation of that astonishing growth in voice and authority of the thinker toward the close of the eighteenth century, of which Romanticism is one facet. The rise of the intellectuals' fourth estate went *pari passu* with a new magic of the mind. We all too readily regard the claims of poet-artists like Blake (who dissolved body into imagination or soul)[135] as being at cross-purposes with those thinkers, such as Priestley, he parodied in *The Philosopher in the Moon.* Yet in fact they are all of a piece, as Peacock's satires show.[136] "When I was young," wrote Théophile

133. E. B. Tylor, *Primitive Culture* (1871), quoted in H. Jennings, *Pandaemonium* (London: A. Deutsch, 1985), 325.

134. For different dimensions see J. Benthall, *The Body Electric* (London, 1976); P. A. Cantor, *Creature and Creator: Myth-making and English Romanticism* (Cambridge: Cambridge University Press, 1984).

135. Man has no Body distinct from his soul;
for that call'd Body is a portion of
the Soul discerned by the five Senses,
the chief inlets of Soul in this age.
Energy is the only life, and is from
the Body; and Reason is the bound or
outward circumference of Energy.
Energy is External Delight.

Quoted in J. Lindsay, *William Blake: His Work and Life* (London: Constable, 1978), 100. For Blake on the body see F. Frosch, *The Awakening of Albion* (Ithaca, N.Y.: Cornell University Press, 1974).

136. Cf. Mr. Flosky on "the morbid anatomy of black bile" in *Nightmare Abbey,* in *The Novels of Thomas Love Peacock,* ed. D. Garnett (London: R. Hart-Davies, 1948), 376.

Gautier, "I could not have accepted as a lyrical poet anyone weighing more than ninety-nine pounds."[137] Yet this romanticization of consumption as the dematerializing disease only echoes Sydney Smith's complaint that a certain man "had not body enough to cover his mind decently with, his intellect is improperly exposed."[138]

Improperly exposed intellects may come a bit near the bone. My coverage here is somewhat skimpy. I haven't touched on the countless layers of ambivalence and contradiction in representations of mind/body relations—for example, to note just one instance, the fact that the pre-Victorian rise of delicacy, when servants were being permitted less and less direct contact with their betters, occurred at precisely the time when man-midwives were being let into women's bedrooms for the first time, to touch the most private, the most delicate parts of all.[139]

Yet what I have attempted is to suggest that in our understanding of the mind/body relation, the view from the body has been neglected. There is far more in the relationship than regular histories of faculty psychology, the philosophy of mind, or of psychiatry allow. In particular, mind/body relations must be understood within specific contexts of use determined by particular problems and cultural configurations. The detailed histories remain to be told.[140]

137. Quoted in S. Sontag, *Illness as Metaphor* (London: Allen Lane, 1979); cf. S. Mcleod, *The Art of Starvation* (London, 1981).

138. *A Memoir of the Reverend Sydney Smith* ed. Lady Holland (London: Longman, Brown, Green, and Longmans, 1855), 1: 258.

139. John O'Neill, *Five Bodies: The Human Shape of Modern Society* (Ithaca, N.Y., and London: Cornell University Press, 1985), 23.

140. See L. Stone, *Family, Sex and Marriage in England, 1500–1800* (London: Weidenfeld and Nicolson, 1977); E. Shorter, *A History of Women's Bodies* (London: Allen Lane, 1983). For proto-Victorianism see P. Fryer, *Mrs. Grundy: Studies in English Prudery* (London: Dobson, 1963); M. Jaeger, *Before Victoria* (London: Chatto and Windus, 1956); E. J. Bristow, *Vice and Vigilance* (Dublin: Gill and Macmillan, 1979); M. Quinlan, *Victorian Prelude* (New York: Columbia University Press, 1941); E. Trudgill, *Madonnas and Magdalens* (London: Heinemann, 1966). For the midwife as sexual threat see Roy Porter, "A Touch of Danger: The Man-Midwife as Sexual Predator," in *Sexual Underworlds of the Enlightenment*, ed. G. S. Rousseau and Roy Porter (Manchester: Manchester University Press, 1987).

THREE

Locke, Hume, and Modern Moral Theory: A Legacy of Seventeenth- and Eighteenth-Century Philosophies of Mind

Philippa Foot

> 'Tis one thing to know virtue, and another to conform the will to it. In order, therefore, to prove, that the measures of right and wrong are eternal laws, *obligatory* on every rational mind, . . . [w]e must also point out the connexion betwixt the relation and the will . . .
>
> —DAVID HUME, *Treatise of Human Nature*[1]

Most philosophers writing today would be surprised to be told that their own philosophical psychology had anything much to do with that of late-seventeenth- and early-eighteenth-century philosophers. No one indeed denies that interest in the philosophy of this period is still very great and not at all declining, if only because in metaphysics Locke's theory of primary and secondary qualities, and his theory of real essences, are widely discussed; and in moral philosophy Hume is a commanding, even dominating, figure, whose arguments we can never quite satisfactorily refute. The philosophies of mind of these two great empiricists has, however, come to seem more than a little quaint. We are no longer interested in the attempt to show the origin of psychological concepts in simple ideas or impressions presented in experience; and Wittgenstein has taught us to regard with suspicion the belief, firmly held by both Locke and Hume, that each person knows only from his own introspection what it is to think, to feel, or to desire.[2]

1. David Hume, *A Treatise of Human Nature* (1739–40), ed. L. A. Selby-Bigge, 2d ed., ed. P. H. Nidditch (Oxford: Clarendon Press, 1978), book III, part i, section 1, p. 465. All subsequent references to Hume's *Treatise* are to this edition.

Where there are problems about the availability of works quoted in this paper, I have occasionally given alternative references, enclosed in square brackets.

2. See Ludwig Wittgenstein, *Philosophical Investigations* (1953), trans. G. E. M. Anscombe (New York: Macmillan, 1968), passim, but especially sections 243 ff., and, e.g., 316, 412, 551, 580, 587. Also part II, xiii.

In this paper I will argue that although we have, it is true, rejected a great deal of the philosophical psychology of Locke and Hume, there is a part of it which we still more or less take for granted. If the debt is little acknowledged, this may be because it has come to appear to many simply as incontrovertible, uncontentious truth. I am thinking here of a part of the philosophy of mind which belongs to the theory of volition and thus to the theory of action; and not surprisingly it is in the related field of moral theory that its influence appears. I will describe the views of Locke and Hume on the subject of the determination of action, showing how these theories affected their own (very different) moralities. I will point out an underlying similarity in their philosophies of action which made it impossible for either of them to give a proper account of moral motivation, and will suggest that our own thinking on the subject of moral judgment would be improved if we made a more radical break with Locke and Hume.

To begin, then, with this part of the philosophical psychology of John Locke. What is interesting in this connection is his account of the determination of action by desire; there are several other parts of the Lockean philosophy of *mind* and *self* which are relevant to modern theories of ethics, as for instance his doctrine of self-identity, or again his theory of free will; but these I will set aside. Naturally, however, Locke's theory of the determination of the will to action must be seen in the context of his general empiricist epistemology. What Locke is out to do, in the theory of action as elsewhere, is to measure the reach of the understanding and to show that we can account for all our knowledge in terms of experience and the combination of ideas in the mind. He insists that all our concepts can be seen as combinations of simple ideas given to us by sense and by reflection, "sense" being the operation of our sense organs, and "reflection" the reflexive movement that we make in order to observe the operations of our minds.

Where, we may ask, do mental elements such as desires and emotions belong in this scheme of things? To Hume they would be impressions of reflection; but the structure of Locke's theory of mind is rather different. Desires and emotions are, he says, modifications of the simple ideas of pleasure and pain; and he classifies these as being not only ideas of reflection but also ideas of sense. What Locke means by this is that pleasure and pain can *arise* either from the senses (as when fire warms

In writing of modern philosophy I confine myself throughout to philosophy of the modern analytic school. It is absolutely necessary to deal with this separately from, e.g., phenomenology.

or burns us) or alternatively from thoughts that bring joy or grief. He makes his position quite clear in a sentence from Book II of the *Essay concerning Human Understanding*:

> By Pleasure and Pain, I must be understood to mean of Body or Mind, as they are commonly distinguished; though in truth, they be only different Constitutions of the Mind, sometimes occasioned by disorder in the Body, sometimes by Thoughts of the Mind.[3]

And again, writing of "Delight and Joy on the one side; and Torment and Sorrow on the other," he says that "to speak truly, they are all of the Mind; though some have their rise in the Mind from Thought, others in the Body from certain modifications of Motion."[4]

Such is the framework into which Locke's account of the antecedents of volition has to fit. He believes that this is how we obtain the simple ideas of pain and pleasure; and it is around pleasure and pain (which he identifies with happiness and unhappiness) that his theory of action revolves.

Turning now to the considerable complexities of this theory we may be glad to find one proposition which he unambiguously and consistently endorsed. Locke held the belief that later came to be known as "psychological hedonism," according to which all action is in some way directed toward pleasure or the avoidance of pain. For all his scorn for Hobbes and his tendency to play down any Hobbesian influence in his own work, he had in fact taken over Hobbes's belief that human nature is under the governance of two masters, pleasure and pain. It is true that Locke had freed himself entirely from Hobbes's materialist account of the origin of these elements of our experience, giving thoughts and bodily states an equal power to produce them. It is also true that Locke was much more liberal than Hobbes in his recognition of the diversity of objects in which men might take pleasure.[5] Nevertheless he says

3. John Locke, *An Essay concerning Human Understanding* (1690), ed. Peter H. Nidditch (Oxford: Clarendon Press, 1979), book II, chapter xx, section 2, p. 229. All subsequent references to Locke's *Essay* are to this edition. Since Nidditch retains the original spelling, capitalization, and italics of the fourth edition of 1700, quotations from the *Essay* in the present paper are not uniform in appearance with the extracts from other writings available only in modernized form. I have chosen to use Nidditch's edition in spite of this, because it is widely available, and very much the best.

4. Locke, *Essay,* II xxi 41, p. 258.

5. In a short undated paper "Thus I Think" Locke had given, in a catalogue of lasting pleasures: health, reputation, knowledge, and "doing good." Lord King, *The Life and Letters of John Locke* (1829), 2d ed. (London, 1830), 2:120 [3d ed. (London: Bohn's Standard Library, 1858), 306–307].

explicitly, and repeatedly, in the *Essay* both that uneasiness and satisfaction determine the will and that good and evil "are nothing but Pleasure or Pain, or that which occasions, or procures Pleasure or Pain to us."[6] In the Journal for 1676 he writes

> The Mind finding in itself the ideas of several objects which, if enjoyed, would produce pleasure, i.e. the ideas of the several things it loves, contemplating the satisfaction which would arise to itself in the actual enjoyment or application of some one of those things it loves and the possibility or feasibleness of the present enjoyment, or doing something toward the procuring the enjoyment, of that good, observes in itself some uneasiness or trouble or displeasure till it be done, and this is what we call desire.[7]

Psychological hedonism as such gives a certain general characterization of the objects of desire; but it leaves a good deal undetermined. For in itself it says nothing about whether or not an agent always seeks the greatest possible balance of pleasure over pain, taking future as well as present experiences into account. This was something about which Locke changed his mind between the first edition of the *Essay*, published in 1690, and the second edition of 1694, the latter being echoed by the third and fourth. Between the first and second editions he abandoned the doctrine that the will was always determined by "the greater good in view."

> To return then to the Enquiry, *what is it that determines the Will in regard to our Actions?* And that upon second thoughts I am apt to imagine is not, as is generally supposed, the greater good in view: But some (and for the most part the most pressing) *uneasiness* a Man is at present under. This is that which successively determines the *Will*, and set us upon those Actions, we perform. This *Uneasiness* we may call, as it is, *Desire*; which is an *uneasiness* of the Mind for want of some absent good.[8]

And again:

> It seems so establish'd and settled a maxim by the general consent of all Mankind, That good, the greater good, determines the will, that I do not at all wonder, that when I first publish'd my thoughts on this Subject, I took it for granted; and I imagine, that by a great many I shall be thought more excusable, for having then done so, than that now I have ventur'd to recede from so received an Opinion. But yet upon a stricter enquiry, I

6. Locke, *Essay*, II xxviii 5, p. 351.
7. W. von Leyden, *John Locke: Essays on the Law of Nature* (Oxford: Clarendon Press, 1954), 265–272. For the importance of this long journal entry, see ibid., 264.
8. Locke, *Essay*, II xxi 31, pp. 250–251.

am forced to conclude, that *good,* the *greater good,* though apprehended and acknowledged to be so, does not determine the *will,* until our desire, raised proportionably to it, makes us *uneasy* in the want of it.[9]

These two quotations come from the considerable material added by Locke in the second edition of the *Essay* and repeated with minor changes in all subsequent editions. In this emendation, sections 28 to 60 of book II, chapter xxi, replace sections 28–38 of the first edition, and although much of the text of the first edition appears in the later editions, it appears in a subsidiary role. Philosophically speaking, the change is significant. For Locke now introduces and discusses at length the subject of *desire,* which had been barely mentioned in the first edition.[10] Moreover he now gives to desire the principal role in the determination of the will. Not that he goes back on his psychological hedonism: what happens is rather that *desire* is introduced as a piece of intermediary mechanism, operated on by present pleasures and pains and by the thought of future pleasure and pain, and itself having the power to produce volition or will.

By this means Locke hopes to solve the problem known since Antiquity as the problem of *akrasia* or incontinence. In the first edition he had tried to explain the problem away in terms of mistakes about the good, saying in words reminiscent of Plato's *Protagoras* that present pleasures and pains appear larger than those of the future on account of their proximity.[11] But in later editions he admits that men may indeed know the better and choose the worse:[12]

Let a Man be never so well perswaded of the advantages of virtue . . . yet till he *hungers and thirsts after righteousness*; till he feels an *uneasiness* in the want of it, his *will* will not be determin'd to any action in pursuit of this confessed greater good; but any other *uneasiness* he feels in himself, shall take place, and carry his *will* to other actions.[13]

9. Locke, *Essay,* II xxi 35, pp. 252–253.

10. See Locke, *Essay,* Nidditch's note to p. 248, line 8.

11. Plato, *Protagoras* 356c4–8, 357a5–b3.

12. Locke, *Essay,* II xxi 35, p. 254.

13. Locke, *Essay,* II xxi 35, p. 253. There is, however, a different view, or at least a different use of the term "desire," to be found in *Some Thoughts concerning Eduation,* a work which Locke put together, from notes written nearly a decade before, at the time when he was revising the *Essay* for the second edition. There Locke opposes desire to reason, apparently identifying desire with immediate inclination or appetite. See *Some Thoughts concerning Education,* sections 33 and 38; James L. Axtell, *The Educational Writings of John Locke* (Cambridge: Cambridge University Press, 1968), 138 and 143.

Desire, Locke tells us, is uneasiness: the idea of desire is a modification of the simple idea of pain: a modification because the idea of desire implies a sufficient degree of pain to determine the will to action.

The first thing we must ask about this newly stressed mechanism is whether Locke thought it the universal determinant of the will. He explicitly says in several places that without uneasiness there is no volition, as in the passage last quoted. And although there is a sentence in which he says that "the *will seldom* [my italics] orders any action, nor is there any voluntary action performed, without some *desire* accompanying it," the context suggests that he is here contrasting the operation of "uneasiness" alone with "uneasiness" forming part of passions such as anger or jealousy.[14] There is, however, a stronger reason for saying that Locke does not consistently affirm that volition is always caused by desire. For in book II, chapter ii, section 30, where he wants to distinguish *desire* and *will,* he actually gives examples in which he says "the *Will* and *Desire* run counter."

> A Man, whom I cannot deny, may oblige me to use persuasions to another, which at the same time I am speaking, I may wish may not prevail on him. In this case, 'tis plain the *Will* and *Desire* run counter. I will the Action, that tends one way, whilst my desire tends another, and that the direct contrary. A Man, who by a violent Fit of the Gout in his limbs, finds a doziness in his Head, or a want of appetite in his Stomach removed, desires to be eased too of the pain of his Feet or Hands (for where-ever there is pain there is a desire to be rid of it) though yet, whilst he apprehends, that the removal of the pain may translate the noxious humour to a more vital part, his will is never determin'd to any one Action, that may serve to remove this pain.[15]

In consistency Locke should not have suggested that desire can tend in one direction and will in another, but rather that there may be two desires, of which one determines the will to a movement which the other opposes. What he needs to show, in order to prove that will and desire are distinct, is that there can be a desire without a corresponding action, which does not of course imply that there can be actions without a corresponding desire.

Locke's usual line from the second edition forward is that volition and hence action are universally determined by uneasiness, that is, by desire. The only important rider that he adds is that when several desires have arisen, "the greatest and most pressing" does not always determine the

14. Locke, *Essay,* II xxi 39, pp. 256–257.
15. Locke, *Essay,* II xxi 39, p. 250.

will. For the mind has the power to suspend the execution and satisfaction of any of its desires, giving us "opportunity to examine, view, and judge, of the good or evil [i.e., the effect on our happiness] of what we are going to do."[16]

To support his account of the antecedents of action Locke has to try to show that whenever we act, or want to act, the volition is triggered by "uneasiness." In book II of the *Essay,* chapter xxi, from section 31 onward, this is just what he sets out to do. I think we can disentangle his arguments more or less as follows.

Locke wants to show that the *object* of desire is always pleasure, either positive enjoyment or else the negative pleasure of "indolency" or relief from pain. He also wants to show, however, that it is only when we are uneasy at the absence of pleasure that we have a desire and are thereby moved to action. So he has to explain how uneasiness comes into the picture in every instance in which we try to gain pleasure or avoid pain. He must consider the cases in which we wish to continue present pleasure or get rid of present pain, and also the determination of the will by the ideas of future pleasures and pains.

Where present pain is concerned he seems to see no difficulty, clearly believing that this pain, being itself an uneasiness, itself represents desire. And he also insists that the removal of a present pain is necessarily a condition of our happiness.[17] What is more difficult for him is to say where uneasiness comes in when we want a present pleasure to continue, and Locke is here driven to the expedient of saying that we are anxious at the thought that the pleasure will end.

> So that even in *joy* it self, that which keeps up the action, whereon the enjoyment depends, is the desire to continue it, and fear to lose it . . . [18]

Future pleasures and pains he deals with in the first place by simply asserting (as in the passage about thirsting after righteousness which was quoted earlier) that until we *feel uneasy* at the prospect of pleasure sacrificed or penalty incurred, we shall not be turned away from present enjoyments and ease. But he also relies heavily on examples that seem to bear out his point.

> [L]et a Drunkard see, that his health decays, his Estate wastes; Discredit and Diseases, and the want of all things, even of his beloved Drink, at-

16. Locke, *Essay,* II xxi 47, p. 263.

17. John Colman, *John Locke's Moral Philosophy* (Edinburgh: Edinburgh University Press, 1983), 217 stresses this point.

18. Locke, *Essay,* II xxi 39, p. 257.

> tends him in the course he follows: yet the returns of *uneasiness* to miss his Companions; the habitual thirst after his Cups, at the usual time, drives him to the Tavern. . . .'Tis not for want of viewing the greater good . . . but when the *uneasiness* to miss his accustomed delight returns, the greater acknowledged good loses its hold, and the present *uneasiness* determines the *will* to the accustomed action . . . [19]

Such examples cannot really show the nature of desire to be uneasiness, and one has to admit that Locke's theory is confusing and confused. Nevertheless Locke shows his genius in fastening on a connection that is deep, and hard to understand. For who can deny that there is some very interesting conceptual connection between *pain, uneasiness,* and *desire*? What Locke says cannot be right; but one may doubt whether anyone else has yet been able to give the true account of this fascinating subject.

The important question from our present point of view is how Locke's theory of action is related to his moral theory, and it is to this that I now turn. As a moral philosopher he has had very little lasting influence; and this is perhaps not surprising. His moral theory is a very curious blend of hedonism and rationalism, held together only by an explicit and often repeated appeal to the existence of God. As we shall see, his account of the determination of action seemed to force him toward something of this kind.[20]

In the *Essay concerning Human Understanding* Locke claims that moral propositions can be known with certainty. He is emboldened to claim the status of a science for morality largely by the similar way in which his theory of knowledge treated moral and mathematical ideas. Unlike the ideas of material substances such as gold, these ideas are "adequate." There is, in such cases, no reference to unknowable "real essences" independent of the mind, and so we can have demonstrative knowledge in morals as we can in mathematics. In the fourth book of the *Essay* Locke gives several examples of moral propositions which can be known with certainty (by intuition and demonstration), as for instance that

19. Locke, *Essay,* II xxi 35, pp. 253–254.

20. Von Leyden wrote that "Locke's hedonism and certain other views held by him in his later years made it difficult for him to adhere wholeheartedly to his doctrine of natural law" (*Essays on the Law of Nature,* 14). John Colman, however, sees no inconsistency here, and in my opinion he is right. There is no reason why one should not be a rationalist about moral knowledge and a hedonist about the motive to moral action, so long as one is ready to rely on God to annex pleasure to the right actions either in this world or the next. See Colman, *John Locke's Moral Philosophy,* 235.

"*Where there is no Property, there is no Injustice,*"[21] or "*Murther deserves Death.*"[22] Complex ideas such as that of property or murder could be analyzed like those of mathematics. Since such ideas were "their own archetypes," we could know the real and nominal essences of *property* or *murder* at the same time.[23] Locke denies, moreover, that these moral propositions are merely verbal, since the same ideas with a different name annexed to them would still carry the same implications.[24] Nevertheless, he believed that the examples which he gave of demonstrable moral propositions were of very little use without a further demonstration which would show why anyone had an *obligation* to act in one way rather than another; and this, he thought, required a knowledge of the laws which God had given to men. In the short piece called "Of Ethics in General" published by Lord King in his *Life and Letters of John Locke,* Locke had said that all the knowledge of virtue and vice which man had attained by the analysis of the complex ideas of morality found in different societies would amount to little unless we could "show the inferments that may draw us to virtue and deter us from vice."[25]

Those who only give definitions

> whilst they discourse ever so acutely of temperance or justice, but show no law of a superior that prescribes temperance, to the observation or breach of which law there are rewards and punishments annexed, the force of morality is lost, and evaporates only into words, disputes, and niceties. . . . Without showing a law that commands or forbids them, moral goodness will be but an empty sound, and those actions which the schools here call virtue or vice, may by the same authority be called contrary names in another country; and if there be nothing more than their decisions and determinations in the case, they will be still nevertheless indifferent as to any man's practice, which will by such kind of determinations be under no obligation to observe them.[26]

Looking for the source of obligation Locke finds it in laws of various kinds, which he classifies under the headings of Divine law, the civil law,

21. Locke, *Essay,* IV iii 18, p. 549.
22. Locke, *Essay,* IV iv 8 p. 566.
23. See, e.g., Locke, *Essay,* IV xii 7 and 8, pp. 643–644.
24. Locke, *Essay,* IV v 9, pp. 566–567.
25. "Of Ethics in General," section 6, in King, *Life and Letters,* 2d ed., 2:127 [3d ed. (1858), 310]. Von Leyden dates this paper to the late 1680s when Locke was organizing chapters for the first edition of the *Essay.*
26. "Of Ethics in General," section 9, in King, *Life and Letters,* 2d ed., 2:129–130 [3d ed. (1858), 311–312].

and "the Law of *Opinion* or *Reputation*."[27] The sanctions of each kind of law can provide motives to good behavior, and in the *Essay* he calls them all "*Moral Rules,* or Laws."[28]

> Good and Evil, as hath been shewn . . . are nothing but Pleasure or Pain, or that which occasions, or procures Pleasure or Pain to us. *Morally Good and Evil* then, is only the Conformity or Disagreement of our voluntary Actions to some Law, whereby Good or Evil is drawn on us, from the Will and Power of the Law-Maker; which Good and Evil, Pleasure or Pain, attending our observance, or breach of the Law, by the Decree of the Lawmaker, is that we call *Reward* and *Punishment*.[29]

The terms "virtue" and "vice" are, he observes, applied to actions merely to mark their conformity with a particular set of mores. Nevertheless the law which God has given to man "whether promulgated to them by the light of Nature, or the Voice of Revelation" is

> the only true touchstone of *moral Rectitude*; and by comparing them to this Law, it is, that Men judge of the most considerable *Moral Good* or *Evil* of their Actions; that is, whether, as *Duties, or Sins,* they are like to procure them happiness, or misery, from the hands of the ALMIGHTY.[30]

And earlier he had distinguished natural and moral good, saying that "moral good . . . is that which produces pleasure of a particular kind, namely the pleasure with which God rewards certain acts which he considers desirable."[31]

To discover our moral obligations we must, therefore, discover the will of God, and as the words quoted above suggest, Locke is uncertain in his mind as to whether we can know our obligations by the light of reason or not.[32] Yet in the *Essay*, book IV, he insists on placing morality

> *amongst the Sciences capable of Demonstration*: wherein I doubt not, but from self-evident Propositions, by necessary Consequences, as incontestable as those in Mathematicks, the measures of right and wrong might be made out, to any one that will apply himself with the same Indifferency and Attention to the one, as he does to the other of these Sciences.[33]

27. Locke, *Essay,* II xxviii 7, p. 352.
28. Locke, *Essay,* II xxviii 6, p. 351.
29. Locke, *Essay,* II xxviii 5, p. 351.
30. Locke, *Essay,* II xxviii 8, p. 352.
31. "Of Ethics in General," section 8, in King, *Life and Letters,* 2d ed., 2:128 [3d ed. (1858), 311].
32. For discussion of this question see von Leyden, *Essays on the Law of Nature,* 51–58, and P. J. Abrams, *John Locke: Two Tracts on Government* (Cambridge: Cambridge University Press, 1967), 85–86.
33. Locke, *Essay,* IV iii 18, p. 549.

Immediately before this passage Locke had written of "the *Idea* of a supreme Being, infinite in Power, Goodness, and Wisdom, whose Workmanship we are, and on whom we depend; and the *Idea* of our selves, as understanding, rational Beings"[34] as the elements from which this demonstration might proceed. And the same kind of suggestion is made, in an amplified form, in a passage from the *Essays on the Law of Nature,* written some thirty years before the *Essay concerning Human Understanding,* and first printed in W. von Leyden's translation from the Latin, in 1954.[35]

It seems that Locke continued to believe that it would be possible to produce a demonstrative science of morality, and that he even hoped to derive moral laws such as "Love thy neighbour as thyself" from the existence of God and from human nature. But although he was asked to do so by Molyneux and others, he never did produce anything of the kind.

Molyneux wrote:

> One thing I must needs insist on to you, which is, that you would think of Obleidging the World with a Treatise of Morals, drawn up according to the Hints you frequently give in Your Essay, Of their Being Demonstrable according to the Mathematical Method.[36]

And Locke replied:

> Though by the view I had of moral ideas, whilst I was considering that subject, I thought I saw that morality might be demonstratively made out, yet whether I am able so to make it out, is another question. Everyone could not have demonstrated what Mr. Newton's book hath shewn to be demonstrable: but to shew my readiness to obey your commands, I shall not decline the first leisure I can get to employ some thoughts that way unless I find what I have said in my essay shall have stir'd up some abler man to prevent me, and effectually do that service to the world.[37]

34. Ibid.

35. "But what it is that is to be done by us can be partly gathered from the end in view for all things. For since these derive their origin from a gracious divine purpose and are the work of a most perfect and wise maker, they appear to be intended by Him for no other end than His own glory, and to this all things must be related. Partly also we can infer the principle and a definite rule of our duty from man's own constitution and the faculties with which he is equipped. For since man is neither made without design nor endowed to no purpose with these faculties which both can and must be employed, his function appears to be that which nature has prepared him to perform" (von Leyden, *Essays on the Law of Nature,* 157).

36. Letter of 27 Aug. 1692, *The Correspondence of John Locke,* ed. E. S. de Beer (Oxford: Clarendon Press, 1976), vol. 4, letter 1530.

37. Letter of 26 Sept. 1692, ibid., vol. 4, Letter 1538.

Locke's moral theory was flawed by this failure to do what he claimed could be done, and even more by his need to appeal to theology to explain moral obligation and the motivation to act morally. He himself said:

> That Men should keep their Compacts, is certainly a great and undeniable Rule in Morality: But yet, if a Christian, who has the view of Happiness and Misery in another Life, be asked why a Man must keep his Word, he will *give* this as a *Reason*: Because God, who has the Power of eternal Life and Death, requires it of us. But if an *Hobbist* be asked why; he will answer: Because the Publick requires it, and the *Leviathan* will punish you, if you do not. And if one of the old *Heathen* Philosophers had been asked, he would have answer'd: Because it was dishonest, below the Dignity of a Man, and oposite to Vertue, the highest Perfection of humane Nature, to do otherwise.[38]

Locke is, therefore, vulnerable to the criticism brought against him, or at least against doctrines such as his, by Richard Price in *A Review of the Principal Questions in Morals* first published in 1758.

Price there wrote:

> Those who say, nothing can oblige but the will of God, generally resolve the power of this to oblige to the annexed rewards and punishments. And thus, in reality, they subvert entirely the independent natures of moral good and evil; and are forced to maintain, that nothing can *oblige*, but the prospect of pleasure to be obtained, or pain to be avoided. If this be true, it follows that *vice* is, properly, no more than *imprudence*; that nothing is right or wrong, just or unjust, any farther than it affects self-interest; and that a being, independently and completely happy, cannot have any moral perceptions. . . .
>
> But to pursue this point farther; let me ask, would a person who either believes there is no God, or that he does not concern himself with human affairs, feel no *moral obligation*, and therefore not be at all *accountable*? Would one, who should happen not to be convinced, that virtue tends to his happiness here or hereafter, be released from every *bond* of duty and morality? Or would he, if he believed no future state, and that, in any instance, virtue was against his *present* interest, be truly *obliged* in these instances, to be wicked?—These consequences must follow, if obligation depends entirely on the knowledge of the will of a superior, or in the connection between actions and private interest.[39]

38. Locke, *Essay,* I iii 5, p. 68.

39. Richard Price, *A Review of the Principal Questions in Morals,* ed. D. D. Raphael (Oxford: Clarendon Press, 1974) [printed also in D. D. Raphael, *British Moralists* (Oxford: Clarendon Press, 1969), 2:162–163].

In spite of criticisms such as this, Locke's idea of a demonstration of morality received some favorable notice in the eighteenth century.[40] Nowadays, however, it seems to be generally agreed that Locke's moral theory is not of the same great interest as his political theory, or his views on such topics as substance, personal identity, and the perception of the external world. Hence, no doubt, the fact that in spite of the interest and vast influence of his political philosophy, Locke's moral philosophy is now rather little read.

By contrast, modern readers are as much concerned with Hume's moral writings as with his epistemology. His moral theory is extensively and intensively studied, and if one had to cite the foremost influence on contemporary ethics one might reasonably name David Hume. Hume's position is therefore quite different from Locke's so far as influence is concerned. Moreover they have sharply contrasting moral theories. In ethics Locke was a rationalist, claiming as we have seen that morality could be a demonstrative science on a par with mathematics. Hume stood on the other side of the great divide that came to separate moral philosophers in the eighteenth century into two schools: the adherents of reason in ethics and of moral sense.[41] He derided Wollaston's attempts to show immorality as a kind of falsehood, and argued against those who like Samuel Clarke saw moral judgment as the perception of eternal and immutable relations of fitness which the intellect could grasp.[42] In his own moral epistemology Hume insisted that morality was "more properly felt than judg'd of,"[43] and said that we could never understand the *practical* nature of morality until we saw that virtue aroused a feeling of pleasure in our minds. In his theory of the "artificial virtues" Hume developed a far more sophisticated system than did eighteenth-century "sentimentalists" such as Shaftesbury and Hutcheson, who had been content to give the sentiment of benevolence as the mainspring of moral

40. See Kenneth MacLean, *John Locke and English Literature of the Eighteenth Century* (New Haven: Yale University Press, 1936), 162 ff.

41. Bishop Butler's attempt to compromise is expressed in the sentence from his *Dissertation of the Nature of Virtue* (1726) in which he refers to "a moral faculty: whether called conscience, moral reason, moral sense, or divine reason; whether considered as a sentiment of the understanding, or a perception of the heart, or, which seems the truth, as including both." *The Works of Joseph Butler*, ed. W. E. Gladstone (Oxford: Clarendon Press, 1896), 1:399 [*Butler's Fifteen Sermons and A Dissertation*, ed. T. A. Roberts (London: S.P.C.K., 1970)].

42. William Wollaston, 1660–1724. Samuel Clarke, 1675—1729. For criticism of Wollaston, see Hume, *Treatise*, III i 1, p. 461. For his opposition to theories such as Clarke's see, especially, *Treatise*, III i 1, pp. 463–470.

43. Hume, *Treatise*, III i 2, p. 470.

action; and he insisted that the peculiarly *moral* sentiments arose only on an objective and disinterested view of "qualities useful or agreeable to ourselves or others."[44] Nevertheless, in the end, it was by feeling not thinking that we distinguished virtue and vice.[45]

Given this sharp contrast between the moral philosophies of Locke and Hume, it may seem strange to link their names as legators to modern theories of ethics. Nevertheless this is just what I meant to do.

Like his predecessor, Hume had a philosophical theory of the antecedents of action. Like Locke, he put out a general deterministic thesis, saying that men's actions were invariably caused by "their motives, temper and situation."[46] But he too went beyond such indefinite statements of determinism, which left the causes of action more or less open, and told a tale about the specific and universal antecedents of voluntary action. For Locke this invariable antecedent had been "an uneasiness." Hume rejected this idea and put forward a suggestion that gave him more room to maneuver; he said that the active element in our psychological makeup, ultimately responsible for all our intentional actions, was "passion," and this was a more compendious term than Locke's "desire."

Hume's theory of reason and the passions, with reason "perfectly inert" and the passions active, with reason the slave and passion the master, is too well known to need description here.[47] It was of course a pillar of his antirationalist, sentimentalist morality; for how, he asked, could anything as cool and detached as reason have the active tendency that so clearly belonged to morality? How could reasoning, whether about ideas or about matters of fact, give that impetus toward one *end* rather than another on which all human action must be based? The import of this theory and the connection between Hume's psychology and his ethics is easy to see, because Hume put the link between moral judgment and action at the center of his moral philosophy and made it one of his grounds for the rejection of rationalism in ethics.

> According to the principles of those who maintain an abstract rational difference betwixt moral good and evil, and a natural fitness and unfitness of things, 'tis not only suppos'd, that these relations, being eternal and

44. Anthony Ashley Cooper, third Earl of Shaftesbury, 1671–1713. Francis Hutcheson, 1694–1746.

45. See Hume, *Treatise,* iii i 2, passim, and *An Enquiry concerning the Principles of Morals,* 1751, Appendix I, "Concerning Moral Sentiment."

46. Hume, *Treatise,* II iii 1, p. 404.

47. See, especially, Hume, *Treatise,* II iii 3, pp. 413–418; and III i 1, pp. 457–459.

> immutable, are the same, when consider'd by every rational creature, but their *effects* are also suppos'd to be necessarily the same; and 'tis concluded they have no less, or rather a greater, influence in directing the will of the deity, than in governing the rational and virtuous of our own species. These two particulars are evidently distinct. 'Tis one thing to know virtue, and another to conform the will to it. In order, therefore, to prove, that the measures of right and wrong are eternal laws, *obligatory* on every rational mind, 'tis not sufficient to shew the relations upon which they are founded: We must also point out the connexion betwixt the relation and the will; and must prove that this connexion is so necessary, that in every well-disposed mind, it must take place and have its influence; tho' the difference betwixt these minds be in other respects immense and infinite.[48]

Hume's theory of action itself is, however, complex and in places even its outline is blurred. What did he mean by a "passion"? What was the relation between passion and desire? What part, if any, did pleasure and pain play in the determination of volition? Was Hume, like Locke, a psychological hedonist? How did he think that men were motivated when they acted morally?

Some of these questions can be answered with confidence. For Hume a passion may either be an "aversion or propensity," in which case it is itself a desire, and a motive to action, or it may be some other "sentiment" or "emotion" or "feeling" such as love or hatred or pride. The second kind of passion can cause action, by a process which Hume describes at great length; but as critics have noted Hume does not think that particular desires are involved in the idea of, for instance, love and hate.[49] Moreover there are some passions, such as hope, that have no special connection with action. It is the two passions of aversion and propensity that are the universal determinants of action.

Beyond characterizing desire in terms of propensity and aversion, Hume does not tell us what kind of experience desiring is, and it would of course have been against his principles to attempt to convey by description the content of the simple impression we receive by introspection and can know only through this experience. But it is clear that all connotation of tempestuousness has gone from the word "passion" as Hume uses it, particularly when he is thinking about desire. As is well known, he even goes so far as to speak of "certain calm desires and tendencies, which, tho' they be real passions, produce little emotion in the

48. Hume, *Treatise,* III i 1, p. 465.

49. See Patrick Gardiner, "Hume's Theory of the Passions," in *David Hume,* ed. David Pears (London: Macmillan, 1963), and Pall S. Árdal, *Passion and Value in Hume's Treatise* (Edinburgh: Edinburgh University Press, 1966), chap. 3.

mind," and are "more known by their effects than by the immediate feeling or sensation," giving as examples "benevolence and resentment, the love of life, and kindness to children."[50] The idea that some desires may be known by their effects rather than by a state of mind revealed to introspection is, clearly, a point on which Hume differs from Locke, and we shall have occasion to say more about this later on.

So far Hume's doctrine is fairly clear; but interpretation is more difficult when we try to say how he conceived the connection between propensity and aversion on the one hand and pleasure and pain on the other.[51] It is a much-debated question whether Hume was some kind of psychological hedonist or not.[52] What is certain is that he did not think that all action was self-interested. He disapproved of Hobbes and Locke for their "selfish system of morals,"[53] and he asks in the final paragraph of the essay on self-love which forms Appendix II to the *Enquiry concerning the Principles of Morals* why there should be difficulty in conceiving that

> from the original frame of our temper, we may feel a desire of another's happiness or good, which, by means of that affection, becomes our own good, and is afterwards pursued, from the combined motives of benevolence and self-enjoyment.[54]

Thus Hume denies that everything we do is actuated by self-interest. But nor did Locke think that—if self-interest is to mean the pursuit of perceived maximum advantage to oneself. We earlier described Locke as a psychological hedonist because he thought that every agent sought some pleasure for himself, or to avoid some pain, in whatever he did. And Hume certainly speaks at times as if he believed this too. Nevertheless there is a passage in the *Treatise* in which Hume explicitly disavows any form of psychological hedonism, saying that

> [b]eside good and evil, or in other words, pain and pleasure, the direct passions frequently arise from a natural impulse or instinct, which is perfectly unaccountable.[55]

50. Hume, *Treatise,* II iii 3, p. 417. As Árdal points out (*Passion and Value,* 94), a calm passion is one so experienced on most, not necessarily all, occasions.

51. Hume talks more about pleasure, whereas Locke is driven by his theory of the nature of desire to place the emphasis on pain.

52. See Árdal, *Passion and Value,* 69–79.

53. Hume, *Enquiry concerning the Principles of Morals,* Appendix II, ed. L. A. Selby-Bigge, 2d ed. (Oxford: Clarendon Press, 1902), 296.

54. Ibid., 302.

55. Hume, *Treatise,* II iii 9, p. 439.

Moreover, as Páll Árdal has stressed, even when pleasure or pain is thought by Hume to be involved in the causal explanation of a desire, pleasure or pain need not be the end the agent wants to attain.[56]

Hume was not, we should conclude, a psychological hedonist. Nevertheless pleasure and pain come in at a critical point in his moral philosophy. For it is clear that he believed himself to have solved the problem of linking moral judgment to the will, by insisting that the perception of virtue consisted of a *pleasant* sentiment or feeling.

> Nothing can be more real, or concern us more, than our own sentiments of pleasure and uneasiness; and if these be favourable to virtue, and unfavourable to vice, no more can be requisite to the regulation of our conduct and behaviour.[57]

Even here, however, it seems most unlikely that what Hume meant was that we are motivated to act virtuously by the wish to obtain pleasure from the contemplation of our own virtuous acts. Hutcheson, who was one of the chief influences on Hume's moral thinking, had argued against philosophers who tried to reduce morality to self-interest by supposing that we have "a secret sense of pleasure arising from reflection upon such of our own actions as we call virtuous, even when we expect no other advantage from them" and that we are motivated to act virtuously "to obtain this pleasure which arises from reflection upon the action." [58]

The question of how Hume did understand the role of pleasure and pain in moral motivation has not so far as I know been satisfactorily answered, and commentators seem oddly incurious about the matter. Hume seemed to assume that what was thought of *with* pleasure tended to be pursued, and perhaps this is a correct idea. It has appeared, though in a curious form, in our own century in the philosophy of G. E. Moore, but has not to my knowledge lately received the attention it deserves.[59]

I hope that I have by now said enough to show in outline what Locke believed, and what Hume believed, about the antecedents of voluntary

56. Árdal, *Passion and Value,* chap. 3, and especially p. 73.

57. Hume, *Treatise,* II i 1, p. 469.

58. Francis Hutcheson, *An Inquiry into the Original of our Ideas of Beauty and Virtue* (1725), 4th ed. (Glasgow, 1738; new printing, 1772), 96. Printed also in D. D. Raphael, *British Moralists,* vol. 2, sec. 305.

59. G. E. Moore, *Principia Ethica* (Cambridge: Cambridge University Press, 1903), chap. 2, sec. 27, p. 42. We should, perhaps, think again, in the light of Wittgenstein's later philosophy, about expressions such as "How good it would be to do such and such."

action. I have tried to show how they differed both in these theories of action and in their moral philosophy; and it is now time to change to the other tack. For the thesis of this paper is that there is a common mistake in their philosophies of action. I want to show that neither of them could give a proper account, within their own theories, of the part which *reason* plays in determining human choice.

The subject of reason and action, which I have just introduced into this discussion, is nothing grand or recondite. I am simply referring to the familiar fact that human beings often do do what they do because it seems the *reasonable* thing to do. Sometimes a process of reasoning is involved, as when we decide "I should do such and such," or say "So I'll do such and such" as the conclusion of one of these bits of practical reasoning. Like speculative reasoning (ordinary nonpractical reasoning by deduction or induction) this kind of practical reasoning has premises and conclusions. In other cases, however, we act *on* a reason or *for* a reason, without having been through any reasoning. Practical reasoning is then in the background, in that it may be appealed to if an argument is required.

My charge against Locke, and against Hume, is that the *type* of explanation of action which is their stock-in-trade cannot accommodate actions done for a reason. I want to say that they cannot give a true account of prudential action, when we act in a certain way for reasons connected with our own future happiness. Nor can they correctly describe even the most common cause of doing something because it is thought that that will be the cause or enabling condition of our getting something that we already want.

Let us first consider prudential action, and think again about Locke's account of the case where someone renounces present pleasure to avoid later distress. What Locke says, and must in consistency say, is that we will act prudently only if an "uneasiness" arises at the thought of the future evil or loss which present indulgence will bring. Thus we act as reason bids us only if we *find ourselves* with the relevant desire. We have as it were to *wait and see* whether the thought of the future does or does not have the *effect* of arousing the uneasiness in us. And even though Locke thinks that we have the power to suspend action and again contemplate the future, this is only to say that we can if we like give the desire *more time to appear.*

To see how little this kind of theory can accommodate reason-based action, and how strange it really is, we have only to observe that it must allow as a possibility that someone who is told that he *should* do something, like giving up drinking, on prudential grounds, might reply that he felt no uneasiness at the thought of his future suffering and therefore could not be expected to do what we advised; as if the necessary mental mechanism was not in place. And if this does not seem strange enough, it should be remarked that the same response would be possible in the other case originally mentioned as one in which reason determines action. For why should it not be given where the reason for action is of the means-end or instrumental kind, related to a present felt desire? For example, suppose that someone had a headache (and so far as that goes, an uneasiness and a Lockean desire to get rid of it) but when told that an aspirin would relieve his condition he waited to see whether he wanted an aspirin. "You should take an aspirin," we say to him, but although he does believe that that would cure the headache he says that unfortunately he finds in himself no desire to do the thing.[60] What really happens is just that he says to himself something like "My headache is awful. An aspirin would do the trick. So I need to go upstairs to get one," *and goes.* In other words, a piece of practical reasoning leads to action. Or perhaps he just goes upstairs without *reasoning,* but could give the desire to get rid of the headache as the *reason why* he went. In neither case do we think of inventing a special desire directed toward going upstairs as an antecedent of the journey. It is enough that reason tells the agent to go. And the question is why in the other type of case we are inclined, with Locke, to invoke a desire for our future good when we obey the dictate of reason which tells us not to drink.

What is at issue here is the supposed requirement for a certain kind of story about how all action comes about. And it is easy to see that on this point Hume and Locke are in agreement, in spite of the differences in the exact story that they tell. Where Locke puts in uneasiness, Hume puts in "passion" as the necessary antecedent of action, so that it is in terms of passions that he will have to explain how men act (as we say) for a reason in curbing their immediate impulses on prudential grounds. Notoriously, Hume himself even denies that prudential action has any special connection with rationality. "'Tis not contrary to reason," he says, "to prefer even my own acknowledg'd lesser good to my greater."[61] The desire for our own good is just one "passion" among others, and its operation is mistaken for the working of reason only because, like reason, it is "calm" and makes very little disturbance in the mind. So much for

60. It would, of course, be quite wrong to say that if the desire did not materialize, the agent would conclude that he did not want to get rid of the headache after all. It is not a question of desires materializing, but of acting on reasons.

61. Hume, *Treatise,* II iii 3, p. 416.

Hume's account of the first "prudential" example, described above (and rightly described) as one case of the determination of action by reason.

Turning now to the other example, where the practical reasoning or the reason for acting was of the instrumental or means-end kind, one finds Hume much more aware of the problem of fitting this into the general theory than Locke had been.

> 'Tis obvious, that when we have the prospect of pain or pleasure from any object, we feel a consequent emotion of aversion or propensity, and are carry'd to avoid or embrace what will give us this uneasiness or satisfaction. 'Tis also obvious, that this emotion rests not here, but making us cast our view on every side, comprehends whatever objects are connected with its original one by the relation of cause and effect. Here then reasoning takes place to discover this relation; and according as our reasoning varies, our actions receive a subsequent variation. But 'tis evident in this case, that the impulse arises not from reason, but is only directed by it.[62]

Hume sees that he needs something to be the dynamic antecedent of the action (in our example, the action of going upstairs) and says that it is the original passion which is at work, having spread itself, by an association of ideas traveling along the relation of cause and effect, to the thing that is to be done. And his use of the word "directed" suggests the image of a force, like a spring of water, or the movement of a body, which is guided in a particular direction.

Now there is something right in this case about his insistence on the relevance of the "original emotion," to the action taken, because *in this kind of case* what we are talking about is the rationality of taking means to something desired. But I suggest that he is wrong in thinking that a story was needed about *how* the desire for the end energizes the agent to adopt the means. Instrumental reasoning to the fulfillment of a desire is one of the forms of practical reasoning; and that is all that needs to be said about how the action comes about. If physiologists or psychologists have some story to tell about causality *on experimental grounds* that is, of course, a different matter. But it is not because we know anything of this kind that we are tempted by the kind of theory of action given by Locke and Hume.

That we are tempted by this kind of theory—that modern philosophers often make the same mistake that I have tried to identify in Locke and Hume—is a main thesis of this paper. But at this point I can imagine that protests will go up. Surely, it will be said, we are *not* nowadays in-

62. Hume, *Treatise,* II iii 3, p. 414.

clined to accept that part of the philosophical psychology of the late seventeenth and early eighteenth centuries which has to do with the determination of action by desire. Indeed, it may be thought that we accept very little of it, particularly now that Wittgenstein has taught us to see as problematic the idea of contents of the mind known to each person only by his own introspection.[63] It is true that contemporary philosophy of mind is radically different from that of Locke and Hume.[63] Nevertheless, with a few notable exceptions, contemporary philosophers share the assumption which I have pointed out as being common to Locke and Hume. To be sure, it is usual now to think of desires as dispositions rather than as introspectible contents in the mind, and they are therefore treated as underlying conditions rather than things that occur in the mind immediately before volition. But as we noticed earlier, Hume thought that some of his calm passions might be "more known by their effects than by the immediate feeling or sensation." The point to be stressed is that even if Hume had thought of desires as underlying dispositions, this would not have saved him from the mistake which I am claiming to find in Locke, Hume, *and* most present-day philosophers. For an account of how reason affects action which is in terms of underlying dispositions is still a causal account. Given a dispositional theory of desire, someone who was told to stop drinking for the sake of his health could still say that he did not *find* in himself the desire for health, now conceived as an underlying condition, a disposition to seek his own good.[64]

My point is that where practical reason is concerned no such causal story is needed to show how action comes about. Practical reasoning, with its counterpart in the giving of reasons for choosing one course of action rather than another, is a kind of operation on a par with speculative reasoning. And it is as odd to ask for a causal account of one as of the other. When someone says that Socrates is mortal on the ground that all men are mortal and Socrates a man, philosophers do not invent a causal story about how his belief comes about. Few would suppose, in the case of speculative reasoning (whether deductive or inductive), that after asserting the premises the reasoner *finds himself* with a belief in the

63. See n. 2 above. As far as I know, Wittgenstein never refers to Locke, but in his later philosophy he often attacks a theory of language, as well as certain propositions in the theory of mind, which are almost exactly those which Locke, in particular, put forward.

64. Barry Stroud and others seem to me to be mistaken in thinking that Hume's account of desire can be radically improved by replacing it with a dispositional theory. See Barry Stroud, *Hume* (London and Boston: Routledge and Kegan Paul, 1977), 167–169.

conclusion, as if by a causal mechanism which he might always discover not to have worked. What I am pointing out is that it would be just as strange, in the case where action is in question, for someone to say that unfortunately he did not have the desire which would lead him to act in accordance with reason. One may of course bemoan the fact that what reason tells us to do (like morning exercises) has so little appeal on its own, and one might try to increase its appeal by some means or other. But this is not the ordinary way that practical reasoning works; on the contrary, it is an expedient adopted as a substitute for practical reason.

What the foregoing pages have shown is that Locke and Hume, however much they differed in detail, both gave an account of the genesis of voluntary action which is questionable. For both of them tried to find a type of antecedent which invariably preceded volition; and the argument of the last few paragraphs has suggested that this was a mistake that made it impossible for either of them to take proper account of one most important type of human activity, namely acting on a reason. Looked at from this point of view the differences between the two philosophers' theories of action seem slight, while their common presupposition leaps to the eye. Moreover, the implications of this seventeenth- and eighteenth-century empiricist philosophy are very important indeed. It is no exaggeration to see here one of the chief influences on the subjectivist, emotivist, and prescriptivist moral philosophies of our own time, and one of the long-term aims of the present inquiry is to oppose such theories by striking at their roots.[65]

To try to give some idea of the shift of perspective that would be involved in giving up the Lockean and Humean point of view, one should remark first of all that what is at issue is the possibility of a certain kind of explanation of human action. If Locke and Hume were right, the explanation of every action would involve an antecedent event or

65. C. L. Stevenson's *Ethics and Language* (New Haven: Yale University Press, 1944) is the book that most explicitly expresses this kind of ethical system; but it is arguable that most moral philosophers in the analytic school are still deeply influenced by such ideas. G. E. M. Anscombe is a notable exception, as well as Paul Grice and John McDowell. See G. E. M. Anscombe, *Ethics, Religion and Politics: Collected Philosophical Papers,* vol. 3 (Minneapolis: University of Minnesota Press, 1981); idem, *Intention* (Oxford: B. Blackwell, 1957; 2d ed., Ithaca, N.Y.: Cornell University Press, 1963); P. H. Grice, "Reply to Richards," in *Philosophical Grounds of Rationality: Intentions, Categories, Ends,* ed. R. Grandy and R. Warner (Oxford: Clarendon Press, 1986); J. McDowell, "Are Moral Requirements Hypothetical Imperatives?" *Proceedings of the Aristotelian Society Supplementary Volume* 52 (1978): 13–30; J. McDowell, "Virtue and Reason," *The Monist* 62 (1979): 331–350. There is also some pioneering work on the subject of action and desire in Thomas Nagel, *The Possibility of Altruism* (Oxford: Clarendon Press, 1970), chap. 5.

condition such as Locke's *uneasiness* or Hume's *aversion or propensity*. If they are wrong, there is no need to search for any such feature of every situation in which voluntary action takes place; though of course such things can be taken into account wherever they really are found. Someone may do something because he is hungry, because he finds a certain course of action attractive, or because he simply wants to do that thing. He may, however, do it because he has some reason to do it: it is a necessary step to something that he now desires; he realizes that he will be in for trouble later if he does not do it; someone has given him an order; the action falls under a rule. These are explanations of his action, and in spite of the possibility of rationalization (in the everyday sense of unconsciously inventing reasons) we should say that what he gives is normally the correct explanation of why he does what he does. That is to say that the explanation is in terms of reasons, and any suggestion that a different account must be given is a philosopher's prejudice. People operate with practical reason as they operate with speculative reason. It is as wrong to invent a parallel process involving psychological causes in one case as in the other.

It is easy to see how moral theory is affected by these considerations about the explanation of action by reasons. For Hume's challenge, which dominated his account of the perception of virtue and vice, has come also to dominate our own thoughts about moral judgment. Hume had insisted, as in the famous passage placed as the motto at the head of this paper, that morality was practical, serving to produce action, and must be shown as such. Modern theories of moral judgment tend to take this challenge very seriously, and to meet it by fixing on some determinant of action, such as feeling or attitude, whose presence is taken to be a condition of the correct use of moral language; thus introducing a subjective element into the account. On the principles suggested in the present paper there is, by contrast, no need to look for any such thing. No such element need come into the explanation of action as motivated by the thought of reasons. And the way is open for a simpler account of the necessarily practical character of morals. For undoubtedly those who have successfully been taught morality see moral considerations as reasons for action. We do not have to look for something special in the way of "moral motivation" to see how it can be that they do things, on many occasions, because morality so dictates.

Nor is it hard to see on these principles that morality is *necessarily* practical; which is to say not that people always act morally (which of course they do not) but rather that there is a conceptual link between morality and action. To show just how this is true is a more complex matter, and it is no doubt hard to get it quite right. Perhaps it is enough here to suggest that a moral system necessarily involves some kind of rules, and to point out that a rule belongs to our armory of *practical* linguistic devices. If someone should insist that it is not necessarily *rational* to obey any and every rule, this observation should be welcomed and not taken as any objection to what has been said. For what I have been trying to do is not to produce some kind of justification of morality—of the making and keeping of moral rules—as a rational human enterprise, in contradistinction to the invention of duelling rules or the more byzantine varieties of etiquette. Nor have I tried to show that someone who acts for a moral reason acts for a *good* reason. What has been in question is rather a clear view of the way in which morality motivates action, and above all a rejection of the kind of story which, in consistency with their own philosophy of mind, Locke and Hume had to tell.

PART TWO

Mind and Body in Practice: Physiology, Literature, Medicine

FOUR

Thomas Willis and His Circle: Brain and Mind in Seventeenth-Century Medicine

Robert G. Frank, Jr.

In the autumn of 1663, a middle-aged, and now moderately successful, Oxford physician took up his pen to write an "Amico Lectori Praefatio." He wanted to explain to his prospective readers how he had occupied his two years past, and how he had come to write the more than 450 quarto pages of *Cerebri anatome* that followed. Academic responsibilities and a disillusionment with his own speculativeness had led him to publication. His position as Sedleian Professor of Natural Philosophy demanded that he lecture twice a week on, as he put it, "the Offices of the Senses, both external and also internal, and of the Faculties and Affections of the Soul, as also of the Organs and various provisions of all these." He had, he said, thought of "some rational Arguments for that purpose, and from the appearances raised some not unlikely Hypotheses, which (as uses to be in these kinds of businesses) at length accrued into a certain System of Art and frame of Doctrine." Yet "when at last the force of Invention [had been] spent," the lecturer reconsidered these things seriously, and "I awaked at length sad, as one out of a pleasant dream." He realized that "I had drawn out for my self and auditors a certain Poetical Philosophy and Physick."[1]

Indeed, if this Clark Library series promises to show us anything, it

1. Thomas Willis, *Cerebri anatome: Cui accessit nervorum descriptio et usus* (London, 1664), sig. a1v. This and all subsequent citations to the *Cerebri anatome* are to the quarto edition of 1664, not to the octavo printing in the same year. Quotations in English are based upon the translation by Samuel Pordage, "Of the anatomy of the brain" [separately paginated], in Thomas Willis, *Practice of physick* (London, 1681), 53. In all cases the English translation has been checked against the Latin original, since there are occasional discrepancies.

is that problems of "mind and body" have exercised the "force of Invention" of numerous thinkers in the Enlightenment, and that "rational Arguments" derived from "appearances" do most certainly "accrue" into systems of "Doctrine."

Yet our physician, Thomas Willis, felt that there was a way out of this dilemma. The contemplation of the mind and its faculties need not lead invariably to "Poetical Philosophy." He felt that he himself had entered upon a "new course," independent both of the "Received opinions of others," and of the "guesses" of his own mind. He would believe only "Nature and ocular demonstrations."

> Therefore thenceforward I betook my self wholly to the study of Anatomy: and as I did chiefly inquire into the offices and uses of the Brain and its nervous Appendix, I addicted my self to the opening of Heads especially, and of every kind, and to inspect as much as I was able frequently and seriously the Contents; that after the figures, sites, processes of the whole and singular parts should be considered with their other bodies, respects, and habits, some truth might at length be drawn forth concerning the exercise, defects, and irregularities of the Animal Government; and so a firm and stable Basis might be laid, on which not only a more certain Physiologie than I had gained in the Schools, but what I had long thought upon, the Pathologie of the Brain and nervous stock, might be built.[2]

This was a bold enterprise indeed: to believe that systematic anatomy of the brain, especially of the comparative sort, would lead to discovering patterns of function and dysfunction, and that these in turn would illuminate the cluster of subjects that launched Willis in the first place—the nature of senses and the faculties of the soul.

Yet it turned out to be an enterprise that, in the eyes of Willis's contemporaries and successors, was both highly productive and very successful. *Cerebri anatome* (1664) was just the first of Willis's books on the nervous system and its attributes. Following soon thereafter was the *Pathologiae cerebri* (1667),[3] then a defense of his views on the neural origins of hysteria and hypochondria (1670),[4] and *De anima brutorum*

2. Willis, *Cerebri anatome,* sig. a2r; "Anatomy of the brain," 53.

3. Thomas Willis, *Pathologiae cerebri, et nervosi generis specimen: In quo agitur de morbis convulsis, et de scorbuto* (Oxford, 1667); translation by Pordage as "An essay of the pathology of the brain and nervous Stock: In which convulsive diseases are treated of," in Willis, *Practice of physick* [separately paginated].

4. Thomas Willis, *Affectionum quae dicuntur hystericae & hypochondriacae pathologia spasmodica vindicata, contra responsionem epistolarem Nathanael Highmore, M.D.: Cui accesserunt exercitationes medico-physicae duae. 1. De sanguinis accensione. 2. De motu musculari* (London,

(1672).[5] These more than 1,400 quarto pages all arose explicitly out of his work at Oxford. The neurological works were embedded in, and made up the largest part of, an oeuvre that occupied an honored place in late-seventeenth- and eighteenth-century medicine. Willis's individual treatises went through numerous editions in his own lifetime. His works were rapidly translated into English in the 1680s, and his *Opera omnia* went through eleven editions between 1676 and 1720.[6] They continued to be highly influential through the 1770s, and in the 1820s the neuro-anatomist Karl Friedrich Burdach had many good things to say about Willis's work on the brain.[7] In the twentieth century, even after his investigations have ceased to have an active scientific influence, Willis is still widely known among neuroscientists, and he attracts a steady stream of biographers and commentators.[8] Certainly then, in any discussion of "mind and body" in the Enlightenment, Willis should command our attention.

Here I wish to examine, not effects, but origins. How is a highly im-

1670). The response to Highmore has not been translated; the other two tracts appear as "Of the accension of the blood" and "Of musculary motion" in Willis, *Practice of physick* [separately paginated].

5. Thomas Willis, *De anima brutorum quae hominis vitalis ac sensitiva est, exercitationes duae. Prior physiologica ejusdem naturam, partes, potentes & affectiones tradit. Altera pathologica morbos qui ipsam, & sedem ejus primarium, nempe cerebrum & nervosum genus afficiunt, explicat, eorumque therapeias instituit* (Oxford, 1672); the Pordage translation is Thomas Willis, *Two discourses concerning the soul of brutes, which is that of the vital and sensitive of man. The first is physiological, shewing the nature, parts, powers, and affections of the same. The other is pathological, which unfolds the diseases which affect it and its primary seat; To wit, the brain and nervous stock, and treats of the cures* (London, 1683).

6. Consider for a moment the numbers and distribution of Willis's individual writings: *Diatribae duae,* fifteen editions in the period 1659–1687, published at London, Amsterdam, Geneva, Paris, The Hague, and Middelburgh; *Cerebri anatome,* eight editions in 1664–1683, published at London, Amsterdam, and Geneva; *Pathologiae cerebri,* eight editions in 1667–1684, published at Oxford, London, Amsterdam, and Geneva; *Affectionum,* four editions in 1670–1678, published at London, Leiden, and Geneva; *De anima brutorum,* eight editions in 1672–1683, published at Oxford, London, Amsterdam, Lyon, and Cologne; *Pharmaceutice rationalis,* parts I and II, eleven editions in 1674–1680, published at Oxford, London, Amsterdam, The Hague, Lyon, Geneva, and Cologne. After Willis's death the most common way of bringing out his writings was as an *Opera omnia* or an edition abridged from it, either in Latin or in English; between 1676 and 1720 there were sixteen such editions, published at London, Geneva, Lyon, Amsterdam, Cologne, and Venice.

7. Cf. the praise for Willis in Antoine Portal, *Histoire de l'anatomie et de la chirurgie* (Paris, 1770–1773), 3:86–105, and A. Meyer, "Karl Friedrich Burdach on Thomas Willis," *Journal of the Neurological Sciences* 3 (1966): 109–116.

8. Since the 1920s, articles on Willis have appeared at the rate of about four to eight per decade; the exception is the 1960s, in which thirty-three articles and books on Willis were published, many of them prompted by the tricentennial of *Cerebri anatome.*

portant set of results and ideas created? Specifically, how does one work on the problem of brain and mind in the context of seventeenth-century medicine and culture? I use the phrase "work on" quite deliberately, because my primary focus is the process of creation, not the results.

I would like to explore this creative process by asking three interrelated sets of *how* questions. How biographically? What is the trajectory of a man's life that brings him to a point of creativity, and what is the constitution and integration of the elements of that life such that he creates a product in a unique way? How operationally? What are the social and scientific circumstances under which the work is carried out, and how do these circumstances relate to the essential nature of the product? How intellectually? In what ways does a scientist approach his subject, and deal with it, so as to produce new ideas and results? Since the object of Willis's inquiry was the brain and nervous system, neuroanatomy necessarily enters into the discussion; but its entry is subservient to my larger aim of showing Willis and his circle at work. I am not concerned here with a complete description of Willis's neuroanatomy and neurophysiology. Nor do I wish to judge in what ways his work anticipates, or fails to anticipate, the concepts of the twentieth-century neurosciences. I ask, rather, how one constructs a system of brain and mind, three hundred years ago, in the absence of what we flatter ourselves by calling the necessary tools and insights of modern science.

WILLIS'S PATH TO THE BRAIN

Willis is in many ways very apt for such purposes of exemplification. He was no great genius. Rather, he was an ordinary man in extraordinary times. He lived through a revolution and a reaction. His life straddled the transition between late-Renaissance and early-Enlightenment England, and he lived it successfully in two contrasting spheres of academic reclusion and worldly bustle.

Willis was born in 1621 near Oxford, and stayed in the shadow of its spires for almost half a century, moving to London only in 1667, where he died in 1675.[9] In his early life he was surrounded by the traditional

9. To date, the only full-length biography is Hansruedi Isler, *Thomas Willis: Ein Wegbereiter der modernen Medizin, 1621–1675* (Stuttgart: Wissenschaftliche Verlagsgesellschaft, 1965); this was translated, with additions, by Isler, *Thomas Willis, 1621–1675: Doctor and Scientist* (New York: Hafner, 1968). The late Kenneth Dewhurst has been the scholar most active in writing about Willis over the past two decades. Much biographical material is contained in the long introductions to his editions of Willis manuscript material: *Thomas Willis's Oxford Lectures* (Oxford: Sandford, 1980), 1–49; *Willis's Oxford Casebook (1650–52)*

verities of crown and church; then, when King confronted Parliament, the world was, in Christopher Hill's phrase, turned upside down. Like many, he fought for the Royalist cause between 1643 and 1646, maintained a secret opposition through the Commonwealth period, and was elated at the Restoration. Nor did Willis possess unusual qualities of personal magnetism. He was merely honest in speech and conservative in mentality. With typical earthiness, John Aubrey tells us that Willis was of "middle stature: darke red haire (like a red pig)," and "stammered much."[10] Antony Wood called him simply "a plain man, a man of no carriage, little discourse, complaisance, or society."[11] What was there about his life that brought him to the enterprise of grounding mental phenomena in neural tissue? His biography, which has been reasonably well explored, contains scattered bits of evidence that bear upon the origins of his neurological work.

Willis was first and last a clinician. He began practicing medicine at Oxford about age 24, and continued his profession daily until the week of his early death at age 54. The greater part of his first book in 1659 applied ideas of fermentation to explain fevers,[12] and his last, the *Pharmaceutice rationalis* of 1674, was an omnium-gatherum of his clinical judgments and prescriptions.[13] He was a successful practitioner, but this came only slowly. As a young doctor in the late 1640s he hustled for pa-

(Oxford: Sandford, 1981), 1–59. A useful synoptic view of Willis's life and scientfic ideas is Robert G. Frank, Jr., "Thomas Willis," in *Dictionary of Scientific Biography* (New York: Charles Scribner's Sons, 1970–), 14: 404–409.

10. *"Brief Lives," Chiefly of Contemporaries, Set Down by John Aubrey, between the Years 1669 & 1696,* ed. Andrew Clark (Oxford: Clarendon Press, 1898), 2: 303.

11. Anthony Wood, *Athenae Oxonienses: An Exact History of All the Writers and Bishops Who Have Had Their Education in the University of Oxford,* new ed., ed. Philip Bliss (London: Rivington, 1813–1820), vol. 3, col. 1051.

12. Thomas Willis, *Diatribae duae medico-philosophicae, quarum prior agit de fermentatione sive de motu intestino particularum in quovis corpore; altera de febribus, sive de motu earundum in sanguine animalium. His ascessit dissertatio epistolica de urinis* (London, 1659). The three treatises are paginated separately, so I shall refer to them as *De fermentatione, De febribus,* and *De urinis.* All were translated by Pordage as "Of fermentation," "Of feavers," and "Of urines" [separately paginated], in Willis, *Practice of physick.* In this, as in other works of Willis for which more than one edition was published in Willis's lifetime, one must exercise caution in using the Pordage translation; it sometimes contains intercalated sentences, paragraphs, or even sections that are not found in the first edition.

13. Thomas Willis, *Pharmaceutice rationalis. Sive diatriba de medicamentorum operationibus in humano corpore [Pars I]* (Oxford, 1674); translation by Pordage as "Pharmaceutice rationalis, Part I," in Willis, *Practice of physick.* Thomas Willis, *Pharmaceutice rationalis . . . Pars secunda* (Oxford, 1675); translation by Pordage as "Pharmaceutice rationalis, Part II," in Willis, *Practice of physick.*

tients on market days in neighboring towns, and a clinical notebook kept in 1650 shows a practice that was certainly not booming.[14] But by 1657 he had acquired enough skill, patients, and financial security to marry, and the Restoration set his career firmly on the upward path. By the early 1660s he was buying properties in Oxford, and just before his departure from there he had the highest income in the town.[15] The move to London brought more success and, as Wood noted, "in very short time after he became so noted, and so infinitely resorted to, for his practice, that never any physician before went beyond him, or got more money yearly than he."[16]

But Willis was successful in more than simply monetary terms. He was a remarkable clinical observer. His characterizations of epidemics were particularly acute; he reported in detail the first English outbreak of war typhus among the Oxford troops in 1643, cases of plague in 1645, measles and smallpox in 1649 and 1654, and influenza in 1657. He also recorded what seems to be the first reliable clinical description of typhoid fever. For a variety of other clinical descriptions, his works contain in each case the *locus classicus*: myasthenia gravis; the distinction between acute tuberculosis and the chronic fibroid type; the first clinical and pathological description of emphysema; extrasystoles of the heart; aortic stenosis; heart failure in chronic bronchitis; emboli lodged in the pulmonary artery; the first European to note the sweet taste of the urine in diabetes mellitus.[17] Overall, he was a moderate in therapy[18] and seems—at least as reflected by his writings—to have had no great knowledge of Galen or Hippocrates. Throughout his life, his abiding interest was his patients, not learned medicine.

In addition to being an acute but conservative physician, he was also

14. Aubrey, *"Brief Lives"* 2: 303. Cf. Dewhurst, *Willis's Oxford Casebook,* where Willis notes seeing only forty-six separate patients in 1650; many, however, were seen more than once, and it seems most likely that Willis did not record all of his cases.

15. On Willis's growing wealth and acquisition of properties, see Dewhurst, *Willis's Oxford Lectures,* 9–12, 14–18, 20–26; *Willis's Oxford Casebook,* 41–42, 55–56.

16. Wood, *Athenae,* vol. 3, col. 1051.

17. See, for example, the selections from Willis's writings in Ralph H. Major, *Classic Descriptions of Disease* (Springfield, Ill.: Charles C. Thomas, 1932), 121–124, 133–136, 192–194, 534–536, 541–545, 591–593. A good overview of Willis's clinical accomplishments is R. Hierons, "Willis's Contributions to Clinical Medicine and Neurology," *Journal of the Neurological Sciences* 4 (1967); 1–13.

18. Willis's practice, as it appeared to his contemporaries, is reflected in the diary-like commonplace books of his younger Oxford contemporary, John Ward; see Robert G. Frank, Jr., "The John Ward Diaries: Mirror of Seventeenth-Century Science and Medicine," *Journal of the History of Medicine and Allied Sciences* 29 (1974): 147–179.

a staunch churchman. He seems originally to have been destined for holy orders, but the Civil War derailed his clerical career. He maintained his strong Anglicanism throughout the interregnum, and his residences at Oxford, both when he lived in Christ Church and in Beam Hall, were used regularly for sub-rosa worship. His friends during this period included John Fell (whose sister he married), Gilbert Sheldon, John Dolben, and Richard Allestree; after the Restoration these four became, respectively, the Bishop of Oxford, the Archbishop of Canterbury, the Archbishop of York, and the Regius Professor of Divinity as well as the Provost of Eton.[19] Willis was especially close to Fell and Allestree; not only did Richard Allestree take a course in chemistry from Willis, but his brother James, the printer, brought out Willis's first four books.[20]

Willis's religion, although not at all theological, was more than merely a matter of friends and politics. He gave to the poor all the fees he earned on Sundays. He went to church daily, and when he found that his London practice precluded midday worship, he paid a priest at St. Martin's in the Fields to read prayers early and late, for such as he, who could not otherwise attend. Characteristically, he endowed this position in his will. As Wood said, he "left behind him the character of an orthodox, pious, and charitable physician."[21]

This orthodoxy squared with his early philosophical education. He had matriculated at Oxford in the boom years of the mid-1630s, proceeding to the B.A. in 1639, and to the M.A. in 1642.[22] At that time the colleges were throwing up new buildings with abandon to accommodate the thousands who, largely for social reasons, wanted a traditional uni-

19. Wood, *Athenae,* vol. 3, cols. 1049–1050; Anthony Wood, *The History and Antiquities of the University of Oxford,* ed. and trans. John Gutch (Oxford: For the editor, 1796), 2: 613; Cf. the brief obituary by John Fell which was appended to the *Pharmaceutice rationalis . . . Pars secunda,* sig. b3v-b4r; "Pharmaceutice rationalis, Part II," sig. A2v-A3r.

20. Richard Allestree was reputed to be the author of *The causes of the decay of Christian piety* (London, 1668), and on the copy in the Bodleian Library is the anonymous note that "Dr. Allestree was author of this book, and wrote it in the very same year wherein he went thro' a course of chymistry with Dr. Willis, which is the reason why so many physical and chymical allusions are to be found in it": *Dictionary of National Biography* 15: 87, under entry "Pakington". Other than purely conventional figures of speech, there are medical or chemical references in *Causes* at pp. 4–5, 29, 58, 75, 118–119, 122, 253. James Allestry, Richard's brother, published Willis's *Diatribae duae* (1659), *Cerebri anatome* (1664), *Pathologiae cerebri* (1667), and *Affectionum* (1670).

21. Wood, *Athenae,* vol. 3, col. 1053.

22. Joseph Foster, ed., *Alumni Oxonienses: The Members of the University of Oxford,* 1500–1714 (Oxford: Parker, 1891–1892), 4: 1650. Willis matriculated from Christ Church, 3 March 1636/7; B.A., 19 June 1639; M. A., 18 June 1642.

versity education.[23] The curriculum was still highly Scholastic, and was organized around the two medieval elements of lectures and disputations.[24] Especially in the years between the B.A. and the M.A., Willis would have studied traditional natural philosophy, geometry, and astronomy. He would have dutifully read his Aristotle, absorbing what he was later to call "those vain figments," the Peripatetic forms and qualities.[25] Although Willis is often—and rightly—portrayed as one of the new breed of savant that the seventeenth century created, he was certainly perceived by his contemporaries as intellectually reliable enough that, in 1660, through the influence of Sheldon, he was elected Sedleian Professor at £120 per annum.[26]

Physician, pillar of the church, Scholastic—described thus far, Willis would hardly seem an innovator. How did he come to his reputation as a master of brain anatomy and theoretician of the soul? His portal of entry, I would argue, was originally not anatomy, as one would expect, but a subject more appropriate to the humble prescribing medico: chemistry. As early as 1648, when he still lived in bachelor rooms in Christ Church, he joined with another Anglican perforce turned physi-

23. On the growing popularity of the English universities see Mark H. Curtis, *Oxford and Cambridge in Transition, 1558–1642* (Oxford: Clarendon Press, 1959); Kenneth Charlton, *Education in Renaissance England* (London: Routledge and Kegan Paul, 1965); Hugh Kearney, *Scholars and Gentlemen: Universities and Society in Preindustrial Britain, 1500–1700* (Ithaca, N.Y.: Cornell University Press, 1970); Lawrence Stone, ed., *The University in Society* (Princeton: Princeton University Press, 1974). In the 1540s Oxford admitted about 40 B.A.s and 20 M.A.s each year; by the 1620s this had grown to the extent that about 400 new students came to Oxford each year, of whom an average of 240 would proceed to the B.A., and about 150 to the M.A.; see Robert G. Frank, Jr., "Science, Medicine and the Universities of Early Modern England: Background and Sources," *History of Science* 11 (1973): 194–216, 239–269, especially 213. For the physical growth of the colleges in the pre–Civil War period, see the *Victoria History of the County of Oxford,* ed. H. E. Salter and M. D. Lobel (London: Institute of Historical Research, 1954), 3:96, 102, 115–116, 127–128, 169–170, 216–217, 240–242, 272–274, 283–285, 289.

24. The relation between statutory forms and scholastic content at an English university is brilliantly set forth in William T. Costello, *The Scholastic Curriculum at Early Seventeenth-Century Cambridge* (Cambridge, Mass.: Harvard University Press, 1958). On the relation of science to the scholastic format, see Frank, "Science, Medicine and the Universities," 200–207.

25. For a description of the arts curriculum at Oxford in the late sixteenth and early seventeenth century, see Andrew Clark, *Register of the University of Oxford,* vol. 2 (1571–1622), part 1 (Oxford: Oxford Historical Society, 1887).

26. The documents on Willis's election are in the Oxford University Archives, "Registrum Convocationis, 1659–1671," reverse codex f. 4r-v.

cian, Ralph Bathurst, in preparing chemical compounds.[27] His case notes of 1650, although largely Galenic in framework, show him edging toward chemical explanations of blood composition. Take, for example, the phenomenon of diffused pains; Willis thought they were due to an "acrid salt."[28] By 1652 Willis was one of an inner circle of eight Oxford virtuosi who, according to Seth Ward, had "joyned together for the furnishing an elaboratory and for makeing chymicall experiments wch we doe constantly every one of us in course undertakeing by weeks to manage the worke."[29] Willis's neat accounts of money "laid out at Wadham coll" for chemical apparatus and supplies, written in the back of one of his surviving casebooks, no doubt dates from his rota of managing "the worke." It was no mean operation; the expenses up to that point totaled almost twenty-five pounds, at a time when a college fellow was paid three pounds a years to tutor a young gentleman in Oxford.[30] As Willis came to know other virtuosi, such as John Wilkins and Robert Boyle, his reputation as a chemist spead.[31] The London projector Samuel Hartlib recorded in November 1654 that

> Dr. Wellis [sic] of Dr. Wilkins acquaintance a very experimenting ingenious gentleman communicating every weeke some experiment or other to Mr. Boyles chymical servant, who is a kind of cozen to him. He is a great Verulamian philosopher, from him all may bee had by meanes of Mr. Boyle.[32]

27. See the letters of John Lydall from Oxford in 1649 referring to "Mr. Willis our Chymist," extracted and explicated in Robert G. Frank, Jr., "John Aubrey, F.R.S., John Lydall, and Science at Commonwealth Oxford," *Notes and Records of the Royal Society of London* 27 (1973): 193–217, especially 196–198, 213.

28. Dewhurst, *Willis's Oxford Casebook,* 109; other references of a chemical bent are on pp. 82, 83, 98, 110, and 119.

29. Seth Ward to Sir Justinian Isham, 27 February 1652, in H. W. Robinson, "An Unpublished Letter of Dr. Seth Ward Relating to the Early Meetings of the Oxford Philosophical Society," *Notes and Records of the Royal Society of London* 7 (1949): 68–70.

30. Dewhurst, *Willis's Oxford Casebook,* 153–154.

31. Wilkins was installed as Warden of Wadham in April 1648 (Wood, *History and Antiquities* 2: 570), although given their difference in politics, they may not have gotten to know each other until their common experience in William Petty's club about 1650. Cf. Robert Boyle to Ralph Bathurst, 14 April 1656, where he sends his service "to Dr. Willis, Dr. Ward, and the rest of those excellent acquaintances of yours, that have been pleased to tolerate me in their company" (Thomas Warton, *The life and literary remains of Ralph Bathurst, M.D.* [London, 1761]. pp. 162–164).

32. Samuel Hartlib, "Ephemerides" [diary-like commonplace books], 1654, ff. WW-WW 7–8, Harlib Papers, Sheffield University Library. The Hartlib Papers are quoted by the kind permission of their owner, Lord Delamere.

By June 1656 Willis had completed his first chemical work, "De fermentatione"; he circulated it among his fellow scientists in Oxford, and word of it even reached London.[33] In late 1658 he appended to it some additional tracts on fevers and on urines, and published the whole as *Diatribae duae medico-philosophicae* (1659).[34] The book attracted much attention not only in Willis's coterie but in London and abroad.[35] To his local reputation as an adept, Willis thereby added an international one as a theoretician of the spagyric art.

Since Willis's ideas about the animal and human body were built upon his chemistry, one must understand something about it in order to see how he approached problems of brain function. All bodies, he believed, were composed of five "principles": spirit, sulphur, salt, water, and earth. The last two were traditional Aristotelian "elements," while the first three were modifications of Paracelsian "principles"—in his chemistry, as in most other things, Willis was always the compromiser between ancients and moderns.

But unlike Aristotelians and Paracelsians, Willis did not believe that the five principles were names for homogeneous substances; rather, they were labels for *categories of particles.* All spirit particles, for example, shared the property of being highly subtle and active. They were always

33. Hartlib, "Ephemerides," 1656, f. 48–48–3, where Hartlib noted that Willis was "a leading and prime man in the Philosophical Club at Oxford," who "hath written a treatise De Fermentatione," which John Aubrey commended highly. Robert Wood, who was at Oxford from 1640 to 1656, and a year younger than Willis, wrote to Hartlib: "If the Booke you write of de Fermentatione be Mr Willis his of Oxford, I am confident it is an excellent peece, having formerly seen some sheets of his upon ye subject, when we met at a Club, at Oxford" (Wood to Hartlib, 9 February 1658[/9], Hartlib Papers, Bundle XXXIII (1)).

34. Cf. *A Transcript of the Registers of the Worshipful Company of Stationers, from 1640–1708* (London: Privately printed, 1913–1914), 2: 207, where the *Diatribae duae* was licenced on 26 November 1658.

35. On 16 December 1658, Hartlib thanked Boyle for sending a copy of Willis's *Diatribae duae* from Oxford, and noted of the London chemist Frederick Clodius that his "chemical son's head and hands are much taken up with animadversiones on Dr. *Willis's* book, he having very clear reason and experiences to dislike very many particulars in it: but, no doubt, of this he will write himself" (Hartlib to Boyle, in *The works of the Honourable Robert Boyle,* ed. Thomas Birch, 2d ed. [London, 1772], 6: 115–116). Three months later Robert Wood wrote from Dublin: "A frend from Oxford has sent me Mr. Willis his much approved Booke de Fermentatione, so yt though I shall not now need yours . . . yet I shall still value your intentions as highly as I do the booke it selfe" (Wood to Hartlib, 2 March 1658[/9], Hartlib Papers, Bundle XXXIII (1)). Boyle also passed on a copy to John Beale in Herefordshire: cf. Samuel Hartlib to John Worthington, 26 June 1659, *The Diary and Correspondence of Dr. John Worthington,* ed. James Crossley (Manchester: Chetham Society, 1847), 1: 135.

attempting to fly out of an object, and had to be bound to other, heavier particles. But because not all spirit particles were of identical size and activity, they could not all fly away at the same time. "Spirit," for Willis, described a population of particles with common characteristics and activities, but which, like individuals that made up a species, were not necessarily identical.

The other four elements were conceived in a similar manner. Sulphureous particles were rather less active than spirit, but they too were capable of flying away. Less subtle than spirit, they were more vehement and unruly. With a little motion, they produced maturation and sweetness; with more motion, heat; with the maximum motion, the body dissolved into flames. Salt was of a more fixed nature than the previous two; it bestowed solidity on things, and retarded their dissolution. The two last principles served as passive matrices for the active ones. If particles of earth predominated, then the substance was solid; if those of water, it was liquid. Willis could, then, look at a biological substance like blood, or a part of the brain, and conceive of it as a heterogeneous population of particles, of varying types, and varying motions. Particles of different principles could combine with each to produce "copula"—spirito-sulphureous, salino-sulphureous, and so forth—which combined the chemical properties of their constituent parts.[36]

Note, though, what Willis had done. He had created a corpuscular matter-theory, and its correlate chemistry, in a way that differed from classical atomism, which did not allow matter to have properties in and of itself. His youth, the 1630s and 1640s, had been a time of revival, and reworking, of Epicurean corpuscular theories.[37] René Descartes had made particles of matter in motion the basis of his supremely influential *Principia philosophiae* (1644).[38] Although Descartes's mechanistic explanations applied to animal bodies appeared only in his posthumous *De l'homme* (1664), many of his physiological ideas were expounded earlier by his Dutch disciples, Henrik de Roy (Henricus Regius) in his *Fundamenta physices* (1646) and *Fundamenta medica* (1647), and Cornelis

36. Willis, *De fermentatione*, 1–17; "Of Fermentations," 1–8. The Pordage translation includes material added in later editions.

37. On the problems and sources of early modern atomism and the corpuscular philosophy, see Kurd Lasswitz, *Geschichte der Atomistik vom Mittelalter bis Newton* (Hamburg: Leopold Voss, 1890); Marie Boas, "The Establishment of the Mechanical Philosophy," *Osiris* 10 (1952): 412–541; Robert Hugh Kargon, *Atomism in England from Hariot to Newton* (Oxford: Clarendon Press, 1966).

38. René Descartes, *Discours de la méthode* (Leiden, 1637); *Principia philosophiae* (Amsterdam, 1644); *De l'homme* (Paris, 1664).

Hooghelande in his *Cogitationes* (1646).[39] Marin Mersenne's brand of mechanism was most clearly delineated in the *Cogitata physico-mathematica* (1644).[40] Pierre Gassendi's massive three-volume *Animadversiones in decimum librum Diogenis Laertii* (1649) established him as the leading spokesman for, and interpreter of, Epicurean atomism as applied to science.[41] Gassendi's was the most highly ramified of the corpuscularian philosophies. According to him, there was only matter and the void. Matter was of one type, and it was only the varying size and figure of the atoms, and their concretion into second-order particles called moleculae, that constituted perceived differences in matter.[42] In page after double-columned page, Gassendi went on to show how light, color, sound, odors, rarity, density, perspicuity, opacity, subtility, hardness, smoothness, fluidity, humidity, and ductility—all could be transposed out of the Aristotelian categories of essences and substantial forms, into the matter-and-motion categories of the atomistic conceptual scheme.[43]

Willis was familiar with much of this literature, and explicitly cites Descartes, Regius, Hooghelande, Mersenne, and Gassendi. Yet he preferred a corpuscularian chemistry in which particles, although of possibly differing activities, had inherent properties by which they could act. In this version, he said, chemistry could demonstrate the principles of natural philosophy, whereas the "Epicurean hypothesis" only supposes them.[44]

However, Willis did not come by his corpuscularianism merely in the library. It was nonexistent in his casebook of 1650, well established in the *De fermentatione* of 1656, and grew into efflorescence in his works written in the 1660s. Whence came such an intellectual trajectory? I

39. Henrik de Roy, *Fundamenta physices* (Amsterdam, 1646) and *Fundamenta medica* (Utrecht, 1647); Cornelis Hooghelande, *Cogitationes, quibus Dei existentia et animae spiritualitas, et possibilis cum corpore unio, demonstrantur; necnon brevis historia oeconomiae corporis animalis proponitur, atque mechanice explicatur* (Amsterdam, 1646).

40. Marin Mersenne, *Cogitata physico-mathematica in quibus tam naturae quam artis effectus admirandi certissimis demonstrationibus explicantur* (Paris, 1644). On Mersenne see the excellent study by Robert Lenoble, *Mersenne; ou, La naissance du mécanisme* (Paris: Vrin, 1943).

41. Pierre Gassendi, *Animadversiones in decimum librum Diogenis Laertii* (Lyon, 1649); on Gassendi's atomism see Bernard Rochot, *Les travaux de Gassendi sur Epicure et sur l'atomisme, 1619–1658* (Paris: Vrin, 1944), and Lasswitz, *Geschichte der Atomistik* 2: 126–188.

42. Gassendi, *Animadversiones* 1: 222–236.

43. Ibid., 236–362.

44. Willis, *De fermentatione,* 4; "On fermentation," 2. The English translation includes a remark that if anyone were to say that the chemical and atomical schemes can be brought together, he would not disagree; but he will leave it to those more clever than he to devise or dream philosophy.

would argue that it was rooted in Willis's experiences in informal scientific groups that met at Oxford in the 1650s and 1660s. Among the participants in these groups were men like William Petty, Robert Boyle, and John Wallis, all of whom we know were, from their Continental contacts and reading, particularly interested in Gassendian atomism.[45] Willis worked with men like these by being a member of no fewer than five such groups that met over the period from about 1648 to 1667.[46] The first was a small chemistry group with Ralph Bathurst and John Lydall that worked at Trinity and Christ Church about 1648–1649.[47] The second was organized by William Petty from late 1649 to early 1652, at his lodgings over an apothecary shop in the High Street. The third convened, from the early 1650s to about 1657, at Wadham College under the auspices of John Wilkins, its Warden. It was by far the largest and most well-organized of the groups, and provided part of the nucleus for the founding of the Royal Society in London in 1660. The fourth group met rather more sporadically at Robert Boyle's lodgings in the High Street, from late 1657 to late 1659, and from July 1664 to April 1668. And the last was Willis's own, largely of physicians and chemists, that met at Beam Hall, in Merton Street, from the late 1650s up to Willis's departure to London in 1667.[48]

Through each of these groups in which Willis participated there were continuities and discontinuities of membership. Younger men became interested in scientific topics, and were brought into activities, while

45. For evidence of the popularity of the French and Dutch mechanists among Oxford scientists, see Robert G. Frank, Jr., *Harvey and the Oxford Physiologists: Scientific Ideas and Social Interaction* (Berkeley, Los Angeles, London: University of California Press, 1980), 92–93.

46. For a survey of Oxford scientific groups in the 1650s and 1660s, see ibid., 43–89; also Charles Webster, *The Great Instauration: Science, Medicine and Reform, 1626–1660* (New York: Holmes and Meier, 1976), 153–178.

47. Frank, "John Aubrey," 196–198.

48. On the venues, membership, and activities of the Petty, Wilkins, and Boyle clubs, see Frank, *Harvey and the Oxford Physiologists,* 52–57, and the sources cited in the notes on pp. 312–314. Willis's membership in these groups is recorded in the following sources: Bodleian Library, MS. donat. Wood 1, pp. 1–3; John Wallis, *A defence of the Royal Society* (London, 1678), 8; John Wallis's autobiography (1697) in *Peter Langtoft's chronicle,* ed. Thomas Hearne (Oxford, 1725), 1: clxiii–clxiv; Wood, *History and Antiquities* 2: 633; Thomas Sprat, *The history of the Royal-Society of London, for the improving of natural knowledge* (London, 1667), 52–58; Aubrey, "*Brief Lives*" 2: 141; participant in the "resurrection" of Anne Green, see [Richard Watkins], *Newes from the dead,* 2d ed. (Oxford, 1651), 1–8; Walter Pope, *The life of the right reverend father in God Seth, Lord Bishop of Salisbury* (London, 1697), 29.

others moved away from Oxford or lost interest. Most of all, these shifting constellations gave rise to numerous cooperative research projects. The ethos was one not of discussion and debate but of experimentation, trial, and manual exploration. Again and again, clusters of investigators served as helpmates, audience, and witnesses in one another's scientific work.

This then was the constellation of elements in Willis's life at the time of the Restoration, the six kinds of conceptual and social raw material out of which one shaped an approach to the relation of brain and soul. They reflected the many sides of the newly elected professor of natural philosophy: Willis the clinician of increasing acuity and fame; Willis the staunch Royalist and devout Anglican; Willis the man of traditional philosophical education, recently placed into an endowed professorship; Willis the enthusiastic experimental chemist; Willis the afficionado of corpuscular philosophies; and Willis the ever-active member of Oxford scientific circles.

ORIGINS OF A NEUROLOGICAL RESEARCH PROGRAM

Yet even given all of this, in 1660 there was no inevitability to Willis's future interest in the brain; it arose as a fortuitous concourse—a phrase beloved by the atomists—of incitement and opportunity.

As he himself noted in his "Praefatio," the incitement was his new responsibilities as a teacher. What were those duties? The Laudian statutes, adopted in the 1630s but codifying the practices of previous decades, specified them quite clearly. During the Michaelmas, Hilary, and Easter terms, each about eight weeks in length, Willis was to read to the bachelors of arts at 8:00 A.M. on Wednesdays and Saturdays. For failing to read a lecture, the professor incurred a fine of ten shillings (about $200 proportionally today), whereas the B.A.s were to be fined fourpence (perhaps $6) for failure to attend. His lectures were to be drawn from a list of Aristotle's works: *De physica, De caelo, Meteorologica, De generatione et corruptione, De anima,* and the *Parva naturalia.*[49] The first four fall into the category of the physical sciences, while the last two might properly be called psychology. It was not a modest province of knowledge; Willis's teaching obligations covered two of the eight cate-

49. John Griffith, ed., *Statutes of the University of Oxford Codified in the Year 1636 under the Authority of Archbishop Laud, Chancellor of the University* (Oxford: Clarendon Press, 1888), 36–37.

gories into which Aristotle's total surviving works could be distributed.

Such were the statutory injunctions. But in good English fashion, at Oxford the statutes were venerated more in the breach than the observance. By the 1650s the Savilian Professors of Astronomy and Geometry—Willis's fellow club members John Wallis and Seth Ward—were teaching the ideas of Copernicus and Kepler, defending the "Atomicall and Magneticall" hypotheses, and in general feeling free, as Ward and John Wilkins put it, to "discent" from Aristotle, "and to declare against him."[50] Willis did no less. He was naturally drawn more to the psychological side of his bailiwick than to the physical, so he chose to honor the statutes by lecturing within the general subject area with which *De anima* and the *Parva naturalia* dealt: the principles animating vegetable and animal life, the senses and sensation, memory, sleep and dreams. That he exercised his freedom from the very beginning can be seen in a passing reference in a commonplace book of a medical student; John Ward, of Christ Church, noted in February 1661 that "Dr. Willis is now reading about ye succus nervosus," and that the professor doubted that the nerve juice actually exercised its reputed nutritive function.[51] Willis's lectures went on to include the nature of life, sensation, movement, narcotics, nutrition, convulsions, epilepsy, hysteria, sleep and wakefulness, nightmare, coma, vertigo, paralysis, delirium, phrensy, melancholia, mania, stupidity, the cerebrum, the cerebellum, and nerve fibers. In fact, it seems that wherever Willis encountered an interesting observation or result, it might well end up as part of his teaching; in 1664 his protégé, Richard Lower, observed an interesting anatomical arrangement in the stomach of a ruminant, and Willis was, as Lower reported to Boyle, "so taken with it" that he wanted to "make a lecture of it the next term."[52] Such freedom within statutory constraints allowed Willis to shape his teaching to reflect his own interests, which were largely chemical and medical. Exactly the opposite happened once he left Oxford, and paid a deputy to discharge his obligations as Sedleian Professor; in 1669 George Hooper was overseeing disputations on such subjects in the physical sciences as "Whether the Medicean stars are

50. [Seth Ward], *Vindiciae academiarum* (Oxford, 1654), 2, 28–30, 32, 45–46; quotation from p. 2, which was written by John Wilkins.

51. John Ward, diary-like commonplace books, 16 vols., in the Folger Shakespeare Library, Washington, D.C. MSS. V.a. 284–299; hereafter cited as Ward, "Diary." Quotation is from Ward, "Diary," VIII, f. 39v. See also Frank, "The John Ward Diaries," 153–154.

52. Richard Lower to Robert Boyle, 24 June 1664, in *The works of the Honourable Robert Boyle,* ed. Thomas Birch, 2d ed. (London, 1772), 6: 474.

the moons of Jupiter? Affirmative," and "Whether a vacuum can exist? Negative."[53]

We know Willis took such a biological approach and covered such neurological subjects, because abstracts of some of his lectures have survived in the form of student notes—notes that are of particular interest and significance both for their content and for their auditors. Most probably in the late 1661 or early 1662, Lower attended some of the Sedleian lectures and wrote out notes on them. In November 1662 Lower then made a transcription of some of the topics and sent it on to Robert Boyle, who was in London at the time.[54] About 1664 Lower also lent his notes to his fellow member of Christ Church, John Locke, who abstracted them into a commonplace book.[55] Even though Lower's notes themselves have not survived, we have, therefore, overlapping extracts among the Boyle Papers at the Royal Society,[56] and in John Locke's manuscripts at the Bodleian Library.[57] The link between the two became clear to me in 1969. I had read the extracts in Locke's commonplace book at Oxford. A few weeks later, while paging through thirty volumes of Boyle Papers in London, I came across an anonymous fascicle of Latin notes on medical topics. As I glanced through them, it struck me that they covered some of the same topics as the Locke notebook. A few hours' work comparing the text with the Locke extracts, and the handwriting with known samples of Oxonians, yielded the answer: this was Willis's work, and Lower was the writer.[58]

Clearly the Sedleian lectures, although Willis expressed some dissatisfaction with the early versions of them, were not treated by his circle of friends simply as a *réchauffé* of old ideas for adolescents. Nor were they.

53. *The Life and Times of Anthony Wood, Antiquary, of Oxford, 1632–1695, Described by Himself*, ed. Andrew Clark (Oxford: Clarendon Press, 1891–1900), 2: 161.

54. Lower to Boyle, 26 November 1662, *Works* 6: 465.

55. Bodleian Library, Oxford, MS. Locke f. 19, pp. 1–68 passim.

56. Royal Society of London, Boyle Papers, XIX, ff. 1–35.

57. The Locke manuscripts are described in P. Long, *A Summary Catalogue of the Lovelace Collection of the Papers of John Locke in the Bodleian Library* (Oxford: University Press, 1959) and in "The Mellon Donation of Additional Manuscripts of John Locke from the Lovelace Collection," *Bodleian Library Record* 7 (1964): 185–193. The existence of Locke's notes from Willis's lectures was first discovered by Kenneth Dewhurst, "Willis in Oxford: Some New MSS," *Proceedings of the Royal Society of Medicine* 57 (1964): 682–687.

58. When the late Dr. Dewhurst expressed an interest in editing the Willis lectures in MS. Locke f. 19, I called his attention to the complementary MS in Boyle Papers. Dewhurst's edition and translation of, and commentary on, the merged MSS appeared as Dewhurst, *Willis's Oxford Lectures*. I cite the lectures in that form unless there is a particular reason to refer back to the original Locke and Boyle manuscripts.

They contained many original and stimulating ideas—ideas that not only provided a program for neurological research but represented significant changes from Willis's very much more conventional earlier concepts. For example, in his casebook of the early 1650s he had attributed hypochondria to a faulty spleen and accepted the uterine origins of hysteria.[59] By the time he began lecturing, however, he had come to trace both to the brain.[60] Similarly with mania and "phantasy"; in the casebook Willis's descriptions reflect the traditional medical explanations,[61] whereas a decade later he had brought both of these conditions into the orbit of the nervous system.[62] In the lectures, then, Willis clearly outlined neurological explanations that, with only a few exceptions, he was to flesh out over the succeeding decade.[63] But one must also be aware of how skeletal this corpus originally was. The corpuscular details were very rudimentary. But even more significantly, Willis's explanations for brain function were insufficiently grounded in a firm and detailed knowledge of anatomy.

It is important, therefore, that we see clearly the academic, philosophical, and rather traditional origins of Willis's neurological research program, as well as its original incomplete state, because together they explain why a set of medical treatises should show a seemingly unmedical concern with the soul and its properties. Willis's medical practice over the previous fifteen years had provided him with an ever-increasing wealth of clinical experience, but no incentive whatsoever to analyze that experience systematically with respect to a long-standing tradition of thinking about the mind/body problem. But Willis, sincere in all things, took seriously his professorship, and the statutory injunctions about its subject matter. He confronted his own medical experience and ways of thinking about the physical world with the distinctly nonmedical and nonanatomical tradition of Aristotelian psychology—and these lectures were the result. Perhaps as important for the end result, Willis had to deliver his thoughts to an audience that included a number of his scientific cronies. One can hardly imagine a stronger incentive to casting the old psychology into new terms.

59. Dewhurst, *Willis's Oxford Casebook,* 67, 93, 95.

60. Dewhurst, *Willis's Oxford Lectures,* 87–92; Willis, *Pathologiae cerebri,* 144–193; Willis, "Pathology of the brain," 76–102.

61. Dewhurst, *Willis's Oxford Casebook,* 127, 145.

62. Dewhurst, *Willis's Oxford Lectures,* 66, 82, 96, 98, 122, 130–134.

63. Dewhurst, *Willis's Oxford Lectures,* has correlated the topics of the lectures with the treatment of the same subjects later in *Cerebri anatome, Pathologiae cerebri,* and *De anima brutorum.*

I wish to argue further, however, that incitement was not of itself sufficient to get this new research program off the ground. Opportunity was needed as well. In the midst of an ever-busier practice, and lecturing responsibilities, Willis would most likely have had little chance to remake the speculations expressed in his Sedleian lectures, had he not been helped by a near-perfectly complementary collaborator: Richard Lower.[64] Ten years younger than Willis, Lower had come from both a higher social background and a better preliminary education than his mentor: respectively, the Cornish gentry and England's best public school of the period, Westminster School in London. In 1649 Lower had come up to Willis's old college, Christ Church, collected his B.A. and M.A. in due order,[65] and supervised students as the college's Censor in Natural Philosophy from 1657 to 1660.[66] He became interested in medicine in the early 1650s and started practicing about 1656. He soon thereafter began to work "under the directions of Dr Thomas Willis, to whose favour he recommended himself, by assisting him in his anatomical dissections."[67] Lower continued to practice as Willis's junior medical partner until he left Oxford in 1665.[68]

64. For Lower's life and scientific activities, see Frank, *Harvey and the Oxford Physiologists,* passim, but especially 64–65, 174–220, and the sources therein cited. The best brief overview of Lower's life is Theodore Brown, "Richard Lower," *Dictionary of Scientific Biography* 8: 523–527.

65. Lower was elected into a Studentship from Westminster in 1649 and seems to have come to Oxford then, although he did not actually matriculate until 27 February 1651; he proceeded to the B.A. on 17 February 1653 and to the M.A. on 28 June 1655 and accumulated his degrees of B. and D.Med. on 28 June 1665, just before leaving Oxford: Foster, *Alumni Oxonienses* 3: 943. It was not unusual for fellows of colleges to practice before formally taking their degrees.

66. Chapterbook (1649–1688), pp. 77, 88, 104, Chapter Archives, Christ Church, Oxford. Lower also served as Praelector in Greek for 1656–57. Occupying one of the positions as a Student (the equivalent of a Fellow in other colleges), he rose in seniority within Christ Church until about 1662, when he reached the top of those not in orders. Then, having as he said to Boyle insufficient "favour or friendship" to obtain one of the two physician's places in the college, he could not keep his Studentship. He did, however, continue to occupy rooms in the college. See Richard Lower to Robert Boyle, 24 June 1664, *Works* 6: 474.

67. *Biographia Britannica* (London, 1747–1766), vol. 5, col. 3009.

68. For example, in September 1662 Willis and Lower treated one of John Locke's tutees; Willis got a one-pound fee, and Lower ten shillings: Bodleian Library, MS. Locke f. 11, f. 24r. Lower was sent out to the country—once as far as Cambridgeshire—to attend Willis's patients: Richard Griffith, *A-la-mode phlebotomy no good fashion* (London, 1681), 171. On the return journey of one such trip into Northamptonshire in April 1664 Lower discovered the medicinal character of the waters of Eastrope, Oxfordshire, near King's Sutton, which he and Willis then promoted as a local spa: *Wood, Life and Times* 2: 12.

But Lower's real interest, as suggested by the activity that brought him together with his mentor, was not so much clinical medicine as anatomy and physiology. He seems to have had an inveterate itch to cut things up. The first surviving piece of evidence about his scientific interests, written by John Ward in his commonplace book about October 1660, pictures him vividly: "Mr. Lower cut a doggs windpipe and let him rune about: hee had a week so: he could note smell but would eat any thing I was told."[69] Lower's curiosity naturally expressed itself in exploring the detailed structure, the precise workings of a living thing. As his later work on the heart, *Tractatus de corde* (1669), showed, he had little interest in broader questions of matter-theory and principles of life. His was a reputation as a dissector and vivisector; his friend, Anthony Wood, was not at all surprised to arrive at Lower's rooms in Christ Church one Sunday morning and find him busily dissecting a calf's head.[70] Lower's personality fit his avocation. He seems to have been anti–High Church, politically a Whig, temperamentally exacting, and—if later testimony is to be credited—inclined to be arrogant about his scientific knowledge.[71]

Willis, a contrast in personality and background, equally contrasted with Lower in having no such eager knife. Before 1660 he actively pursued chemistry but did little anatomy. Of fifty patients whose treatment is recorded in his casebook from the early 1650s, ten died, and on only one was a cursory postmortem performed; even in that case the phrasing of the notes seems to hint that it was a surgeon, not Willis, who did the necropsy.[72] Although the only official university teaching post in anatomy, the Tomlins Readership, changed hands several times during Willis's residence in Oxford, there is no indication that he sought the position.[73] His first book, the *Diatribae duae medico-philosophicae* of 1659, reports no postmortems, and of the numerous scattered references to Willis to be found in published works, diaries, and correspondence be-

69. Ward, "Diary," VII, f. 83r.

70. Wood, *Life and Times* 2: 4.

71. Frank, *Harvey and the Oxford Physiologists,* 283 and sources cited there.

72. In Dewhurst, *Willis's Oxford Casebook,* deaths are recorded on pp. 74, 80, 91, 97, 100, 105, 118, 122, 127, 132. The only postmortem was carried out on F. Symmons (118); the phrasing seems to imply that Willis only did the chemical examination of fluids:

> In the dead body it was found that the lungs were floating in a large quantity of water which was enclosed in the saepta of the thorax.
>
> Moreover when we evaporated some of this water with slow heat on sand there was, in the bottom of the vessel, a residuum like mucus or flour porridge and whites of egg, viscous and smelling adominably.

73. On the Tomlins Readership, see Wood *History and antiquities* 2: 883–884.

fore 1660, only one links him to an anatomical proceeding. This is the renowned "resurrection" of Anne Green in December 1650, in which Petty, Willis, Bathurst, and others assembled to dissect the body of a hanged convict, only to find the proposed cadaver very much alive.[74] But on this occasion it was not Willis but Petty, a skilled dissector trained in Leiden, who took the lead.[75]

But Lower's presence at Oxford, and especially in Willis's coterie, provided the opportunity. Lower reported the start of the project in a letter to Boyle in January 1662:

> The doctor was not at leisure till of late to make those dissections of the brain, which he hoped; but at length we have had the opportunity of cutting up several, and the doctor, finding most parts of the brain imperfectly described, intends to make a whole new draught thereof, with the several uses of the distinct parts, according to his own fancy, seeing few authors speak any thing considerable of it.[76]

Thus began an intense period of dissections in which "no day almost past over without some Anatomical administration; so that in a short space there was nothing of the Brain, and its Appendix within the Skull, that seemed not plainly detected, and intimately beheld by us."[77] Entire "hecatombs" of animals, Willis said, were slain in the anatomical court.[78] They dissected not only human cadavers but horses, sheep, calves, goats, hogs, dogs, cats, foxes, hares, geese, turkeys, fishes, and even a monkey. The indefatigable worker was Lower, the "edge of whose Knife and Wit" Willis gratefully acknowledged for assistance in "the better searching out both the frames and offices of before hidden Bodies."[79] Others of the club helped out. John Wallis, the mathematician, and a longtime club member, participated in some of the initial dissections.[80] The physician Thomas Millington and the mathematician Christopher Wren, both con-

74. The incident is described in [Watkins], *Newes from the dead,* 2d ed. (Oxford, 1651), 1–8. Petty also described the resurrection in a letter to Samuel Hartlib, 16 December 1650: Hartlib Papers, Bundle VIII (23).

75. Petty was appointed Tomlins Reader on 31 December 1650, about two weeks after the Anne Green affair. His anatomical work at Oxford is reflected in volume 3 of the Petty Papers (now at Bowood House, Calne, Wiltshire), which contain his medical and anatomical lectures at Oxford c. 1650–1652. For details, see Frank, *Harvey and the Oxford Physiologists,* 101–103.

76. Lower to Boyle, 18 January 1661[/2], *Works,* 6: 462.

77. Willis, *Cerebri anatome,* sig. a2v; "Anatomy of the brain," 53.

78. Ibid., sig. A4r and 51.

79. Ibid., sig. a2v and 53.

80. Wallis's presence at a brain dissection is mentioned in Lower to Boyle, 18 January 1661[/2], *Works* 6: 463. Cf. also John Wallis to Henry Oldenburg, 17 February 1673, *The*

temporaries of Lower's at Westminster, and by then at All Souls, "were wont frequently to be present at our Dissections, and to confer and reason about the uses of the Parts." Millington especially was Willis's sounding board, to whom he proposed almost daily his "Conjectures and Observations."[81] Within ten months Lower could send to Boyle the extracts of Oxford lectures, and report that the "doctor hath now perfected the anatomical part likewise, but being not satisfied in some things," might not soon be induced to publish.[82] By April of 1663, however, Willis and Lower were "wholly diverted" with more dissections, which were "very near finished" because Willis intended to put the book into the press by midsummer.[83] Within the next few months Wren had, as Lower reported to Boyle, "drawn most excellent schemes of the brain, and the several parts of it, according to the doctor's design," and Willis was resolved "to print his anatomy forthwith."[84] Lower carried the same news personally to London in July. He missed presenting Willis's service to Boyle, but told his old Westminster schoolfellow Robert Hooke that Willis's book "is within a little while to come forth, and he added, that Dr. Wren had drawn the pictures very curiously for it."[85] A "little while" and "forthwith" were faster in the seventeenth century than today, and the book came out six months later.

To those wishing to assign credit for the *Cerebri anatome,* the role of Lower especially has posed some problems. Anthony Wood, in his capsule biography of Willis, noted of the *Cerebri anatome*: "Whatsoever is anatomical in that book, the glory thereof belongs to the said R. Lower, whose indefatigable industry at Oxon produced that elaborate piece."[86] Twentieth-century scholars have noted that Lower was a frequent drinking chum of Wood,[87] that Wood later had a land dispute with Willis,[88]

Correspondence of Henry Oldenburg, ed. and trans. A. Rupert Hall and Marie Boas Hall (Madison: University of Wisconsin Press, 1965–), 9: 466, in which Wallis shows an intimate knowledge of Willis's *Cerebri anatome.*

81. Willis, *Cerebri anatome,* sig. a3r: "Anatomy of the brain," 54.

82. Lower to Boyle, 26 November 1662, *Works* 6: 465.

83. Lower to Boyle, 27 April 1663, *Works* 6: 466.

84. Lower to Boyle, 4 June 1663, *Works* 6: 466.

85. Robert Hooke to Robert Boyle, [3 July 1663], *Works* 6: 487.

86. Wood, *Athenae,* vol. 3, col. 1051; see also the comment to similar effect in Wood's biography of Lower, ibid., 4: 297.

87. Dewhurst, *Willis's Oxford Lectures,* 13, 32. Wood's references to eating or drinking with Lower are in Wood, *Life and Times,* vol. 1: (1657) 230; (1658) 259; (1659) 266, 267, 279, 284; (1660) 313, 318, 321, 327; (1661) 405, 410; (1662) 428, 430, 444, 450; (1663) 471, 474, 477, 486, 487, 501, 503, 507; vol. 2: (1664) 1, 2, 4, 6, 8, 12, 14, 15, 23, 24; (1665) 27, 31, 33, 35, 37, 40, 43; (1666) 71, 73, 76; (1667) 99.

88. Dewhurst, *Willis's Oxford Lectures,* 33.

and finally that Wood's judgment was taken almost word for word from one of Henry Stubbe's blasts against the Royal Society.[89] They have therefore tended to discount Lower's participation in the research and to credit Willis with everything.[90] Such a judgment is untenable and unnecessary. Stubbe and Wood were admirers of both Willis and Lower and merely wished to recognize the interdependence of the two.[91] In reality, the collaborative relationship was quite complex. Clearly Willis provided the impetus; from the very beginning Lower's letters remarked how "the doctor" suggested, and participated in, this or that aspect of the brain dissections.[92] Moreover, Willis's concepts seem to have directed the interpretation of the findings, as for example when Willis showed Lower "several times" how the dissections supported "his opinion of the use of the cerebellum for involuntary motion." Similarly with the medullary and cortical parts of the cerebellum, and the origins of the optic nerves.[93] The degree of collaboration could vary from day to day. Lower often wrote in letters of dissections, postmortems, and experiments that

89. The argument of the biased testimony of Wood was first made by Sir Charles Symonds, "The Circle of Willis," *British Medical Journal* (15 January 1955), i, 119–124, especially 121. It has been accepted by: William Feindel, "Thomas Willis (1621–1675)—The Founder of Neurology," *Canadian Medical Association Journal* 87 (1962): 289–296, especially 289; and Isler, *Willis* [1968], 33–34. Wood's phrase was taken almost verbatim from Henry Stubbe, *The plus ultra reduced to a non plus* (London, 1670), 95, where Stubbe is attempting to refute Joseph Glanvill's claim of anatomical novelties to be found in Willis's *Cerebri anatome*. Stubbe wrote further that Willis did not lack abilites but that because of his great practice, he did not have leisure to attend the dissections. All that Willis contributed, Stubbe heard, was the "discourses and conjectures" upon Lower's anatomical deductions; these were ingenious, but they were not inventions in the sense that Glanvill wished to claim.

90. Dewhurst, *Willis's Oxford Lectures,* 13.

91. For most of his career, Stubbe was a great admirer of Willis. See for example, his praise for, and use of, Willis's ideas in: *The Indian nectar; or, A discourse concerning chocolata* (London, 1662), dedication to Willis, sigs, a2r-v, whom he calls second only to Harvey, pp. 124–125; *The miraculous conformist* (Oxford, 1666), prefatory epistle to Willis, sigs. A2r-A3v, pp. 14, 18–19, 29; *Legends no histories* (London, 1670), 64–65, 79; *An epistolary discourse concerning phlebotomy* ([London], 1671), 8, 44–48, 110, 114–115, 119, 172–240. Moreover, even in *The plus ultra reduced,* 178, Stubbe was willing to grant that Willis did "propose new matter for improving the discoveries, and put Dr. Lower upon continued investigation, thereby to see if Nature and his Suppositions did accord; and although that many things did occur beyond his apprehension, yet was the grand occasion of that work, and in much the Author." Stubbe had an excellent collection of medical books, which included all the works of Willis and Lower, and many of Boyle's: cf. British Library MS. Sloane 35, ff. 6r, 8r, 9r, 12r–13r, 15r, 16r, 17r–18v, 20r.

92. Lower to Boyle, 18 January 1661[/2], *Works* 6: 462, 463; Lower to Boyle, 4 June 1663, ibid., 467, 468; Lower to Boyle, 24 June 1664, ibid., 470–471.

93. Lower to Boyle, 18 January 1661[/2], ibid., 462, 463.

"we" did. In other circumstances he mentioned times when "I tried an experiment for Dr. *Willis*."[94] On yet other occasions he reported instances of his own dissections and experiments, although these are almost invariably not on the nervous system. Willis and Lower, at least, seem to have been quite clear about the mutually distinct, but symbiotic collaborative roles that they occupied. Willis needed Lower's results and continuing efforts as much as Lower needed Willis's direction, facilities, and literary follow-through. And both needed Wren's drawings, which visualized and encapsulated the highly detailed written description in the text.

It is important to realize this cooperative nature of the *Cerebri anatome*, and to a lesser extent Willis's later work, because such origins explain the recurring puzzlement that commentators have felt when confronted with his books. They are vocal in their praise of the accuracy of the anatomy and the quality of the illustrations, are intrigued by the localizations proposed, are repelled by the fancifulness of the hypothetical mechanisms described, are befuddled by the corpuscular language in which they are expressed, and are bemused by the therapies counseled.[95] It always seems as if Willis is trying to do too much. But if one views Willis's neurological works as products rather of many minds, each with a different forte, then the reason for this synthetic quality becomes clear. Indeed, given the history of small-scale cooperative ventures in research at Oxford, the very model upon which the Royal Society was originally founded, this synthetic quality should be expected.

THE SOUL ON THE DISSECTING TABLE

Thus far I have characterized the biographical trajectory from which Willis's neuroanatomy and neuropsychiatry arose, and the process through which his research program was launched and carried forward within his Oxford circle. What did Willis and his confreres do once they attempted to put the *animus* under the dissecting knife? What were the axioms, the assumptions, the heuristic principles—the *moves*, or *tactics*—through which a new view of brain and soul was worked out? By assumptions or principles, let me reiterate, I do not mean his specific conclusions in neuroanatomy, neurophysiology, or neuropsychiatry, although I will have occasion to look closely—albeit selectively—at these

94. Lower to Boyle, 24 June 1664, ibid., 470.

95. Even one of Willis's admirers, Isler, speaks of "the combination of epoch-making scientific ideas and discoveries with reckless speculation and overt nonsense which is typical of Willis' books" (*Thomas Willis* [1968], 106).

concepts.[96] I mean instead his *ways of reasoning* in order to reach those conclusions. Seldom does Willis set these out explicitly, with a full and clear explanation. They must rather be extracted from his actual processes of reasoning, as they are laid out in his lectures and books.

The first such principle was a methodological one: the initial and seemingly thoroughgoing separation of what later generations would call "mind" into two kinds of soul, the *rational* and the *animal.*[97] Willis took the outline of this distinction most immediately from Gassendi, although he argued that it had also been held by St. Jerome and St. Augustine among the ancients, and Henry Hammond among his own

96. For detailed discussions of one or another aspect of Willis's ideas in neurology and neurophysiology, see the following (arranged chronologically); Jean Vinchon and Jacques Vie, "Un maître de la neuropsychiatrie au XVIIe siècle: Thomas Willis (1662[sic]–1675)," *Annales médico-psychologiques* 86 (1928): 109–144; Donal Sheehan, "Discovery of the Autonomic Nervous System," *Archives of Neurology and Psychiatry* 35 (1936): 1081–1115, especially 1085–1089; Paul F. Cranefield, "A Seventeenth-Century View of Mental Deficiency and Schizophrenia: Thomas Willis on 'Stupidity or Foolishness,'" *Bulletin of the History of Medicine* 35 (1961): 291–316; Raymond Hierons and Alfred Meyer, "Some Priority Questions Arising from Thomas Willis's Work on the Brain," *Proceedings of the Royal Society of Medicine* 55 (1962): 287–292; Alfred Meyer and Raymond Hierons, "A Note on Thomas Willis's Views on the Corpus Striatum and the Internal Capsule," *Journal of the Neurological Sciences* 1 (1964): 547–554; Raymond Hierons and Alfred Meyer, "Willis's Place in the History of Muscle Physiology," *Proceedings of the Royal Society of Medicine* 57 (1964) 687–692; Raymond Hierons and Alfred Meyer, "On Thomas Willis's Concepts of Neurophysiology," *Medical History* 9 (1965): 1–15, 142–155; Edwin Clarke and C. D. O'Malley, *The Human Brain and Spinal Cord* (Berkeley and Los Angeles: University of California Press, 1968), 158–162, 333–390, 388–390, 472–474, 582–585, 636–640, 723–726, 775–779; Isler, *Thomas Willis* [1968], 88–141, 148–182; Kenneth Dewhurst, "Willis and Steno," *Analecta medico-historica* 3 (1968): 43–48; Elvira Aquiola, "La lesion nerviosa en la obra de Th. Willis," *Asclepio* 25 (1973): 65–93; Yvette Conry, "Thomas Willis, ou la premier discours rationaliste en patholgie mentale," *Revue d'histoire des sciences* 31 (1978): 193–231; John D. Spillane, *The Doctrine of the Nerves: Chapters in the History of Neurology* (New York: Oxford University Press, 1981), 53–107; Kenneth Dewhurst, "Thomas Willis and the Foundations of British Neurology," in *Historical Aspects of the Neurosciences,* ed. F. C. Rose and W. F. Bynum (New York: Raven, 1982), 327–346; Adolf Faller, "Die Präparation der weissen Substanz des Gehirns bei Stensen, Willis und Vieussens," *Gesnerus* 39 (1982): 171–193; Richard U. Meier, "'Sympathy' in the Neurophysiology of Thomas Willis," *Clio medica* 17 (1982): 95–111. Hierons and Meyer [1965] has a very full bibliography and provides the best entrée into the older literature on Willis's neuroanatomy and neurophysiology.

97. Although the notion of the corporeal soul was adumbrated partially in the Sedleian lectures, it was not stated clearly until the *Cerebri anatome.* See Dewhurst, *Willis's Oxford Lectures,* 125–129; Willis, *Cerebri anatome,* 133–134, 253; "Anatomy of the brain," 95, 130; Willis, *De anima brutorum,* sig. A2r-v, b1v-b4v, pp. 1–16; *Soul of brutes,* sig. A2v, A3v-A4v, pp. 1–6.

98. Willis, *De anima brutorum,* sig. A2v, pp. 7–8. 115–119; *Soul of brutes,* sig. A2v, pp. 4, 40–42.

contemporaries.[98] According to this distinction, the characteristics of the rational soul were relatively straightforward: it reasoned and judged; it was immortal and possessed by man alone.[99] The animal soul, which he also called the corporeal soul, or *anima brutorum,* was possessed by both man and the animals, and in the case of man was subservient to the rational soul.[100] Logically, the distinction between the two was sharp and clean. In actuality, as we shall see, the corporeal soul came to take on a complexity of meaning and function such as to infringe significantly on the autonomy of the rational soul.

Was this supposition of a corporeal soul merely a ruse, a quasi-Cartesian device to avoid confrontation with church authorities? The very piety of Willis's life should refute any implication of devious intentions. Nor did the church see danger; his three major neurological works, the *Cerebri anatome,* the *Pathologiae cerebri,* and *De anima brutorum,* were dedicated to Sheldon, his good friend, patient, and Archbishop of Canterbury. Each book carried the "Imprimatur" of the highest scholarly and religious official of the University of Oxford, the Vice-Chancellor; in two of these cases, that was Willis's brother-in-law, John Fell. Willis's attachment to the distinction between the rational and the corporeal soul arose rather, I believe, from his pressing desire to see man in a way that squared with his own experience as a clinician and scientist. For years he had looked at patients and seen bodies capable of multifarious derangements, of which the most interesting seemed to stem from the brain. Yet to see most of these functions and dysfunctions as proceeding from the traditional, unitary, soul was repugnant to his belief that anatomy could be pictured in chemical, corpuscular terms and could be manipulated by treatment for the benefit of the patient. Moreover, if one ascribed all human mental phenomena to the rational soul, then diseases of the body could be thought to derange that which was immortal in a human being: his reason and will. This verged on blasphemy. Indeed, Willis felt strongly that the dignity of the rational soul was actually vindicated by believing in its corporeal servant.[101] I am led to conclude that the *anima brutorum,* if it served as a device for any purpose, functioned to give meaning to Willis's integrated life as devout churchman, clinician, and scientist.

Willis conceived the corporeal soul, in its turn, to be composed of two parts: the vital soul lodged in the blood, and the sensitive soul seated in

99. Willis, *De anima brutorum,* sigs. b3v–b4r, pp. 96–99, 110–124; *Soul of brutes,* sig. A4r, pp. 32–33, 38–44.

100. Willis, *De anima brutorum,* 87–109; *Soul of brutes,* 29–38.

101. Willis, *De anima brutorum,* 2; *Soul of brutes,* 2.

the nervous system.[102] For our purposes here we need know about the vital soul only that Willis conceived it as a kind of "flame" in the circulating blood, which was fed by the nitrous, active particles from the air absorbed in respiration. Through a mutual agitation of these nitrous aerial particles with the sulphureous, spirituous, and saline particles of the blood—a process which Willis more and more firmly identified as a "fermentation"—the vital soul generated heat, assimilated digested food, and maintained the body parts.[103] In contradistinction, the sensitive soul consisted of the movement and agitation of particulate animal spirits within the brain and nerves. It was linked to the vital soul because these particles of animal spirits in the nervous system were extracted from the most subtle and active spirits of the blood.[104] The sensitive soul lodged in the nervous system was the part of the corporeal soul most directly subservient to the rational soul, since it was only through the sensitive soul that sensation and movement could take place.

The second implicit axiom of Willis's neurological reasoning related these subtle and active particles of animal spirit to the perceived differences of anatomical texture in the nervous system, and in turn correlated these textural differences with differences in function. Willis emphasized, as few did before him, that the substance of the nervous system was of three distinct types: the gray cortical masses (both cerebral and cerebellar), the white medullary structures, and the long, thin peripheral nerve bundles. He and his collaborators noted the consistent way in which blood vessels encased both cerebral and cerebellar cortices, running inward, and deduced that this first type of texture, cortex, must therefore serve to separate animal spirits from the blood for use by the nervous system.[105] The image that recurred again and again in interpreting this anatomical relationship was the chemical alembic: the cortex "distilled" the finest spirituous particles out of the blood.[106] The second set of neural elements, the deeper, white, medullary structures, whether

102. Willis, *Cerebri anatome,* 133–134; "Anatomy of the brain," 95; Willis, *De anima brutorum,* 9–33, 69–70; *Soul of brutes,* 4–7, 22.

103. The concept of the vital soul was mentioned briefly in *Cerebri anatome,* 133; "Anatomy of the brain," 95, but was not developed fully until *De sanguinis accensione* in 1670, and *De anima brutorum,* 12–72; *Soul of brutes,* 6–23.

104. The sensitive soul seems to have been the first of these linked concepts to emerge in any clarity: Dewhurst, *Willis's Oxford Lectures,* 67, 125–129, 132; Willis, *De anima brutorum,* 72–77; *Soul of brutes,* 23–24.

105. Dewhurst, *Willis's Oxford Lectures,* 63; Willis, *Cerebri anatome,* 109–113, 125–126, 187–194; "Anatomy of the brain," 87–89, 92, 110–113; Willis, *De anima brutorum,* 72; *Soul of brutes,* 23.

106. Willis, *Cerebri anatome,* 83–84; "Anatomy of the brain," 79.

of cerebrum, brain stem, or cerebellum, received the animal spirits and provided the tracts and labyrinths within which these particles exercised their functions.[107] The third part of the nervous system, the peripheral nerve structures such as cranial nerves, spinal nerves, and the nerve plexi linked to the brain, all served as grand highways for the action of the spirits to be propagated over a long distance. Although all three textures of the nervous system were solid, this was no impediment to the movement of subtler particles. They could flow through the liquid/solid matrix that was created by the grosser classes of particles, such as earth and water. Although Willis himself does not use the image, one can visualize the relationship as a stream of water flowing through a solid mass of gravel. Certainly Willis had this picture in mind when he thought of the peripheral nervous system; he had examined cut cross-sections of nerves and always found them solid, but felt that spirits could percolate through the nerve none the less.[108]

The image of spirituous particles residing in a differentiated neural matrix has a link to Willis's third underlying principle of neurological explanation: the belief—one that became more and more explicit through the sequence of his writings—that effects within the nervous system could be carried out by two different, and complementary, kinds of activity, mechanisms that I wish to designate as "particle flow" and as "wave propagation." Although Willis nowhere explains these mechanisms in a systematic way, they were assumed again and again in his explanations of function and dysfunction.

In the first, particle flow, he pictured spirits physically moving, streaming from one part of the nervous system to another. The net movement was from center, where the spirits were generated, to the periphery, where they were slowly consumed in muscular motion.[109] But within this net flow there could be transitory local reversals. What was sleep, Willis asked in his lectures of the early 1660s, but the movement of spirits to their proper places in cerebral and medullary tissues, where they rested; he used an elaborated version of the same explanation a decade later in *De anima brutorum*.[110] This overall flow of particles also

107. Dewhurst, *Willis's Oxford Lectures,* 65–66; Willis, *Cerebri anatome,* 126–130, 153–155; "Anatomy of the brain," 92–94, 101; Willis, *De anima brutorum,* 72–73; *Soul of brutes,* 23.

108. Willis, *Cerebri anatome,* pp. 236–244; "Anatomy of the brain," pp. 125–128.

109. Dewhurst, *Willis's Oxford Lectures,* 54–55, 72; Willis, *Cerebri anatome,* 248–251; "Anatomy of the brain," 129–130; Willis, *Pathologiae cerebri,* 1–21; "Pathology of the brain," 1–12.

110. Dewhurst, *Willis's Oxford Lectures,* 96, 100; Willis, *De anima brutorum,* 234–244; *Soul of brutes,* 87–91.

accounted for how derangements within the blood could eventually make themselves felt in the brain. For example, beginning with his Sedleian lectures, Willis argued quite consistently that hysteria was caused by heterogeneous particles in the blood that infected the animal spirits in the brain with unstable and explosive copula; these wayward particles were then carried through the nerves to muscles and to visceral organs, and rendered the movements of those organs convulsive. He denied that the womb had anything essential to do with hysteria. Indeed, this neural rather than uterine cause for the disease explained why men could suffer it also, and why postmortems showed the wombs of hysterical women to be perfectly normal.[111]

Willis's second mechanism of neural effects, wave propagation, depended equally on the particulate nature of the animal spirits. How, one might ask, were sensations carried so quickly into the brain, and incitements to movement carried so rapidly out to the periphery? Willis solved this problem by proposing that such messages traveled as propagated percussion waves within the fluid mass of particulate animal spirits which, when the brain was active, was maintained at a certain requisite tension. Originally in the lectures the notion appeared simply as a suggestion that spirits in external senses, when agitated by some object, communicated their motion through the nerves to the brain, "just like a stone thrown into a pond causes ripples."[112] But by the *De anima brutorum* the concept had developed into a highly ramified and clever device capable of explicating complex phenomena of touch, hearing, sight, and triggering of muscle contractions.[113] The concept could explain why, although sensation and movement required their own proper end organs, the same nerves, and hence the same animal spirits, could carry out communication between center and periphery; the wave fronts going into and out of the brain passed through each other unimpaired, like intersecting ripples on a pond.[114]

The image of messages coursing through nerves brings us to Willis's fourth working principle: that the remarkable spatial differentiation of the brain must be correlated with an equally deep differentiation of function. Willis clearly conceived of all brains as composed of three parts: 1) the cerebrum, with its underlying medullary mass, which he called the corpus callosum; 2) the medulla oblongata and the spinal

111. Dewhurst, *Willis's Oxford Lectures,* 77–78, 87–91; Willis, *Pathologiae cerebri,* 144–165; "Pathology of the brain," 76–87.

112. Dewhurst, *Willis's Oxford Lectures,* 100.

113. Willis, *De anima brutorum,* 154–165; *Soul of brutes,* 55–60.

114. Willis, *De anima brutorum,* 156; *Soul of brutes,* 56.

marrow; and 3) the cerebellum with its associated structures. His ideas for the functions of these structures, especially the cerebrum and the cerebellum, appeared first in his lectures, and although elaborated in the three subsequent books, did not change greatly. He believed that the cerebrum and its underlying structures served the voluntary functions, especially those of memory and imagination. Memory, being largely a matter of storage, was the province of the cerebral cortex. The huge, seemingly irregular mass of the cortex in man, with its many gyri and sulci—the mounds and recesses—was well suited to the capacious memory and free association of images that was characteristic of humans.[115] The cerebellum, in contrast, had an orderly, determinate, and almost clock-like structure, which would seem to be designed for some function distinct from that of the cerebrum. This function, he concluded, was the supply and direction of animals spirits for involuntary acts, like heartbeat, respiration, and digestion. Therefore the cerebellum had close access to cranial nerves, especially to the vagus, which went out to all parts of the body.[116]

In the elaboration of Willis's ideas on the differing functions of the cerebrum and cerebellum one can see clearly at work a further axiom: that the comparative anatomy of the nervous system could be a powerful tool in explicating its functions.[117] This *anatomia comparata,* as Willis called it in *Cerebri anatome,* was not only a philosophical desideratum but a practical and technical one as well. Human heads were difficult to find. Moreover, the large bulk of the human cerebrum was a hindrance to seeing the true relations of structures. Animals, in contrast, especially the dog, calf, sheep, and hog, made for easier dissections. More important, the study of animal brains threw the essential features of human brains into clear relief.[118] Willis noted, for example, that the shape, size, and laminar structure of the cerebellum was very much the same in many animals. This fitted neatly with the notion that any animal,

115. Dewhurst, *Willis's Oxford Lectures,* 66, 138–143; Willis, *Cerebri anatome,* 123–126; "Anatomy of the brain," 91–93.

116. Dewhurst, *Willis's Oxford Lectures,* 66–67, 102–103, 145–149; Willis, *Cerebri anatome,* 41–48, 176–233; "Anatomy of the brain," 67–69, 108–125; Willis, *De anima brutorum,* 346–348; *Soul of brutes,* 142–143.

117. Willis, *Cerebri anatome,* 3–5; "Anatomy of the brain," 56.

118. Remarks on Willis's use of comparative anatomy are scattered throughout the secondary sources, but see Robert S. Dow, "Thomas Willis (1621–1675) as a Comparative Neurologist," *Annals of Medical History,* 3d series, 2 (1940): 181–184, and especially William F. Bynum, "The Anatomical Method, Natural Theology, and the Functions of the Brain," *Isis* 64 (1973): 444–468, which contains an acute and penetrating analysis of Willis's use of anatomical findings.

whether fish or man, had an irreducible set of involuntary functions that had to be directed by the cerebellum.[119] Conversely the cerebrum. It had many fewer gyri in quadrupeds, indicating less capability for memory and learning. In cats, Willis noted, the cerebral cortex showed a fixed and simple pattern of foldings, which indicated that the animal did not learn easily, remembered little, and lived largely by instincts. In even lesser animals like fowl or fish, the cerebral surface was plain and even, indicating action even more dominated by instinct, and an inability to learn activities of more than one type.[120] A similar kind of argument could be constructed regarding the underlying cerebral medullary parts—all of which Willis comprehended under the term "corpus callosum." They were, he noted, much more highly developed in man. This served to provide ample paths for the movement and interaction of spirits that carried memory, and which thereby gave rise to imagination and appetite.[121]

These kinds of comparative reasoning occurred again and again in Willis's writings. It was a form of argument which was made possible only by accumulating a rich trove of evidence, from which one could then pluck out the specific set of comparisons to make a point. Here Willis could make the fullest use of Lower's talents while they were both at Oxford, and those of his later anatomical collaborators in London: Lower's younger Christ Church contemporary, John Masters, and the more rough-and-ready surgeon, Edmund King. King was one of Willis's favorite consulting surgeons, and Masters was a medical protegé and younger associate much as Lower had been a few years earlier.[122] These latter two provided many of the animal dissections—including those of such invertebrates as an earthworm, oyster, and lobster—that Willis used to bolster his arguments in *De anima brutorum.*[123]

Moreover, the comparative argument was one based firmly in the tradition of natural theology, which was very strong in the Oxford clubs. Again and again in their works, John Wilkins, Robert Boyle, and Willis himself had argued that dissecting a wide range of animals conduced to

119. Dewhurst, *Willis's Oxford Lectures,* 64, 148–149; Willis, *Cerebri anatome,* 74, 181–182, 223–226; "Anatomy of the brain," 76, 109, 122.

120. Dewhurst, *Willis's Oxford Lectures,* 138; Willis, *Cerebri anatome,* 125; "Anatomy of the brain," 92.

121. Dewhurst, *Willis's Oxford Lectures,* 97–98, 134–135; Willis, *De anima brutorum,* 81–82, 249–253; *Soul of brutes,* 26–27, 93–95.

122. Willis, *De anima brutorum,* sig. b4v; *Soul of brutes,* sig. A4v. John Master was about fifteen years younger than Lower: see Foster, *Alumni Oxonienses* 3:986.

123. Willis, *De anima brutorum,* 33–56; *Soul of brutes,* 7–17.

knowing more fully the power and majesty of the Creator.[124] Whether one beheld "a Flea, a Louse, or a Mite" through a microscope, or like Boyle, spent many hours "conversing with dead and stinking Carkases," one had joy "in tracing in those forsaken Mansions, the inimitable Workmanship of the Omniscient Architect."[125]

Willis's use of comparative anatomy to assign functions to the cerebrum and cerebellum illustrates a sixth underlying heuristic principle of Willis's neurology: he tended to explain function as sequential processing—or at the least, sequential action—within the nervous system. Consider, for example, his scheme for the main flow of information between cerebrum and the rest of the body. Sensory impressions—whether they were optic species, sound vibrations, or the sense of touch—were, he thought, carried to the area under the cerebrum that he called the corpora striata. There an inward perception arose. If the impression was carried farther forward into the corpus callosum, then imagination resulted. If the impression went on even farther to the cortex, and impressed its character there, then a memory of that sense impression was created; this memory could be recalled by having the image carried back to the corpus callosum.[126]

In most cases Willis saw this sequential action as corporeal changes taking place under the direction of the rational soul. The particles, in their movements and vibrations, could be guided by will. But in some cases, portions of the chain could be activated without other parts. For example, in an oft-cited passage, Willis remarked that impressions could strike the corpora striata, and cause a reciprocal action of the animal spirits out toward the periphery, without the brain—and therefore consciousness—being aware of it. When we have a pain or irritation in our sleep, we move our hand to it and rub, even though we have no consciousness of the event. Willis was describing what was later to be known as the scratch reflex—a description that contains a better and clearer idea of the general notion of a reflex than the earlier hypothetical

124. On the natural theology of Wilkins and Boyle, see Frank, *Harvey and the Oxford Physiologists,* 56, 93–97; cf. Willis, *Cerebri anatome,* sigs. A3v–a1r; "Anatomy of the brain," [51–52]; Willis, *De anima brutorum,* 98–99; *Soul of brutes,* 34.

125. Matthew Wren, *Monarchy asserted* (London, 1659), sig. A7v-8r, for the quotation about microscopy in the Wilkins group; Robert Boyle, *Some considerations touching the usefulnesse of experimental naturall philosophy* (Oxford, 1663), First Part, Essay I [written c. 1648–1650], 5.

126. Dewhurst, *Willis's Oxford Lectures,* 65–67, 134–135, 138–139; Willis, *Cerebri anatome,* 133–139; "Anatomy of the brain," 95–96; Willis, *De anima brutorum,* 76; *Soul of brutes,* 25.

mechanism of Descartes.[127] Or, he wrote, if an impression was carried beyond the the corpus callosum, striking the cortex, it could raise not only the appropriate memories but associated ones as well, giving rise to fantasies that combine memories in ways not intended by the will.[128]

Both localizations of functions, and determinate processing paths, were in turn grounded in Willis's belief that the nervous system acted only through defined tracts within its solid parts. Such a principle was obviously true in the peripheral nervous system; no message could be carried outside of the clearly delineated nerves that went to muscles in arms and legs. But Willis seems to have felt that a similar principle was true within the brain and spinal cord as well. Beginning with his lectures, he wrote often of the animals spirits "carving out" tracts by their movements, or repetitive actions being caused by spirits flowing along the same paths.[129] This belief had several implications. For one, he could vigorously reject the idea that any path-directed functions could take place in a watery medium. He thereby dismissed out of hand the classical notion that sensation, imagination, and memory could be lodged in the set of ventricles deep within the brain, and therefore in the cerebrospinal fluid with which they were filled.[130] Such a traditional physiological belief was possible when the soul was thought to exercise its functions through unitary and spatially nondifferentiated faculties. But such a scheme could not work when a corporeal soul consisted, as Willis believed it did, in the orderly movement of particles, which had to act in a given place, at a given time. Even assuming that the traditional Galenic localizations in the ventricles had been based on a corpuscular philosophy, such particles within a liquid would not have any constraints upon their motions, so they could not carry out any directed actions. Thus, they could not constitute a soul.

In applying all these principles to construct a picture of the relationship between brain and soul, postmortem examinations occupied an important and interesting, although sometimes anomalous, position. Once he and Lower started their systematic dissections in 1662, Willis was quite anxious to find as many cases as he could in which visible brain

127. Dewhurst, *Willis's Oxford Lectures,* 74, 134; Willis, *Cerebri anatome,* 137; "Anatomy of the brain," 96.

128. Dewhurst, *Willis's Oxford Lectures,* 119, 134–135; Willis, *Cerebri anatome,* 137; "Anatomy of the brain," 96.

129. Dewhurst, *Willis's Oxford Lectures,* 55, 67; Willis, *De anima brutorum,* 72–74, 77; *Soul of brutes,* 23–25.

130. Dewhurst, *Willis's Oxford Lectures,* 139–141; Willis, *Cerebri anatome,* 139–143; "Anatomy of the brain," 96–98; Willis, *De anima brutorum,* 325; *Soul of brutes,* 133.

pathology could be correlated with symptoms, and hence the defective function could be localized. The surviving Sedleian lectures mention about eight such postmortems,[131] and in one letter of Lower to Boyle in mid-1663, he reported the results of four recent ones.[132] More were mentioned in *Cerebri anatome* and *Pathologiae cerebri*, and Willis was most successful in bringing them into *De anima brutorum*. In other words, it seems that the more seriously and precisely he explored the mind/brain interaction, the more he was led to seek confirmation of his speculations in postmortem examinations.

Such evidence was most unequivocal and useful when the findings dealt with the cerebral circulation. In a number of cases, for example, Willis and Lower found an obstructed carotid artery going to the brain. Yet because of the anastomosing ring of arteries at its base, which still goes by the name of the "circle of Willis," the flow of arterial blood to neural tissue had been maintained.[133] Similarly in apoplexy. Although many medical writers attributed such symptoms to an obstruction of blood flow to the brain, Willis could show that the postulated postmortem findings did not always occur.[134]

Postmortems could also be used to show that diseases which Willis believed were neurological, and which traditional medicine attributed to other organs, were not due to the widely reputed causes. Willis opened a "noble gentleman" who was "much afflicted with scurvy," a disease thought to be caused by the spleen. Yet the postmortem showed that organ free from fault, which Willis took to vindicate his own notion that a taint in the blood had been distilled into the nervous juice and thereby been carried throughout the man's system.[135] In his lectures Willis rejected the notion that phrenzy was caused by an inflammation of the meninges, and paraphrenzy by a similar sepsis of the diaphragm. He had, he said, found inflamed meninges in three or four necropsies, and inflamed diaphragms in two, but in all these cases the patients had shown no signs of phrenzy or paraphrenzy during their lifetimes.[136]

The most logically desirable cases—those in which a clear brain lesion correlated with impaired function—were also the hardest to find. In his lectures Willis argued for the corpora striata as the primary sensorium by noting that in those "who suffer or have died from paralysis, I have

131. Dewhurst, *Willis's Oxford Lectures*, 86, 108, 115–116, 120, 141.
132. Lower to Boyle, 4 June 1663, *Works* 6:466–468.
133. Ibid., 467; Willis, *Cerebri anatome*, 95; "Anatomy of the brain," 83.
134. Willis, *De anima brutorum*, 372–391; *Soul of brutes*, 153–161.
135. Willis, *Pathologiae cerebri*, 219; "Pathology of the brain," 177.
136. Dewhurst, *Willis's Oxford Lectures*, 120.

often observed that these corpora are affected: they become flaccid and their striae are almost obliterated."[137] In the *Pathologiae cerebri* he reported opening the body of a gentlewoman who had been troubled with hysterical distempers; the womb seemed faultless, but her nerve plexi—Willis meant here the sympathetic ganglia—appeared pathologic.[138]

Just as pathological findings allowed Willis to deduce the function of a part from its visible malfunctions, so might he and his colleagues have approached the functions of the brain by using experimentation—one investigates the functions of structures by intervening manually to create a new circumstance, even an artificial pathology. Certainly there was no lack of experimental skill in one or another of the Oxford groups; Lower, Boyle, Hooke, and Wren were among the best, as their contemporaneous work on circulation and respiration showed.[139] Yet the only experimental work on the brain that Willis and his coterie carried out was to investigate the cerebral circulation by injecting ink, and other colored materials, into the blood vessels.[140] Why not, one is tempted to ask, test the proposed functions for parts of the brain by performing ablation experiments on animals? Such experiments, performed routinely throughout the nineteenth century, required no technology that could not have been found in seventeenth-century Oxford.[141] But it would have required both a more finely honed set of operative skills, and a laboratory environment in which dozens of such experiments could be carried out, the animals nursed back to health, and the results observed and evaluated in a systematic way. Seventeenth-century physicians, even skilled dissectors like Lower, were not surgeons; and surgeons were not scholars interested in such questions as the functions of various parts of the brain. Nor were back rooms in an Oxford college, or in a prac-

137. Dewhurst, *Willis's Oxford Lectures,* 141; Willis, *Cerebri anatome,* 158–159; "Anatomy of the brain," 102.

138. Willis, *Pathologiae cerebri,* 84; "Pathology of the brain," 45.

139. See Frank, *Harvey and the Oxford Physiologists,* 90–223 passim.

140. Cf. the experiments on cerebral circulation described in Lower to Boyle, 4 June 1663, *Works* 6:467; also the similar experiments in Willis, *Cerebri anatome,* 13–14, 60–63, 94–95; "Anatomy of the brain," 59, 72–73, 82–83. For commentary on the discovery of the circle of Willis, see: Sir Charles Symonds, "The Circle of Willis," *British Medical Journal* (15 January 1955), i, 119–124; Alfred Meyer and Raymond Hierons, "Observations on the History of the 'Circle of Willis,'" *Medical History* 6 (1962): 119–130; Charles N. Swisher, "The Centripetal and Centrifugal History of the Circle of Willis," *McGill Medical Journal* 33 (1964): 110–124.

141. By far the best introduction to experimental techniques of ablation, and what they were capable of revealing, is Max Neuburger, *The Historical Development of Experimental Brain and Spinal Cord Physiology before Flourons,* translated and edited, with additional material, by Edwin Clarke (Baltimore: Johns Hopkins University Press, 1981).

titioner's house, true laboratories. Experimental neurophysiology had in large part to wait for the time of men like Magendie and his successors, skilled operators within institutional settings where they did not have to squeeze their science into the odd or slack moments of a practitioner's career.

Finally, I should like to point out the very noteworthy way in which Willis systematically attempted to convert diseases that had long been thought to be caused by the blood, viscera, or even supernatural agents, into diseases of the nervous system. Hysteria, hypochondria, headache, lethargy, somnolency, coma, nightmare, vertigo, apoplexy, paralysis, delerium, phrenzy, melancholy, mania, foolishness, epilepsy and a wide array of convulsive diseases, even gout, scurvy, and colic—all were seen by Willis as diseases of the nervous system. For each he constructed an explanation using the assumptions and heuristic principles that I have tried to tease out in the foregoing pages. On each he brought to bear his collection of case descriptions and—especially in the later works—recommended medicaments. In a very real sense, this last of Willis's intellectual tactics brought him back full circle, back to the concerns of practical medicine with which he had begun his career as a young physician of twenty-four.

The foregoing list of approaches and assumptions could quite easily be expanded to include a half a dozen more, each used by Willis in an idiosyncratic and creative way to construct his own explanations of brain function. It is worth reviewing the ones I have chosen to illuminate, just to see how powerful and attractive they are: the concept of the corporeal soul, divided between its vital and sensitive functions; the assignment of different categories of functions to different neural textures; the proposed mechanisms of communication within the nervous system both by particle flow and wave propagation; the concept that spatial differentiations were correlated with functional differences, especially a division between voluntary and involuntary functions; the clever use of comparative anatomy; the conceptual device of sequential processing; the assumption of defined tracts within the brain; the multifaceted use of postmortem findings; and the way in which he orchestrated all of these to bring large numbers of disease states into the neurological orbit. In his intellectual bag of tricks, Willis had more than enough tools to fit together the collection of evidence in the way that he wanted.

Within his own particular circle of natural philosophers in Oxford, such a synthetic approach was appreciated by physicians and nonphysicians alike. In 1666 Samuel Parker, a close friend of Ralph Bathurst, managed to work into such an unlikely topic as the preexistence of souls an account of Willis's findings on the linkage of brain and heart via the intercostal nerves.[142] Robert Sharrock, in a sermon on the resurrection, digressed to discuss Willis's neurological theories, especially the functions of the corpus striatum and the corpus callosum.[143] Beyond Oxford, Willis's books were touted in the Europe-wide correspondence of Henry Oldenburg,[144] and extolled in reviews in his newly founded *Philosophical Transactions,* the world's first scientific journal.[145]

But I suspect that after Willis's death in 1675, and those of his colleagues in the 1680s and 1690s, Willis's books exerted their direct effects primarily upon doctors. They were, after all, fundamentally anatomical works, unlikely to draw the casual attention of the gentleman, litterateur, or academic philosopher. They contain a massive amount of detail, and a plethora of conjectural mechanisms that the passage of time might easily render suspect. Hence, I would venture, their relative lack of prominence in nonmedical writings. Willis—then, as now—was a writer whose reputation was greatest among those whose professional or technical backgrounds most fitted them to understand the details that he tried to synthesize.

There is, however, an indirect route through which Willis's influence may have been carried forward well into the late eighteenth century. In a widely read article, G. S. Rousseau has suggested not only that Willis's findings served as an important background source for Locke's *Essay concerning human understanding* but that his assumption of sensory phenomena delimited to the brain and nerves was, as filtered through Locke, an important trope in the development of the fiction of sensibility

142. Samuel Parker, *A free and impartial censure of the Platonick philosophie,* 2d ed. (Oxford, 1667), 194–195.

143. Robert Sharrock, *De finibus virtutis Christianae* (Oxford, 1673), 114–115.

144. From 1659 to 1674 Oldenburg recommended Willis's books to savants such as Pierre Borel, Samuel Sorbiere, Henri Justel, Adrien Auzout, and Jean Baptiste Duhamel in France, Christiaan Huygens in the Netherlands, Johann Hevelius, Johann Michaelis, and Martin Vogel in Germany, Erasmus Bartholin in Denmark, and John Finch, Lorenzo Magalotti, Marcello Malpighi, and Francesco Travagino in Italy; in some cases he even arranged to send on copies. See A. Rupert Hall and Marie Boas Hall, eds. and trans., *The Correspondence of Henry Oldenburg,* 13 vols. (Madison, Wis., and London: [various publishers], 1965–1986), 1:225–227, 230–231, 240–242, 266–267, 355; 2:142–143, 301–305, 632; 4:135–137, 148–149, 173–174, 537–539; 8:17–20, 168–170, 430, 529–531, 548–549; 9:36–39, 108–109, 499–500; 10:6–8, 283–284, 296–297, 337, 432, 540–541.

145. Willis's *Diatribae duae* and *Cerebri anatome* appeared before the *Philosophical transactions* was started by Oldenburg in March 1665. *Pathologiae cerebri* was reviewed in *Philosophical transactions* 2 (6 January 1667/8): 600–602; *Affectionum,* ibid. 5 (25 March 1670): 1178; and *De anima brutorum,* ibid. 7 (20 May 1672); 4071–4073.

and sentiment within English literature from the time of Samuel Richardson in the 1740s.[146] It is a fascinating insight that is still, to my knowledge, unexplored—perhaps because it falls between the stools of the literary historian, the medical historian, and the historian of philosophy.

MEDICINE, MATTER, SOUL, AND BRAIN

I have focused my attention upon the origins of Willis's neurological oeuvre. In looking at that body of work from three different perspectives—biographical, social/institutional, and intellectual—I have tried to distinguish those elements in each picture that most account for the peculiar ensemble of characteristics that his neurological writings ended up displaying. Mine is an activity akin to that of some scientists who study the nervous system itself. Twentieth-century neuroanatomy and neurophysiology have come to see the brain as an amalgam of structures and functions, accreted by evolution over hundreds of millions of years: a mammalian brain is layered upon a reptilian brain, upon which in turn has overgrown a primate and human brain. Much about that human brain and its action can be learned, it is believed, by probing those structures and functions that lie hidden both by the depths of neural space and the continuum of evolutionary time. So does a developmental, or "genetic" (in the old sense of that word), explanation tell us much about Willis's work.

His elaborate system of facts and ideas was clearly driven by medicine. Willis's clinical practice provided him with the basic conundrums that had to be solved. Solve them he did, at great length and, seemingly, to the satisfaction—or at least stimulation—of the physicians of his own and succeeding generations. Moreover, I would argue, it was the very richness of that experience that forced him to conceive of more and more of the mind's functions in neural terms. For a philosopher, it was relatively easy to conjure with terms such as "reason," "judgment," "passion," "sensation," or "volition," because a philosopher need take into account only his own introspective experience, and the rationalized accounts of other individuals' similar introspective experience. He has a purified universe of normal phenomena with which to deal. Not so the physician. Because the clinician must cope with derangements, the

146. G. S. Rousseau, "Nerves, Spirits, and Fibres: Towards Defining the Origins of Sensibility," in *Studies in the Eighteenth Century, III: Papers Presented at the Third David Nichol Smith Memorial Seminar, Canberra, 1973,* ed. R. F. Brissenden and J. C. Eade (Toronto and Buffalo: University of Toronto Press, 1976), 137–157; reprinted with a postscript in *The Blue Guitar* (Messina) 2 (1976): 125–153.

pathological rather than the normal, his universe of phenomena is in no way so delimited. Every neurological or psychiatric patient is beyond the normal in his or her own particular way. Moreover, the doctor must react to these derangements, and not merely just study them. To react, he must have reasons for his therapies. And to have reasons, he must believe that the processes he treats exist in an objective and deterministic way. Willis's hundreds of pages of conjectural mechanisms provided that basis for the clinician. Indeed, they were intended to do so; both the *Pathologiae cerebri* and the *De anima brutorum* were consciously arranged so that, after the anatomical and physiological explanations of each disease, there were almost interminable discussions of useful therapies and recommended medicaments.

Such a system of medicine was bound together by Willis's picture of the nervous system seen in corpuscular and chemical terms. I use the term "picture" advisedly, because Willis seems to have had an extraordinarily visual apprehension of the conjectural mechanisms he spun out at such great length. He could almost see the particles of spirit, sulphur, and salt arrayed through nerve tracts, combining and disjoining, migrating and percussing. His intense interest in practical chemistry had, over the years, created in him an intellectual eye that really saw what his own biological ones could not. The fact that his matter-theory was both chemical and corpuscular made this possible. When needed, he could conceive of "heterogeneous copula" that gave rise to convulsions or fantasies, and whose atoms had real, and differing properties, from a similar copula made up of other sorts of atoms. Classes of matter could be seen as having inherent chemical properties and resultant forms of action. Conversely, when he needed his particles to act like so many billiard balls as they transmitted an impulse up or down a nerve, that property of mere mass and incompressibility was also open to him. The two sides of corpuscular chemistry not only met the methodological desiderata of fashionable philosophy but squared with the diversity and reality of those messy, colorful, smelly, and indisputably real properties of substances that the kitchen chemist could pulverize, mix, melt, crystallize, sublime, distill, and otherwise manipulate with his own very dirty hands.

The initial outline of conceptual categories that bound together brain and mental phenomena was taken from Scholastic philosophy. The notion of sites for perception, imagination, memory, and the concept of the common sensorium that mediated them, were standard issue in early-seventeenth-century Oxford. Willis knew them and had been trained up on them—the more so since he was originally destined for the church, and completed much of his preparation for that career at a time before political ideology and philosophical innovation called Scholastic philsophy into doubt. But by temperament he was no philosopher. Speculator, yes; metaphysician, no. Only the impetus of standing in the Natural Philosophy room in the Schools Quadrangle twice a week, and having to say something about the soul, forced him to do so in a way that was consistent with his clinical background and chemical beliefs. He could elaborate a vision of the soul—or rather of many souls—that had probably been gestating through the 1650s, when he was both toiling physician and clandestine high churchman.

But speculation, if it was not to be "poetical philosophy," had limits. Willis knew already the boundaries imposed by clinical experience and chemical/corpuscular matter-theory. He had still to seek the limits imposed by anatomy. To find them, he had to use hands other than his own. Whereas Willis took the lead in clinical experience and chemical expertise, Lower did so in sheer anatomical exuberance. He reveled in the messy details of human and animal structure in a way unexcelled in the Europe of his time, much less in Oxford. Lower could do so because he had neither extensive practice, nor chemical agenda, nor systematizing incentives or inclinations—the very elements that were to give organization and structure to the multitudinous facts that his knife laid bare. It was Lower's anatomy that provided the basis for that handful of clever ways in which Willis, using this device and that, one trick now and yet a different one later, constructed a system of relations between brain and mental phenomena.

In the scientific terms of the late twentieth century, almost all of those detailed constructions end up being judged wrong. In standard accounts, Willis is remembered for his positive contributions to neuroanatomy, not for his "fantasies" about how the brain worked. Yet his ideas are "wrong" in ways which, to me as a historian, are highly appealing. They are beguiling because, once one digs down under the particular explanations of particular diseases or functions, one sees at work a person capable of coordinating large amounts of detailed information, while trying to find general patterns in the chaos.

In the end, Willis is appealing because most of all he wanted to *understand.* He wanted to feel that when he saw a patient in hysteria, or participated in a postmortem, or discussed an animal dissection, or performed a chemical experiment, he was seeing simply different aspects of the same unified world. Not for him the more limited and austere satisfaction of knowing merely that he had contributed some small part to knowledge. Willis, like so many other thinkers in the seventeenth century, wanted to encompass a total set of explanations. He started from a position of differentiating sharply between the independent rational soul and the corporeal soul. Yet by the time he was through, he had explored a multitude of ways in which perception, apprehension, understanding, memory, and their relations to the entire body, were dependent in seemingly most complex ways upon that body itself, and preeminently upon its nervous system. The rational soul, by contrast, remained that aloof and—at least in Willis's thought—undifferentiated piece of internal immortality, almost completely and sometimes even woefully dependent upon the environment of information and preconditions created for it by the nervous system. Indeed, when one started with clinical experience, seasoned it with a large portion of corpuscular chemistry, and mixed it with generous quantities of anatomical inquiry, it would be hard to imagine any other outcome.

Yet for all its mistakes in retrospect, Willis's system was a concoction with great appeal to the medical practitioners of succeeding generations, precisely because of this mixture. He has been condemned by some twentieth-century psychologists for having so firmly started medicine down the road of seeking behavioral explanations in neurological terms. But perhaps that was exactly what the early modern physician felt he most needed. And before one dismisses such medical influence as trivial, it is well to remember that in the Enlightenment, as even today, it was the physician, not the philosopher or litterateur, who was confronted almost daily with practical problems in the relations of body and "mind." In many ways, Anthony Wood spoke on Willis an epitaph of more complex meaning than he knew, when he wrote:

> When at any time he is mention'd by authors (as he is very often) it is done in words expressing their high esteem for his great worth and excellency, and placed still, as first in rank, among physicians. And further also, he hath laid a lasting foundation of a body of physic chiefly on hypotheses of his own framing.[147]

147. Wood, *Athenae*, vol. 3, col. 1051.

FIVE

Running Out of Matter: The Body Exercised in Eighteenth-Century Fiction

Carol Houlihan Flynn

To save Samuel Richardson from his hypochondriac tendency "to Rotundity and Liquor," the tireless and by now notorious Dr. George Cheyne prescribed a wonderful machine called "a chamber horse." Actually a chair "set on a long board, which must have acted like a joggling board, supported at both ends and limber in the middle, with hoops to brace the arms and a footstool to support the feet," the horse promised "all the good and beneficial Effects of a hard Trotting Horse except the fresh Air." Since the horse "rides double better than single," Cheyne suggested that Richardson hire "an Amenuensis and dictate to him riding on the new Chamber Horse."[1] The image of plump Richardson, that sentimental traveler of the imagination, jogging cautiously back and forth in a motion designed to get precisely nowhere is a fascinating one.

1. T. C. Duncan Eaves and Ben D. Kimpel, *Samuel Richardson: A Biography* (Oxford: Oxford University Press, 1971), 63–64; *The Letters of Doctor George Cheyne to Samuel Richardson* (1733–43), ed. Charles F. Mullett (Columbia, Mo., 1943), 26–27. In "Mysticism and Millenarianism: The 'Immortal Dr. Cheyne,'" in *Millenarianism and Messianism in English Literature and Thought, 1650–1800*, ed. Richard Popkin (Leiden: Brill, 1988), 81–126, G. S. Rousseau considers the shape of Cheyne's life as England's leading "nerve doctor" in light of his millenarian and mystical activities. Lester King finds Cheyne to be the "Mirror of Eighteenth-Century Medicine," in the *Bulletin of the History of Medicine* 48 (1974): 517–539.

I would like to thank Sheila Emerson, Miriam Hansen, Peter Linebaugh, Felicity Nussbaum, and Claude Rawson for their readings of this essay. Richard Wolfe and his staff at the Countway Library, Harvard Medical School were especially helpful to me. I am particularly grateful to George Rousseau for his careful interest in this subject, and his bibliographic and critical advice.

The chamber horse, a most material hobbyhorse designed to exercise the all too solid flesh as well as the "hyppish," depressed spirits, would appear to be just the thing to satisfy the writer's need to escape from himself. ("As to my health," he confessed in a letter, "I write, I do anything I am able to do on purpose to carry myself out of myself; and am not quite so happy, when, tired with my peregrinations, I am obliged to return home.")[2] The exercise would also provide a physical stimulation, a pleasant sensation accompanying the imaginary peregrinations. As Francis Fuller, a passionate advocate of the "Power of Exercise," noted, riding increases the velocity of circulation and exalts the spirits while it "gives the Solid and Nervous Parts a grateful Sensation, which in some cases is not contemptible," as well as a "Sence of Tingling and Heat."[3]

Cheyne also recommended an "imaginary" vehicle to exercise Richardson's generally low spirits. Since Richardson was a "hyp" who exacerbated his physical disorders by worrying, he needed a "hobbyhorse" to occupy and divert his tortured mind. Diversion, mental as well as physical, was essential to the treatment of nervous disorders. "It seems to be absolutely impossible," Cheyne argued in *The English Malady,* "without such a Help, to keep the Mind easy, and prevent its wearing out the Body, as the Sword does the Scabbard; it is no matter what it is, provided it be but a *Hobby Horse,* and an Amusement, and stop the Current of Reflexion and intense Thinking, which Persons of weak Nerves are aptest to run into."[4]

2. *Correspondence of Samuel Richardson,* ed. Anna Laetitia Barbauld (London, 1804), 3: 190–191.

3. Francis Fuller, *Medicina Gymnastica: or, A Treatise Concerning the power of Exercise, with Respect to the Animal Oeconomy; and the Great Necessity of it in the Cure of Several Distempers* (London, 1705), 43–44, 260. Fuller's book went through nine editions by 1777. Addison recommends him in *The Spectator,* no. 115, 12 July 1711 (ed. Donald F. Bond [Oxford, 1965], 1: 473–474), for his description of the mechanical effects of riding, adding that "for my own part, when I am in Town, for want of these Opportunities, I exercise my self an Hour every Morning upon a dumb Bell that is placed in a Corner of my Room, and it pleases me the more because it does every thing I require of it in the most profound Silence." George Cheyne mentions Fuller in *The English Malady; or, A Treatise of Nervous Diseases of All Kinds* (London, 1733), 176.

4. *The English Malady,* 181–182. Cheyne is using the word "hobbyhorse" to denote "a favorite pursuit or pastime," but the word itself also suggests more literal, physical play as "a stick with a horse's head which children bestride as a toy horse" and as the figure of a horse employed in morris dancing or on the stage. The word was also used throughout the seventeenth century to suggest foolish, wanton, and lustful behavior, and connoted wanton prostitution (see the *Oxford English Dictionary*). Michael DePorte, in *Nightmares and Hobbyhorses: Swift, Sterne, and Augustan Ideas of Madness* (San Marino, Calif.: Huntington Library, 1974) writes at length on the idea of the hobbyhorse.

Cheyne's faith in both machines, material and imaginary, testifies to a widespread interest in the ways body and spirit intersect. While investigating the possibility of treating disorders of the soul mechanically and externally, writers against the spleen approached the body as a physical space affected by a spirit in need of diversion. Cheyne and his numerous medical colleagues set out to treat a disease known as the English Malady, that psychosomatic disorder also known as the Hypochondriack Disease, the Hyp, Hysteria, Melancholy, and the Spleen.[5] Their theories, however, had significant implications not only for medical and psychiatric practitioners but for creative writers in the process of developing the novel. Medical theorists and early English novelists were committed in their different ways to sustaining, and at times inventing, modes of feeling to sustain vitality and to cheat, if not conquer, death.

Writers against the spleen concentrate on the necessity for provocation, stimulation, and diversion in their ironically fatal battles against closure. In his recent study of narrative "design and intention," Peter Brooks argues that "plot is the internal logic of the discourse of mortality." Like so many commentators on the novel form, Brooks prefers to begin his studies with the "golden age of narrative," when "the advent of Romanticism and its predominantly historical imagination"[6] ex-

5. An early helpful survey of literature of melancholy is C. A. Moore's "The English Malady," in *Backgrounds of English Literature, 1700–1760* (Minneapolis: University of Minnesota Press, 1953), 179–235. L. J. Rather provides an excellent discussion of the idea of hypochondria in *Mind and Body in Eighteenth-Century Medicine: A Study Based on Jerome Gaub's De Regimine Mentis* (London, 1965). In his edition of John Hill's *Hypochondriasis: A Practical Treatise on the Hypo* (London, 1776; reprint, Los Angeles: William Andrews Clark Memorial Library, University of California, 1969, as no. 135 of the Publications of the Augustan Reprint Society), George Rousseau provides a useful introduction to the melancholy disease and makes significant connections between "nerves" and the discourses of sensibility in "Nerves, Spirits, and Fibres: Towards Defining the Origins of Sensibility," in *Studies in the Eighteenth Century, III,* ed. R. F. Brissenden and J. C. Eade (Toronto and Buffalo: University of Toronto Press, 1976. Reprinted in *The Blue Guitar* (Messina) 2 (1976): 125–153; continued by Rousseau's invaluable theoretical study of "Discourses of the Nerve," in *Literature and Science as Modes of Expression,* ed. Frederick Amrine (Dordrecht: Kluwer, 1989), 29–60. John Mullan productively discusses the relationship between melancholy and the cult of sensibility in "Hypochondria and Hysteria: Sensibility and the Physicians," *The Eighteenth Century: Theory and Interpretation* 25 no. 2 (1984): 141–177.

6. Peter Brooks, *Reading for the Plot: Design and Intention in Narrative* (New York: Alfred Knopf, 1984), 22, xii. Swift proleptically treats the "modern" condition of the writer who cannot stop writing in *A Tale of a Tub,* where his hack confesses to be "now trying an Experiment very frequent among Modern Authors; which is, to *write upon Nothing;* When the Subject is utterly exhausted, to let the Pen still move on; by some called, the Ghost of Wit, delighting to walk after the Death of its Body. And to say the Truth, there seems to be no Part of Knowledge in fewer Hands, than That of Discerning *when to have*

pressed itself through relatively well made plots. By determining the nineteenth-century novel with its emphatic devotion to regularized form as the model, the critic can then read into the twentieth century's suspicion of plot and its short-circuiting of the satisfying ending a tragicomic progress toward the modern condition. A reading of the eighteenth-century novel, however, makes such an analysis highly problematic, for from the start, the novel resisted the sort of determinancy, the "sense of an ending" modernists like to depart from.

Early novelists, like medical writers against the spleen, were searching for ways to come to terms with a mortality becoming all too pressing in a secularized world. While the medical therapists warn against the dangers of solidification, for to allow one's juices to grow stiff and solid is to harden into death itself, the writers of fiction resist ending their narratives, often fictionalized peregrinations, with digressions, anachronistic disruptions, parodic tailpieces that turn upon themselves, and metaleptic misspellings. In novels and treatises alike, their authors frequently locate themselves in their texts as sufferers of the malady they are trying to control; indeed, the writing becomes the cure as long as it goes on. And since to end it is textually, and sometimes literally, to die, writers against the spleen are most reluctant to lay down their pens. Sterne most notoriously refuses to end his *Sentimental Journey,* which doesn't even get his narrator to Italy and collapses his *Life and Opinions of Tristram Shandy* into a "COCK and a BULL," but he merely exaggerates a tendency for strategic digression shared by his less obvious colleagues. Cheyne issues and reissues compulsive directives designed to alter most radically his reader's diet, Nicholas Robinson rewrites his prescription against consumption to cure the spleen, while Smollett resumes his adventures of picaresque Ferdinand Count Fathom within the sentimental pages of *Humphry Clinker.* Richardson, when not astride his hobbyhorse, writes and rewrites the longest works of fiction in his language, taking each new edition of his novels as an occasion to "improve" most compulsively novels that by virtue of their fluid state never really end.

Done. . . . The Conclusion of a Treatise, resembles the Conclusion of Human Life, which hath sometimes been compared to the End of a Feast; where few are satisfied to depart." Not ready to leave his reader, Swift's writer will only agree to "pause awhile, till I find, by feeling the World's Pulse, and my own, that it will be of absolute Necessity for us both, to resume my Pen" (ed. A. C. Guthkelch and D. N. Smith [New York, 1968], 208, 210). The classic "modern" discussion of closure can be found in Frank Kermode, *The Sense of an Ending* (Oxford: Oxford University Press, 1966). More to the point of the "providentially patterned" eighteenth-century novel is Melvyn New's "'The Grease of God': The Form of Eighteenth-Century Fiction," *PMLA* 91, no. 2 (1976): 235–243.

This essay will first examine the protean nature of "the Spleen" itself, both organ and condition, and follow this exploration with a discussion of the therapeutic "Power of Exercise" so celebrated by most writers on the spleen. I will then consider in some detail the significance of mental and physical exercises in the work of Smollett and Sterne, while intimating the broader theoretical implications of their literary attempts to run, jump, and swing out of matter. Usually regarded as formidable opposites, the splenetic Dr. Smelfungus provoking sentimental Yorick into postures of sweet benevolence, they both address the same problem, the dilemma of the spirit being contained by matter that will inevitably betray. Their narrative strategies are designed to frustrate the logical end of their discourse, fictional closure that represents physical death. Since both writers suffered from the same fatal condition, consumption, their attempts to run out of matter take on an urgency less obviously shared by their contemporaries. Attempting to escape the logic of plot, they pushed metaphors into a reality charged with an all-too-understandable desire.

In his *Essay of Health and Long Life,* George Cheyne announces "The *Grand Secret* and Sole Mean of Long Life." It is

> to keep the Blood and Juices in a due State of Thinness and *Fluidity,* whereby they may be able to make those Rounds and Circulations through the animal Fibres wherein Life and Health consist, with the fewest Rubs and least Resistance that may be.

Unfortunately, Cheyne complains, in spite of all effort, in a process "*Mechanical* and *Necessary,*"

> Time and Age will *fix* and *stiffen* our *Solids.* Our original Frame and Make renders this unavoidable and necessary. As in the greater World, the Quantity of the Fluids is Daily lessening and decreasing; so in our *lesser* World after a limited Time, the Appetite and Concoctions failing, the *Fluids* are lessened and spent on the continual Repairs of the Solids, and thereby lose their Nature, and become firm and hard.[7]

Cheyne's model man, contained by the limitations of his own frame, is a familiar one to readers of eighteenth-century medical texts. Radical practitioners would try to revitalize the fluids themselves through blood transfusions. In his *History of Health and the Art of Preserving It,* James MacKenzie reports tales of "old, decrepid and deaf animals" that "had their hearing, and the agility of their limbs, restored by the transfusions

7. George Cheyne, *An Essay of Health and Long Life* (London, 1724), 220–221.

of young and healthy blood into their veins," and cites the cure of a young man "of an uncommon lethargy" restored to health by the blood of a lamb. Another thirty-four-year-old man was cured "of an inveterate and raging phrenzy" by transfusions of calves' blood, but when the bowels of Baron Bond, son to the first Minister of State in Sweden, mortified after a transfusion, MacKenzie's enthusiasm dwindles. Let us cheerfully submit to "that happy state for which we were originally intended," he suggests, echoing the necessarily philosophical conclusions other physicians were drawing. In his attempt to understand the "hardening process," Claude-Nicolas Le Cat decided that our growth turned inward. The only way to escape solidification would be to continue to grow outward, becoming in the process a giant. It is growth itself, Marat acknowledged, that destroys life.

It is one thing to be philosophical, to shrug with grudging acceptance at the wisdom of Buffon's aphorism that "La vie est un minotaure . . . elle devore l'organisme,"[8] but it is another thing entirely to be human—that organism being devoured. All the while medical writers chasten themselves for seeking relief from their impossible condition, they tend to play, nonetheless, at improving it. To do this effectively, they need the proper material, a place that allows room for at least imaginary relief. The spleen provided just the place: that shadowy mysterious organ with no obvious function offering a locus of anxiety and of hope, a place both real and unreal to theorize over, a place to exercise the imagination. The spleen's significance depends upon its obscurity, its subtle texture "remote not only from the Senses but likewise from the Reach of human Understanding . . . Eternally hid[den] from us."[9] Just this obscured quality lends to the subject of melancholy its fascination. Its remote inaccessibility creates poetic license for fantastic speculations about the true nature of the cave of the spleen. Not until the time of Freud's unconscious would a place both imaginary and real receive such attention.

Bernard Mandeville, a physician as well as moral philosopher, is most blunt about the instability of the "meaning" of the spleen in his *Treatise on Hypochondria*. His dialogue format opens up his discourse to the con-

8. James MacKenzie, *The History of Health and the Art of Preserving It* (Edinburgh, 1758), 432–436; John McManners, *Death and the Enlightenment* (Oxford: Oxford University Press, 1981), 113–114. Gerald J. Gruman discusses the century's interest in blood transfusions in *A History of Ideas about the Prolongation of Life: The Evolution of Prolongevity Hypotheses*, Transactions of the American Philosophical Society, vol. 56, pt. 9 (Philadelphia, 1966), 82–83.

9. B. Mandeville, M. D., *A Treatise of the Hypochondriack and Hysterick Diseases in Three Dialogues*, 3d ed. (London, 1730; 1st ed. 1711), v.

tradictory opinions about a disease that he purports to treat. Thus, when his melancholy sufferer Misomedon, inspired by the works of Thomas Willis, compares his model of the body to a still that "exalts in the nature of a Ferment" the earthy and muddy part of the blood that must be "cooked" in the spleen before it rises to circulate, his physician Philopiro listens to his theory only to deride it. "These *Similes* . . . are very diverting for People that have nothing else to do," he sneers. "We are altogether in the Dark, as to the real use" of the spleen, he argues, quite sensibly, but then contradicts his skepticism by offering his own rather poetic theory of animal spirits to explain Misomedon's attacks of hypochondria. Nimble, volatile messengers "fly through all the *Mazes* and *Meanders*" and "beat through all the Paths, and hunt every Enclosure of the Brain in quest of the images we want." Philopiro can almost feel their labors as he calls them up in his own imagination, those obliging sylphs darting between mind and body sometimes bewildered in the search until they light by chance upon the looked-for image. Overly active spirits produce too much cogitation, causing scholarly melancholia and a bad case of indigestion.

Philopiro's airy discourse irritates Misomedon, who reminds his doctor that animal spirits are just as metaphoric as his own disparaged model of the body and as Willis's still. Hedging at first, arguing that their existence has never been "controverted," Philopiro suddenly gives up his argument by acknowledging that truth is not the point. The animal spirits are not necessary "real," but they are useful metaphorically "to express the Instruments of Motion and Sense." As long as the body guards its secrets, the abstraction of body can be manipulated through a discourse that actually depends upon speculation and ambiguity.[10]

Just this ambiguity complicates medical treatment of a condition both imaginary and real. The disease manifests itself physically in palpably understood symptoms; yet these symptoms, also attributed to the mind, become part of a larger system that defines its sufferer's idea of his or

10. Mandeville, *Treatise*, 95–98, 115, 136, 160–162. In *Ideas of Life and Matter: Studies in the History of General Physiology* (Chicago: University of Chicago Press, 1969), Thomas Hall discusses Thomas Willis's idea of "Life as a Subjugated Flame" (1: 312–325). Cheyne expresses a similar, rather pragmatic skepticism about the existence of the animal spirits in *The English Malady*, seeming to dismiss the likelihood of their being more than an idea based upon "the readiest Resemblance the *Lazy* could find to explain *Muscular Motion by*. . . . On such a slender and imaginary Similitude, the Precarious *Hypothesis* of *Animal Spirits* seems to be built." Cheyne ultimately suggests that "the Notion of *animal Spirits* is of the same Leaven with the *substantial Forms* of *Aristotle*, and the *coelestial System* of *Ptolemy*" (74–75, 85).

her culture. The spleen becomes for the eighteenth century the inevitable disease resulting from the complexities of urban, "civilized" life that literally makes people sick. It becomes part of the neurotic discontent Freud would find impossible to disconnect from the civilization he would not be able to live without. Even as he enumerates the pains of London, that "greatest, most capacious, close, and populous City of the *Globe,*" stinking with the "Ordure of so many diseased, both intelligent and unintelligent Animals; the crouded Churches, Church-yards and Burying-places, with putrifying Bodies, the *Sinks, Butcher-Houses, Stables, Dunghils, & c.,*" Cheyne nonetheless depends upon the impossible system that makes his profession necessary. As he observes, it was, after all, the luxury and disease of the Egyptians, Greeks, and Romans that provoked them to study sacred Physick to remedy their own evils. Once a people cultivate the polite and ingenious arts, they follow by developing "Physick to any tolerable Degree of Perfection" to cure their most civilized ills.

Melancholy becomes therefore a responsibility, but also a privilege, a sign of the status of its sufferer. It is not even clear that melancholy can—or should—be resisted. "Virtue and Happiness are literally and really Cause and Effect,"[11] Cheyne remarks, suggesting that health is something the gentle reader can achieve through labor and learning. Yet ironically, most treatises insist upon the over-determined nature of the melancholy "type." Lively, quick-witted, acutely sensitive, profoundly obsessive sufferers of the spleen are cursed with imaginations that certify their worth. Even while the reader is exhorted to break out of the splenetic condition, the end result, health, looks at best dull and unattractive. Naturally "healthy" people are the laborers, the poor, doltish owners of "callous" organs of sensation, "*Ideots, Peasants* and *Mechanicks,*" incapable of wit.[12] "Slow and heavy thinking" secures "drowsy thick-scull'd Fellows . . . from becoming hypochondriacal, as those, who cannot Write, from being pillory'd for Counterfeiting other People's Hands,"[13] Mandeville suggests, making melancholy a condition as natural and as personal as one's signature, a privileged symbol of class. To lose the morbid sensitivity in question is to lose a certificate of worth. Cheyne, celebrating his own delicate sensibility, wonders how "One shall suffer more from the Prick of a *Pin,* or Needle, from their extreme Sensibility, than others from being run thro' the Body; and the *first* Sort,

11. Cheyne, *The English Malady,* 55–56, 26.
12. Cheyne, *Essay of Health and Long Life,* 160.
13. Mandeville, *Treatise,* 237–238.

seem to be of the *Class* of . . . *Quick-Thinkers*." More ominously, he believes that "some rational Creatures" of the hardy variety "would suffer less in being finely butcher'd than a strong *Ox*, or *red Deer*."[14]

Cheyne, particularly, in tract after tract, edition after edition, seems dedicated to dwell on the condition that he resists yet calls up each time he describes it. His own personal story, "The Case of the Author," borders on farce as he painstakingly describes his own fall into and out of varying degrees of health always precarious. Cheyne's narrative violently alternates between complacency and self-loathing as his body "swell'd to an enormous size" when it was not "melting away like a *Snow-ball* in Summer." Cheyne seems driven to illustrate the irremediable nature of a body he is still determined to cure as he keeps trying to find an impossible balance between states of excess. Wasted away by fever, he suffers from an appetite so insatiable that "I suck'd up and retained the *Juices* and *Chyle* of My Food like a *Sponge*," growing in the process "*plump, fat*, and *hale* to a wonder; but indeed too fast." An "extreme Case," Cheyne balloons up at one point to over thirty-two stone and is "forced to ride from Door to Door in a Chariot even here at *Bath*; and if I had but an Hundred Paces to walk, was oblig'd to have a Servant following me with a Stool to rest on," while he is curing others of his own radically unstable disease. Cheyne considers himself recovered through "extraordinary Remedies," but his discourse, lurching between states of extremity, dwelling obsessively upon the times that his body became "*tumified, incrusted*, and *burnt* almost like the Skin of a *roasted Pig*," suggests a fundamental instability that preoccupies writer and reader alike. Characteristically, in closing his "case," to demonstrate his sound health, Cheyne describes exultantly his latest disaster. After being thrown out of a chariot and falling on his head, suffering a dreadful wound in the temple, after his eyebrows are shaved off, after being bled, Cheyne reports with enthusiasm his miraculous recovery, an event that barely survives the violence of his prose.[15]

In writing their attacks against the spleen, our authors almost guarantee their splenetic states, for axiomatically those most prone to attacks of melancholy are scholars, those weak, sedentary, and studious martyrs who wear away their eyes and their digestive tracts in their pursuit of

14. Cheyne, *The English Malady*, 366; George Cheyne, *Essay on Regimen* (London, 1740), 71.

15. Cheyne, "The Case of the Author," in *The English Malady*, 330, 342–343, 351, 360–361.

phantom truth.[16] Ramazini, a physician who carefully categorized the industrial diseases typical of professions as various as the cleaners of jakes, the bearers of corpses, nurses and footmen, horse coursers and midwives, addressed with great seriousness the diseases of "learned Men," as "slothful and idle in their Body, as they are active in their Mind and Brain." Suffering from bad digestion and constipation, "hard students . . . by Reading and Writing with their Head and Breast bent, compress the Stomach and Pancreas," strain their eyes, cripple their hands, and deprive their brain of its tone.[17] Forgetful of their bodies, scholars abuse it through neglect while they spend too much time thinking on subjects—like melancholy—that seize their imagination. While "People of lower Fortunes labour under such a Variety of Necessities . . . that they have not time stedfastly to think on one thing," scholars, relieved from tedious "Necessity," demonstrate "strong Symptoms of a labouring Imagination" as they "revolve long upon the same Ideas."[18]

To cure the spleen, practitioners prescribed diets, vomits, purges, and empiric courses of physick. One course of advice often contradicted another, but most treatises agree on one principle: the power of exercise. To move the animal spirits, to open up the great sensorium, one must move the body itself. "The difference between the lowest, most abject, and the highest, most elevated natural Capacities must depend upon the different Degree of Motion coming to the Seat of the common Sensorium," Nicholas Robinson argued. Robinson wonders just why the solids need to be roused, why they grow sedentary and effete, incapable

16. In *The History of Health* MacKenzie advises the studious and contemplative to "endeavour to repair by their temperance, regularity, and care, what is perpetually impaired by their weakness, situation and study" (416–417). In *Essay of Health and Long Life,* Cheyne suggests that the "*Weak, Sedentary* and *Studious,* should frequently *shave* their Head and Face, *wash* and *scrape* their Feet, and *pare* the Nails of their Toes" (228). In "The Art of Preserving Health," John Armstrong advises the scholar "to stand and sit by turns / As Nature prompts," warning that "o'er your leaves / To lean for ever, cramps the vital parts, / And robs the fine machinery of its play" (bk. IV, 11. 80–83, *Poetical Works* [Edinburgh, 1781], 67).

17. Bern. Ramazini, *A Treatise on the Disease of Tradesmen, to which they are subject by their particular Callings,* trans. and ed. Dr. James (London, 1740), 269, 273. Ramazini finds that mathematicians, "abstracted from the Senses, and cut off in a manner from all Commerce with the Body," are "almost all stupid, slothful, lethargic, and perfect Strangers to human Conversation, or the Business of the World," while writers tend to suffer most from constant sitting, "perpetual motion of the Hand in the same manner," and constant attention and application of the mind (286, 400).

18. Mandeville, *Treatise,* 220; Nicholas Robinson, *A New System of the Spleen, Vapours, and Hypochondriack Melancholy: Wherein All the Decay of the Nerves, and Lowness of the Spirit, are Mechanically Accounted for* (London, 1729), 22.

of sending the precious fluids to the extreme parts of the body, and decides that it all has to do with the Fall. God makes good in every case "that Sentence he pronounc'd against disobedient Man, that in the Sweat of his Face, he should eat his Bread."[19] Since "civilized" melancholics do not literally need to labor for food that their servants gather and prepare, they needed to be forced into a course of bodily exercise.

Mandeville presents a typical course of exercise in his prescription for a greensick, melancholy maiden. After being awakened before 6:00 A.M.,

> let her be swung for half an Hour, then eat her Breakfast and get on Horseback for at least two Hours, either gallopping or trotting as much as her Strength will permit her. Immediately after this let her be undrest, and by some Nurse or other chafed or dry-rubb'd for a considerable time, 'til her Skin looks red and her Flesh glows all over: Let her begin to repeat the same Exercise about Three in the Afternoon, and after supper keep upon her Legs two Hours before she goes to Bed. The Swing I speak of may be made after what manner your Daughter fancies most; that which they call a Flying-horse, makes a very agreeable motion, but if she be apt to be giddy, she may swing in a Chair, or other Seat to which she is fasten'd; otherwise a Rope tied with both Ends to a Beam is sufficient.[20]

Mandeville outlines here the course of exercise promoted by Francis Fuller, M.A., author of *Medicina Gymnastica,* once a sufferer from "giddiness" but now grown hale and hearty after following Dr. Sydenham's regimen of exercise.[21] Fuller argues that the body "improves by Exercise, and acquires by frequent Motion an Ability to last the longer." Exercise particularly increases the animal spirits, aids the digestion, enriches the blood, and stimulates an increased velocity of the circulation.

The idea of exercise was not in itself new or startling for the eighteenth-century reader. Considered one of the six "non-naturals" fundamental to proper health, it, like civilization and its discontents, went back at least to the Greeks. Fuller defers to Hippocrates and Galen

19. Robinson, *System of the Spleen,* 32–33; see also Nicholas Robinson, *A New Method of Treating Consumptions: Wherein all the Decays Incident to Human Bodies, are Mechanically Accounted for* (London, 1727), pt. 1, 202. In *Primitive Physick: or, An Easy and Natural Method of Curing Most Diseases* (London, 1747), John Wesley argued that exercise was "intimated by the Great Author of Nature, in the very Sentence that intails Death upon us. 'In the Sweat of thy face shalt thou eat bread till thou return unto the Ground'" (v). John Dussinger provides an excellent introduction to the idea of the sensorium in "The Sensorium and the World of *A Sentimental Journey,*" *Ariel* 13 (1982): 3–16.

20. Mandeville, *Treatise,* 305.

21. Fuller reported that he suffered from "Giddiness," and in an attempt to recuperate drank Bath Waters so long that he was "scarce able to go about without Staggering like a Drunken Man" (*Medicina Gymnastica,* 256).

when he recommends his "modern" method to lovers of the ancients, and alludes to Asclepiades, inventor of the "Lecti Pensiles," hanging beds, which served as swinging cradles to soothe ancient hysterics.[22] But while the benefits of exercise had become a commonplace, once the body became matter difficult if not impossible to transcend, exercise itself offered a more urgently sought solution to the problematic mortal condition. Emphasizing the mechanical nature of the body, theories of exercise could appeal to a materialistic sensibility, while at the same time offering a way to achieve "Sympathy *betwixt* the Soul *and* Animal Spirits." Thus a therapist like Richard Browne, in his *Medicina Musica: Or a Mechanical Essay on the Effects of Singing, Musick, and Dancing, on Human Bodies,* might argue for mechanical results, but he promises as well a rhapsodic response to the "mighty Power and Energy of Musick" and movement that should displace fears of bodily containment. Fuller more prosaically, but no less confidently, prescribes horseback riding for the vigorous victim of melancholia. The "true Hysterick Colick" is best soothed by the "Use of a Chaise, or light Calash . . . convenient for Women . . . wherein the sick Person may at once enjoy the Convenience of a Cradle, and the Vehemence of Exercise."[23] Cold baths, swinging, and applications of the "flesh-brush"—wielded by a vigorous servant—should enliven the most debilitated.

The ideal goal of exercise is to strengthen the constitution. By stimulating the "animal spirits," one "may come to the strength of a *Tartar*."[24] But in fact, most of the exercises recommended depend more upon the health and vigor of surrogate bodies "moving" their master or mistress. Motion becomes that which is done to one's body by the agency

22. Fuller, *Medicina Gymnastica,* 13–21, 236–237. As James Work notes in glossing Sterne's use of the term, "Non-Naturals" is "A term formerly used by physicians to indicate the six things which because they do not enter into the composition of the body are not 'natural' yet which are essential to animal life and health and which by accident or abuse often cause disease: air, meat and drink, excretion and retention, sleep and waking, motion and rest, and the affections of the mind" (Laurence Sterne, *The Life and Opinions of Tristram Shandy, Gentleman,* ed. James Work [New York: Odyssey Press, 1940], 76). Melvyn New's note on the non-naturals is very helpful: *The Life and Opinions of Tristram Shandy, Gentleman,* ed. Melvyn New and Joan New (Gainesville: University Presses of Florida, 1978–1984), 2:121–122. (All further quotations will be from the Florida edition.) In "The 'Six Things Non-Natural': A Note on the Origins and Fate of a Doctrine and a Phrase," *Clio Medica* 3 (1968): 337–347, L. J. Rather suggests that by the eighteenth century the term itself would seem inappropriate, certifying Tristram's own complaint that "the most natural actions of a man's life should be call'd his Non-Naturals" (*TS* 1:84).

23. Richard Browne, *Medicina Musica* (London, 1729), 7, 121; Fuller, *Medicina Gymnastica,* Fuller, 50–52.

24. Fuller, *Medicina Gymnastica,* 118.

of another. Adam's curse, to earn daily bread by the body's daily sweat, seems to have been redistributed to fall more often than not upon the stronger, coarser backs of his poorer children. As the proverb went, We are all Adam's Children, but Silk makes the Difference.[25] While exercise was valued for its benefits, it was also distrusted for its coarsening, often debilitating side effects. In *An Account of the Effects of Swinging,* James Carmichael Smyth, measuring the effect swinging has on pulmonary cases, makes a clear distinction between exercise and motion. Exercise is muscular action, an exertion of the locomotive powers of the body "to increase the force and frequency of the heart's contraction, the velocity and momentum of the blood, the quickness of the breathing, and the heat, irritability and transpiration of the whole body." While exercise may temporarily increase strength and vigor, "when continued beyond a certain time, [it] induces lassitude, debility, and languor."[26] (Ramazini had earlier observed the running footmen's tendency to "have a Swelling in the Spleen: for the loose Substance of this Organ receives more Blood, upon the violent Motion, than it discharges." Even more alarming was the tendency for "Horse-Coursers or Grooms, and those who ride Post" to become frigid and impotent: "the Strength of the Loins and the genital Parts is dissolved by the continual Shaking and Jogging.")[27] Motion, however, rather than exercise, can provide the benefits of exercise without the "agitation, or succession of the body." Smyth considers three sources of motion beneficial to pulmonary patients: sailing, swinging, and aerostation. The last-named is "a method of conveying an animal with great velocity through the atmosphere, without the smallest exertion of its own powers, or even consciousness of motion." The advantage of this violent form of transportation is that it would provide the maximum opportunity for a "change of air," since a quick succession of air so necessary to health depends upon the "velocity with which the body moves through it." But Smyth prudently forbears catapulting pulmonary patients through the air: as "the expence and hazard attending such experiments precludes this from being applicable to the

25. A London Proverb of 1732 as cited by Peter Linebaugh in his forthcoming study of eighteenth-century social and criminal history, *The London Hanged.*

26. James Carmichael Smyth, *An Account of the Effects of Swinging, Employed as a Remedy in the Pulmonary Consumption and Hectic Fever* (London, 1787), 17–18. Smyth argues that swinging offers the benefits of sailing recommended so highly by the ancients in cases of consumption, without the detrimental effect of sea air. "The change of air . . . a quick succession of air, owing to the velocity with which the body moves through it, is best obtained by swinging" (12).

27. Ramazini, *Disease of Tradesmen,* 224 (misnumbered 252), 229.

purposes of medicine or of common life, they must always remain more a matter of curiosity than of use."[28]

When Fuller and Smyth prescribe their jogging and swinging machines, they are attempting to work externally on the spirit as well as the body, by diverting and disrupting the natural tendency of their patient's progress toward depression, toward "solidification," toward, not just metaphorically, death itself. If, as Robinson suggested, "the labouring [melancholic] Imagination revolve[s] long on same Ideas," it must be interrupted from its obsessive revolution. As Fuller noted, briskness of motion "must take a Man off from close Thinking," for "there is nothing like Hurrying the Body, to divert the Hurry of the Mind." Even "the Perception of a Pain, may be in some Measure interrupted by a swift Motion, for that Perception cannot strike so strong at such a time." Motion becomes displacement, a way of staving off perceptions that turn morbid, since "a Man that should set himself to Muse on a full Gallop, would think but very incoherently."[29] Just this planned incoherence generates narrative strategies of digression, disruption, and disjunction in the eighteenth-century novel.

Eighteenth-century novels are, as a rule, scrambled, jogging, rocking narratives that resist interiority while refusing to end. They tend, in fact, to embarrass critics dedicated to the rise of a more regularized generic form. Sterne is the greatest violator of what formalists like to think of as generic imperatives to close a matter that has been opened. But he just makes obvious what Defoe, Richardson, Smollett, Cleland,

28. Smyth, *Effects of Swinging,* 17–19.

29. Fuller, *Medicina Gymnastica,* 162–163, 272. Sterne provides a good example of the therapeutic benefits of equestrian diversion in *Sentimental Journey* when Yorick, pensively considering the dead ass he has just seen on the road, is jostled out of his lamentation by his postillion, who will "go on tearing my nerves to pieces till he has worked me into a foolish passion, and then he'll go slow, that I may enjoy the sweets of it. The postillion managed the point to a miracle: by the time he had got to the foot of a steep hill about half a league from Nampont,—he had put me out of temper with him—and then with myself, for being so" (*A Sentimental Journey through France and Italy by Mr. Yorick,* ed. Gardner Stout [Berkeley and Los Angeles: University of California Press, 1967], 143).

30. Answering his own provocatively posed question, "Did Sterne Complete *Tristram Shandy?*" Wayne Booth argued that Sterne consciously and coherently completed his text, carefully tying his major episodes together: *Modern Philology* 48 (1951): 172–183. R. F. Brissenden disagrees with his argument in "'Trusting to Almighty God': Another Look at the Composition of *Tristram Shandy,*" in *The Winged Skull: Papers from the Laurence Sterne Bicentenary Conference,* ed. Arthur H. Cash and John M. Stedmond (Kent, Ohio: Kent State University Press, 1971), 258–268.

Goldsmith, and even Fielding were doing.[30] Various "sources" of the novels are often successfully invoked to explain the road trips that most fictional characters seem to be taking. Pilgrimages, heavenly and familial, picaresque assaults on bourgeois sensibility, romance quests, post-Edenic forced marches through life into death are all, with good reason, appreciated for their bearing on the early English novel. I would like, however, to consider the disruptive principle of motion itself as prod and brake, as a principle of narrative progression sustaining a movement whose logical ending is narrative closure, physical death. Like medical theorists writing against the spleen, the novelists are grappling with the same materiality, the same "limitations of frame" that force the most well-plotted life to end.

This principle of motion disallows sustained interiority. To avoid closure, one must keep moving and keep on the superficies of things. Inside is where the maggots lurk, where the vital spirits solidify, harden, and die. Do not loll in bed too long, warns Robinson writing on the spleen, for "these overlong Interruptions with Self, so weaken the Springs of the finest Animal Fibres, on which the Exercise of [intellectual] Faculties depend."[31] To escape and to conquer self, one must keep moving, but ironically to move with purpose is to reach one's destination. Enter the swing, the chamber horse, the journey itself as disruptive agents of motion that exercise the body and soul physically and sentimentally, extending feeling to text that sustains vitality and displaces matter.

Swinging doesn't get you anywhere. That is its point, illustrated with great delicacy by Fragonard,[32] whose erotic appreciation of that moment of desire when all is possible, when body itself has not inserted its own unidealized and often contradictory demands, makes clear just what the swing can and cannot do. In a swing, one enters new air only to be drawn back into the old, and while it is theoretically possible to escape the power of gravity itself between states of up and down, the swinger is nonetheless forced into another just as demanding rhythm that only looks effortless. A certain urgency enters into the most idyllic scene of swinging from the awareness that to stop moving is to fall into the matter at hand.

31. Robinson, *System of the Spleen,* 335. In *Essay of Health and Long Life,* Cheyne also warned against the dangers of "*lolling* and *soaking* in *Sheets,* anytime after one is distinctly awake." The practice "*thickens* the Juices, *enervates* the Solids, and *weakens* the Constitution" (84).

32. "The Swing," The Wallace Collection.

After Mandeville's physician prescribes his course of exercise to cure the greensick maiden, her father asks, quite sensibly, "But might not Marriage be as effectual as all these Exercises?"[33] His question gets to the masturbatory point of swinging, its eroticized avoidance of conjugal connections that indeed get you somewhere, get you married, get you pregnant, get you tied to complications of matter itself. When Fragonard's lady of the swing stops moving between yes and no, she will fall into that matter which is, pictorially, her destiny, just as when Smyth's pulmonary patients step down from their swings, their pulses will reassert their tedious talent at measuring an illness better evaluated on the ground. Fuller compared quite tellingly the motion of the soothing chaise to that of a cradle, for the cradle, simulating the undulating motion of the womb itself, keeps its fragile occupant safe from the real motion outside that will, naturally, propel it into life leading into death. To swing is figuratively not to die.

The swinger also engages in a mock death, by flirting with the idea of falling off. Recall Mandeville's warning against giddy daughters mounting their lofty flying horses, as well as Fuller's appreciation of the "Vehemence of Exercise" the undulating chaise could provide.[34] Even as therapists describe the safety features of their apparatus, they seem to be introducing elements of danger. And on occasion, the apparatus is designed to be dangerous, to induce—therapeutically—terror.

Jerome Gaub discusses the therapeutic uses of pain in his two essays on regimen, *De regimine mentis.* In the first essay (1747), he refers obscurely to the power of stimulants "that stir up the humors, excite the nerves, and inflict pain," and calls attention to the benefits of water therapy in hysterical cases. "The frightful torment that the near loss of life from suffocation inflicts on the mind" might be a "terrible remedy indeed but one hardly to be exceeded in efficacy by any other when an unsound mind is to be helped by the effects of a bodily change." Gaub becomes more specific in his prescription of "Terror as a Therapeutic Agent" in his second essay (1763), where he calls for "a machine that will inspire extreme terror, and submersion of such duration and frequency that life itself is put in hazard and doubt arises when the man is withdrawn whether he is quite dead or can still be revived." Even arthritis can be relieved by terror. A certain gouty patient "whose hands

33. Mandeville, *Treatise,* 307. Philopiro answers, Yes, but adds that the marriage might fail, making two people unhappy instead of one, and "may but half Cure the Woman, who lingering under the Remainder of her Disease, may have half a dozen Children that shall all inherit it."

34. Mandeville, *Treatise,* 305; Fuller, *Medicina Gymnastica,* 50.

and feet had been covered with poultices of milk, flour and turnips in order to relieve the pain," was left unattended. Disastrously, a pig forced its way into the patient's room, and "Attracted by the odor it began to devour the poultice." This rough assault "threw the man to the floor, not without the greatest emotional disturbance but with the result that his pains abated from then on and shortly thereafter entirely disappeared, never to return again."[35] As Fuller noted, "Torture will rouse the Spirits for some time very much,"[36] while Robinson cited with approving wonder the case of an idiotized woman in Cheshire "that had been subject to Fits of Lunacy for near twenty Years," who recovered "the perfect Use of all her Senses" after fortuitously slipping 150 feet "from the Ridge of a steep Hill."[37]

Through the power of exercise, in bouts of swinging, jogging, bouncing, more radically through shock therapy designed to divert depressed spirits by dunking, whirling, and plunging mad matter into consciousness, writers against the spleen work to create irritation to stimulate the spirits into action, forming "those vivifying secretions" so necessary to sexual and mental vigor.[38] The benefit of irritation is invoked parodically

35. Quoted in Rather, *Mind and Body,* 109–110, 188–189. Rather's commentary is particularly valuable. He cites many examples of remarkable therapeutic procedures. Boerhaave, for instance, described the practice of a practitioner in Holland "so successful that some of the highest men in the country were committed to his care." The patient was treated with consideration and leniency, "but the moment the disorder asserts itself he is seized and soundly beaten. . . . at last his fear of a beating is so great that he puts his madness aside" (193).

36. Fuller, *Medicina Gymnastica,* 9.

37. Robinson, *System of the Spleen,* 67.

38. Wesley recommended that the deranged suffering from raging madness "Keep on the Head a Cap fill'd with *Snow,* for two or three Weeks." Alternatively one could "Set the Patient with his Head under a Great *Water-Fall,* as long as his Strength will bear" (*Primitive Physick,* 79). Illustrations of Joseph Guislain's more orderly methods of shocking his patients into consciousness dramatically extend these earlier ideas, especially those found in *Traité sur l'aliénation mentale et sur les hospices des aliénes* (Amsterdam, 1826). The idea of "irritability" and "sensibility" was particularly significant in the work of Albrecht von Haller, who reported experiments with hundreds of animals to determine which parts were irritable and which sensible. He decided that a part was irritable if it contracted when stimulated, and sensible, if when stimulated the organism demonstrated that it felt pain. Haller concluded that only nerves or organs containing nerve endings were sensible. The preface to the English translation of Haller (taken from Simon Tissot's French translation) discusses the extreme irritability of hysterics and refers the reader to the *Medicinae compendium* (Leiden, 1735–1737) and the *Praxis medicae systema* (Padua, 1752) of "the celebrated Dr. Gorter, to whom the practice of physic is so much obliged," and "the first who has treated expressly of mobility, a disease so frequent and so little known" (*On the Sensible and Irritable Parts of Animals* [London, 1755], xv). Thomas Hall discusses the debate over

by Sterne in his definition of "True Shandeism." Quizzing the readers on the state of their heads—"my own akes dismally"—Tristram boasts that Shandeism "opens the heart and lungs, and like all those affections which partake of its nature, it forces the blood and other vital fluids of the body to run freely thro' its channels, and makes the wheel of life run long and chearfully round" (1:401).[39] Less sanguine, but cursed with the same "akeing head," bent on opening up the same heart and lungs, Smollett notes in a letter to Dr. William Hunter, foremost surgeon of the age as well as Smollett's physician and friend, that were it not for the "Stings" of his Grub Street Friends, his "Circulation would have stopped of itself" to leave him "stupefied with ill Health, Loss of memory, Confinement, and Solitude."[40] Eager to "increase the motion of the machine, to *unclog the wheels of life* and now and then to take a plunge amidst the waves of excess,"[41] Smollett clarifies more than Sterne the mixed nature of "excess" and motion in his delineation of a search for health that depends as much upon cranky irritation as it does upon Sterne's voyeuristic sentimental moments. But significantly, in their sentimental quests, both writers disrupt, digress, and mobilize narratives to "move" readers into keeping their fictions, through the exercise of reading, alive.

Their desire to extend their lives through paper into a community of feeling readers is not surprising. Both suffered from consumption, a physical condition often connected specifically to the melancholia feared

Haller's concept of irritability (*Ideas of Life and Matter* 1:396–404). R. F. Brissenden considers Haller's influence on the sentimental movement in *Virtue in Distress: Studies in the Novels of Sentiment from Richardson to Sade* (New York: Barnes and Noble, 1974). In her forthcoming study of sensibility, Ann Van Sant makes compelling connections between the language of scientific experimentation and the language of the sentimental novel.

39. Roy Porter discusses Sterne's medical history as a consumptive in "Against the Spleen," in *Laurence Sterne: Riddles and Mysteries,* ed. V. G. Myer (London: Vision; Totowa, N. J.: Barnes and Noble, 1984), 84–98. Porter's extensive footnotes are particularly helpful. Max Byrd is sensitive to Sterne's splenetic race against death in his critical study, *Tristram Shandy* (London, 1985). Sterne specifically discusses his method of writing "against the spleen" in volume 4, "in order, by a more frequent and a more convulsive elevation and depression of the diaphragm, and the succussations of the intercostal and abdominal muscles in laughter, to drive the gall and other *bitter juices* from the gall bladder, liver and sweet-bread of his majesty's subjects, with all the inimicitious passions which belong to them, down into their duodenums" (*TS* 1:360).

40. *The Letters of Tobias Smollett,* ed. Lewis M. Knapp (Oxford: Oxford University Press, 1970), 133.

41. *The Expedition of Humphry Clinker,* ed. Lewis M. Knapp (Oxford: Oxford University Press, 1966), 339.

TRAITE

SUR

L'ALIÉNATION MENTALE

ET SUR

LES HOSPICES DES ALIÉNÉS.

PAR

JOSEPH GUISLAIN,

MÉDECIN à GAND.

OUVRAGE COURONNÉ ET PUBLIÉ PAR LA COMMISSION DE SURVEILLANCE MÉDICALE DANS LA PROVINCE DE NORD-HOLLANDE, SÉANT à AMSTERDAM.

TOME SECOND.

A AMSTERDAM,
CHEZ J. VAN DER HEY ET FILS,
et
LES HÉRITIERS H. GARTMAN.
1826.

Pl. 1. From Joseph Guislain, *Traité sur l'aliénation mentale et sur les hospices des aliénés* (Amsterdam, 1828).

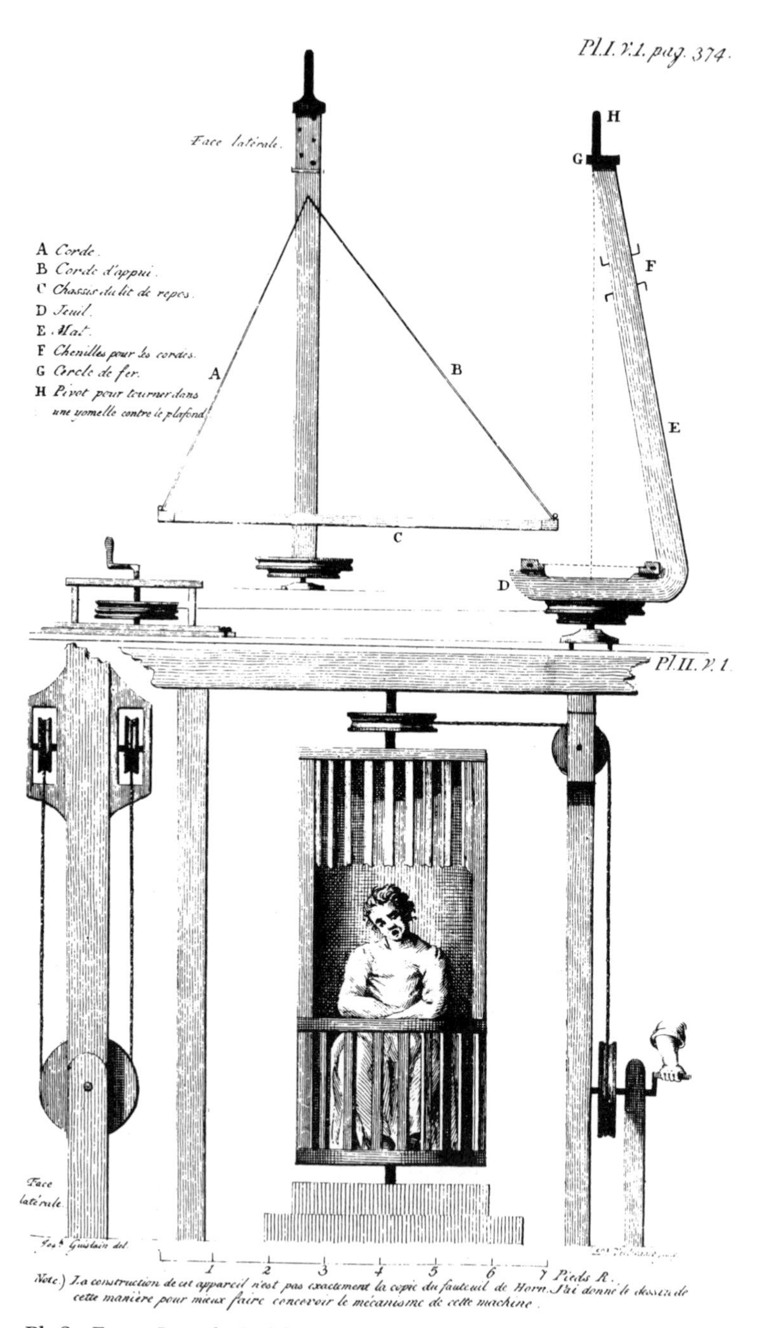

Pl. 2. From Joseph Guislain, *Traité sur l'aliénation mentale et sur les hospices des aliénés* (Amsterdam, 1828).

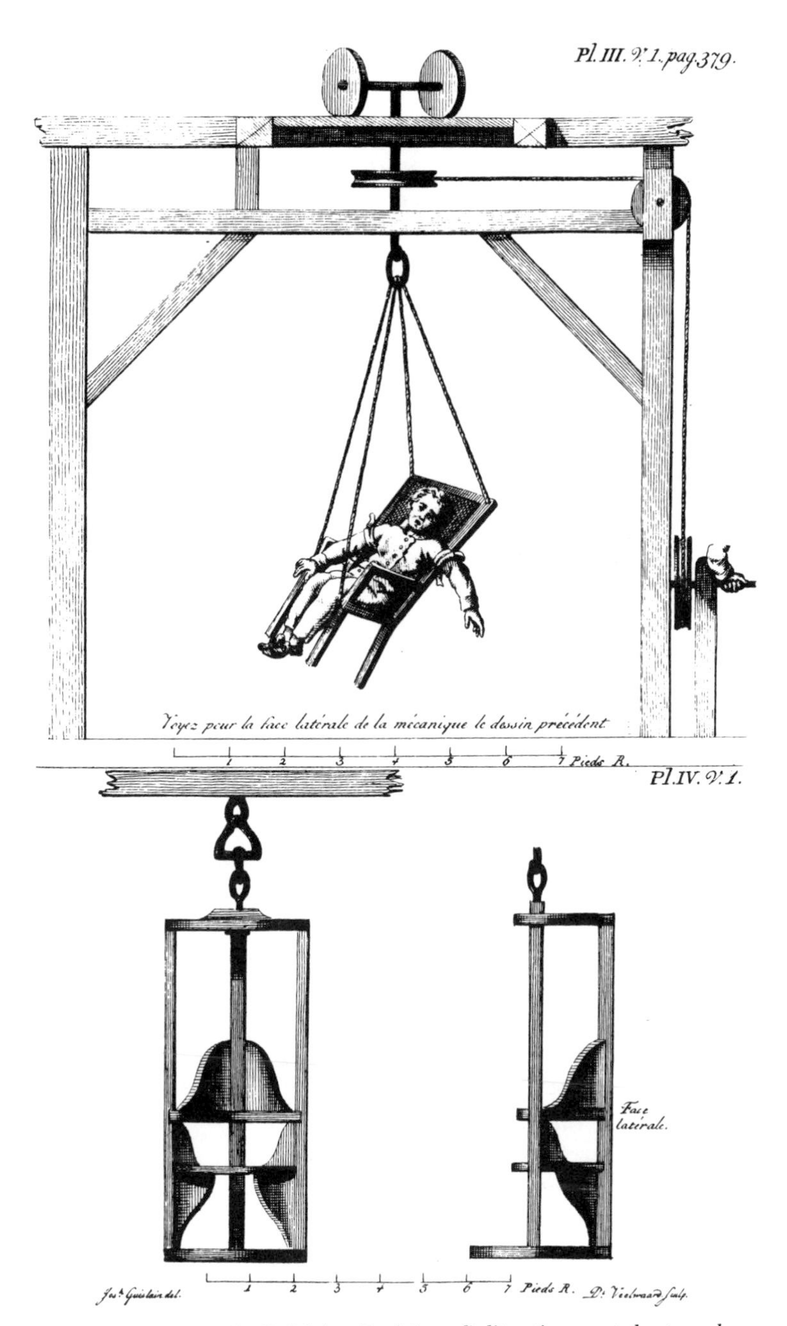

Pl. 3. From Joseph Guislain, *Traité sur l'aliénation mentale et sur les hospices des aliénés* (Amsterdam, 1828).

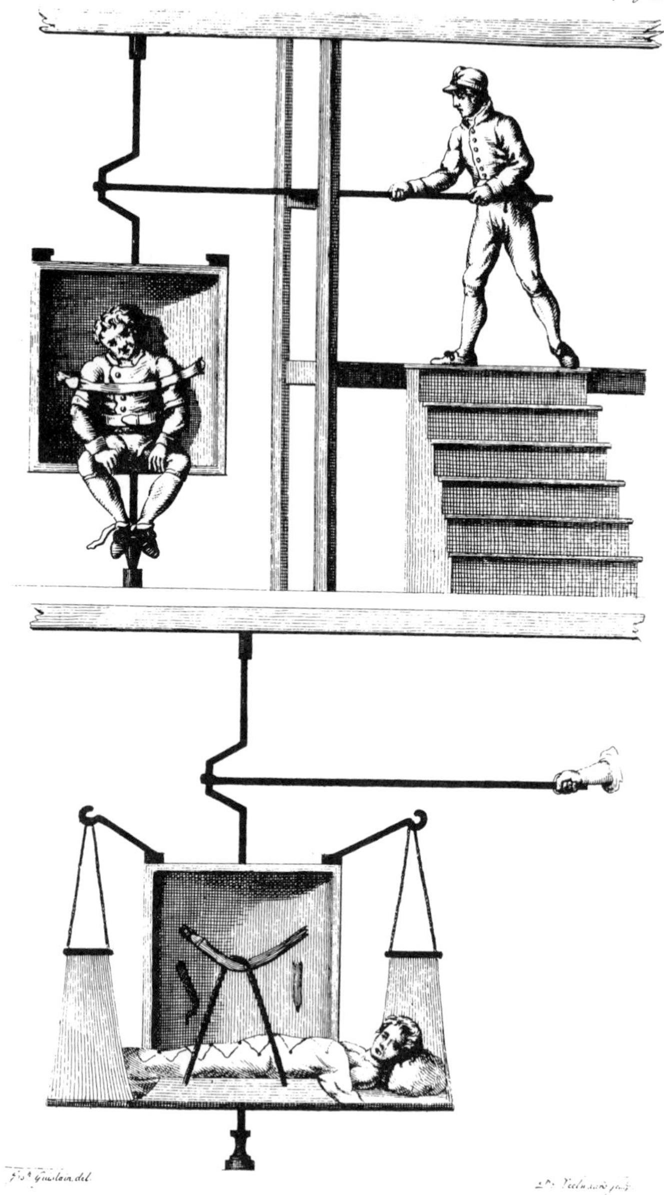

Pl. 4. From Joseph Guislain, *Traité sur l'aliénation mentale et sur les hospices des aliénés* (Amsterdam, 1828).

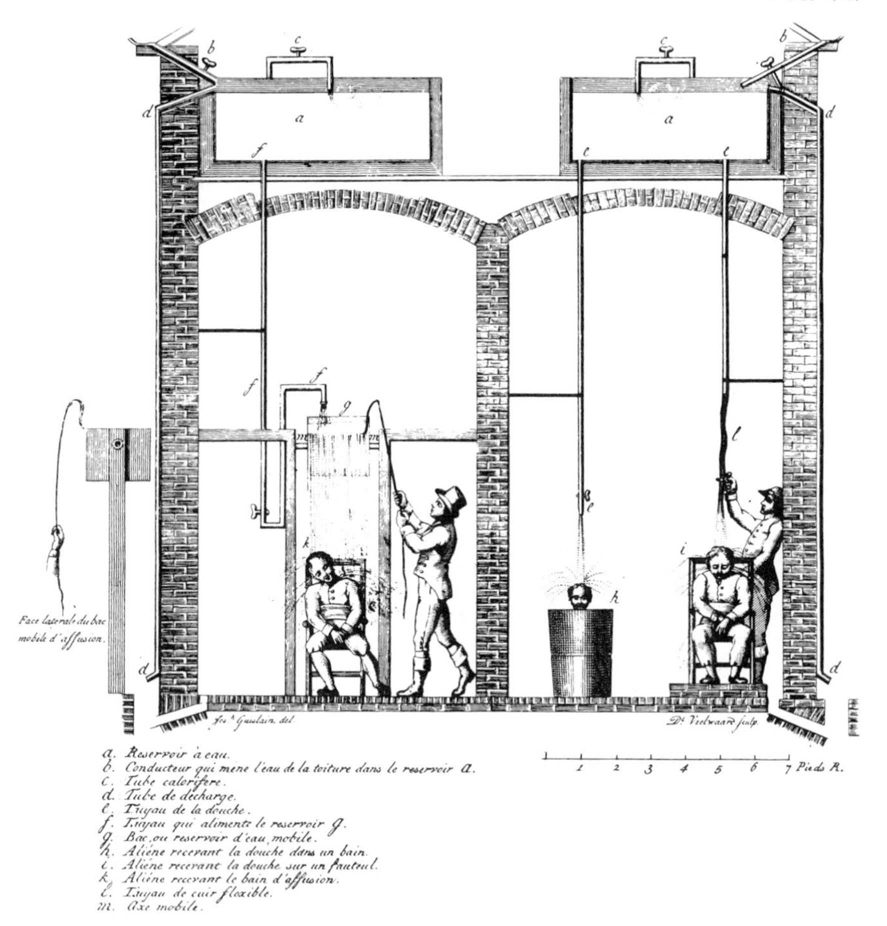

Pl. 5. From Joseph Guislain, *Traité sur l'aliénation mentale et sur les hospices des aliénés* (Amsterdam, 1828).

to depress the necessary animal spirits;[42] both wrote, in critically different ways, against the spleen; and both died of their "natural" condition shortly after completing (or rather refusing to complete) their most obvious attempts to run out of the matter that finally contained them. It is time to look at their fictional strategies.

"Fabricating at great rate" his *Sentimental Journey,* Sterne guarantees a correspondent that the work "shall make you cry as much as ever it made me laugh—or I'll give up the Business of sentimental writing—& write to the body."[43] He reveals in this boast the edgy, nervous relationship he has to a method of writing that ironizes the tears he wrings from his subject, the body he is always displacing in language. To write "to the body" is to approach it directly and follow its course into death. Its progress is sure, Sterne makes clear as he quantifies the blood he coughs up while tracing the source of his discontent. Engaging in "hectic watchings" (1:104) (the term is a tubercular one), born into a "scurvy world" (1:8), Sterne turns body into a text that must be interrupted to keep it from ending, for the straight plot line of gravity can only lead into closure most fatal.

The act of writing itself creates physical communion with problematic flesh. Preparing to describe Walter Shandy's grief over Tristram's crushed nose, the writer enters this part of his story "in the most pensive and melancholy frame of mind, that ever sympathetic breast was touched with," his "nerves relax" and he feels "an abatement of the quickness of [his] pulse." His cautious composure, so different from "that careless alacrity with it, which every day of my life prompts me to say and write a thousand things I should not," seems to be associated with the seriousness of his subject. More typical are

> the rash jerks, and harebrain'd squirts thou art wont, *Tristram,* to transact it with in other humours,—dropping thy pen,—spurting thy ink about thy table and thy books,—as if thy pen and thy ink, thy books and thy furniture cost thee nothing. [1:254]

Is the ink Sterne's blood, costing indeed something, sign of his transubstantiated text? Or merely ink? Flesh and blood, paper and words

42. Nicholas Robinson seems to treat the two conditions as one, offering the same advice to sufferers of the spleen that he gives to consumptives. Most works addressing the melancholy condition make continuous connection between "low" spirits and consumption, while often linking the psychosomatic attacks of the spleen to the physical manifestations of scurvy and consumption.

43. *Sentimental Journey,* 19–20.

commingle violently as Sterne throws fair sheets of text into the fire and, for relief, "snatch[es] off [his] wig" to throw it perpendicularly upward, defying the gravity he writes against (1:350).

Writing against the spleen to extend, in the process, his own life, Sterne, through exertion, comes up against the very problem he is trying to solve, for in exercising his vital animal spirits, he is also, in his rash transactions, spurting his ink, his energy, his life's blood about the room. "In writing," Ramazini noted, "the whole Brain with its Nerves and Fibres are highly tense, and a Privation of their due Tone succeeds."[44] Writing, like study, is, after all, bloody work. Witness the trials of Uncle Toby, displacing his wound through hard study guaranteed to feed the flames of melancholia as he pursues the intricate mazes of the labyrinth promising "this bewitching phantom, KNOWLEDGE . . . O my uncle! fly—fly—fly from it as from a serpent.—Is it fit, good-natur'd man! thou should'st sit up with the wound upon thy groin whole nights baking thy blood with hectic watchings?" (1:103–104). And how can Toby fly from the knowledge threatening to consume him, a knowledge, not of javelins and bridges and sentry boxes, but the deeper knowledge of "whole nights baking thy blood with hectic watchings" after death? In the text, the answer is clear. Toby must mount his hobbyhorse and ride away from the wound itself.

A hobbyhorse. Not an overlooked vehicle to be sure, but one, I think, more directly connected to Sterne's narrative strategies and one closer to Cheyne's chamber horse than to "hobbies" emptied of the physicality they promise. Sterne employs his hobby to move, lurch, jerk, and jog the matter of his text across a page that is alarmingly substantial, and he does so to exercise spirits that are too active for a badly decomposing "real" body.

Sterne's own mythologized equestrian escapades suggest a violent propensity for movement, just what, after all, the doctors prescribe. Writing from Montpellier, he complains that the "Thiness of the pyrenean Air brought on continual breaches of Vessels in my Lungs, & with them all the Tribe of evils insident to a pulmonary Consumption—there seem'd nothing left but gentle change of place & air." "Gentle," however, is a word that becomes altered by the movement itself, and once Sterne puts himself into motion, "having traversed the South of France so often that I ran a risk of being taken up for a Spy, I . . . jogg'd myself out of all other dangers."[45] Wildly excursing with a mad wife who thinks she

44. Ramazini, *Disease of Tradesmen,* 401.

45. *The Letters of Laurence Sterne,* ed. Lewis Perry Curtis (Oxford: Oxford University Press, 1965), 205.

is the Queen of Bohemia, demoniacally racing across Crazy Castle sands,[46] he violates therapeutic prescriptions for moderate exercise just as thoroughly as his morbidly energetic race against death flaunts Nicholas Robinson's sound admonition to his consumptive patients. "All the dejecting Passions should be banish'd," Robinson advises, "and Objects only admitted that may create gay, merry and chearful Scenes. . . . I should think it highly detrimental, too much to play with the gloomy Prospects of Death, unless manifest Symptoms appear of his approaching Dissolution."[47] It would be, I imagine, difficult not to gag on such banal bromides. Sterne shows no signs of swallowing the discourse of cheerful moderation. His gaiety will crack at its edges as he perversely calls up "gloomy Prospects of Death" (37–38), two of them, impenetrable black monuments to Yorick's mortality, only to flaunt them, to exorcise their spirit through a brisk, cracked energetic course of exercise.

Resurrecting "poor Yorick" at will, Sterne jerks his invincible—because already dead—character across fictive landscapes that strain beneath the weight of curvetting, frisking hooves. Sentimental travelers "Crack, crack—crack, crack—crack, crack," across France (2:599), and on domestic ground are prone to take "a good rattling gallop," to risk routinely life and limb in order to arouse the appropriate spirit:

> Now ride at this rate with what good intention and resolution you may,—'tis a million to one you'll do some one a mischief, if not yourself—He's flung—he's off—he's lost his seat—he's down—he'll break nis neck—see! [1:356]

46. In *Scrapeana* (York, 1792), John Croft reports that Elizabeth Sterne imagined herself the Queen of Bohemia. To amuse her, "and induce her to take the air," "Tristram, her husband . . . proposed coursing, in the way practised in Bohemia; for that purpose he procured bladders, and filled them with beans, and tied them to the wheels of a single horse chair. When he drove madam into a stubble field, with the motion of the carriage and the bladders, rattle bladder, rattle; it alarmed the hares, and the greyhounds were ready to take them" (22, as cited in David Thomson, *Wild Excursions: The Life and Fiction of Laurence Sterne* [New York: McGraw-Hill, 1972], 123). Arthur Cash finds this to be "one of the least trustworthy stories about Sterne" (*Laurence Sterne: The Early and Middle Years* [London: Methuen, 1975], 286), but something in it rings true. Wilbur Cross states that of all the pastimes that "took Sterne out of doors, none pleased him quite so much" as "racing chariots along the sandy beach" near Crazy Castle "'with one wheel in the sea'" (*The Life and Times of Laurence Sterne* [New Haven: Yale University Press, 1925], 1:121).

47. Robinson, *Consumptions* pt. 2, 48.

Motion, not ripeness, is all. Ripeness must, in fact, be interrupted, for to ripen is to rot. Growth becomes in nature death—unless the natural channels are diverted. Tristram knows that, as he compulsively displaces his origins, pushing them always beyond his own comprehension, short-circuiting in the process his logical narrative end.

To escape the real problems of body, the quarts and gallons of blood that Tristram decides not to measure, Sterne sets up several diversionary strategies. To escape being "killed" by kind questions addressed to the nature and location of his wound, My Uncle Toby displaces his corporeal state through military maneuvers. Trim, his surrogate, in love and war, one of those accommodating "body servants" so necessary to exercise the vital spirits, makes it possible for Toby to swing between states of benevolence and bloody gore as he races his hobbyhorse from the Bowling Green to Dunkirk and back again without getting anywhere at all. Walter, less tactile, depends upon auxiliary verbs to move the soul, that great sensorium of verbal connections:

> Now the use of the *Auxiliaries* is, at once to set the soul a going by herself upon the materials as they are brought her; and by the versability of this great engine, round which they are twisted, to open new tracks of enquiry, and make every idea engender millions. [1:485]

Aided by the auxiliary yet active parts of speech not unlike accommodating servants willing to administer brisk rubbings of the flesh-brush for their mistress's own good, Walter sets the great white bear dancing across the page to not quite end another book:

> A WHITE BEAR! Very well. Have I ever seen one? Might I ever have seen one? Am I ever to see one? Ought I ever to have seen one? Or can I ever see one?
>
> Would I had seen a white bear— (for how can I imagine it?) If I should see a white bear, what should I say? If I should never see a white bear, what then?
>
> If I never have, can, must or shall see a white bear alive; have I ever seen the skin of one? Did I ever see one painted?—described? Have I ever dreamed of one?
>
> Did my father, mother, uncle, aunt, brothers or sisters, ever see a white bear? What would they give? How would they behave? How would a white bear have behaved? Is he wild? Tame? Terrible? Rough? Smooth?
>
> —Is the white bear worth seeing?—
>
> —Is there no sin in it?
>
> Is it better than a BLACK ONE? [1:487]

Walter's final question exposes the absurd limits to his own system, promising endless discourse, newly opened tracks of inquiry that would "make every idea engender millions" of words going absolutely nowhere, ending up in tautological exercises that, nonetheless, "set the soul a going by herself" and keep, in the process, the wheel of life running "long and chearfully round" (1:401).

Tristram compulsively pursues motion for its own sake. "So much of motion, is so much of life, and so much of joy . . . that to stand still, or get on but slowly, is death and the devil," he claims, rejecting Bishop Hall's desire for heavenly rest. "*Make them like unto a wheel*" becomes not a "bitter sarcasm" made against the restless spirit of fallen man, but a benediction allowing, however mechanically, transcendence. "I love the Pythagoreans . . . for their . . . '*getting out of the body, in order to think well.*' No man thinks right whilst he is in it" (2:592–593).

Tristram travels by coach, by hobbyhorse, and by sentimental chance, depending, when particularly weary, upon sturdy surrogates to move his dangerously hardening soul. To get out of the body, Sterne depends upon moving his and his reader's soul mechanically, but also pathetically, by allowing a sentimental escape from the hard realities of life. Auxiliary agents of feeling, body servants as indispensable as Trim, will become in *Sentimental Journey* necessary for the sentimental commerce Yorick conducts.[48] Just as the White Bear carried into and out of Walter's discourse calls attention to the arbitrary, fragmentary nature of any discourse, so the isolated, often inconclusive sentimental tales filling both novels emphasize their transitory, yet necessary, quality. Tristram, in fact, highly recommends the pitiful Maria piping her sorrows as a good sentimental side trip to Yorick, the sentimental traveler in search of emotional and motional diversion. Maria's madness and pathos is just the thing to exercise the spirits and rouse the soul.[49] Feelings, the property of patients genteel enough to suffer from the spleen, are expensive to sustain and will continue to depend, sentimentally, largely upon the sufferings of other, hardier souls valued for their compliance and visibility.

48. In his "Preface" written in the Desobligeant, Yorick decides that "the balance of sentimental commerce is always against the expatriated adventurer: he must buy what he has little occasion for at their own price—his conversation will seldom be taken in exchange for theirs without a large discount—and this, by the by, eternally driving him into the hands of more equitable brokers for such conversation as he can find, it requires no great spirit of divination to guess at his party" (*Sentimental Journey,* 78–79).

49. The pitiful condition of LeFevre also serves to rouse Toby from his sickbed. Most of the sentimental incidents in both *TS* and *SJ* seem designed to elicit a short, strong response that will invigorate its feeling spectator.

All these side trips, all this openness to the pleasing sensation of disruption, prohibits narrative coherency. That is, in fact, the point. Tristram "so complicate[s] and involve[s] the digressive and progressive movements, one wheel, within another, that the whole machine, in general, has been kept a-going;—and what's more, it shall be kept a-going these forty years, if it pleases the fountains of health to bless me so long with life and good spirits" (1:82). In the hectic spirit, he sets out to move through time and space Dr. Slop, Obadiah, Uncle Toby, Corporal Trim, Yorick, Walter, and himself—and on occasion, that inveterate lover of coach travel, Aunt Dinah, players all in his "dance . . . song . . . or . . . concerto between the acts" of birth and death.

Compulsively calling attention to the seams and struts of his narrative, Sterne makes clear with cloying irritation the effort it takes *not* to be splenetic. If I were to choose a kingdom, Tristram muses, let it be filled with "hearty laughing subjects." The Rabelaisian dream of a "body politick as body natural" as body laughing is poignantly undermined by his salute to the reader he takes leave of "till this time twelve-month, when (unless this vile cough kills me in the meant time) I'll have another pluck at your beards" (1:402). Not only does his own body natural intrude upon his vision of "subjects" with the "grace to be as WISE as they were MERRY," but his assertion of authority reveals even more the unlikely nature of his fictional structure. His hearty subjects must laugh, humorists subject to a regimen of joy that strains against its imperative. Crack, crack—crack, crack—crack, crack—watch the "characters" prance and paw as they course across a narrative designed to get them nowhere. The less nimble need to be occasionally carted off the stage, for movement, not direction, is all. "Getting forwards in two different journies together, and with the same dash of the pen," playing parlor tricks with time and space as he walks across the marketplace of Auxerre with my father and my uncle Toby just as he enters Lyons with a "post-chaise broke into a thousand pieces . . . moreover this moment" rhapsodizing on the banks of the Garonne (2:621–622), Sterne exhausts the reader with his frantic attempts at capering in the Shandy manner.

By denying his vehicle, his text, stability, by "breaking it up into a thousand pieces," Sterne collapses it finally in a "COCK and a BULL." Strategies of interruption and digression energize—hectically—a discourse that can even mobilize "auxilary verbs" to "open new tracks of enquiry, and make every idea engender millions." But in the case of the wonderful dancing bear, such multiplication is essentially nongenerative. The bear moves through the text, but doesn't get anywhere—he doesn't even make sense. New tracks of inquiry lead to dead ends that require yet another detour. Thus Tristram multiplies his own activity textually: "I have three hundred and sixty-four days more life to write just now, than when I first set out; so that instead of advancing, as a common writer, in my work with what I have been doing at it—on the contrary, I am just thrown so many volumes back" (1:341). Advancing, and then "thrown back," the writer swings back and forth between birth and death, between those "acts" that threaten closure. The swinger escapes time, escapes death, as long as he can sustain movement ultimately as sterile as Walter's recalcitrant bull. For there is, within the text itself, a resistance to the cracks and jerks and jogs and pokes that creates a hectic, masturbatory exhaustion of the "animal spirits" Sterne tries to resuscitate. The irritability that Sterne wants to transform into "good humor" reveals the strains of sublimation. Smollett, less rarefied, makes more apparent the pains and pleasures of exercising a body resisting inevitable consumption.

As a practicing physician as well as a splenetic patient, Smollett knew too well his "bad state of health." Smollett describes his condition in terms that would be found in most texts dealing with not only "the spleen" but "consumption." He suffers from "an asthmatic cough, spitting, slow fever, and restlessness, which demands a continual change of place, as well as free air, and room for motion."[50] It may very well be that his professional knowledge inspired his most professional defenses against his own disease. His desire for displacement, his attempt to turn matter into text, can be seen most vividly in his letter to Dr. Fizes, noted professor of medicine at the University of Montpellier. Although he was actually staying at Montpellier, Smollett, however curious to "know the opinion" of the celebrated doctor, could not bring himself to consult the local "Boerhaave" in the flesh. The "great lanthorn of medicine is become very rich and very insolent; and in proportion as his wealth increases, he is said to grow the more rapacious," he reports, deciding that such unsavory demonstrations of both character and deportment "left [him] no desire to converse with him." Instead, Smollett resolved "to consult with him on paper" (88). On paper, Smollett retains control of his case, his story of a disease that can be only what he allows into his

50. Tobias Smollet, *Travels through France and Italy*, ed. Frank Felsenstein (Oxford: Oxford University Press, 1981), 64. Further references will be cited in the text. Felsenstein suggests that the "the abrasiveness and bad temper which characterize many of Smollett's remarks seem to have had a more immediately therapeutic effect than the medicinal remedies proffered him. There is something positively curative to be found by venting his spleen" (xi). John Sena considers "Smollett's Persona and the Melancholic Traveler," *Eighteenth-Century Studies* 1 (1965): 353–369.

text. Body disappears altogether while Smollett anachronistically resists the growing medical practice of hands-on examination.[51] By refusing to see—and be seen by—his physician, Smollett hides behind words to remain free to invent his adversary's response to his condition. "The professor's eyes sparkled at the sight of the fee," he reports (93), imaginatively invading the consulting room he refuses to visit.

Smollett scrupulously reports the symptoms of his hectic, perhaps consumptive constitution—in Latin. The language of medical discourse is perfectly appropriate, but its utilitarian generality is precisely what allows him to quibble about Fizes's diagnosis. For when Fizes answers Smollett's letter—in French—to diagnose Smollett's condition as a slow fever with probable tubercules in suppuration on the lungs, "a circumstance which we should have ascertained, had the nature of the spitting been described in the case" (96), suggesting a consumptive condition, the patient turns a medical consultation into a linguistic contest. Forget Smollett's ailing body, the professor does not "understand Latin." Promising not to make any remarks upon "the stile of his prescription, replete as it is with a disgusting repetition of low expressions," Smollett nonetheless feels the need to "point out to [Fizes] the passages in my case which he had overlooked" in his original Latin descriptions. His objections reveal his understandable desire to arrest in prose the course of his disease.

> *I cannot think there are any tubercules on my lungs,* as I never spit up purulent matter, nor anything but phlegm or *pituita* in colour and consistence like the whites of eggs. *Sputum albumini ovi simillimum. I imagine, therefore,* that my disorder was originally owing to a sudden intermission of bodily exercise, intense application of the mind, and a sedentary life which hath relaxed the whole fibrile system, and that now it may be called a *pituitary,* not a *purulent* consumption. [English italics mine]

Imaginings aside, Dr. Fizes read Smollett's revised description, stood by his diagnosis, and invited him to come the next morning to his house "if [he] had any doubts . . . and he would resolve them." Still avoiding contact, Smollett sent in his place twelve livres wrapped in a note most equivocal:

51. Stanley Reiser, *Medicine and the Reign of Technology* (Cambridge: Cambridge University Press, 1978), discusses the ways that the modern medical technology affected the patient's sense of autonomy. Once the physician was able to examine the patient's body as material disconnected from its owner's narrative, the patient became less the subject than the object of examination.

It is not without reason that *Mons.r Fizes* enjoys such a large reputation. I have no doubts remaining; thank Heaven and *monsieur Fizes*. [98–101]

Not surprisingly, the doctor pocketed the livres, proving to Smollett his venality, allowing him even further room to rage against the diagnosis. Besides, Fizes did not prescribe exercise, Smollett's favorite remedy against the spleen. For that lapse in therapy alone, Fizes's interpretation of Smollett's shadowy, Latinized body could be disregarded.

Smollett's real body was another matter. "I was not at all pleased with the famous statue of the dead Christ in his mother's lap, by Michael Angelo," he reports, projecting onto a statue the symptoms he vigorously denied at Montpellier. "The figure of Christ is as much emaciated, as if he had died of a consumption" (255). Consumption must be resisted with energetic jolts of motion triggered by jerks, jolts, and splenetic bursts of irritation. Searching for health, Smollett follows a course of exercise violently charged. His travelers seldom jog along complacently. Here is his description of the difficulty he encounters "pulling off" a companion's boots after a day on the road:

the marquis's boots . . . were . . . so loaded with dirt on the outside, and so swelled with the rain within, that he could neither drag them after him as he walked, nor disencumber his legs of them, without such violence as seemed almost sufficient to tear him limb from limb. In a word, we were obliged to tie a rope about his heel, and all the people in the house assisting to pull, the poor marquis was drawn from one end of the apartment to the other before the boot would give way: at last his legs were happily disengaged, and the machines carefully dried and stuffed for next day's journey. [306]

Reducing body to mechanized matter, Smollett turns his subject man into the objectified "homme machine,"[52] an entity possessing, and being possessed by, detachable parts that need to be "dried and stuffed" overnight. In the process, he also calls attention to the pains of movement, and paradoxically, the pleasures those pains afford. He seems to delight in such fleshly battles. Sentimental battering only increases the animal spirits. Here he is splenetically approaching Florence, certain he is being waylaid by villainous servants to a solitary, "bad" house only five miles from his appropriate destination. Enraged, he and his wife, "up to the ancles in mud," set out against prudent advice to walk to Florence:

52. The classic discussion of man the machine can be found in Aram Vartanian's edition of Julien Offray de La Mettrie, *L'Homme Machine: A Study in the Origins of an Idea* (Princeton: Princeton University Press, 1960).

> Behold us then in this expedition; myself wrapped up in a very heavy great-coat, and my cane in my hand. I did not imagine I could have walked a couple of miles in this equipage, had my life been depending; my wife a delicate creature, who had scarce ever walked a mile in her life. . . . The night was dark and wet; the road slippery and dirty; not a soul was seen, nor a sound was heard: all was silent, dreary, and horrible. I laid my account with a violent fit of illness from the cold I should infallibly catch, if I escaped assassination, the fears of which were the more troublesome as I had no weapon to defend our lives. While I laboured under the weight of my great-coat, which made the streams of sweat flow down my face and shoulders, I was plunged in the mud, up to the mid-leg at every step; and at the same time obliged to support my wife, who wept in silence, half dead with terror and fatigue.

Not only does Smollett reach Florence, but he arrives "with great satisfaction . . . from a conviction that my strength and constitution were wonderfully repaired . . . fully persuaded that the hardships and violent exercise . . . had greatly contributed to the re-establishment of my health" (286–289).

When Smollett "increase[s] the motion of the machine, to *unclog the wheels of life*; and now and then take a plunge amidst the waves of excess in order to case-harden the constitution" (*HC*, 339), he practices a harder version of the sentimentality Sterne plays at. His sentiments can, indeed must, hurt to be felt, and provoke in the process a motion that depends upon irritability. "It was happy for me that I had a good deal of resentment in my constitution, which animated me on such occasions against the villainy of mankind," Roderick Random crows, "and enabled me to bear misfortunes otherwise intolerable." His, and Smollett's other frequent travelers could not drag their bodies across his pages without "inveigh[ing] with great bitterness" and "boiling with indignation."[53]

The spleen pushes traveler Smollett across France, invigorating his discourse on the trials of hazarding "cold, damp, dark, dismal, and dirty" inns where one inevitably encounters "disobliging and rapacious . . . auwkward, sluttish and slothful . . . lazy, lounging, greedy, and impertinent" churls along the way. His version of "sentimental commerce" works on the principle of underpayment. While Sterne explains complacently that properly distributed livres smooth the roughest, stoniest path, Smollett provokes the hardships that reward his notorious resistance to accommodation.

53. *The Adventures of Roderick Random,* ed. P. -G. Boucé (Oxford: Oxford University Press, 1979), 242.

> The best method I know of travelling with any degree of comfort is to allow yourself to become the dupe of imposition, and stimulate their endeavors by extraordinary gratifications. I laid down a resolution (and kept it) to give no more than four and twenty sols per post between the two postillions; but I am now persuaded that for three-pence a post more, I should have been much better served, and should have performed the journey with much greater pleasure. [328–329]

But what is the point of comfort and pleasure? Resentment, not pleasure, animates and "case-hardens" the constitution.

The animating principle of irritation and hardship is most vividly illustrated in Roderick Random's encounter with the marching regiment of Picardy. He meets a party of soldiers and their wives and children dancing together, "unbending and diverting themselves . . . after the fatigue of a march."

> I had never before seen such a parcel of scare-crows together, neither could I reconcile their meagre gaunt looks, their squalid and ragged attire and every other external symptom of extreme woe, with this appearance of festivity.

Random joins their band only to learn that it is the hunger, thirst, and fatigue that drives them forward. "So much chased with the heat and motion of my limbs that in a very short time the inside of my thighs and legs were deprived of skin," he proceeds "in the utmost torture." The plumpness of his constitution inhibits his progress, and he envies the withered condition of his comrades "whose bodies could not spare juice enough to supply a common issue, and were indeed proof against all manner of friction." The "miserable wretches, whom a hard gale of wind would have scattered through the air like chaff," bear toil that his softer, juicier flesh cannot endure. Literally marching and dancing "out of matter," the soldiers have refined their flesh into an efficient marching machine that runs not on the "onions, coarse bread, and a few flasks of poor wine,"[54] but on motion itself.

Smollett's texts depend upon this principle of motion. His heroes are notorious for pushing through episodes so random that endings, when they turn up, seem suspiciously parodic. Even *Humphry Clinker,* with its "country dance" of weddings, moves past closure toward an unstable text studded with "turds," "crutches," "mattermoney," slick with the "grease of God" (333, 335, 352). Tabitha and Win have the last words

54. *Roderick Random,* 244–245. Significantly, when Yorick witnesses a farmer's family dance after their simple meal of lentil soup, bread, and wine, he beholds "*Religion* mixing in the dance" of "Grace" (*Sentimental Journey,* 283–284).

in language that unravels the "fatal" conjugal knots (346) ostensibly designed to tie up loose ends. Matthew Bramble begins his first letter to his physician "as lame and as much tortured in all my limbs as if I was broke upon the wheel" (5), and ends, like Sterne's sentimental wheel, rolling through a narration designed to circulate the spirits and strengthen the constitution. Such exercise, however, depends upon agents of exercise and feeling to free Bramble from his sedentary, vaporous, claustrophobic state.

Searching for health, Bramble struggles for strategies against the melancholia threatening to overwhelm him. Bramble suffers from a spleen that does not animate so much as it depresses his failing spirits. "When his spirits are not exerted externally," Jery notes, "they seem to recoil and prey upon himself" (49–50). The narrative by prescription demands exteriority, and, as Robinson, Cheyne, and Fuller recognized, depends upon a constant disruption designed to displace morbid consciousness. Painfully aware of the therapeutic benefits of exercise, Bramble nonetheless cannot free himself from the "vapour-pit" of his "inchanted" condition. If he "take[s] the air a-horseback" the way Fuller would have him do, he will be "stifled with dust or pressed to death in the midst of post-chaises, flying machines, waggons, and coal-horses," while climbing the Downs would only fatigue him to death. Having "made divers desperate leaps at those upper regions," he always falls "backwards," swinging dangerously between states of nervous despair (64).

Enter Humphry Clinker, physical surrogate, whose bare—lily-white—posteriors guarantee his physical strength while testifying to his ultimate gentility as well as Matthew Bramble's potency. As bastard auxiliary, Clinker literally moves Bramble through the text. An invigorated Bramble becomes persuaded "that in a raw, moist climate, like this of England, continual exercise is as necessary as food to the preservation of the individual" (327). To reach this point, however, Bramble must be taken up in the faithful Clinker's arms "as if he had been an infant of six months," carried ashore out of a violent stream, and bled "farrier style" back into life (313). A firm believer in the efficacy of cold-water baths and plunges into the sea,[55] Smollett, in spite of his own muscular assertions, falls back on the agency of a sentimental agent of feeling, a "staunch auxiliary,"

55. Felsenstein discusses Smollett's "pet theory" of the benefits of cold-water bathing, expressed in *An Essay on the External Use of Water* (1752), in his introduction to the *Travels*, xi. G. S. Rousseau considers Smollett's interest in cold-water bathing in his chapter "Smollett and the Eighteenth-Century Sulphur Controversy," in *Tobias Smollett: Essays of Two Decades* (Edinburgh, 1982), 144–157.

who rouses him into sensibility. Yes, "plunge amidst the waves of excess," yes, "*unclog the wheels of life,*" but whilst moving the constitution, be sure to have a hardy surrogate standing by to resuscitate waterlogged bodies and repair broken chaises. Affirmation swings back into an ironic awareness of the cost of living, of assigning the body and mind to a course of exercise that requires two bodies—one to be moved and one to do the moving.

In this last novel, close to death, Smollett splits himself into various characters designed to displace his own end. Mr. S., for instance, a sweeter Smollett, dispenses solid tokens of benevolence to a circle of dependents that only certify his patience and tolerance. His remarkable presence extruding from the real matter of Smollett's historically doctored reality disrupts the narrative almost as violently as Ferdinand Count Fathom's appearance, an extraliterary event that breaks out of the confines of Smollett's last novel. Both characters radically confuse conventions of narrative order as they insist upon their right to invade fictional time and space. Dr. S. forces his reader to regard Smollett the writer of splenetic fictions as a man of feeling; Ferdinand Count Fathom interrupts the narrative of *HC* to unsettle in the process the fictional notion that novels actually have a beginning and an end, for if their heroes keep turning up, where is the form designed to contain them?

Of all of Smollett's last characters, Lismahago, the disaffected Scot who cannot go home again, seems to speak for the once and perhaps always Scottish Smollett exiled to die in Leghorn from the disease he would not name. He is alienated not only from his homeland but from his body, representing most violently an attenuated physicality, pieced together as he is with parts not worn down but pared away by Indians after his scalp. A "caricatura" of his mortality, "the limbs and the muscles—every toe denot[ing] terror" (300), Lismahago enters the novel so dead to the present that his Scottish relations think he is an ancestral ghost. Yet through sheer, relentless energy enlivened by splenetic argumentation for and against almost every opinion Matthew Bramble holds dear, he triumphs over death itself in tableau. Adopting "the impressions of fear and amazement so naturally, that many of his audience were infected by his looks," he plays Pierot pursued by a Harlequin Skeleton, his horror endowing him "with such praeternatural agility as confounded all the spectators" in "a lively representation of Death in pursuit of Consumption" (347). In this dramatization, running out of matter becomes comically, and triumphantly, imperative.

The imperative, however, costs something, the cost of the spectacle of irritations that must be "felt" by the reader if it is to be sustained.

Sentimentality seems to require larger and grander "theatres of pain" on which to exercise the vital animal spirits necessary to set the soul in motion. Sterne's voyeuristic contemplation of spectacles of suffering, Smollett's splenetic dependence upon irritation, suggest a need for pain sensationally realized that becomes even more excessively apparent in more intentionally erotic texts. Richardson's teasing, extended modesty in offering over the course of one thousand pages Clarissa's rape to his reader only to withhold for almost two hundred pages more the victim's own shadowy version of the spectacle itself is completely and almost immediately overturned by Cleland's use of Fanny Hill's body as an always reliable theater of pain and pleasure, and culminates in the mass tableaux of orgiastic mayhem Sade designs to provoke the most exquisitely numbed feelings. The more spectacular the sexual encounters, the more fragmented and episodic their diverting, provocative representations. Experience becomes in these narratives something essentially incomplete, depending upon the instantaneous force of a feeling that becomes so painful that it must be denied, for to be experienced fully, it kills. Ironically, the sentimental quest for feeling may interrupt and divert the "natural" process leading into death only to offer more dramatically felt alternatives that might prove fatal. The dangers implicit in attempts to move the soul can be seen in two last sentimental episodes, one fictional, one factual, both dedicated to the sensationalism required to rouse the animal spirits.

The first sentimental episode comes from Cleland's *Memoirs of a Woman of Pleasure.* Fanny Hill and her friend Louisa, "loitering away the time," in search of stimulation, come across the gentle idiot, "*Good-natur'd Dick,*" selling his nosegays for a livelihood. Dick is such a perfect changeling that he can only stammer out "animal ideas." The women, ostensibly testing the rule that idiots are the most well-endowed, enter into a teasing relationship with the idiot Dick that reveals their own desires to provoke consciousness passionately and mechanically. Dick reveals a member astonishing enough to surprise his mistresses, "its enormous head seem'd in hue and size, not unlike a common sheep's heart." More significantly, the idiot Dick, entering the compliant Louisa, feels "the sting of pleasure so intolerable" that he assumes a character of furious consciousness:

> his countenance, before so void of meaning, or expression, now grew big with the importance of the act he was upon . . . his face glowing with ardours that gave all another life to it . . . his whole frame agitated with a raging ungovernable impetuousity, all sensibly betraying the formidable fierceness with which the genial instinct acted upon him.

While he awes the onlooking Fanny into respect, he rends the "torn, split, wounded" Louisa into "the utmost extremity" with "nothing either to fear, or to desire," until she goes "wholly out of her mind . . . now as meer a machine as much wrought on, and had her motions as little at her own command, as the natural himself." Once the "delicious delirium" has past, the idiot loses consciousness to take on an air of "droll, or rather tragi-comic . . . air of sad, repining foolishness, superadded to his natural one of no meaning, and ideotism."[56]

Consciousness, for a time, is made acessible through pain, in this case, Louisa's, transferred—terribly—to the idiot Dick. Cleland would seem here to be extending earlier theories of the therapeutic value of terror into an exchange that is both reciprocal and exploitative. While the lady from Cheshire regains her lost senses after falling 150 feet off a cliff, while Gaub's theoretical patients should benefit from the terrors of water therapy applied to their own minds and bodies, Louisa's idiot Dick gains consciousness from experiencing the pain he inflicts upon a mistress who "true to the good old cause" suffers "with pleasure" and enjoys "her pain." A veritable flesh-brush, an auxiliary designed to move her partner into consciousness of his pleasure, she extends the sentimental moment that depends upon her own pain, more palpably demonstrating the pliability that Sterne would exploit in his portrait of the mad Maria, an only slightly more decorous agent of feeling. Cleland makes even more obvious the role of the flesh-brush in Fanny's adventure with Mr. Barvile, a gentleman "under the tyranny of a cruel taste . . . not only of being unmercifully whipp'd himself, but of whipping others." In this painful encounter in which Fanny is "like a victim led to the sacrifice," Fanny becomes a "theatre of [Barvile's] bloody pleasure," feeling the lashes that Barvile requires to experience potency. Fanny, written into a role of compliance that threatens to be, ultimately, ironic, bears witness to the exertions required to exercise the animal spirits.[57]

Both Barvile and the idiot Dick require strong measures to rouse their sluggish animal spirits, to be provoked into escaping a state of "no meaning" that Dick eventually, with a "droll, or rather tragi-comic" air,

56. John Cleland, *Memoirs of a Woman of Pleasure,* ed. Peter Sabor (Oxford: Oxford University Press, 1985), 160–66. Sabor discusses Cleland's depiction of the "physiology of sexual reactions" in his introduction, particularly mentioning Leo Braudy's study of the connections between Cleland and La Mettrie, "*Fanny Hill* and Materialism," *Eighteenth-Century Studies* 4 (1970): 21–40. The use of the female body as feeling agent is not surprising in the light of Mandeville's rather early discussion of its particularly sensible properties. He found women "more capable Both of Pleasure and of Pain" (*Treatise,* 246).

57. Cleland, *Memoirs,* 143, 152. I consider this phenomenon at length in "What Fanny Felt: Cleland's Experiment in Sentimental Form," *Studies in the Novel,* 19, no. 3 (1987): 284–295.

resumes. The fear of falling into such a sluggish state generated enthusiasm for the most radical therapies. By the late eighteenth century, the auxiliary proved, with a certain degree of danger, to be completely mechanical. In 1791 Franz Kotzwara was discovered "hanging in a house of ill fame in Vine Street, Covent Garden," suspected of having "been making experiments in hanging in the company of some half-drunken women." An anonymous pamphlet, apparently inspired by his predicament, *Modern propensities; or, An essay on the art of strangling, & c.*, warns against, yet celebrates, a mechanical strangulation device designed to stimulate the animal spirits in elderly and antiquated males who might otherwise suffer the disagreeable effects of their mortal condition. Since the natural fear of death vitalizes lagging animal spirits, the author of the pamphlet offers an "external expedient," to suspend his clients "near death" until certain vital emotions are awakened. Promising relief, the advocate of strangulation almost parodies the tracts written against the spleen. In all cases, the vital spirits must be aroused, the great sensorium must be stimulated, and motion becomes a principle of redemption, for to sit still is to die. What is desired is

> that everything which produced irritation in the lungs and thorax [from the sensation of strangulation] produced also titulation in the generative organs: that the blood by such means being impeded in its regular velocity, rushed to the centre, and there formed, by sudden and compulsive operations, a redundancy of those vivifying secretions which animate an invigorate the machinery of procreation.[58]

When the practice of mechanically induced strangulation proved fatal to at least one seeker after vital juices, public curiosity and outrage prompted the trial of the prostitute, Susannah Hill, who was found with Kotzwara's all too material body. (She was acquitted.) Swinging between life and death, fullness and emptiness, motion and closure, Kotzwora violently and radically illustrates the dangerous temptations of the sentimental movement, and reason enough why, at least in the narratives, the motion must never cease. The blood must be kept circulating, the vital vivifying secretions rushing, but if the machinery truly works, animation can lead directly into death. Sterne knew this in his masturbatory deferral of sexual experience, and Smollett seems to have suspected as much as he parodically unravels "fatal" knots to disrupt an inevitably mortal progress. For the uninterrupted narrative becomes, fatally, closed, producing that ultimate end of the plot that must be resisted. At least on paper.

58. Richard J. Wolfe, "The Hang-up of Franz Kotzwara and Its Relationship to Sexual Quackery in Late 18th-Century London," *Studies on Voltaire and the Eighteenth Century*, no. 228 (1984): 53.

SIX

Of Masks and Mills: The Enlightened Doctor and His Frightened Patient

Antonie Luyendijk-Elshout

Fear is the most interesting of the passions.

—TOBIAS SMOLLETT, *Ferdinand Count Fathom,* 1753, 1:21

Of all the sufferings to which the mind of man is liable in this state of darkness and imperfection, the passion of fear is the severest, excepting the remorse of a guilty conscience, which however has much of fear in it, being not solely a tormenting anguish of reflection on the past, but a direful foreboding of the future.

—JAMES BOSWELL, "On Fear," *London Magazine,* November 1777

In a letter form Antonio Sanches in 1747 the distinguished Leiden professor Hironymus David Gaub learned that his friend was ill. Sanches complained about his health[1] and described his deplorable disease, which was intensifying, twisting around like a snake, producing terrible symptoms like a *pudor vitiosum*—a consuming timidity—which curtailed his activities as a court physician in Moscow. Gaub was already aware of Sanches's disease. In a previous letter, written in December 1746, he had advised Sanches to try Peruvian bark, which Gaub, among others, considered to be salutary in nervous diseases. Sanches, however, had tried the bark in vain, and Gaub thought it better for him to leave Moscow and find refuge in a warmer, drier climate. "I am afraid," Gaub wrote, "that the loneliness you are enforced to endure will increase this symp-

1. Letter from Sanches to Gaub, without exact date but probably written in 1747. See S. W. Hamers-van Duynen, *Hieronymus David Gaubius (1705–1780)*: Zijn correspondentie met Antonio Nunes Ribeiro Sanches en andere tijdgenoten (Assen and Amsterdam: Van Gorcum, 1978), 84–91. Sanches (1699–1783) was a Portuguese Jew, recommended by his teacher Boerhaave in 1731 to the Empress Anna Ivanovna. For political reasons he was obliged to leave Russia in 1747, since Anne's successor Elisabeth Petrovna suspected him of practicing his Jewish religion secretly. See David Willemse, "Antonio Nunes Ribeiro Sanches, élève de Boerhaave et son importance pour la Russie," *Janus,* suppl. 6 (1966).

tom and finally it will prevent the daily intercourse with people, even ending into misanthropy. Finally, this illness will destroy the power of the herbs."[2] Loneliness, fear, misanthropy: this was the psychological sequence Gaub suspected, yet fear was a common symptom in patients during the eighteenth century. But for Sanches, fear was a consequence of seeing Russia as a hostile foreign environment, and this uneasy situation left him perpetually anxious and uncertain.

This study explores the various roles played by fear in both the theory and practice of medicine in the eighteenth century. Of particular concern is the presentation of fear by patients to physicians, and the varying interpretations of that fear. I will also review the vast repertoire of serious and experimental therapies employed to cope with fear, the state of the patient's mind and body (considered separately and in union), which few physicians understood.

Not even the medical world could be isolated from the ordinary speculations they had engendered. Preachers and philosophers, painters and actors, physicians and authors: all suffered their own concept of fear and anxiety—and these fears were reflected in their behavior: preacher to congregation, actor to audience, and surely, patient to physician. Frightened people have been variously described in a wide body of eighteenth-century literature. What were people afraid of? Did their fears focus on other things than death, poverty, and war? How did they handle stress and anxiety and how did they express their emotions?

My answers to these questions trace the opinions of young physicians who, even in their earliest dissertations, studied and evaluated anxiety and fear. We shall see how their attention and concern created a revolution in the practice of medicine. These studies have a certain *fraîcheur,* an open-mindedness not often found in accepted textbooks. Moreover, they lead us directly to the important medical opinions of the time delineating fear, and they both reflect and betray the influence of the school and the philosophy that followed. The essence of fear is not easily captured in a brief confession of patient to doctor, and there were few wealthy enough to spend time and money for in-depth consultation. But a few case histories survive, written in the traditional manner and language, and they are most revealing.

By the early eighteenth century, anxiety and extraordinary fear were among the symptoms of insanity, albeit the presence of anxiety in itself was not sufficient to declare a patient insane. Coupled to the physician's

2. Hamers-van Duynen, *Gaubius,* 86. Gaub was attempting to keep the power of the bark from public derogation. Since there were no proven drugs, all forms of placebo needed reinforcement and constant postive feedback.

difficulty in weighing the degree of fear and anxiety is the philosophical (and even semantic) category of madness, a category whose history Michel Foucault brilliantly described almost two decades ago.[3] Foucault's work, as is well known, has been developed and refined by a worldwide flood of publications on the history of lunatic asylums, on the treatment of the insane, and on the biographies of those persons concerned.[4] Thus, my interest concerns not the "grande peur" of madness, as so eloquently described by Foucault, but the fears of ordinary people who suffered from ordinary and common somatic diseases and emotional disturbances, from the *perturbationes animi,* as they were called in the parlance of the time.

One must recognize that the eighteenth-century physician saw as many anxious patients as the physicians of today. He was trained to listen to their complaints, suggest diet and exercise, and prescribe medicines to calm them down. More often it was the surgeon who dealt with truly scared patients—those who had to undergo amputation or other major surgery. Since possibilities of anesthesia were limited, reactions to pain and panic were mixed, and no clear distinction was made between the variety of sensations in the reports of the operation or in learned treatises on the passions of the mind. We would expect to find important answers to our questions about fear in medical treatises, written by either physicians or surgeons who practiced in densely populated areas and major cities of Europe. Medical practice was more limited in the rural districts, where a local surgeon or apothecary more typically kept an open shop, and patients could come for treatment. The complaints of patients from these rural districts rarely reached a doctor of medicine. Peasants often used drugs prepared in the tradition of folk or domestic medicine; a surgeon was visited only in cases of trauma or, if he practiced obstetrics as well, in cases of problems with a delivery. In the country each surgeon had a self-compiled list of medicines. In the Netherlands, for example, the surgeons were not obliged to follow the pharmacopoeia until 1805.[5] There were some books in the vernacular

3. Michel Foucault, *Histoire de la folie a l'âge classique* (Paris: Gallimard, 1972).

4. Small research societies in many countries are active in the history of psychiatry, in part as the consequence of this paradigmatic Foucaldian work. In Belgium and the Netherlands, for example, vast inventories have been made of archives and collections dealing with psychiatric hospitals and lunatic asylums. In Belgium, P. van der Meersch has edited studies on psychiatry, religion, and authority; see *Psychiatrie, Godsdienst en gezag: De ontstaąnsgeschiedenis van de psychiatrie in Belgie als paradigma* (Leuven: Amersfoort, 1984).

5. D. J. B. Ringoir, *Plattelandschirurgijns in de 17e en 18e eeuw* (Diss. Amsterdam; Bunnik, 1977), 101. See also G. B. Risse, R. L. Number, and J. W. Leavitt, *Medicine without Doctors* (New York, 1977).

during the eighteenth century for rural surgeons, some of these being translated pharmacopoeias, but rather little is known about the solitary frightened patients deep in the country. Especially lacking is an understanding of that fear which stems from isolation—the relationship of personal anxiety to the environment.

If we proceeded in this vein, we should soon find ourselves investigating outbursts of mass hysteria, witchcraft, suicides, and riots. Despite the Enlightenment and the rationality it brought with it, a great part of the European population—the poor in the cities and the peasants in the country—was illiterate and hopelessly attached to medical superstition.[6] An example of fear among peasants was recorded by the members of the Académie de la Rochelle in France. In February 1784, only a few months after Montgolfier's experiment, the townspeople were invited by the Academy to be present at a balloon fair, arranged by the local pharmacist. The balloon went up and stayed aloft for about thirteen minutes. When it came down in the open fields where workers were unaware of the event, it was cut to pieces by farmers, who attacked the balloon with their pitchforks. To assuage panic, the town published a pamphlet to explain that the balloon was an experiment, due to natural causes, and not the work of the devil.[7]

PIETY, PATIENTS, AND PASSIONS OF THE MIND

It was early believed that pathological phenomena, such as a state of anxiety, might be a consequence of sin. Metaphysical causes were considered as well: a punishment by God or retribution of debt, which brought the patient into a situation that he needed the assistance of the Church. These interactions between the physical and the metaphysical, between the mind and the body, belonged foremost to the field of moral theology.[8] Doctors were only permitted to give their opinion on the

6. An impressive study of this problem can be found in Michael MacDonald, *Mystical Bedlam: Madness, Anxiety, and Healing in Seventeenth-Century England* (Cambridge: Cambridge University Press, 1981).

7. Jean Torlais, "l'Académie de la Rochelle et la diffusion des sciences au XVIII siècle," *Revue des sciences* 12 (1959): 111–135.

8. G. S. Rousseau, "Psychology," in *The Ferment of Knowledge: Studies in the Historiography of Eighteenth-Century Science*, ed. G. S. Rousseau and Roy Porter (Cambridge: Cambridge University Press, 1980), 175. Rousseau wisely pays attention to religious treatises on the soul by English clergymen, adapted by physicians. The French school of historians (especially *Annales* and the social historians) has been very active in their search for traces of fear in last wills and prayers; see for instance Jean Delumeau in *La peur en occident, XVIe au XVIIIe siècle* (Paris, 1978).

temper of the patient; they were not free to venture upon the psychological analysis of his fear.[9] It would be fruitless to search medical treatises for such psychological evaluation. Instead of analysis, doctors were trained to substantiate evidence on the four tempers, the choleric, melancholic, phlegmatic, and sanguine temper, and to respond to the predisposition of patients for emotional reactions such as fear. They explained the physiology and pathophysiology of these emotional reactions, they described various case histories, but they refrained from explaining the "spiritual fears," in terms of guilt and remorse.

The pious had a different attitude in the acceptance of the emotionally disturbed patients, different in that they invoked religious agents as antecedent to physiological causes. They did not neglect anatomy or physiology: they rather blended the two into an original pietistic model.[10] This was especially true in Halle, Germany, where Pietism was the leading religion. Michael Alberti (1682–1757) rejected any materialistic explanation of disease, certainly for disease in which the mind was involved. Alberti was the son of a pietist minister. After studying theology and afterwards medicine, he became a devoted pupil of Georg Ernst Stahl (1659–1734), the leading professor of medicine in Halle. Alberti's *Specimen Medicinae Theologicae* (1726) was an attack against the Cartesian concepts of Friedrich Hoffmann (1660–1742), who discussed the passions of the mind in his *Medicina Rationalis Systematica* (1716). In the Netherlands, physicotheology became an important field of interest of enlightened Protestantism. It allowed *ratio et experientia* as a tool for searching the causes of natural phenomena, for emotional disturbances as well as for other diseases.[11] So it is likely that we find more open discussions of the emotions in medical treatises written in the Netherlands at the time of Herman Boerhaave (1668–1738) and Hieronymus David Gaub (1705–1780). The differences between the Leiden and Halle Schools will be discussed later in this essay.

9. K. Rothschuh, *Konzepte der Medizin in der Vergangenheit und Gegenwart* (Stuttgart: Hippokrates Verlag, 1978), 67–70.

10. Rothschuh, *Konzepte.* An excellent discussion on the attitude of the patient in pietistic centers in Germany has been given by Johanna Geyer-Kordesch, "Cultural Habits of Illness: The Enlightened and the Pious in Eighteenth-Century Germany," in *Patients and Practitioners: Lay Perceptions of Medicine in Pre-industrial Society,* ed. Roy Porter (Cambridge: Cambridge University Press, 1986), 177–204.

11. J. Bots, *Tussen Descartes en Darwin: Geloof en Natuurwetenschap in de achttiende eeuw in Nederland* (Assen and Amsterdam, 1972), especially 49–60; J. van den Berg, "Theologiebeoefening te Franeker en te Leiden in de achttiende eeuw," *It Beaken: Tydskrift fan de Fryske Akademy* 47 (1965): 181–191.

Fear is one of the most important passions of the mind, as the great novelist quoted in the epigraph intuited at mid-century. These *passiones animi* were a subject of study for philosophers from Aristotle onward, who reduced all passions to pleasure and pain.[12] The philosophers of the seventeenth and eighteenth centuries paid sufficient attention to the emotions and their interaction with the body in order to bring these phenomena into agreement with the new philosophy of René Descartes and the discoveries in anatomy and physiology.[13] This newfound classical series of passions attached to pain and pleasure were *ira* (wrath), *terror* (fright), *metus* (fear), *moeror* (grief), *pudor* (timidity), *spes* (hope), *gaudium* (joy), and *amor* (love). These passions, like the group of six non-naturals, were most popular in medical literature and had been described by Galen.[14] The nine passions received more attention in the course of the eighteenth century, especially through the contribution of Arnulfe d'Aumont in the *Encyclopédie* of Diderot on health and hygiene.[15] A well-balanced mind was important, not only for the pious and the patients but also for the politicians, to keep the people peaceful and in a state of mental health. Although medical students were primarily engaged in the physical bodily changes accompanying the passions, they referred to John Locke's *An Essay concerning Human Understanding* (1690)[16] and to Hume's *A Treatise of Human Nature* (1739), the chapter "On the Passions," for their philosophical backgrounds and understanding of fear. Neither author believed in an inborn ability to reason but accepted experience by way of the external senses at the main source of knowledge. For Hume (1711–1769), the passions were sense perception intercepted by its idea.[17] Hume considered fear a direct passion, an

12. L. J. Rather, "Old and New Views of the Emotions and Bodily Changes: Wright and Harvey versus Descartes, James and Cannon," *Clio Medica* 1 (1965): 1–25.

13. Ibid. Descartes's *Les passions de l'âme* was translated into Dutch in 1659 by J. L. Glazemaker.

14. Air, motion and rest, food and drink, sleep and watch, evacuation and retention, and the passions of the mind. For a contemporary definition see John Harris, *Lexicon Technicum, or, An universal English Dictionary of Arts and Sciences: explaining not only the Terms of Art, but the Arts Themselves* (London, 1736). He describes them as the Non-Natural Things, or the Non-Natural Causes of Diseases. See n. 15.

15. William Coleman, "Health and Hygiene in the Encyclopédie: A Medical Doctrine for the Bourgeoisie," *Journal of the History of Medicine and Allied Sciences* 29 (1974): 399–421. See also L. J. Rather, "The Six Things Non-Natural: A Note on the Original Fate of a Doctrine and a Phrase," *Clio Medica* 4 (1968): 337–347.

16. Sylvana Tomaselli, "Descartes, Locke and the Mind/Body Dualism," *History of Science* 22 (1984): 185–205.

17. David Hume, *A treatise of human nature, being an attempt to introduce the experimental Method of Reasoning into Moral Subjects,* vol. 2, *Of the Passions* (London, 1739).

impression that arises immediately from good or evil, from pain or pleasure.[18] He also attached great value to the power of imagination in this passage from the perception of the virtue or vice to the impression he considered almost identical with the passion. Furthermore, Hume used the term "probability" to change a passion:

> Throw in a superior degree of probability to the side of grief, you immediately see that the passion diffuses itself over the composition, and tinctures it into fear. Encrease the probability and by that means the grief, the fear prevails still more and more, till at last it runs insensibly, as the joy continually diminishes, into pure grief.[19]

This combination of passions or transitions from one passion into the other was also considered by some medical students from Edinburgh, as we shall see. Combining passions suggested a way of psychological analysis and psychological treatment. Hume's enthusiasm for natural philosophy drove him far so as to compare the passions with optical phenomena:

> Are not these as plain proofs, that the passions of fear and hope are mixtures of grief and joy, as in optics it is a proof, that a colour'd ray of the sun passing thro' a prism, is a composition of two others, when as you diminish or increase the quantity of either, you find it prevail proportionally more or less in the composition? I am sure neither natural or moral philosophy admits of stronger proofs.[20]

For the enlightened students, educated by *ratio et experientia,* this metaphor must have been delightful. It is also interesting to notice that ideas of uncertainty in fear are preeminently present in theories of acting. We shall pay brief attention to the concept of fear as it was used in the theater. An actor had to play his part in such a way that his facial expressions and his gestures could be recognized by a large audience. In effect, there were prescriptions for the interpretation of the passions.

A semblance of fear should be expressed by a shrinking of the body; the actor should stand erect, with his arms along his body and his fists closed. His legs should be slightly apart; his eyes should be flickering with a restless glance. He should pace up and down the stage, twisting his fingers, but at the same time keep his shoulders hugged and he should express the uncertainty in his face.[21] These instructions were

18. Ibid., 181.
19. Ibid., 218.
20. Ibid., 219.
21. J. Jelgershuis, *Theoretische lessen over de gesticulatie en mimiek* (*Amsterdam: Meyer/Warnars,* 1827), 150.

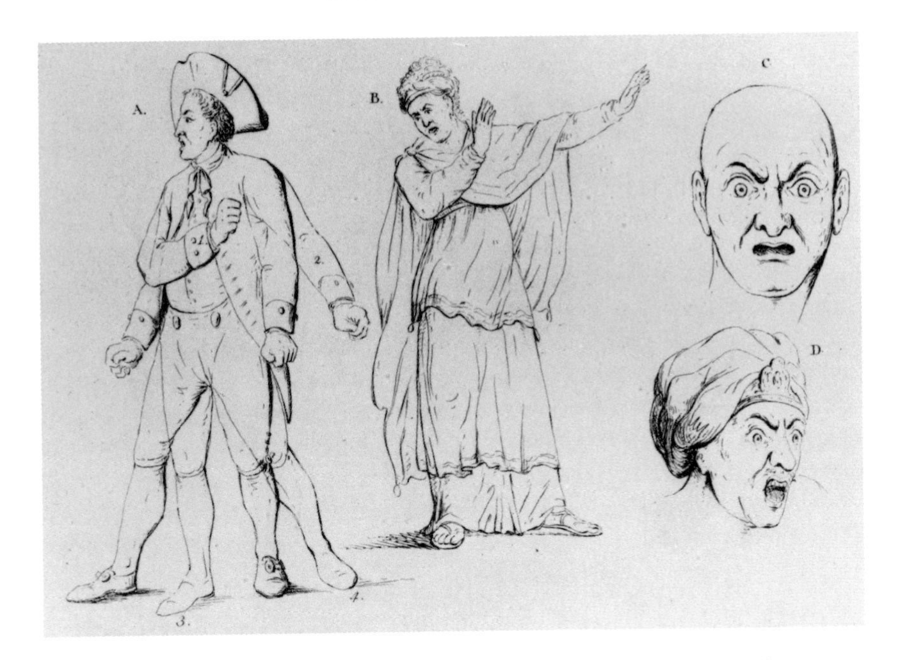

Pl. 6. "Expressions of Fear by Actors," in J. Jelgerhuis, *Theoretische lessen over gesticulatie en mimiek* (Amsterdam, 1827).

partly inspired by the French painter Charles le Brun (1619–1690), who wrote a manual on the way of illustrating the passions.[22] This booklet influenced several Dutch painters including Gerard de Lairesse (1641–1711), who praised le Bruns's work.[23] But the actors were also indebted to Petrus Camper (1722–1789) and Georges Louis Leclerc de Buffon (1708–1788), who paid attention to the physiognomy of the passions from a medical and a biological point of view. Buffon described with great care the changes of the facial expression in various stages of fear, observing the eyes, the eyebrows, the lips, and the opening of the mouth.[24] Petrus Camper tried to explain these changes anatomically, paying tribute to the innervation of the facial muscles and urging his students to notice the changes in the body in general, when they were

22. *Over de afbeelding der Hartstogten of Middelen, om dezelve volkomen te leeren afteekenen,* translated into Dutch by F. Kaarsgieter (Amsterdam, 1703), from the original French version by Charles le Brun, *Conférence sur l'expression générale et particulière* (Paris, 1698).

23. Jelgershuis, *Theoretische lessen,* 130.

24. Buffon's *Histoire naturelle* was published between 1749 and 1789. Part of this impressive work is on the natural history of man. In this study, he described the expressions of passions. *Histoire naturelle,* vol. 20 (Paris, 1799), 177, 183).

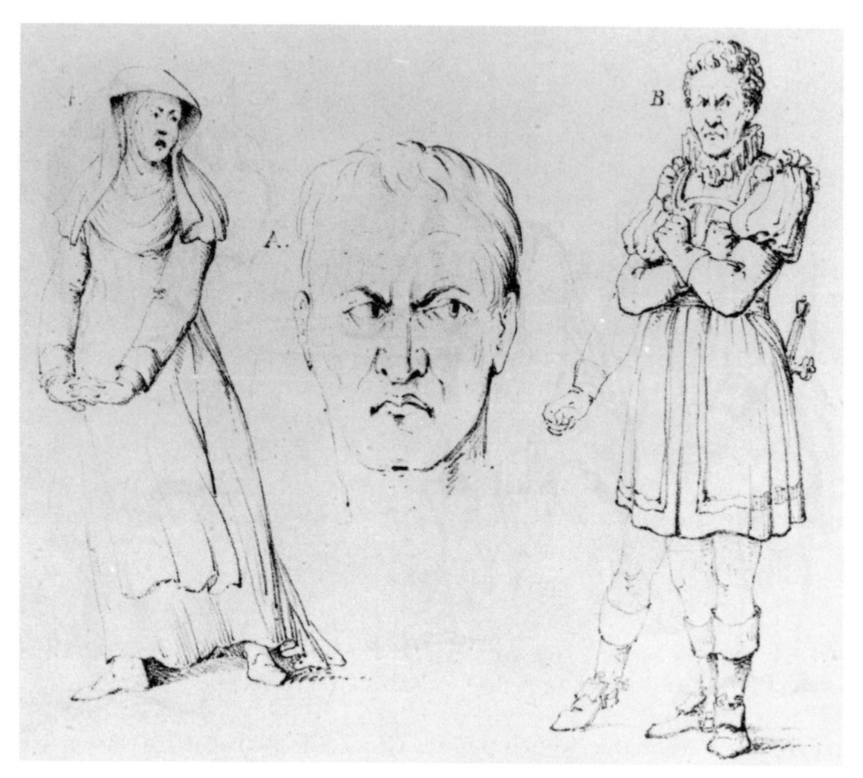

Pl. 7. "Expressions of Fear by Actors," in J. Jelgerhuis, *Theoretische lessen over gesticulatie en mimiek* (Amsterdam, 1827).

describing frightened persons.[25] These facial expressions were also observed by the physicians, who mentioned these signs in their description of the frightened patient. But physicians used a medical interpretation; they were more interested in the physiological explanation of the pale color, the trembling lips, and the shaking knees, than in a lively portrayal of the patients' physionomy. We find these representations in particular in some student dissertations.

FEAR AND ANXIETY IN MEDICAL DISEASE

The main diseases of the time which held anxiety as an underlying symptom were *hypochondria* and *hysteria*. The diagnosis of such a disease

25. P. Camper, "Over de wijze, om de onderscheidene hartstogten op onze wezens te verbeelden" (On the way to depict different passions on our appearances). This lecture

was of great importance for a medical practitioner. The treatment would be lengthy and the patient would need serious attention. If he succeeded in curing the patient, he was considered a successful doctor and he could afford himself a *praxis aurea,* earning much money from usually well-to-do patients. *Hypochondria* thus became an especially fashionable disease. As the Swiss structuralist critic and historian of medicine Jean Starobinski has pointed out, it was closely related to *melancholy,* the classic disease described by Hippocrates, as a neuropsychiatric syndrome with depression, hallucinations, mania, and convulsive crises.[26] The theory of the origin of this disease was humoral: a corruption of the black bile would mix with the blood and act as a poison. Afterward, authors differentiated the signs and symptoms of the disease in various clinical pictures. Galen described three types of *melancholy,* one located in the whole body, one located in the brain, and finally a third type, *hypochondriacum flatulentumque morbum,* a disease in the upper abdomen with flatulence, belching, abdominal pain, and fear.[27]

This last form of *melancholy* became a separate entity, known as hypochondria, described in medical treatises from the seventeenth century onward as a common disease. Among others, Robert Burton (1577–1640), who published his *Anatomy of Melancholy* in 1621, maintained that the boundaries between *melancholy* and *hypochondria* stayed rather vague and held that one was simply a form of the other. The physician accepted patients with an isolated delusion as long as they were socially acknowledged as hypochondriacs. He would treat them with much care, provided they were not too excited or aggressive, only involved in their own world, without causing nuisance to their environment. In the event a patient became agitated by a delirium or a dominating "idée fixe," insanity was suggested, and the patient was sent to an asylum for care. Boerhaave took this idée fixe as the most serious symptom of melancholy, combined with the agitated delirium without fever.[28] *Hypochondria* in the eighteenth century was a disease with a great variety of symptoms

was presented to the pupils of the Academy of Art in Amsterdam in 1774. Published by A. G. Camper in *Redevoeringen van wijlen Petrus Camper* (Utrecht, 1792).

26. Jean Starobinski, "Geschichte der Melancholiebehandlung von den Anfängen bis 1900," *Acta Psychosomatica* (Basel) 4 (1960): 15.

27. E. Fischer-Homberger, *Hypochondrie, Melancholie bis Neurose: Krankheiten und Zustandsbilder* (Bern, Stuttgart, Vienna: Verlag Huber, 1970), 15. The author refers to Galen, *De locis affectis,* liber 3, cap. 10.

28. H. Boerhaave, *Aphorisms,* 1089. The *Aphorismi de Cognoscendis et Curandis morbis in usum doctrinae domesticae* were first published in Leiden in 1709. They were translated into English by J. de la Coste in 1715 as *Boerhaave's Aphorisms concerning the Knowledge and Cure of Diseases.*

of which fear was only one of the complaints. It mainly affected men of all ages, and women after their childbearing period.[29] The patients were afraid of death, afraid of diseases, afraid of being poisoned. Sometimes they were possessed by delusions, such as the impression of a number of frogs hidden in their abdomen or that they were changing into glass figures.[30] This glass delusion is a remarkable phenomenon in the history of psychiatry. It was widespread from the beginning of the seventeenth century up to 1850, when the diagnosis disappeared into a new and different system of nosology.[31] Patients suffering a glass or pottery delusion had one thing in common: an obsessive fear they might break into pieces. They did everything to protect themselves; they were even afraid of being pushed or touched.

The first description of such a delusion can be traced back to the second century. It was described by Rufus of Ephesus. The patient fancied himself to be a "keramon," a large piece of pottery.[32] In another case a Florentine nobleman fancied himself to be an oil vessel, and there are various other cases of the pottery delusion to be found in history.[33] In the book *On the condition and disposition of the human body,* which was published in 1561, the Dutch physician Lieven Lemnius (1505–1568) gave a very exact description of a patient who believed his buttocks to be made of glass.[34] He was afraid to sit down, he thought his buttocks would break and the glass would be scattered all over the floor. This case history was repeated in various textbooks all over Europe. Because of

29. At the Edinburgh Infirmary thirteen cases of hypochondria, of which nine were men and four women, were registered between 1770 and 1800. G. Risse, *Hospital Life in Enlightenment Scotland: Care and Teaching at the Royal Infirmary of Edinburgh,* Cambridge History of Medicine, ed. Charles Webster and Charles Rosenberg (Cambridge: Cambridge University Press, 1986), 153.

30. F. F. Blok, *Caspar Barlaeus: From the correspondence of a melancholic* (Assen and Amsterdam: Van Gorcum, 1976), 110. This book deals with the depression of the eminent scholar Caspar Barlaeus (1584–1648), how he informed his friends of the glass delusion and other signs of his disease, and how his friends reacted to his melancholy. It also gives information on the medical treatment of depressions at the time.

31. A. J. Lameijn, "Wie is van glas? Notities over de geschiedenis van een waan" ("Who is made of glass? Notes on the history of a delusion"), in *Een Psychiatrisch Verleden,* ed. J. M. W. Binnenveld et al. (Baarn: AMBO, 1982) 26–93. A. J. Lameijn is a Dutch psychiatrist who made a profound study on the glass delusion.

32. Lameijn, "Wie is van glas?" 28. See also Hellmut Flashar, *Melancholie und Melancholiker in den medizinischen Theorieen der Antike* (Berlin: de Gruyter, 1966) and Starobinski, "Geschichte der Melancholiebehandlung."

33. See works cited in n. 32. The case was mentioned by the artist Benvenuto Cellini (1500–1571) in his autobiography, first published in 1728. *La Vita* was translated into English in 1771 for the first time.

34. L. Lemnius, *De habitu et constitutione corporis* (Antwerp, 1561), fol. 141v.

the rather grotesque phenomena of the disease, these delusions became a favorite subject for literature and poetic expression. For instance, Constantijn Huygens, the seminal Dutch poet of the early seventeenth century, wrote a poem as early as 1622 on the glass delusion of a hypochondriac.

> Here's one fears everything that moves in his vicinity
> What's wrong? Well every where he's touched is made
> of glass, you see
> The chairs will be the death of him, he trembles at the bed,
> Fearful the one will break his bum, the other smash his head
> Now it's a kiss appeals him, now a flicked finger shocks
> Just as a ship that's gone off course sails, fearful of
> the rocks.[35]

The gloomy aspect of these delusions was the loss of the identity of the patient. Moreover, it could mean an impulse for disorderliness, superstition, or even religious sectarianism.

So even in hypochondria or in the twilight zone of melancholy these delusions were observed with suspicion by the enlightened rationalists, since they disturbed the wordly order of state. Henry More warned in his *Enthusiasmus Triumphatus* (1656) of these perfidious dangers:

> For I shall easily further demonstrate that the very nature of Melancholy is such, that it may more fairly and plausibly tempt a man into such conceits of inspiration and supernatural light from God, then it can possibly do into those more extravagant conceits of being Glasse, Butter, a Bird, a Beast, or any such thing.[36]

In contrast, these delusions were mostly accepted as a part of a fashionable, if somewhat seraphic, disease: "the English Malady, the spleen or the Vapours," in Dr. Cheyne's memorable phrase, as *hypochondria* was known in England and France.[37] The patients were not incarcerated so

35. Blok, *Caspar Barlaeus,* 115. Constantijn Huygens (1596–1687) was a well-known poet and secretary to the Stadholder Frederik Hendrik. The poem was probably composed for Barlaeus.

36. Henry More, *Enthusiasmus Triumphatus* (London, 1662; reprint, Los Angeles: William Andrews Clark Memorial Library, University of California, 1966, as Publication no. 118 of the Augustan Reprint Society), 10. See also H. J. Schings, *Melancholie und Aufklärung* (Stuttgart: Metzler Verlag, 1977), for the tensions between delusions and authorities.

37. Richard Blackmore, *A treatise of the Spleen and Vapours* (London, 1726), 161–162. See also Ilza Veith, "On Hysterical and Hypochondriacal Afflictions," *Bulletin of the History of Medicine* 30 (1956): 233–251. There were a vast number of medical treatises written on hypochondria; for a survey of eighteenth-century treatises on this disease see Fischer-Homberger, *Hypochondrie,* 35–44, also her bibliography.

long as their disease did not develop into the cerebral condition of *melancholy,* which was considered to be a state of insanity.

The hypochondriac might also be vexed by the nightly apparition of an incubus.[38] This is a little monster which sits upon the belly of the patient. The poor victim feels a heavy pressure on his stomach, he lies frightened and paralyzed with wide-open eyes looking at his nasty visitor without being able to move or to scream. Sometimes the monster does not sit on his victim, but is experienced as lying under his body. In that case, it is called succubus, a typical nightmare for a male patient, since either the victim or his physician ascribed a sexual origin for the apparition. The students define the succubus as a consequence of onanism,[39] which was coming under the attention of the physicians at the time. When young women complained about suffering from a nightmare in the shape of an incubus, it was usually considered to be a symptom of suppressed sexual desire. Sometimes the victims are caught by seizures, which dispel after some time. This nightmare has a long history. The incubus was already known to St. Augustin[40] and has been associated with demonic powers. When the belief in demons was on the wane, the incubus continued to harass anxious patients. It was used as a theme in art, the good and the bad nightmare, as painted for instance by the Swiss artist Henry Fuseli in 1781.[41]

The presence of an incubus could also be a symptom of *hysteria,* a condition considered to be the female counterpart of the exclusively male *hypochondria.* This disease had its seat in the womb. Thomas Sydenham (1624–1689) wrote a famous book on the disease, in which he described the womb as "the seat of a thousand evils," suggesting that Hippocrates had already mentioned this fact. *Hysteria* caused headache, anxiety, convulsions, and several disturbances in sensation. The greatest

38. The incubus became a popular theme for medical theses under the influence of the mechanistic explanation of human physiology. In Leiden the first thesis on this subject was defended by a Polish student, Christiaan Maevius, in 1692. In 1734 a Dutch student, Matthaeus Huisinga, presented his *Dissertatio Medica Inauguralis sistens Incubi causas praecipuas,* followed by the Swedish student Tiberius Zacharias Kiellmann in 1739 on the same subject.

39. See on this problem Th. Tarczylo, *Sexe et liberté au siècle des luminères* (Paris: Presses de la Renaissance, 1983).

40. Augustinus, *De Civitate Dei,* liber XV, cap. xxiii. Virgil describes the incubus in the *Aeneid,* 12.908–912 *non lingua valet, non corpore notae sufficient vires; nec vox aut verba sequuntur* (the tongue is powerless, the familiar strength fails the body, nor do words or utterance follow—tr. Mackail).

41. A. M. Hammacher, *Phantoms of the Imagination* (New York: Harry N. Abrams, 1981), 41–46.

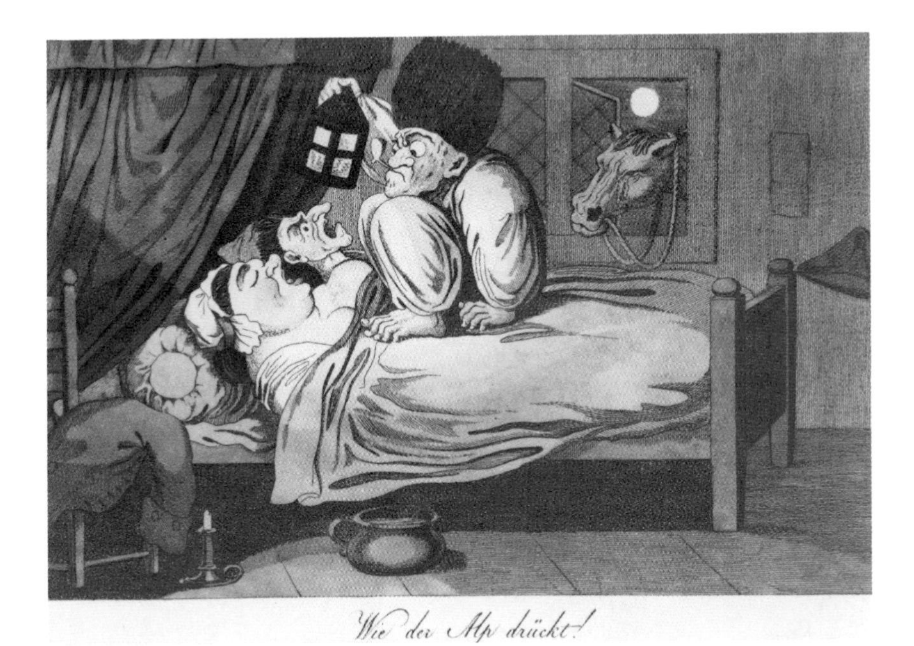

Pl. 8. German cartoon in the manner of Rowlandson, "The Pressure of an Incubus" (ca. 1800).

danger of hysteria was its location; "suffocation of the womb" might affect pregnancy in its early stage and cause serious harm to the embryo. Thomas Sydenham called *hysteria* and *hypochondria* the same disease; the hysterical man, however, was only fully accepted in the nineteenth century, when Jean Marie Charcot analyzed *hysteria* as a neurological disease and traced the signs in both sexes.[42] The frightening symptoms of the disease were usually the changes in body sensations, sometimes followed by convulsions. Gerard van Swieten (1700–1772), professor in Vienna and a true pupil of Boerhaave, ascribed the onset of the disease to emotional breakdown:

> Healthy women, who have been made angry or frightened become anxious, their blood gets upset in the vessels and their heartbeats accelerate. Shortly afterwards, they experience something in their abdomen turning and moving, rising on the left side. As soon as this sensation hits the mid-

42. On hysteria, see Ilza Veith, *Hysteria: The History of a Disease* (Chicago: University of Chicago Press, 1965), especially chapters 7 and 8; idem, "On Hysterical and Hypochondriacal afflictions." Also E. Fischer-Homberger, *Krankheit Frau und andere Arbeiten zur Medizingeschichte der Frau* (Bern, Stuttgart, Vienna: Hans Huber Verlag, 1979).

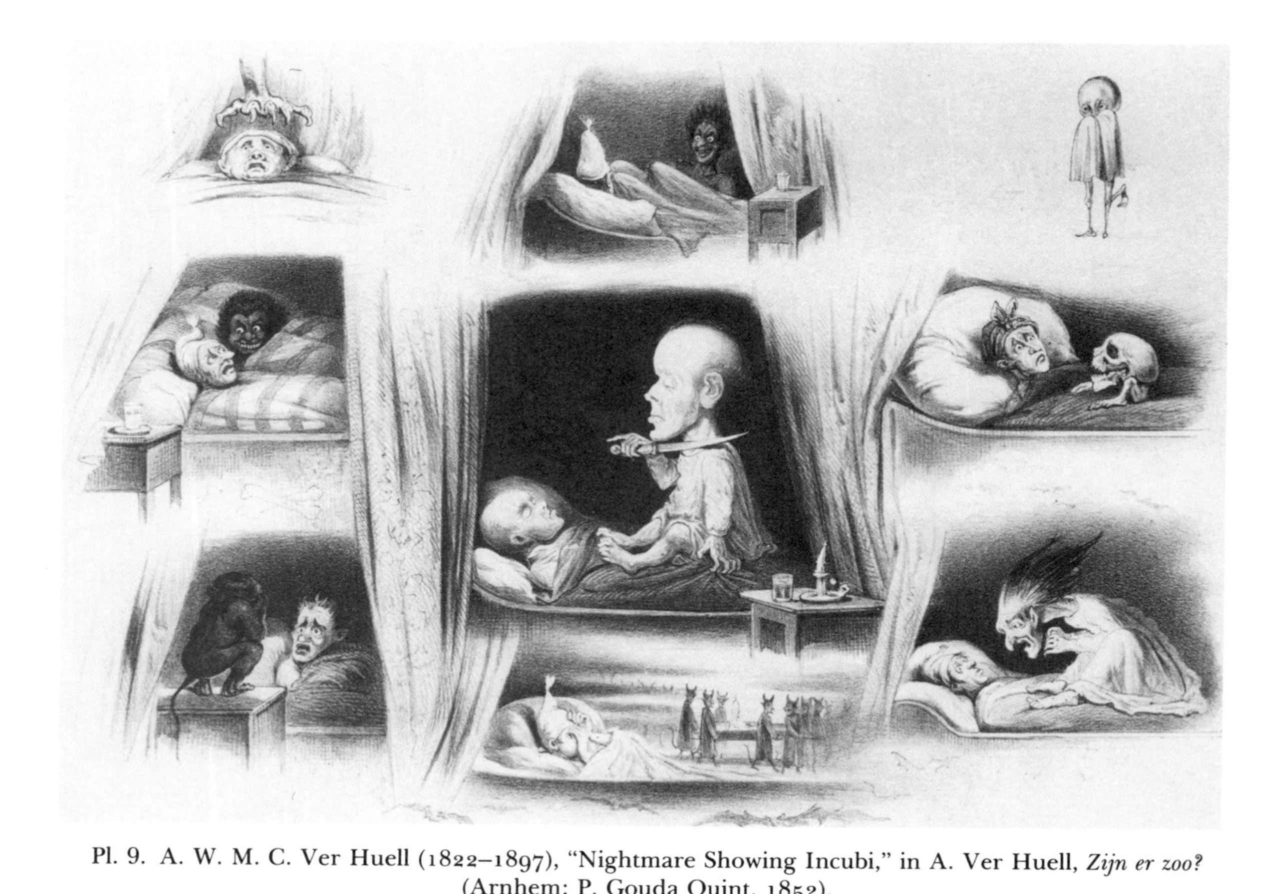

Pl. 9. A. W. M. C. Ver Huell (1822–1897), "Nightmare Showing Incubi," in A. Ver Huell, *Zijn er zoo?* (Arnhem: P. Gouda Quint, 1852).

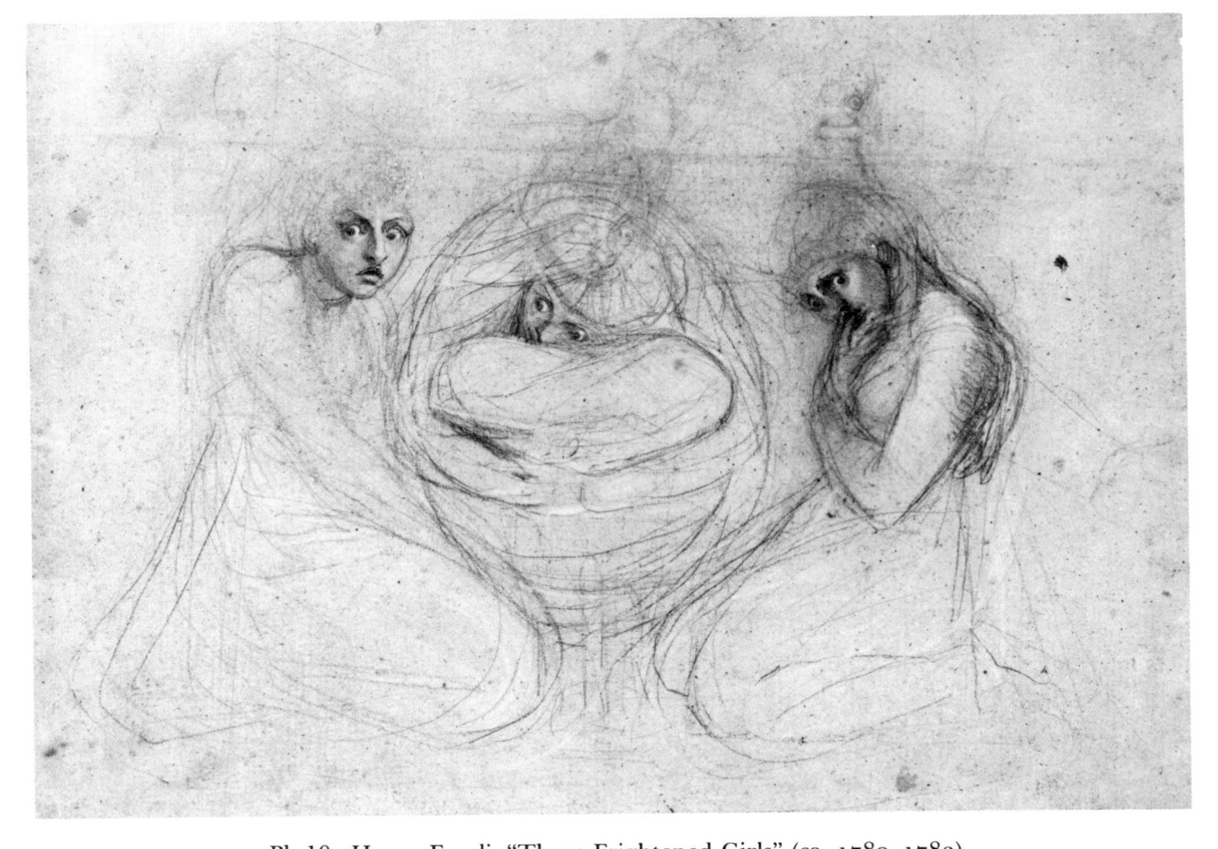

Pl. 10. Henry Fuseli, "Three Frightened Girls" (ca. 1780–1782).

riff, they get a feeling as if they are being strangled. Then they experience a heavy globe in their throat, usually they fall into convulsions.[43]

During the eighteenth century the cause of *hysteria* became firmly rooted in the nervous system. The brain itself was considered to have a high degree of irritability. In addition, patients were believed to have weak cardiovascular and muscular systems: patients fainted easily, even by such light shock as the appearance of a mouse! More serious cases would be accompanied by hysterical paralysis or a disturbed imagination with frightening delusions of devils, making obscene gesticulations. These patients were considered to be possessed by a demon, especially when they had additional symptoms such as a hoarse voice, uttering blasphemy, a tortured face, and a loss of sensibility in certain parts of the body. In these instances the church would be consulted for an exorcism. The more enlightened doctors, however, described these patients as *severe* cases of hysteria and not victims of the Devil. Anton de Haen (1704–1776), a professor in Vienna and a Dutch pupil of Herman Boerhaave, treated several hysterical patients without the interference of an exorcist with good results.[44] In his book *On Miracles* de Haen described his rather drastic therapy on severe cases of presumed demoniacal possession. The patient was put under a cold shower each time she started to curse God and the Empress of Austria or other authorities. Certainly these women suffered, but without necessary documentation we lack a full appreciation of eighteenth-century hysteria. More specifically, there seems to have been no instance of a female George Cheyne or John Hill. That is, the expounders of the condition were, like Cheyne and Hill, males, and except for a few comments about hysteria by women (I do not mean in fiction but in didactic-explanatory statements) the medical literature of hysteria is a male record composed exclusively by males. While this archive defines and describes the condition, its degree of sympathy is often lacking, sometimes for no other reason than that the physician could not penetrate its dynamcis. In fact, the cases of

43. Gerard van Swieten, *Commentaria in Hermanni Boerhaave Aphorismos de Cognoscendis et Curandis Morbis* (Hildburghausen, 1754), 3:416. Ad S 1075 of Boerhaave's *Aphorisms.* See n. 28.

44. See Dieter Cichon, *Antonius de Haens Werk "De Magia"* (1775), Münstersche Beitrage zur Geschichte und Theorie der Medizin no. 5, ed. K. E. Rothschuh, R. Toellner, and Chr. Probst (Münster, 1971). The medicalization of hysteria was very important, since in Austria witchcraft and incantations still were practiced and consequently witches could be burned at the stake! See also A. De Haen, *De Miraculis Liber* (Frankfurt and Leipzig, 1776), 194 for his description of a woman, who was supposed to have been possessed by the devil for eighteen years.

the "hysterical passions," as they were called already in 1667 by Willis[45] and others, give us more insight into the phenomenology of *hysteria* than into the psychology of the suffering women. Furthermore, several of these cases should rightly be considered as the more serious disease, *psychosis,* a true form of insanity.

Besides the diseases *hypochondria* and *hysteria,* or the combined diagnosis, there were various other reasons why patients were continually frightened. As has already been said, we shall not discuss the psychotic fears of the insane patient in this study. Our main interest remains focused on the daily life of men and women who were frightened for some reason and complained about these fears to their family, their friends, or their physician. Such anxieties have been described by scholars in learned treatises and by novelists in literature, but also in a long line of anecdotes, which are repeated again and again from the classical authors like Galen and Pliny onwards. What kinds of fears are mentioned? Besides the fear of the changed bodily sensations in hysteria and hypochondria like the glass delusion, the patients were scared of ghosts, monsters, bed-curtains, mice, earthquakes, explosions, burglars, contagious diseases, and even masks. Both Boerhaave and Tissot believed that masks may be very disconcerting. Tissot referred to Boerhaave in his warnings:

> Mr. Boerhaave discussed various cases of epilepsy in his work, following a sudden fright. Two of these cases were caused by masks. If we compare these with my cases we may say that this type of amusement is not without danger.

Indeed, Boerhaave warned against Twelfth Night parties for children and also against "making faces or grimaces." Even the reflecion of a distorted face in a mirror could frighten a sensible person and provoke convulsions.[46] A false face could frighten not only pregnant women and children but even men. We shall return to this point later on.

45. Thomas Willis accepted already a neurogenic cause of hysteria in 1667. See Veith, *Hysteria,* 133, 134. See also Robert Frank, chapter 4 above.

46. S. A. Tissot, *Traité des nerfs et leurs maladies* (Lausanne, 1778). I consulted part IV from the *Œuvres complètes* (Lausanne, 1790). Tissot describes on p. 392 a case of a child frightened by masked children on the street during a party. The child suffered from diarrhea for some weeks. Tissot refers to Boerhaave on p. 406. See Jacobus van Eems, *Hermanni Boerhaave Praelectiones Academicae de Morbis Nervorum* (Leiden, 1761), 2:801. Boerhaave repeated in his lectures the danger of frightening spectacles and the "homo larvatus," the masked man. See also John Locke, *Some Thoughts concerning Education* (1693) on scaring children with stories on ghosts and monsters. This work was already translated into Dutch in 1697. A French edition was prepared by P. Coste, which was reprinted many times, the fifth edition in Amsterdam in 1743.

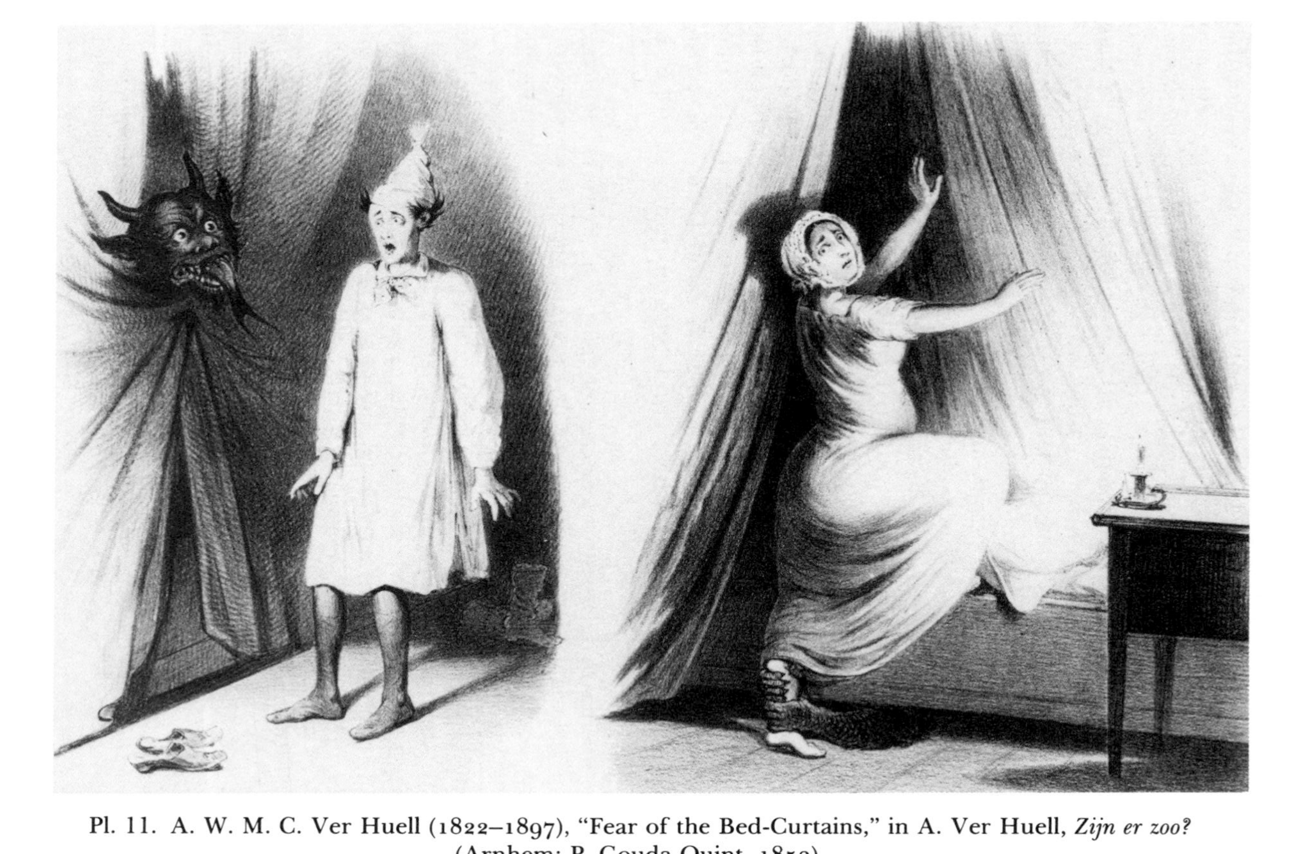

Pl. 11. A. W. M. C. Ver Huell (1822–1897), "Fear of the Bed-Curtains," in A. Ver Huell, *Zijn er zoo?* (Arnhem: P. Gouda Quint, 1852).

But fear and anxiety were most striking in serious affections of the body. It is true, most eighteenth-century studies of anxiety discuss five points of fear accompanying diseases: cardiac origin, an intoxication of the respiratory system, an obstruction of the abdominal tract, different types of fever, and *agonia,* the struggle with death. Anxiety itself was considered to be of physical origin, while fear was primarily a matter of the mind. Great medical thinkers on disease—Morgagni, Hoffmann, Boerhaave, Van Swieten, Gaub—treated all five of these points in their medical manuals with great attention. Yet we must remember that various symptoms in *hypochondria* may have had their origin in physical causes, which were yet to be perceived and understood: such as abdominal cancer or obstruction of the pathways of the bile by pathological changes in the tissue of the liver (cirrhosis). A defect of the cardiac valves was often diagnosed as *hysteria,* as were brain tumors and other neurological diseases. Before introducing some independent theories let us first pay attention to changes in the medical schools, where psychological phenomena were incorporated in the teaching program.

PIETISM, MECHANISM, AND THE SENSORIAL POWERS OF THE BRAIN

At mid-century there were three important medical schools in continental Europe whose leaders held competing medical philosophies: the schools of Georg Ernst Stahl (1659–1734) and Friedrich Hoffmann (1660–1742), both in Halle, Germany, and a third school of Herman Boerhaave (1668–1738) in Leiden. In the schools of Hoffmann and Boerhaave, medicine was practiced on the basis of a mechanical model of the human body. Stahl's system, however, has been labeled *animistic* or vitalistic. In Stahl's concept the soul is the leading power of the organic structure and is directly involved in any behavior of the body.[47] The impact of these schools upon existing medical education fostered order and structure in the teaching program and generated a rational basis for medicine. In the other European countries there was little impact for a complex number of reasons, much too complicated to be

47. On the animistic and vitalistic doctrines of Stahl see L. J. Rather, "G. E. Stahl's Psychological Physiology," *Bulletin of the History of Medicine* 35 (1961): 37–49 and Lester S. King, *The Philosophy of Medicine: The Early Eighteenth Century* (Cambridge, Mass., and London: Harvard University Press, 1978), 143–151. See also G. S. Rousseau's important study of Enlightenment vitalism and Bakhtin in *The Crisis of Modernism: Bergson and the Vitalist Tradition,* ed. Frederick Burwick and Paul Douglas (Cambridge: Cambridge University Press, 1991).

treated at any length here. In France, mechanism as a leading principle was hardly accepted.

In Germany and Leiden the concepts of the mechanistic schools interacted quite peacefully with the animism of Stahl, especially on physiological grounds such as the circulation of the blood, and the idea of *sanitas* (health) as an equal, moderate, and continuous perfusion of the humors through the parts of the body. But there was a difference in therapy: Stahl paid more attention to uncommon drugs, which he used in a sophisticated therapy of the presumed *cacochymia* in the body. *Cacochymia* was a supposed putrefaction of the body fluids, and an important part of Stahl's concept of disease. The main part of the recommended drugs were herbal, mentioned in the *Wurtemberg Pharmacopoeia* (1741).[48] Stahl also accepted more uncommon drugs as *lapis manati* and *cornu cervi*. Lapis manati is a part of an otic bone of *Manatus Australis* (sea cow) and was used in treating spasmodic diseases. *Cornu cervi* (Harts horn), discussed by Stahl in 1690, was a popular antispasmodic remedy in the chemiatric schools. Hoffmann prescribed *alterantia* to change the temper of the blood and the organs.[49] These medicines were based on the corpuscular theories of Robert Boyle's chemistry, related to the Cartesian concept of the crucial ether as a spiritual fluid through the nerves. Boerhaave wanted to act upon the "spissity" (thickness) of the body fluids and to control the density and the laxity of the fibers. His drugs were mainly Galenic and he attached much value to diet and exercise, especially in cases involving the sufferings and passions of frightened patients.[50]

The extraordinary convergence of Pietism in Halle and a concept of the *persona* (the soul inextricably linked with man's individual being) created a new school of medicine which the Germans called "Pastoralmedizin," pastoral medicine.[51] In this concept medicine was the servant

48. See Joachim Petrus Gaetke's dissertation on the general therapy of hypochondriasis, *De Vena Portae Porta Malorum Hypochondriaco-splenetico-suffocativo-hysterico-colico-haemorrhoidariorum* (Halle, 1698), 52–55 (on the portal vein as the gateway to the evils of hypochondria, of smothering of the spleen and the womb, and of hemorrhoids in the colon).

49. On Hoffmann's therapy, see K. E. Rotschuh, *Konzepte der Medizin in Vergangenheit und Gegenwart* (Stuttgart: Hippokrates Verlag, 1978), 247–249.

50. On Boerhaave's therapy, see B. P. M. Schulte, *Hermanni Boerhaave Praelectiones de Morbis Nervorum* 1730–1735, Analecta Boerhaaviana, 2, (Leiden: E. J. Brill, 1959).

51. Wolfram Kaiser and Arina Volker, "Michael Alberti (1682–1757)," *Wissenschaftliche Beiträge der Martin-Luther-Universität* (Halle-Wittenberg) 4 (1982): 9–11. See also Rothschuh, *Konzepte*, 67–70. Michael Alberti was the author of the *Specimen Medicinae Theologicae* (1726).

of faith and godliness. The *conscientia medica,* medical conscience, should always be aware of the agreement of a medical theory with theology. Students of pastoral medicine were to learn how to preserve the *tranquillitas animi*—the mental balance of the patient—a medical approach highly appreciated by evangelists and preachers. Stahl taught that there must be a direct interaction between mind and body and dictated his ideas to his students in the form of deontology: a list of duties including "musts" and "must nots." After digesting this material, students were required to dispute or defend it in dissertation.[52] There are a large number of *propemtica* (introductions) by Stahl which accompany these student works. In these speeches Stahl emphasizes medical ethics; he discusses the role of the physician in medical practice and his responsibility to his patients. For instance, in 1706 when Henricus König presented a thesis *De curatione aequivoca* (On a well-balanced therapy), Stahl gave his propemticon *De temeritate, timiditate, modestia et moderatione medici* (On drastic and reticent, on modest and restrained medical behavior) as an example of variability in an administration of therapy by the physician. Various propemtica such as *De Dissensu Medicorum* (1703) (On the disagreeing doctors), *De Visitatione Aegrorum* (1703) (On the visit of patients), *De Testimoniis Medici* (1706) (On medical reports), *De Constantia Medica* (1707) (On medical steadfastness), *De Auctoritate et Veritate Medica* (1705) (On medical authority and integrity) deal with ethics. Hoffmann went even further and expressed the need for morality in some letters to young doctors. One such letter is on physical *pietas,* which he describes as a spiritual combination of mental and physical health. Thus mental health is only possible as the individual's complete union with, and devotion to, the source of life: God.[53] As such, it may restore physical health in a patient. Stahl stressed this point too in every discussion of the *animi pathemata*: frightened patients might be bled to restore the *temperies* of the blood, but Stahl warned his students that if they wanted to treat

52. A collection of medical dissertations presented to the Halle Faculty is present in the university library a Leiden, dating from 1696–1714. They have been bound in four volumes under the title *G. E. Stahl ii . . . Dissertationes Medicae, tum epistolares tum academicae in unum volumen congestae (Halle,* 1707 *ff.).* This collection also contains dissertations defended under the supervision of Hoffmann, A. O. Goelicke (1671–1744) at Magdenburg, Johann Gottfried Berger (1659–1756) at Wittenberg, and Michael Alberti (1682–1757), just mentioned. The volumes of the collection were more or less haphazardly gathered; there is no introduction and the pages are not indicated, except for the first volume.

53. "Epistola gratularia ad Virum Magnificum, Excellentissimum atque Experientissimum Dn. Bernhardum Barnstorffium," Halle, 1 October 1696, in Stahl, *Dissertationes,* vol. 3. A congratulatory letter was reserved for important inaugurations "more majorum." In this case, it was Bernard Barnstorff, who was Dean of the Rostock University.

patients psychologically, they should be in tune with themselves and tread lightly,[54] rather resorting to *doctrina moralis*.[55] Needless to say, students were not permitted to vent their personal opinions in these dissertations, but their experience allowed some conjecture to avoid explanations of diseases by natural or materialistic causes alone.

The state of medical affairs differed profoundly in Leiden. There, students were free to speculate in their writing, albeit more or less in agreement with the current school philosophy. Calvinism and the hierarchical, mechanistic concept of the body guided by an immortal soul were compatible views on man. In Leiden the concept of medicine remained theoretical and scientific; unlike the students in the Halle school, they paid less attention to moral or spiritual issues, to the physician's duties, or to the noble task (*officium nobile*) of the physician.

At least in part, the difference in medical thinking was due to the introduction of the concepts *irritability* and *sensibility*.[56] The growing importance of the nervous system in physiology focused the attention of scholars on these phenomena. The human body summoned a new view. It became an organism with a mind, which was believed to be responsive to outside influences apart from the pathways of mechanical connections. The mind/body relation became crucial in a different way, as well; more attention was suddenly paid to psychology, education, physiognomy, and medical anthropology. In Leiden, Hieronymus Gaub took the chair after Boerhaave's death in 1738. Gaub's concept of the human body was mechanistic in Boerhaave's sense, but he was also deeply involved in the mind/body discussions then taking place within and without the university, and, especially, in the *pathemata* of the mind,[57] which

54. J. J. Reich, "De Passionibus Animi Corpus Humanum Varie Alterantibus" (Diss. Halle, 1695), in Stahl, *Dissertationes* 1:97. *Temperies,* "inter se mutua proportia," is meant by Stahl as a chemical balance in the blood; *homeostasis* in present medicine.

55. Geyer-Kordesch, "Cultural Habits of Illness" (n. 10 above), 178–204. She considers Pietism an affair of the sentiments. The faithful "feel" themselves pietists. They "feel" God within their heart. (In Calvinism, God is outside, he is the *Arbiter,* a dialogue is possible.)

56. Richard Toellner, "Albrecht von Haller: Ueber die Einheit im Denken des letzten Universalgelehrten," *Sudhoffs Archiv* 10 (1972): 171–182. Albrecht von Haller published in 1750 his famous study on these properties of the parts of the body, especially of the muscles. Since tissue could react to a stimulus, even when it was no longer in contact with the body, irritability and sensibility had a rather autonomous quality.

57. L. J. Rather, *Mind and Body in Eighteenth-Century Medicine* (London: Wellcome Historical Medical Library, 1965). This is an excellent study on Gaub's addresses *De Regimine Mentis, quod Medicorum est*—a great help for any scholar who wants to be informed on the complex material of the mind/body problem in medicine at the time.

became his preeminent study. He inspired Robert Whytt (1714–1766), the Scots Professor of Medicine in Edinburgh, who used Gaub's textbook for teaching purposes.[58] So there became a close teaching connection between Leiden and the Edinburgh school, founded in 1727 on Boerhaave's model, where the interest in psychological phenomena was growing. We may naturally expect to find concepts derived from both schools in Leiden publications, especially in the students' dissertations.

The growing interest in the sensorial powers of the brain was also responsible for a shift in the concept of disease accompanied by fear such as *hypochondria* and *hysteria*, and was especially apparent in the work of Robert Whytt, who declared these diseases to be neurogenic,[59] by which he meant originating in the nervous system. Another important consequence was the popularization of the mind/body subject. S. A. Tissot's (1728–1797) influential book *Traité des nerfs et leurs maladies* (Lausanne, 1778) became especially popular, not least because he gave an extensive survey of case histories on the *animi pathemata*, which were cited by professors of medicine all over Europe. The medical schools at Paris and Montpellier, where mechanistic doctrines never took root, explained virtually *all* emotional disturbances as "crises nerveuses" and looked for chemical changes in the blood and for indigestion.[60] Furthermore, the concept of *sympathy* gained ground again, especially in Montpellier. This "action on a distance," or external aspects of nerve endings acting in a type of vibrational or materialistic sympathy, was entirely condemned by the mechanists, but later in the eighteenth century it captured the interest of all the European physicians. Tissot paid great attention to the action on a distance upon several parts of the body by the distribution of the peripheral nerve. By this distant influence the brain had the sympathy of the stomach (*consensus*), and the concept became very important in physiology and psychology, not only in

58. R. K. French, *Robert Whytt, the Soul, and Medicine,* Publications of the Wellcome Institute of the History of Medicine, n.s., vol. 17 (London, 1969), 151. The textbook is H. D. Gaub, *Institutiones Pathologiae Medicinalis* (Leiden, 1758), which was quite popular. It was translated into English in 1778 by C. Erskine and published by C. Elliot and T. Cadell in London and Edinburgh.

59. French, *Robert Whytt,* 31–45. See also Fischer-Homberger, *Hypochondrie,* 32.

60. Jean Astruc (1684–1766) lectured in 1759 at the Collège Royal. In this lecture, he discussed the causes of hypochondria and hysteria, especially the primary cause of tension of the nerves. See the MS at the Municipal Archives in Middelburg, corr. David Henri Gallandat (1732–1782). On Gallandat, see G. A. Lindeboom, *Dutch Medical Biography: A Biographical Dictionary of Dutch Physicians and Surgeons 1475–1975* (Amsterdam, 1984).

France,[61] where Tissot's influence was considerable, but also in Scotland among Whytt's students.

The consequences for psychotherapy were not obvious. Galenic drugs were still dominant, and as we have seen, Gaub prescribed Peruvian bark and musk for attacks of hysteria or fearfulness.[62] Gaub had a special preparation for his tranquilizing medicine: he combined valerian root with Peruvian bark in a single pill. For hysterical patients his formula was an odorous drink composed of musk, Peruvian bark, and several other herbs. All these herbal and chemical formulas were fine, but they only worked to subdue the hypochondriac's fear. Amelioration required psychological treatment, a subject about which even the young medical students then had suggestions.

PORRIDGE AND RUSSIAN TEA

The following views of the concept "fear" were presented by medical students in their dissertations. Principally, there were three different conceptions: anxiety (*anxietas*), fear (*metus*), and fright (*terror*). The students wrote their treatises in obedience to the philosophical doctrines of the school, but they were encouraged to voice their own opinions; in fact they betray their training ground in a most amusing series of manners. The German students, for instance, were systematic in their discussion of the signs of fear in a patient. They often quote the case histories described by J. N. Pechlin (1644–1692), professor at the University of Kiel in Germany,[63] preferring the tale of the intimidated professor who was so frightened of his students that he would empty his bladder and rectum in a special pot just before he entered the lecture hall. In another

61. Heini Walther Bucher, *Tissot und sein Traité des nerfs: Ein Beitrag zur Medizingeschichte der schweizerischen Aufklärung,* Zürcher medizingeschichtliche Abhandlungen, ed. E. H. Ackerknecht, Neue Reihe, 1 (Zurich, 1958), 44–54. For Whytt's relation to the *consensus,* see the lectured notes of his Edinburgh pupils.

62. See Hamers-van Duynen, *Gaubius* (n. 1 above), 186.

63. J. N. Pechlin, *Observationum Physico-Medicarum Libri tres quibus accessit Ephemeris Vulneris Thoracici et in eam Commentarius* (Observations in physics and medicine in three books, and a comment on the description of a wound in the chest) (Hamburg, 1691), liber III—obs. XVII: "A Metu alvi flexus" (Loss of Faeces, caused by Fear); mentioned by J. J. Monjé, a student from Tübingen who took his degree in Leiden in 1785: *Spec. Medica Inauguralis de animi pathematibus eorum effectibus nec non salutari eorundem in morbis efficacia* (Dissertation on the affliction of the soul and their effects, with (sometimes) salutary efficacy in diseases). See also Abraham Heemskerk, *Dissertatio ethico-medica inauguralis De Animae Pathematum Efficacia in corpus Humanum* (Medical-ethical dissertation on the efficacy of the affliction of the soul upon the human body) (Leiden, 1754). Pechlin is often cited by Gaub in his *De Regimine Mentis* etc.

tale, a preacher lost his urine, when he stood in the pulpit preaching about the miracles by Christ! A Leiden student tells a similar story, this time about a lady who lost her urine each time she went to Holy Communion. Most of the case histories relating to fear involve rather grotesque details verging on the scatological, and they were repeated in medical textbooks and popular handbooks all over Europe during the late eighteenth century.[64]

Among these dissertations the one written by William Clark, an Englishman, stands out.[65] Clark was a devout Christian who eventually settled down as a general practitioner in rural Wiltshire. In his attempt to reconcile observations in medicine with the Christian faith, his dissertation remains more in the tradition of moral theology than a medical argument. Clark first treats the free will of man, which should, he believes, control the emotions. God gave emotions to man as guardians against evil and danger, and should be compared, by analogy, with physical pain as a bodyguard, which alerts the mind in case the body is threatened. But, Clark contends, the physician's duty extends beyond consideration of the patient's temper. Clark's teacher, Boerhaave, had discussed the observations of Sanctorius (1562–1636) in his lecture on imperceptible perspiration.[66] Sanctorius described this imperceptible natural perspiration under different circumstances. He observed that people who were depressed and scared gained weight; they were "heavier" than when they were happy and relaxed. Boerhaave, said Clark, advised his students to restore the perspiration in case of depressed and frightened patients by administering drugs to open the pores, but Clark disagreed. In his opinion, excitement, caused either by fear or anger, should be tempered, not medicated. To be an Englishman meant to be moderate, and moderation was a way to prevent monumental changes in the quality of the body fluids. The best prevention against

64. For instance, Wilhelm Gesenius, *Medicinisch-moralische Pathematologie oder Versuch über die Leidenschaften und ihren Einfluss auf die Geschäfte des körperlichen Lebens* (Erfurt, 1786). The most popular medical book at the time remained S. A. Tissot's *Traité des nerfs et leurs maladies* (Lausanne, 1790); see n. 46.

65. Wiliam Clark (1698–1780) studied medicine under Boerhaave and took his medical degree in Leiden in 1727, writing a dissertation on the influences of the emotions upon the human body (*Dissertatio Medica Inauguralis De Viribus Animi Pathematum in corpus humanum*).

66. Sanctorius published in 1614 his *Ars de Statica Medicina aphorismorum sectionibus septem comprehensa* (Treatise on static medicine contained in seven sections of aphorisms) in Venice. He became one of the founders of the Italian iatromechanical school. The Leiden edition of *Medicina Statica* was published in 1728. Clark refers to Boerhaave's lectures after hearing Boerhaave speak on the insensible perspiration in case of emotions.

these ominous changes (which might provoke water retention) was daily consumption of a rich, English porridge, and a flask of Rhine-wine at night. Thereby Clark drew attention to the relaxing effect of food and drink in a tense patient.

Clark also bore great admiration for the well-known doctor George Cheyne, whose treatise entitled *An Essay on Health and Long Life* was published in 1726.[67] The last paragraph of Clark's dissertation is a long and reverent quotation from a chapter by Dr. Cheyne on the *affectus animi.*[68] Clark's theory of fear may be medical and derived from Boerhaave's lectures, but his main concept lies more in the tradition of moral theology than in moral treatment. His ideology is more involved in faith than in medicine. He accepts Boerhaave's explanation of the physiological phenomenon of fear according to the experiments of Sanctorius, but he objects as follows:

> What is said in Sanctorius' theory on the effect of expected joy and hope, could more justly be applied to the hope and faith of the Christian believers.[69]

It is the *charitas divina* that gives these laws to the *animi pathemata*. Man should listen first to God (Paul,Rom. 2:15): one knows best in his heart. Clark considers disease to be a punishment of God, also a fear. He is aware of physiology and his medicines are meant to calm down an upset stomach, but he resists interfering in the pattern of anxiety by introducing psychological factors or attempting to analyze the patient's fear.

Clark's dissertation on fear differed considerably from one presented in 1738 by another student of Boerhaave, Otto Barckhuysen, a Russian student in Leiden about whom virtually nothing biographical is known.[70] Barckhuysen discussed his idea of *terror* as a sudden, unexpected confrontation with a danger, which resembles our notion of fright or alarm. But he was not inclined to call upon the metaphysical, and was interested neither in the seat of the soul nor in the interaction between body and soul and its relation to God. Barckhuysen also rejected Leibniz's theory

67. In London, 1726, by Strahan, and in Bath by John Leake.

68. He refers to G. Cheyne, *Tractatus de Sanitate Tuenda,* cap. de animi affectis, sec. 22. See on Dr. Cheyne: G. S. Rousseau, "Medicine and Millenarianism: 'Immortal Dr. Cheyne,'" in *Hermeticism in the Renaissance: Studies in Honor of Dame Frances Yates,* ed. Allen Debus and Ingrid Merkel (Cranbury, N.J.: Associated University Press, 1987), 192–230.

69. Clark, *Dissertatio,* 25.

70. Otto Barckhuysen, *Diss. med. inaug. sistens considerationem Terroris Pathologico-Therapeuticam* (Medical dissertation for the doctor's degree, on the pathology and therapy of terror) (Leiden, 1738).

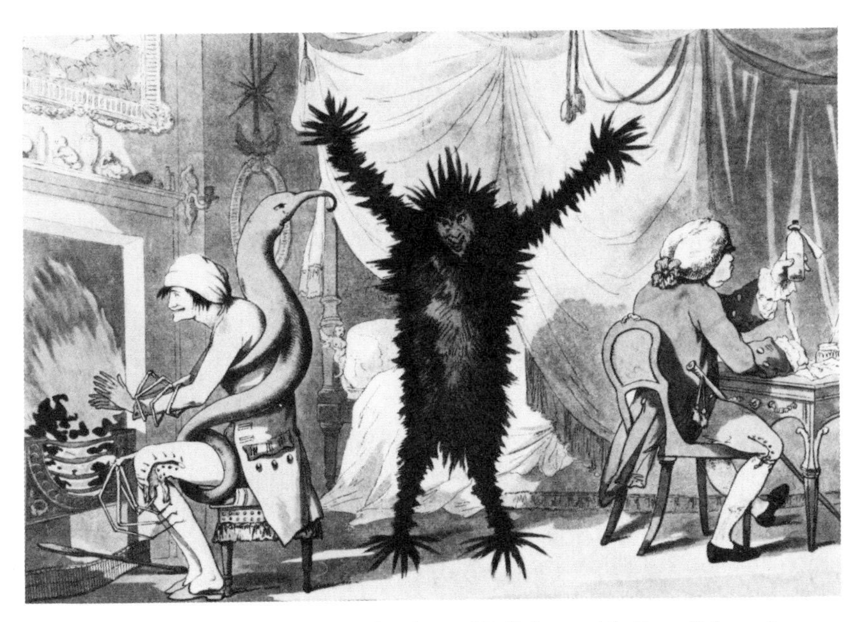

Pl. 12. Cartoon by T. Rowlandson, "Delirium with Fever" (1792).

of a preestablished harmony, which means that he rejected the notion of a perfect clock-like arrangement between body and soul.[71]

Barckhuysen argued that physicians should be direct and practical, should observe the psychological reactions of their patients, and should try to understand the principles of these reactions. Neither philosophers nor moralists should interfere with the treatment of the fearful patient. Barckhuysen provides the example of a merchant who hears the news of a shipwrecking of one of his best ships loaded with merchandise, which partly belonged to some merchant colleagues under his charge. He reasons that the best way to break the catastrophic news to this poor man is to inform him *gradually*—this pace is crucial. If the merchant were to be confronted with the full reality at once, he may become morbidly *terrified,* which can lead in turn to apoplexia or even to sudden death. By contrast, when he is intentionally kept in suspense, merely

71. At the time a dispute raged between Stahl and Leibniz on the agreement. See L. J. Rather and J. B. Frerichs, "The Leibniz-Stahl Controversy—I, Leibniz' Opening Objections to the *Theoria Medica Vera,*" *Clio Medica* 3 (1968): 21–40; "II, Stahl's Survey of the Principal Points of Doubt," *Clio Medica* 5 (1979): 53–67. Leibniz compares the action of the body and that of the soul as the maintenance of a perfect synchronization of two independent clocks.

supposing the ship is missing but having no further news, he naturally becomes a victim of anxiety, which may cause loss of body temperature and perspiration, as described above, accompanied by palpitation of the heart, paleness, and shivering. Slowly induced anxiety is preferable to shock, says Barckhuysen, since the body can then build up a kind of physical resistance to the full impact of the catastrophe. In the meantime the doctors can take care of his comfort. As an ameliorative he suggests some hot Russian tea, carefully prepared from several mixed herbs! Barckhuysen is very proud of his Russian compatriots. Generally speaking, he says, the Russians are not easily frightened; they harden their bodies and minds by swimming in an air hole in the ice, even during the severest cold of wintertime.

Clark and Barckhuysen, both true followers of Boerhaave's doctrines, did not try to analyze the psychological factors involved in the process of fear. They did not define guilt or hallucination, nor did they refine the differences between anxiety and oppression. Mainly, they interpreted all ailments of the psyche as a breakdown of mental processes which allowed for depression and the symptoms of fear and anxiety to surface in response to stress. Moreover, anxiety and fear were used as synonyms for the same state of mind, albeit that most students attributed a corporeal quality to anxiety and a spiritual quality to fear. The difference in the treatises that have anxiety as a subject and those that deal with one or more emotions (*animi pathemata*) lies in the choice of the diseases put forward in the dissertations. For example, anxiety and pain are closely intermingled in the diseases discussed by those students who took *anxietas* as a subject of their studies. Five corporeal examples of anxiety are prominent in these studies: anxiety caused by (1) heart failure, by (2) pulmonary obstruction, by (3) abdominal oppression, by (4) serious affects of the nervous system, and by (5) surgical intervention.[72]

By discussing these five examples of anxiety, the students could test their knowledge of clinical medicine, culminating in a long description of *agonia,* the struggle with death.[73] Moreover, they could demonstrate

72. See Francis Gallis, *Disputatio Medica Inauguralis de Anxietate* (Harderwijk, 1739): he followed Boerhaave's institutions, but his therapy is based on Stahl's doctrines. Dirk Schouten, *Disputatio Medica Inauguralis de Anxietate* (Leiden, 1742): Boerhaavian physiology, Hoffmann's therapy. Isaac Voyer, *Dissertatio Medica Inauguralis de Anxietate* (Leiden, 1769): following Hieronymus David Gaub, *Institutiones Pathologiae medicinalis* (Leiden, 1758), S 683.

73. Prosper Alpinus, *De Praesagienda Vita et Morte Aegrotantium Libri Septem,* ed. H. Boerhaave, emendationes Hier. Dav. Gaubius (Leiden: Ex. off. Isaaci Severini, 1733; editio princeps, Frankfurt, 1601). Boerhaave considered this work of the highest importance for

that they had followed Boerhaave's clinical teaching in the Caecilia hospital as well as his instruction in physiology. With the help of his pupil H. D. Gaub, Boerhaave edited *The prediction of life and death of the diseased* (1733) by the famous Italian physician Prosper Alpinus (1533–1617). The definition of anxiety in this context is: the sad and obstructed perception of the mind or the sensation that our life is fading away.[74] For instance, this feeling of terror is dominant in being choked, in having a perforated stomach, or in the terrible anxiety in rabies. The more subtle feelings of anxiety as experienced in hypochondria or hysteria were of relatively minor concern to these students, whose interest was peaked by more serious diseases. They were most eager to explain these dreadful sensations in terms of iatromechanics. The affliction of the mind was considered to be only a consequence of the disease itself; it was a *consensus* (sympathy) between the brain and the affected organs. This thinking is evident in the medical explanation of the incubus;[75] such a monster does not really exist. It is a product of imagination, caused by oppression of the abdominal area, due to overeating and drinking too much wine. It is a consequence of Newton's laws of gravity, which teach us that the weight of a body presses against another body with a certain force. Thus, the stomach presses against the diaphragm and the diaphragm presses against the heart. By this pressure the circulation to the head becomes obstructed, and the ventricles of the brain become overfilled, the pressure disturbs the animal spirits, and the monster appears in a certain shape to the patient, such as his imagination would allow.

These strict mechanical explanations are also applied to the serious conditions of heart failure, gas poisoning with sulphureous vapors in volcanic eruptions, and the frightening experience of the amputation of a leg. Medical students paid little mind to the workings of the imagination; we must look instead for studies on the *affectus animi,* or on the

the daily praxis of medicine. Prosper Alpinus was a famous physician who became director of the botanical garden at the University of Padua in 1593.

74. "Anxietas est ergo illa tristis, molestaque Mentis perceptio, vel sensus quo putamus vitam destituram esse." See also Schouten, *De Anxietate,* and Gallis, *De Anxietate,* who claim that it is "quasi certamen cum morte" (any anxiety is like a struggle with death). The word *agonia* (Greek) was used in ancient medicine, similar to *angor* in the double meaning of combat and anxiety. See Prosper Alpinus, *De Praesagienda Vita,* lib. III, cap. IV.

75. See Huisinga, *Dissertatio . . . sistens Incubi causas praecipuas* (n. 38 above). He gives a mechanical explanation. The backward position of the head gives an intracranial obstruction of the ventricles, there is no more secretion of the animal spirits, so the body cannot move. The apparition of the incubus is not a matter of metaphysics but a product of imagination.

perturbationes animi—in other words: on the effects of the emotions upon the mind.

MUSIC AND NO-RESTRAINT

In 1735 we find the very first testimony in the Leiden school of a changing interest in the *animi pathemata*. James Goddard, a student from Jamaica, defends under Boerhaave his dissertation *De animi Perturbationibus* (On the disturbances of the mind),[76] in which the beginnings of psychology are discernible. Goddard, already recognized for his work on Descartes, Hobbes, and Locke,[77] was impressed by the series of lectures on diseases of the nervous system presented by Boerhaave between 1730 and 1735. In these lectures Boerhaave gave several explanations of the transmission of emotional disturbances to the different parts of the body. Goddard grew interested in this theme and expanded it, describing several symptoms of body change as a consequence of hidden fear: the voice of the patient changes, it is softer, the stomach suffers from spasm, the pulse becomes smaller and accelerates. He also notes changes in facial expression, the paleness, the restless glance. Goddard provides an amusing picture of anthropological and environmental differences between people with regard to their emotional reactions: Catalans are restrained and do not show their emotions, the French on the contrary are more exuberant. People from the mountains and people living in the plains react differently, as Hippocrates taught. Goddard then deals with inherited traits. An aggressive father will beget a hot-tempered lad, and a funk (stercoraeus) will beget a funk! He believes that passions have a contagious affect: "like laughing faces get moist when crying people come in," or "like a disease strikes as lightning, a sudden emotion can spread easily." According to Goddard, women are

76. James Goddard was born in 1714 in St. Ann, Jamaica. In 1732 he attended Jesus College, Oxford; in 1733 he matriculated in Leiden. Boerhaave took personal care of this dissertation. R. W. Innes Smith, *English-speaking Students at the University of Leiden* (Edinburgh and London, 1932).

77. John Locke's *Some Thoughts concerning Education* (1693) was translated into Dutch in 1698 by Barent Bos in Rotterdam under the title *Verhandeling over de opvoeding der kinderen*. Another Dutch edition was published in 1753 in Amsterdam by K. van Tongerlo and F. Houttuyn. Locke's theories on education were discussed in lectures, probably by Gaub. Thomas Hobbes was following Descartes, but his mechanism and materialism were condemned by the authorities of the church as well as by university professors. Goddard rejects Hobbes's theories from *De Homine* (1657) on the *innata praenotio* (inborn knowledge).

much more susceptible to fear than men, especially when they eat too many sweets.

He also proposes various therapeutic measures against fear. The majority of these prescriptions were already well known and frequently mentioned by the teachers of the schools in Europe. We can find them in all books on *hypochondria,* such as George Cheyne's *English Malady* (1733),[78] which was most popular during the eighteenth century. Physical exercise, fresh air, moderation in the use of alcohol, and a light diet without herbs or fat food. Especially for fear and sadness Goddard recommends the soothing affects of music and traveling, preferably sea voyages, or occupational therapy. We can recognize those advices as being already familiar in the chapters on hygiene in the ancient textbooks. So far as music therapy was concerned, Goddard referred to the *Tusculan Disputations* of Cicero[79] and mentioned Pythagoras's therapy with the violin and songs. Music therapy became popular again in the eighteenth century, especially in those systems of medicine which had a mechanical background: Goddard calls it a *medicamentum amabile* and he points out the use of musical therapy in tarantism, a disease caused by the bite of the tarantula, a spider that was common in harvest time, especially in Italy. He does not discuss the physiology of the cure. Goddard's psychotherapy is partly suggestive; when the physician prescribes remedies, he should emphasize the beneficial effects to be expected from their use. Hope and optimism, bolstered by proper medical guidance, should keep fear at distance. The author does not suggest tranquilizing the patient's mind. Emotions, even fear or grief, are necessary for a healthy life. Life should not be a stagnant pool; the passionless doctrines of any form of Stoicism are unhealthy for the patient.

78. George Cheyne, *The English Malady: or, A Treatise of nervous diseases of all kinds, as spleen, vapours, lowness of spicity, hypochondriacal and hysterical distempers, etc.* (London and Dublin, 1733). On Cheyne, see Rousseau, "Medicine and Millenarianism" (n. 68 above). A popular work called *Hypochondriasis, a practical treatise on the nature and cure of that disorder, commonly called the hype and the hypo* was written in 1766 by John Hill. It was reprinted in 1969 with notes and apparatus by G. S. Rousseau.

79. Goddard refers to *Tusculan Disputations,* liber IV, cap. II. In this chapter Cicero points at the importance of the music of the harp as soothing the emotions. See also H. J. Möller, *Geschichte und Gegenwart musiktherapeutischerKonzeptionen* (Stuttgart: J. Fink Verlag, 1971), 18. Also W. Kümmel, *Musik und Medizin: Ihre Wechselbeziehungen in Theorie und Praxis von 800–1800* (Freiburg and Munich, 1977) as a general survey. Also E. Ashworth Underwood, "Apollo and Terpsichore: Music and the Healing Art," *Bulletin of the History of Medicine* 21 (1947): 639–673. The general idea in the eighteenth century was that music stimulated the vital spirits by the composition of the sound waves, which penetrated into the brain.

Stoicism, as other authors in this book have noticed in its national contexts, was a dominant philosophy in Leiden during the sixteenth and seventeenth centuries. The ancient authors like Seneca, Plautus, Tacitus, and Terence were studied, and the virtues of steadfastness, modesty, and prudence were elements of the neo-Stoic moral philosophy.[80] This morality suggested a strong mind, not sensitive to emotions, and a capacity for self-restraint. Goddard is against this hiding, this repression, of emotions. He opts for a no-restraint therapy: *let the patient scream it out*!

Goddard most likely attended some lectures given by H. D. Gaub, who had been teaching at the university since 1734. In 1747 Gaub presented his well-known address as the vice-chancellor of the university: *De regimine mentis, quod medicorum est* (The management of the mind, as it concerns physicians). It was here that Gaub discussed the interrelationship of mind and body in healthy and mentally confused persons. He made a distinction between minor disburbances of the mind and diseases of the mind, and he pointed out the importance of corporeal defects in mental disturbances. He tried to convince his audience that once these corporeal defects were treated, the mind would be cured as well. At the end of his address, Gaub pleaded that physicians should actively engage in a search for new drugs capable of affecting the mind. Understandably, his lecture created a stir in the Leiden community. Among the audience was Julien Offraye de La Mettrie, whose volume *L'homme machine* appeared that same year. This publication, which included case histories from Gaub's address, was condemned by the intellectual world as being irreligious and materialistic.[81] Gaub received similar charges and was reprimanded for his remarks on the search for mind-altering drugs and for inspiring La Mettrie. To put the matter right, Gaub gave a second address in 1763 on the same subject. In this speech he publicly and emphatically denied any involvement with "the little Frenchman's . . . mechanical man."[82] He pointed out the patient's responsibility for his own emotional disturbances, the harmful effects of emotions upon the body, and the sometimes salutary effects of anger and terror upon a patient. He avoided questions about drugs, warned physicians

80. See Gerhard Oestreich, "Justus Lipsius als Universalgelehrter zwischen Renaissance und Barock," in *Leiden University in the Seventeenth Century: An Exchange of Learning*, ed. Th. H. Lunsingh Scheurleer and G. H. M. Posthumus Meyes (Leiden: Brill, 1975), 180–201.

81. Rather, *Mind and Body* (n. 57 above), 13.

82. Ibid., 115–122. Also quoted by Rather.

of their limitations, and pleaded for a commitment by physicians to treat the "Whole Man."

The scholarly style of both lectures confirms that the Leiden professor had deeply and thoroughly studied the issues. Gaub's influence is quite obvious when we review the following dissertations by two students whose work also inspired the doctrines of the Edinburgh school to emerge. The first treatise was written by Thomas Cogan, who graduated in 1767.[83] The second work was presented in 1777 by twenty-five-year-old Thomas Pemberton.[84] Both students had widely read the books of the contemporary medical schools: Gaub's pathology, Boerhaave's lectures, Haller's physiology, van Swieten's commentaries, Whytt's essays, and Friedrich Hoffmann's medical counsels. Pemberton had also attended a lecture series given by William Cullen. The results of their efforts were tripled. First, both students had a better grasp on the concept of fear, and no longer confused that sensation with others. Second, they understood the theory of inspiring fear in patients as a means to cure them, referring to remarkable case histories of past and contemporary character. Finally, they were alert to the most current and successful psychological achievements.

SHOCK THERAPY AND ANALYSIS OF FEAR: THE ORIGINS OF MODERN TECHNIQUES

Thomas Cogan (1736–1816) defended his dissertation *De Animi Pathematum vi et modo agendi in inducendis vel curandis morbis* (On the

83. Thomas Cogan (1736–1818) was 31 years old when he took his degree in Leiden. He started his career as a minister of the Anglican Church in England, but he became a Unitarian and had to leave his parish in 1762. He went to the Hague, where he served as a minister. When he intended to marry a banker's daughter, he was refused by her father, unless he trained for the medical profession. He got his medical degree at Leiden in 1765 and presented his dissertation in 1767. He defended his thesis under Gaub, saying that he had collected his material from different authors and different schools, but that he thanked his teachers (probably also B. S. Albinus) for their support. It is clear from this study that he wanted to be well informed on the physiology of the mental processes and that he was avoiding explanations in the field of moral theology. In his later work he tried to combine the medical and the moral insights into the problem. His essay *Philosophical Treatise on the Passions* was printed in 1800; in 1802 a second edition followed. Later, he turned fully to moral theology, See *Dictionary of National Biography* (London: Smith and Elder, 1887), vol. 11.

84. Thomas Pemberton was born in 1750. He took his medical degree in Edinburgh and went to Leiden. His father, Eduard, was a friend of Boerhaave. See Innes Smith, *English-speaking Students.*

power of the emotions and their action in causing or curing disease) in 1767. His study is in complete agreement with Gaub's concepts on the disturbances of the mental processes by the *pathemata,* which he describes as perturbations of the mind by the classical emotions: hope, joy, love, shame, anger, fright, fear, and sadness. [85] Cogan discusses each affect in a physiological and a psychological context. He also offers suggestions on how to induce some of these emotions in patients. *Terror* (fright) cannot be medically cured or provoked. But the effect of terror can be produced by inducing a state of shock.[86] Such induced shock has been successful in curing symptoms of depression. It is possible to cure a fever by inflicting terror; even a mute may talk after a shock! A paralyzed patient may suddenly walk, and girls may suddenly start to menstruate. But shock treatment is not indicated for the already frightened patient. Imposed terror will further paralyze a fearful patient: he becomes pale and cold, with trembling lips, his hair rises, and he loses control over his bladder and bowels. His heartbeat accelerates, his pulse becomes rapid and uneven, and he feels pressure (*anxietas*) on his chest.[87] Fear, Cogan states, is the gateway to serious diseases: it agitates the irritability of the nervous system, the capillaries contract, and patients who are living in a continuous state of anxiety may suffer physically. According to mechanical principles, if the contracted capillaries were not supplying the delicate parts of the body with sufficient quantities of blood, irregular cell growth or tumors could result. Cogan cites Van Swieten's remarks on breast cancer in women who live under stress.[88] Fear has other negatives in connection with disease. Frightened people are likely to contract contagious diseases earlier than those who are strong-minded (*fortitudo animae*), as was described by Diemerbroeck's study on an epidemic of the bubonic plague.[89] Cogan offers

85. Spes, gaudium, amor, pudor, ira, terror, metus, moeror—this is the classical series from Galen onward. A systematic description with a classification of the passions was published by Christian Heinrich de Marees, *De Animi Perturbationum in corpus potentia* (Göttingen, 1775).

86. Thomas Cogan, *De Animi Pathematum vi et modo agendi in inducendis vel curandis morbis* (Leiden, 1767), 28.

87. Ibid., 30.

88. G. van Swieten, *Commentaria in Hermanni Boerhaave Aphorismos de cognoscendis et curandis morbis* (Commentaries on Herman Boerhaave's Aphorisms on diagnosing and curing diseases) (Hildburghausen, 1754), 1:495. Van Swieten notes the danger of long-lasting depressions (*affectus animi tristes et biliosi*). These can provoke tumors or change chronic illness into cancer. The case of the breast tumor was described ibid. 1:127.

89. IJsbrand van Diemerbroeck (1609–1674) studied an epidemic of the bubonic plague at Nijmegen in 1636–1637, which he published in 1644 in Arnhem. The book was

a mechanical explanation to describe how fear-based skin eruptions complicate disease: fear causes the skin vessels to contract, limiting the expulsion of contagious material through perspiration, which aggravates skin eruptions. Since eighteenth-century doctors saw many patients with smallpox, Diemerbroeck's observations at the time of a bubonic plague epidemic received new interest and a new underlying theory was considered.

In his psychological analysis of the *anima pathemata* Cogan discusses combinations of the emotions. He describes the effects of proneness to anger (*iracundia*), which produces a grim visage, sleepless nights, and bad appetite, especially in combination with hatred and jealousy.[90] While loneliness produces fear and sadness, a combination of fright, sadness, and anger may drive a person to suicide.[91] Cogan also rejects humoral theories to explain the effects of the emotions upon the body and maintains that all responses are dependent on the system of nervous irritability and sensibility; the patient responds to diverse stimuli with diverse reactions.[92] Here then was a model of psychology that depended exclusively on prescribed notions of mind and body viewed in relation.

But why has the highest *Arbiter Rerum* (God) created the emotions in such a way that they always produce the same phenomena in the human body? Why does anger act so differently from sadness and hope so differently from fear? Cogan also introduces the human element in differing human responses, but he considers the infliction of emotions not only a matter of physics but a consequence of the construction of the society as well.[93] The living-together of people influences the mind. The body reacts on the conflicts in society by the passway of the mind. We

reprinted several times. The idea of fear as a provoking factor for infectious diseases was already known to the ancients.

90. Cogan, *De Animi Pathematum vi,* 35.

91. Ibid. The idea of composed passions of the mind in different combinations is present in Descartes's and Hume's theories. Descartes analyzes the emotions in *passiones primitivae* with the opposite passion, for instance amor-odium, laetitia-tristitia, spes-metus. He refines the emotions further: hope gives safety, fear gives despair, indignation gives wrath. Cogan analyzes more as a physician! But he is an admirer of Descartes, judging by his motto: "Nihil affirmo, nihilque ab ullo credi velim, nisi quod ipsi evidens et invicta ratio persuadebit" ("I affirm nothing, and I would have no one believe anything unless convinced by clear and irrefutable reasoning") (*Principia philosophiae* [Amsterdam, 1644], pars 4, art. 207).

92. Cogan, *De Animi Pathematum vi,* 36. He relies on Robert Whytt, *Physiological Essays, . . . II. Observations on the sensibility and irritability of the parts of men* (Edinburgh, 1755), 2–3.

93. Cogan, *De Animi Pathematum vi,* 38–39.

can notice these changes in the trembling, frightened people who must appear in court, even when they are not guilty. But, Cogan asserts, the human body adjusts itself to the burden of the emotions imposed by society on the mind. It is the physicians' task to take better notice of the mental state of their patients, to find the right way to stimulate the emotion that favors the healing of the disease.[94]

Thomas Pemberton's psychological analysis of *metus* is quite interesting. He states that fantasy, the product of disordered imagination, causes disease, whereas the expectation of an approaching calamity generates fear. He cites David Hume's remark on a man in prison who had just received a death warrant.[95] Pemberton speaks of *terror* (fright), the sudden confrontation with an unexpected danger. There is also *pavor,* the children's fright, as described by John Locke—a consequence of a faulty education by maids and nurses who tell the children stories about ghosts and monsters. *Timor* is the kind of walled-in fear of which the patient is unaware. Pemberton pays particular attention to this form of fear, the tired and sick patient with lower-back pain, weak and slow pulse, and frequent urination. He describes cold and perspiring hands and feet, deep sighs, pale faces, visual disturbances, and inertia as signs of suppressed anxiety.[96] One recognizes in this description the quintessential *neurasthenia,* described in 1880 by George Miller Beard, as the new disease of American civilization,[97] just as *hypochondria* had been the disease of English civilization *par excellence* in Europe during the seventeenth and eighteenth centuries. Pemberton also discusses the fear of earthquakes, of volcanic eruptions, of confrontation with masked men, of burglars, of ghosts, of bed-curtains, of mice, of women, of loneliness, of poison, and of contagious diseases. And he also mentions the use of inflicting *terror* (fright) as a means of therapy.

Aside from the cases described by Pemberton, various textbooks offer grotesque studies using terror in the form of therapy. For instance, the

94. Ibid. Various students use this point of opposite passions in their dissertations. They refer to Sanctorius, *Ars de Statica Medicina,* the chapter on the emotions (sec. 7, aphorism 12). "Ira et spes auserunt timorem, et laetitia moestitiam" (Wrath and hope may chase fear, and joy sadness). For instance, Wilhelmus Ouwens, a Dutch student who got his doctor's degree in Leiden in 1737 on the subject *De Horrore* (On Shivering), 44, and Pemberton, *De Metu,* 59.

95. Pemberton, *De Metu,* 17, citing David Hume, *Of the Passions* (n. 17 above), 190.

96. Pemberton, *De Metu,* 35.

97. George Miller Beard (1839–1883) published in 1880 *A practical treatise on nervous exhaustion (neurasthenia); its symptoms, nature, sequences, treatment.* The concept "neurasthenia" was first published in the *Boston Medical and Surgical Journal* 3 (29 April 1869): 217–220.

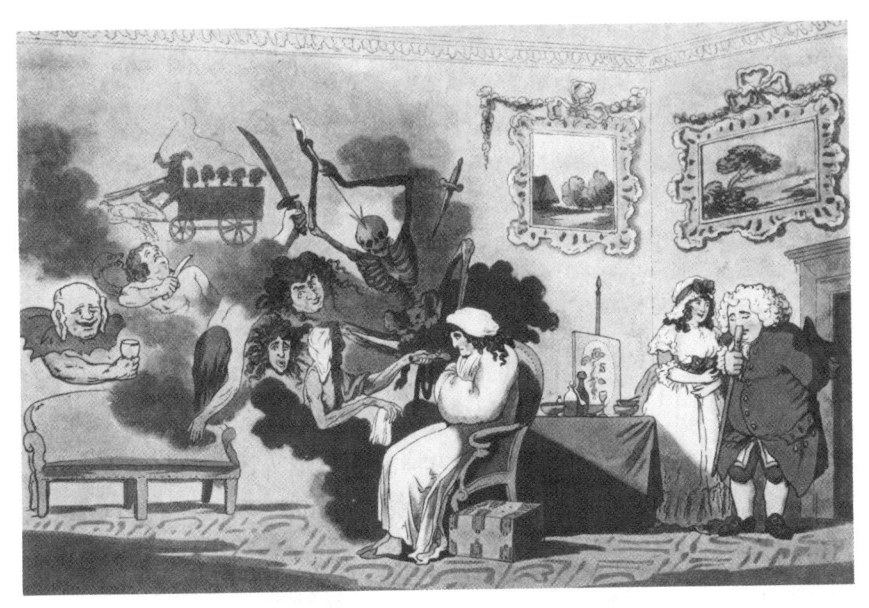

Pl. 13. Cartoon by T. Rowlandson, "Delusion of Persecution" (1792).

well-known case of Herman Boerhaave's action in the orphanage of Haarlem is recorded. In this orphanage a girl fell into convulsions caused by a sudden fright. Gradually the other children developed fear symptoms and one after the other fell to the floor. Boerhaave called all the children into the common room of the orphanage. He had pots prepared with glowing coals. On these pots he put small iron hooks of different configurations. Then he said to the children: "I do not know of any medicine to cure you. But each child be it a boy or a girl, that falls into a convulsion, will be burned with a little hook in his arm." The children were terrified with this prospect and nobody fell down again. Indeed, when one can detach the mind from an idea and replace it by another feeling or by terror, convulsions can be cured.[98]

Pemberton also mentions a case described by Tissot:

98. Pemberton, *De Metu,* 54. This case history was quoted by many authors. It was first described by Boerhaave's nephew Abraham Kaau Boerhaave in his study *Impetum faciens dictum Hippocrati per corpus consentiens philologice et physiologice illustratum* (The so-called Hippocratic arousal, experienced in the body, explained by its philology and physiology) (Leiden, 1745), 355–406. See G. A. Lindeboom, "Boerhaave in het weeshuis," *Nederlands Tijdschrift voor Geneeskunde* 102, no. 1 (1958): 24.

> A Swiss officer refused to be bled since he always fainted at the sight of blood. The commander solved the problem by giving the order: attention! accompanied by a role of the drums. This distraction allowed the officer to be bled without problems.[99]

Two further examples which Pemberton describes come from Schenck von Grafenberg and may be considered "classic" studies of recovery with induced shock:

> A depressed girl refused to obey the physician's orders. The doctor asked her father's permission for a drastic therapy. The doctor went out, undressed, rushed back naked into the room and jumped into the girl's bed. The startled girl jumped from her bed and her depression ended.[100]
>
> An unmarried woman was frightened by a mouse and became subject to a permanent fear of mice. The doctor forced her to put a dead mouse in her lap and again shock acted as a cure.[101]

The lap was, of course, the crucial geographic spot. If the girl could keep it there—as she apparently did, although for what length of time is unknown and unrecounted—close to the uterus, for so long the acknowledged seat of female hysteria, then her dread of mice would be allayed. According to Pemberton, who found the story credible, it was successful. In both cases, the action of the physician held overtones of sexual aggression, which were salutary for the patients. The girl who refused to get up from her bed was probably a virgin. The woman who feared mice was generally fearful and timid. Shock was induced and both were able to reduce their anxieties. In another example of induced terror, Pemberton mentioned a lecture, given by William Cullen on whooping cough in children. Cullen discussed terror as a therapeutic agent, and he mentioned some habits used in folk medicine but not well documented. Children who were suffering long-lasting coughs were

99. Mentioned by S. A. Tissot. See n. 46 above. I found the passage in the German edition *Sämtliche zur Arztneykunst gehörige Schriften . . . übersetzt nach den neuesten Verbesserungen* (Leipzig, 1761), 4:338.

100. Pemberton, *De Metu,* 55. He cited Joannes Schenck von Grafenberg (1530–1598), a famous physician from Freiburg. His book, which contains many case histories, was later edited by his son and reprinted many times. See *Παρατηρήσεων sive observationum medicarum rarum, novarum, admirabilium, et monstrosarum volumen* (Volume of rare, new, remarkable, and strange medical observations) (Frankfurt, 1609), 154: "singulari solertia medici a melancholia asserta" (A case of melancholy, cured by the extraordinary ingenuity of a physician). This book by Schenck was kept as a handbook for medical students in the university library at Leiden, having been acquired in 1618. The call number is 637A1.

101. Pemberton, *De Metu,* 44.

locked into a working mill.[102] The *crepitaculum molare* (the sound of the grinding millstone) would so frighten them that they would overcome their coughing reflex. According to Pemberton, Cullen was not supporting this drastic treatment, he just offered it as a neutral example of the therapeutic effect of terror. Cullen mentioned the mill in his textbook when he discussed the therapy of whooping cough, but he promoted the use of herbal medicines.

Cogan as well as Pemberton had discarded considerably the earlier mechanistic explanations of the interaction between mind and body in cases of anxiety. Both discuss the nervous system as the seat of the disturbances, and they accept the vascular changes only as secondary symptoms. They notice the variation of sensibility of the brain for the stimuli of fear, and, after careful analysis, they record a difference in anxiety-proneness. Pemberton acknowledges that anxiety may underlie other emotional symptoms, such as a general state of depression. But they both use the classic shock agent again, to expel a passion with the opposite emotion. Still, their observations witness a sharp analysis of emotions, and they come very near to modern trends in psychology and even more contemporary ones in psychiatry.[103]

DISCUSSION AND CONCLUSION

Eighteenth-century man, as we have witnessed again and again in this book, was living in a changing world. At the beginning of the age, immaterial forces such as witchcraft and possession by demons, cosmic influences, and hidden sympathies were still evident everywhere, in spite of the growing confidence in reason and experience. But the allegory of the world was fading, fear no longer had a valid alibi. The world picture became mechanized and secularized as well. Newton's empty space had replaced the concentric nine spheres, the harmony of the world around the earth was losing its mysteries and its charm. In this world, eighteenth-century man tried to be "absolute," that is, free from the chains of mystery and fantasy, obedient to reason and understanding. In this world there was no place for human feelings, which should be

102. Ibid., 55. William Cullen, *First lines of the Practice of Physic* (Edinburgh, 1784), vol. 3, S 1423. He mentions "terror" but not the mill.

103. For instance, the modern concept of state and trait anxiety. See Charles D. Spielberger, "Anxiety as an Emotional State," chap. 2 of *Anxiety: Current Trends in Theory and Research* (New York, Academic Press, 1972), 1:23–49.

straightened and dissimulated, or, later in the century, overacted by the heroes and heroines of Romanticism.

Perhaps we cannot call the eighteenth century an age of anxiety with total impunity, but anxiety and fear were extant everywhere just as they are in our time. Then, however, the objects of fear were different and anxiety was not so hidden in complicated psychological jargon as it is today. Furthermore, the anxiety of the patients during their too often incurable illness made a deep impression upon their family and their family doctor. To watch a patient struggling for breath, writhing in pain, bleeding to death, or having one epileptic fit after another is frightening. Incapability of the physician to give relief to the patient and his family is a disgrace for the medical profession. It is small wonder the medical schools paid more tribute to the actual diseases than to the nonfatal symptoms. Most disease was "atrocious,"[104] painful, stinging, lingering, and if the physician was impotent to save the patient from agony and death, he should at least know the underlying pathophysiology of the process. So doctors were most eager to find remedies to give the patient free breath, to relieve the spasms, to stop bleeding, and to avoid epileptic fits and convulsions. In this last category especially, the passions of the mind were taken into consideration.

In eighteenth-century case histories and other medical literature, a remarkable number of patients are mentioned who suffer from convulsions, epileptic fits, or grimaces. In the first half of the century, these pathological phenomena are most often ascribed to fear or to a sudden fright, especially with children. Grimaces and distorted faces must have been observed everywhere, in the streets, in the taverns, in the schools. Why did Boerhaave and Tissot attach so much value to these faces, mentioning them together with false faces and masks? Why was the *homo larvatus* (masked man) such a danger? According to Jean-Jacques Rousseau, there was a great distance between "être" and "paraître," between the inner feelings of man and the social mask he was obliged to wear.[105] Wearing such a social mask entails a precarious and delicate balance for a sensitive nature. But a civilized man had to wear his mask to fit into

104. *Atrocis rarissimique morbi historia altera conscripta ab Hermanno Boerhaave* (Leiden, 1728); *Atrocis, nec descripti prius, morbi historia secundum medicae artis leges conscripta ab Hermanno Boerhaave* (Leiden, 1724). Two case histories of serious diseases, accompanied by pain and anxiety.

105. Lameijn, "Wie is van glas?" 50. J. -J. Rousseau, *Du Naturel de Jean Jacques et ses habitudes: Deuxième Dialogue*, in *Œuvres complètes* (1784), 3:156 ff. In this chapter, Rousseau discussed paintings of well-known men like David Hume. Did the artist portray the man as he really was, or as he wanted to present him to the Paris public?

the new order of optimism and rationalism and to show a firm belief in the order of nature, with its laws and certainties.[106]

By contrast, man was confronted with his own political and social impotence to change the world in which he lived into a more righteous world of a different order. Eighteenth-century sensitive man dreamed of a utopia, even a satirical utopia in which the order of his time was criticized.[107] He was used to his social mask, wearing it invariably—but he should not be confronted with a man wearing a black mask or a false face. Such a man had neutralized the social order, he did not belong to civilization, he was an outlaw, a symbol of disorder and irrationality. The false face could be an omen for a complete destruction of the reality of the people that confronted the mask-wearing figure. There was no longer security and certainty. And certainty was wanted most by the enlightened intellectuals. It was a high topic in medicine.[108]

Diseases in which anxiety caused by an underlying psychological problem was involved became popular in eighteenth-century medicine; they even dominated the daily practice of physicians, as we have seen. No doubt hypochondria and hysteria were the refuge of many uncertain people, who were hiding their problems behind the fig leaves of these diseases. They were ultimately diseases of civilization, as John Hill intuitively warned his readers in his brief but revealing analysis of this cultural phenomenon and as students at almost all universities, both in Europe and on the Continent, wrote in their dissertations: a soft life, high living, late nights, too much studying by the light of a lamp, too much tea or coffee, too much air pollution—these were in their opinion the causes of hypochondria and hysteria.[109]

In spite of the iatromechanical explanation of anxiety and terror and the other passions of the mind, there is no great tendency to analyze fears of patients or to study the psychological differences in their relations before 1740. This was partly due to the authority of the dominant religion, which did not allow physicians to intrude into the psychic problems of the patient, especially when guilt feelings and remorse were

106. Foucault, *Histoire de la folie* (n. 3 above), 392–393. He speaks of "monde illusoir ou s'annonce l'antiphysis."

107. Lameijn, "Wie is van glas?" 51.

108. On "certitudo" in medicine, see Erna Lesky, "Cabanis und die Gewissheit des Heilkunde," *Gesnerus* 2 (1954): 152–182; Pierre Jean George Cabanis (1757–1808), *Du degré de la certitude de la médecine* (Paris, 1798); Petrus Camper's address *De certo medicinae* (Amsterdam, 1758), translated into Dutch and published in *Bijdragen tot de Geschiedenis der Geneeskund* 19 (1939): 87–103.

109. John Hill, *Hypochondriasis, a practical treatise* (London, 1766), 20–21.

involved. Medicalization of psychic problems was not encouraged by the church, which compounded already varying interpretations of the way physicians should deal with patients vexed by fear. In Halle, all efforts were combined to train the students in perfect bedside manners and duties of a physician, but they were instructed to refrain from any attempt to analyze the fear. We may assume that this was also the case in Catholic universities.

Fear as a passion of the mind was more open for discussion in the Calvinist universities of northern Europe, provided the medical professors avoided materialistic interpretation of the mind and did not endanger the doctrine of free will. But the more tolerant attitude of the Calvinists was not enough to allow medical insights into psychic problems to develop. The mechanistic concept of the function of the human body provided a closed and rigid system by which virtually all reactions of the human body to emotions could be explained. The function of the nervous system was of lesser importance; in cases of easily frightened people it was "facile mobile," easy to manipulate.[110] Nerves provoked only the less-startling circulatory changes, which produced the symptoms of fear: paleness, palpitations of the heart, trembling lips, and shaking knees. In contrast, changes in the human body, caused by failure of the circulation of the blood and other mechanistic causes, such as the incubus, could produce a disturbed imagination, resulting in fear or anxiety.

These mechanistic explanations take an important place in medical textbooks throughout the century. No paradigmatic change took place after the introduction of irritability and sensibility into physiology, in spite of the fact that the central nervous system gained more importance. But Haller's *First Lines of Physiology*[111] were carefully studied by William Cullen, and became an important part of the doctrines of the Edinburgh school. Cullen's concept of disease, in which debility of the brain and its connections were discussed, opened a field of interest in psychic phenomena.

> In medical psychology, differing only in a few remarks from that science which is simply called psychology, the actions of the soul or mind are inves-

110. This term was popular with the Leiden students; for instance, William Clark and the students who discussed anxiety used it in their dissertations.

111. The English edition was completed after the Göttingen edition of 1764, annotated by H. A. Warisberg (1739–1808). See *First Lines of Physiology by the celebrated Baron Albertus Haller, M.D. etc., translated from the correct Latin edition printed under the inspection of William Cullen M.D.* (Edinburgh, 1786; reprint, New York and London, 1966, as vol. 32 of Sources of Sciences).

tigated. A more elegant subject, and more worthy of attention, can not be imagined, than the thinking principle in man.

So read a passage in the *First Lines of Physiology* which was most welcome to the students.[112] Moreover, as we have seen, the Leiden school of H. D. Gaub was open to all new achievements in the field of psychosomatic medicine. When Gaub was appointed professor of chemistry in the medical faculty in 1734, he was cooperating closely with Boerhaave in preparing the edition of Prosper Alpinus's work on the prediction of life and death in illness.[113] Boerhaave presented his lectures on nervous diseases between 1730 and 1735. As we know from L. J. Rather's work, the mind/body relation was more in the picture of the medical teaching from that time on. So James Goddard, the first student in Leiden who tried to discuss the psychology of the passions of the mind, found that the ears of the professors of the medical faculty were open. In the attempts made by Gaub and his students to pay more attention to the psychology of fear, many case histories were reproduced from ancient medicine on. These studies, often characterized as "grotesques," were brought forward as examples of diseases resulting from a sudden fright or the use of *terror* as a therapeutic agent.

In this respect we must recall Cogan's study of the treatment of psychic diseases, as well as William Cullen's report on folk medicine in England, where a child with whooping cough was locked into a mill. In Yorkshire, it was long the practice of mothers to cure whooping cough by putting their children through the hoppers of a mill.[114] Inducing fright in a patient may overcome a reflex, as Pemberton demonstrated in his review of Boerhaave's treatment of a case of mass hysteria in the Haarlem orphanage. But the probabilities of using an electric shock to cure a patient who was haunted by an "idée fixe," or a delusion, did not come into practice before *1800*, when Giovanni Aldini (1762–1834) published his experiments with electric shocks administered to mentally ill patients.[115]

Millstones and rotating instruments as a treatment for agitated patients became popular again at the end of the century. Erasmus Darwin (1731–1802) suggested rotation for a patient suffering from fever, "so as to whirl him round with his head most distant from the center of mo-

112. *First Lines* 2:38.

113. See n. 73 above.

114. Samuel X. Radbill, "Whooping Cough in Fact and Fancy," *Bulletin of the History of Medicine* 13 (1943): 33–52.

115. Giovanni Aldini, *Essay théorique et expérimental sur le galvanisme* (Paris: Fournier, 1804).

tion, as if he lay across a millstone."[116] Darwin considered any form of severe emotional disturbance, even madness, to be accompanied by fever. He suggested diminishing the "sensorial power" by spinning the fever out of the body.[117] Since millstones were not available to the average practicing physician, a rotating bed or chair might be used. Darwin's rotation idea was elaborated and actually applied in practice by Joseph Cox (1762–1822). It became a regular treatment for mentally disturbed patients owing to the work of the Belgian psychiatrist Joseph Guislain (1797–1860), who designed several rotating chairs for his patients.[118] Just the appearance of these frightening instruments aroused fear among those who were to undergo this treatment.

The mill as therapeutic instrument may be understood as a straw in the wind announcing a new period in the history of mankind—not merely the beginnings of the Industrial Revolution, which would bring new instruments for medical treatment and diagnosis, but the force of the new psychology. Moreover, there were few, frightening, and almost demonic powers, if one can call them by this name, such as the steam engine, electricity, the new chemical formulas of materials yet unknown. Fear of new technology would arise as engineering marched ahead and would continue as one of the great menaces of our time. In this respect, Pemberton's reference to Cullen's lecture on the use of a mill to cure a child's whooping cough strikes us as a prophecy. Time will tell how prophetic it really was.

116. Erasmus Darwin, *Zoonomia; or The laws of Organic Life* (London, 1794–1796), 2:608.

117. Ibid. 578.

118. Joseph Cox used a rotating chair: *Practical Observations on Insanity* . . . (London, 1804–1814). I did not consult this work. Joseph Guislain pays full tribute to Darwin for the idea of rotation: see *Traité sur l'aliénation mentale et sur les hospices des aliénés* (Amsterdam, 1826), 1:374, discussed by Flynn in chap. 5 above.

PART THREE

The Politics of Mind and Body: Radical Practitioners and Revolutionary Doctors

SEVEN

States of Mind: Enlightenment and Natural Philosophy

Simon Schaffer

The voice of the Devil:

All Bibles or sacred codes have been the cause of the following Errors:

1. That Man has two real existing principles: Viz: a Body & a Soul.
2. That Energy, call'd Evil, is alone from the Body; & that Reason, call'd Good, is alone from the Soul.
3. That God will torment Man in Eternity for following his Energies.

—WILLIAM BLAKE, *The Marriage of Heaven and Hell*, 1790–1793

If it were possible to find a method of becoming master of everything which might happen to a certain number of men, to dispose of everything around them so as to produce on them the desired impression, to make certain of their actions, of their connections, and of all the circumstances of their lives, so that nothing could escape, nor could oppose the desired effect, it cannot be doubted that a method of this kind would be a very powerful and a very useful instrument which governments might apply to various objects of the utmost importance.

—JEREMY BENTHAM, *Panopticon; or, The Inspection-House*, 1787–1791

THE PRISON OF THE BODY

The relationship between mind and body provides graphic political images of knowledge and power. The slogans composed by Blake and Bentham in the early 1790s are good examples of this imagery. Blake wrote against "the notion that man has a body distinct from his soul." He said that this false notion bred a self-imposed imprisonment of the mind: "man has closed himself up, till he sees all things thro' narrow chinks of his cavern." Political liberty went hand in hand with spiritual liberty. The destruction of the Bastille was figured as the action of

Abbreviations:

Bowring: John Bowring, ed., *The Works of Jeremy Bentham*, 11 vols. (Edinburgh, 1838–1848).

Rutt: John T. Rutt, ed., *The Theological and Miscellaneous Works of Joseph Priestley*, 25 vols. (London, 1817–1832).

liberating energies in the human mind. So, pastiching Emmanuel Swedenborg's visionary cosmology, Blake proposed a new Code, the "Bible of Hell" directed against old penology and old morality: "Prisons are built with Stones of Law, Brothels with bricks of Religion." Bentham also proposed a new Code to replace old penology and morality, and he also represented this radical reform through an appeal to the relation of bodies and minds. He claimed that in his Panopticon a remakable architectural arrangement of bodies allow the possibility of the "power of mind over mind." In this visionary building, a concentric ring of cells was to be arranged around a central guard tower and a chapel. From the tower, the warden could survey every denizen of the "inspection house" but would always remain invisible to these inmates. The plan was to be fitted to prisons or factories, schools or workhouses—in short, any model polity that demanded the supervisory power of an "invisible eye." The members of such a polity were to be governed through the complete management of their atmosphere and their surroundings. The Panopticon relied on the link between the bodily situation of its inhabitants and their state of mind. The right distribution of light, air, and space prompted the right associations: every inmate would "conceive himself" to be under constant surveillance.[1]

The Panopticon was an "enlightened" project, concerned with rational order and moral reform, deriving its authority from the natural philosophical understanding of the work of the mind. Spectacularly unsuccessful in reformed Britain, the scheme was initially drafted for the enlightened despotism of Russia and greeted with rapture in Revolutionary France. It has always invited allegorical interpretation. Its author helped himself to the language of a secularized theology: the Panopticon combined "the apparent omnipresence of the inspector (if divines will allow me the expression)" with "the extreme facility of his real presence." He told his Girondin admirer J. P. Brissot that it was "a mill for grinding rogues honest and idle men industrious," and yet confessed in private that it was "a haunted house." For William Hazlitt, the Panopticon was a "glass beehive," a scheme marked by luminous clarity, impractical idealism, and deadly obsession. Edmund Burke was even more scathing: "there's the keeper, the spider in the web." Recent com-

1. William Blake, *Complete Writings*, ed. Geoffrey Keynes (Oxford: Oxford University Press, 1972), 154, 151; Bowring, 4:66, 79, 40. For Blake and Swedenborg, see Mona Wilson, *The Life of William Blake* (Oxford: Oxford University Press, 1971), 56–60; for Blake and the Revolution, see David V. Erdman, *Blake: Prophet against Empire*, 3d ed. (Princeton: Princeton University Press, 1977), 175–197.

mentators, no less critical, have found that Bentham's vision provides fruitful evidence of Enlightenment mentality. Bentham has been castigated for the pursuit of crass commercial gain under the mask of disinterested reform, thus damning the motives of future generations of his utilitarian disciples. He has been celebrated as the author of a "symbolic caricature of the characteristic features of disciplinary thinking in his age." Under the inquiring gaze of Michel Foucault, the Panopticon has been transformed into the ideal type of a "microphysics of power," "at once a programme and a utopia," whose disciplinary strategy of surveillance and individuation marked the birth pangs of the human sciences. Precisely because of this exemplary history, the Panopticon and its author's career provide important clues to the concerns of a reforming philosophy of mind and body in the age of reason.[2]

The concerns of the reforming philosophers connected a model of the right role to be performed by expert intellectuals and a picture of mind and body. The Panopticon was a sign of a reconstructed discipline, both a new way of exercising power and a new form of knowledge. Foucault argued that this discipline was accompanied by the emergence of "the modern soul." Displaced from Christian theology, this soul was at once the site at which power was to be exercised and the object of which knowledge was to be produced. Hence Foucault's characteristically gnomic remark about the relationship between the subject of the enlightened philosophy of mind and the regimes of corporeal discipline these philosophers proposed: "the soul is the effect and instrument of a political anatomy; the soul is the prison of the body."[3] More prosaically, the account of the mind produced by Bentham and his colleagues directly confronted established religion and moral philosophy. Apparently

2. Bowring, 4:45; Bentham to Brissot, [1791], in Bowring, 10:226; for the "haunted house" see Bowring, 10:250; for Hazlitt, see William Hazlitt, *The Spirit of the Age* (1825; London: Henry Frowde, 1904), 12–13; for Burke, Bowring, 10:564. For commentary on the Panopticon, see Gertrude Himmelfarb, "The Haunted House of Jeremy Bentham," in *Victorian Minds* (New York: Alfred Knopf, 1968), 32–81; Michael Ignatieff, *A Just Measure of Pain: The Penitentiary in the Industrial Revolution, 1750–1850* (London: Macmillan, 1978), 113. For Michel Foucault on "panopticism," see his *Discipline and Punish: The Birth of the Prison* (Harmondsworth: Penguin Books, 1979), 200–209; "The Eye of Power," in *Power-Knowledge: Selected Interviews and Other Writings*, ed. Colin Gordon (New York: Pantheon Books, 1980), 146–165. For comments on Foucault's account, see Michelle Perrot, ed., *L'impossible prison: Recherches sur le système pénitentiaire au XIXe siècle* (Paris: Seuil, 1980); Martin Jay, "In the Empire of the Gaze: Foucault and the Denigration of Vision in Twentieth-Century French Thought," in *Foucault: A Critical Reader*, ed. D. Couzens Hoy (Oxford: Blackwell, 1986), 175–204.

3. Foucault, *Discipline and Punish*, 29–30.

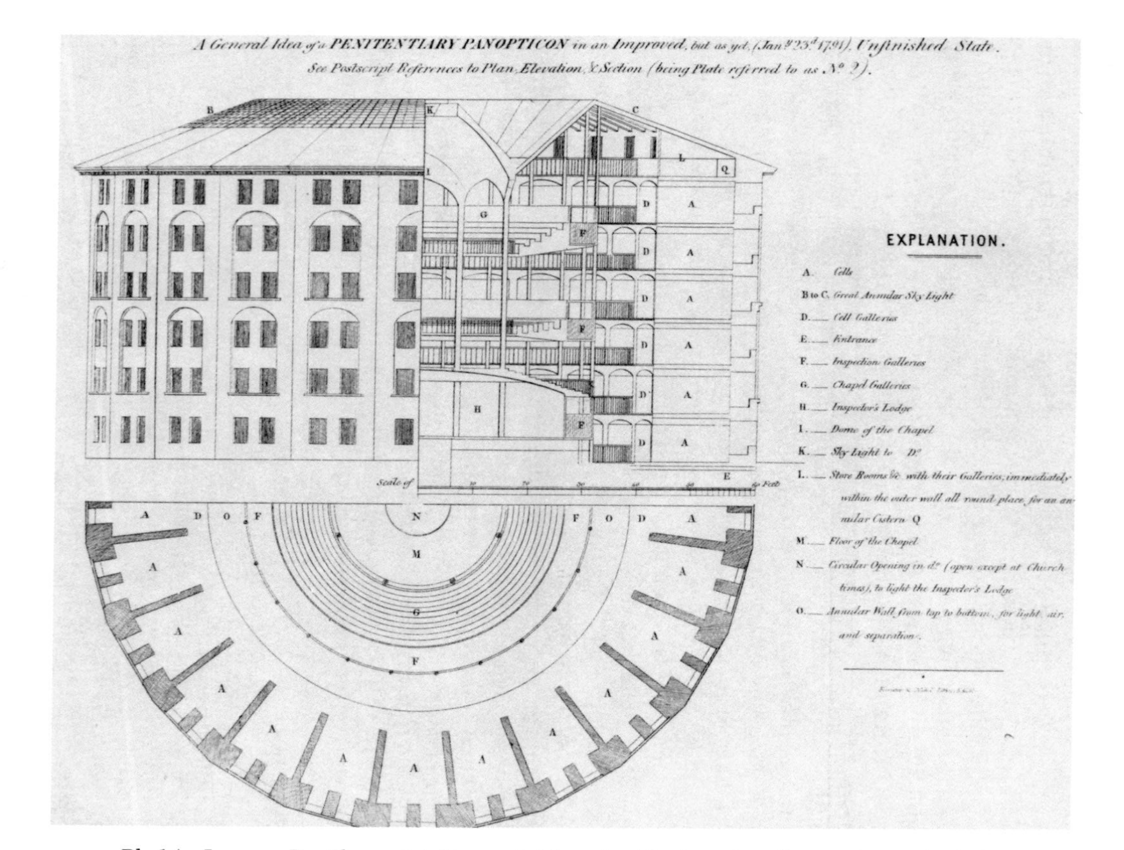

Pl. 14. Jeremy Bentham, "A General Idea of a Penitentiary Panopticon" (1787).

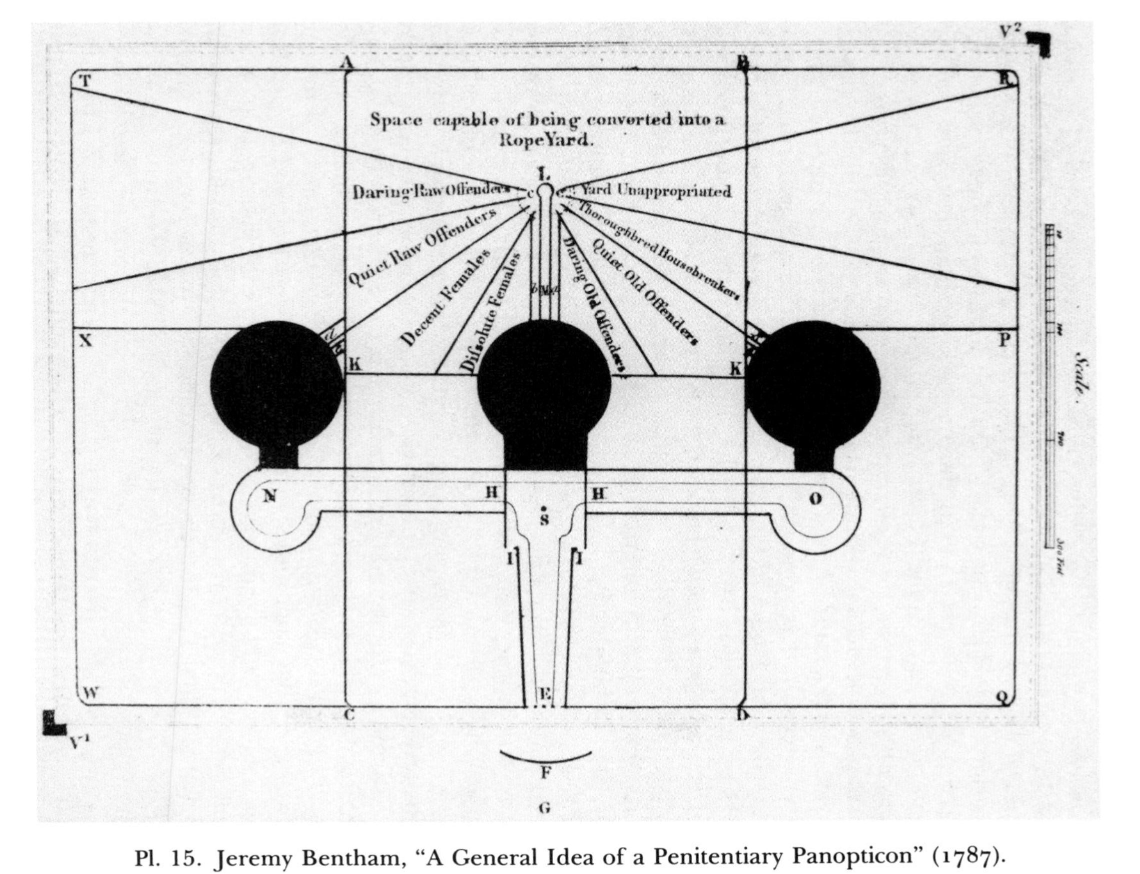

Pl. 15. Jeremy Bentham, "A General Idea of a Penitentiary Panopticon" (1787).

abstruse exchanges on the immortality of the soul, the possibility of thinking matter, and the character of human motivation carried explicit political resonances. Traditional guardians of moral conduct were to be displaced by philosophers who knew the material sources of passions and interests. Materialist philosophy was allied with a natural philosophical inquiry into the activity of matter and life. It was also allied with reformist projects for the redistribution of authority in the social order.

To provide an example of this network of alliances, a case is taken from the work of some English clerics and lawyers in the 1770s. As Foucault suggested, "these tactics were invented and organised from the starting points of local conditions and particular needs." In this paper, the locale is provided by the work of Joseph Priestley, a dissenting minister at Leeds until 1773 and subsequently the Earl of Shelburne's librarian at Bowood House in Wiltshire until 1780, and of Bentham himself, working in London as a legal writer until he became Shelburne's client in 1781. The connections between these men play an important part in my argument. The "Bowood group," of whom Bentham and Priestley were members, with others such as Richard Price and Samuel Romilly, was later to be identified as a key source of subversive ideas by anti-Jacobins in the 1790s. The enterprise connected with Shelburne, organized under the banner of economic and philosophical reform, provides a convenient site from which to investigate the links between natural philosophy, epistemology, and reforming civil philosophy at this period. While at Bowood, Priestley composed a lengthy series of texts that criticized contemporary philosophies of mind, notably those developed in Scotland by Hume and the Common Sense school, and offered a challenging materialist account of moral philosophy and of mind and body, based on the theories of David Hartley and Priestley's views of proper religion. At the same time, Priestley was actively engaged in political and religious campaigning for civil reform and the emancipation of dissent. Shelburne also provided Priestley with support for his research in pneumatic chemistry, which was inaugurated just before the move to Bowood. Similarly, it was during this period that Bentham began his composition of an ambitious series of texts on political and legal reform and his search for influential backing for these schemes, of which the Panopticon was the most celebrated. The admiration of Benthamite disciples and the hostility of conservative critics have often obscured the process through which these visionary proposals were formed. It will be emphasized that the utopian character of the work mounted by Priestley and Bentham at this period is a significant aspect of their campaigns. Priestley's strong commitment to a millenarian vision of humanity's future, and Bentham's extraordinary dreams for that future—and his part in it—are among the more striking aspects of their knowledge of civil society and of natural order. The reformers were visionaries because to change the state they had to change minds.[4]

This paper is divided into five sections. The first explores an ambiguity in the sense of "enlightenment" as it was used in late-eighteenth-century Britain. During the 1790s, in particular, conservative critics of radicals and reformers argued that the "light" of these philosophers was indistinguishable from the "illumination" of occult mystics and enthusiasts. They pointed out a peculiar feature of the social organization of the reformers, the Masonic club or secretive association of like-minded members of the intelligentsia. The anti-Jacobins then argued that this social form promoted a subversive form of knowledge: the dangerously ambitious account of mind which materialist *philosophes* used to explain and defend the deeds of the Revolution. The ambiguity of "enlightenment" depended on the ambiguity of reformist philosophy, a knowledge that promised both freedom and discipline. Conservatives interpreted this freedom as anarchy and this discipline as tyranny. Radicals promised a world of free individuals who would pursue the dictates of reasoned self-interest. In contemplating Foucault's analysis of the Panopticon, Jacques Léonard has pointed out that "utilitarian rationalization and political rationalism go together; one must pause here over masonic philosophy: the mason builds and frees."[5] The conservative attack on the visions of the reformers suggests a promising line of inquiry into the interests of their philosophy. In particular, it suggests a link between the social forms of patronage and association and the philosophy which the reformers espoused. The second section of the paper documents the local setting of the work of Priestley and Bentham in the 1770s and 1780s, when they were working closely with Shelburne on schemes

4. For Foucault on the local context, see "The Eye of Power," 159. For Bentham and the Bowood group, see Charles W. Everett, *The Education of Jeremy Bentham* (New York: Columbia University Press, 1931), 122–132; Mary P. Mack, *Jeremy Bentham: An Odyssey of Ideas, 1748–1792* (London: Heinemann, 1962), 370–404. For politics and the Bowood group, see Elie Halevy, *The Growth of Philosophic Radicalism* (1928; London: Faber and Faber, 1972), 145–150; John Norris, *Shelburne and Reform* (London: Macmillan, 1963), 83–85, 250–253; Derek Jarrett, *The Begetters of Revolution: England's Relationship with France, 1759–1789* (London: Longmans, 1973), 130–135; D. O. Thomas, *The Honest Mind: The Thought and Work of Richard Price* (Oxford: Clarendon Press, 1977), 142–148; Albert Goodwin, *The Friends of Liberty: The English Democratic Movement in the Age of the French Revolution* (London: Hutchinson, 1979), 101–106.

5. Jacques Léonard, "L'historien et le philosophe," in Perrot, *L'impossible prison*, 9–28 at 19. Compare Reinhart Koselleck, *Krise und Kritik* (Munich: Karl Albert, 1959), chap. 2.

for reform in philosophy, religion, and politics. It is suggested that there were important connections between the immediate concerns of this period and the apparently utopian schemes which the reformers proposed. In particular, work on the natural philosophy of the powers of matter, pursued both by Priestley and Bentham in the 1770s, is shown to be an important source for ideas about the progress of society. The link between natural philosophical and social reform lay in a new doctrine of pneumatics, of the behavior of matter and spirit.

In the third section of the paper, this connection is explored in some detail, and it is argued that work in pneumatic chemistry provided powerful resources for an understanding of the way the mind worked and the true doctrine of the soul. Priestley's experimental philosophy and the way he suggested experimenters should work generated a materialist philosophy of mind and a reconstruction of the orthodox model of the soul. The two final sections of this paper examine the consequences of this materialism. Such a philosophy of mind and of soul involved the development of what can be called a "counter-theology," a vision of the future of humanity which relied on a reform of the understanding of human nature. This understanding argued against dualism, removed the division between body and soul, and made mind an object of philosophical inquiry and reform. Mind could become such an object because it was supposed to be material. Philosophical materialism suggested an appropriate role which these intellectuals should follow, that of the medical manager, the expert equipped with an understanding of what Bentham named "mental pathology." So reforming philosophy posed as a therapy. Alongside their account of current social ills, both Priestley and Bentham wrote histories that explained how society and philosophy had developed. These histories simultaneously explained the source of error and suggested ways of correcting it. Social and philosophical error were due to "fictions," corrupt illusions generated by the interests of those in power. The right philosophy of mind and body would discriminate between the real and the fictional by distinguishing between the material and immaterial. Because both writers saw a link between the current social order and the current crisis of philosophy, they supposed that a future of improvement would be marked by a future of rational triumph. The last section of the paper connects this reformed philosophy of mind and this counter-theology with the visionary character of the reformers' project. While philosophical materialism deprived subjects of the illusory hopes of a spiritual world to come, it affirmed a certain future of advance in the social order. The exemplary deaths of Priestley and Bentham dramatized their attitude to this prospect. Reform would continue under the guidance of expert managers armed with the right account of mind and body and thus the ability to cure the diseases of the body politic. In the nineteenth century, followers of this reforming philosophy developed new disciplines that sought to survey the mental and bodily habits of the subjects of the state. It is concluded that these new disciplines shared much of the utopianism and ambition of the "enlightened" philosophers of the 1770s.[6]

ENLIGHTENMENT AND ILLUMINATION

Enlightened philosophers grew up in a world of spirits. Priestley recalled that when he was a child in Yorkshire in the 1730s, "it was my misfortune to have the idea of darkness, and the ideas of malignant spirits and apparitions, very closely connected." He also described the "feelings . . . too full of terror" prompted by his strict Calvinist education: "in that state of mind I remember reading the account of the 'man in an iron cage' in the *Pilgrim's Progress* with the greatest perturbation." Bentham had very similar memories about his upbringing in Essex twenty years later: "this subject of ghosts has been among the torments of my life," he wrote, while Bunyan was again a source of fear: "the devil was everywhere in it and in me too." No doubt this captures a conventional view of "enlightenment": reason destroyed the world of spirits and liberated humanity from superstition. Priestley's "remembrance . . . of what I sometimes felt in that state of ignorance and darkness," he revealed, "gives me a peculiar sense of the value of rational principles of religion." His fears were well known to Bentham, who reminisced about the "sensation more than mental" produced in Priestley by the name of a spirit "too awful to be mentioned." Commenting on his own reading of *Pilgrim's Progress,* Bentham exclaimed "how much less unhappy I should have been, could I have acknowledged my superstitious fears . . . now that I know the distinction between the imagination and

6. For materialism and eighteenth-century natural philosophy, see Aram Vartanian, *Diderot and Descartes: A Study of Scientific Naturalism in the Enlightenment* (Princeton: Princeton University Press, 1953); Robert E. Schofield, *Mechanism and Materialism: British Natural Philosophy in an Age of Reason* (Princeton: Princeton University Press, 1970); John Yolton, *Thinking Matter: Materialism in Eighteenth Century Britain* (Oxford: Blackwell, 1983). For Bentham on "mental pathology," see *Introduction to the Principles of Morals and Legislation* (1789; Oxford: Clarendon Press, 1876), vii; Bowring, 1:304–305. For Bentham on "fictions," see Bowring, 1:235; C. K. Ogden, *Bentham's Theory of Fictions* (London: Kegan Paul, Trench, Trubner, 1932); Ross Harrison, *Bentham* (London: Routledge and Kegan Paul, 1983), 24–46.

the judgement!"[7] This image of enlightenment has proved remarkably robust. Historians of natural philosophy have documented the processes whereby spiritual powers hitherto attributed to divine will or immaterial substances were made immanent in matter and subjected to reasoned experimentation. Enthusiasm was tamed: the mad were confined and their claims to inspiration referred either to somatic causes susceptible to medical treatment or to mental disturbance that needed moral therapy. Spirits no longer walked: astrologers were made the butt of the wits and ghost stories a matter of titillation rather than juridical process. It is suggested that these processes touched both the godly and the dissolute. Philip Doddridge, founder of the dissenting academy where Priestley studied, lectured his pupils on the astrologers, who "may as justly be punished as those who keep gaming houses brothels, &c." Yet he warned that some spirits were real: "Seeing there is something in the thought of such agents as these which tends to impress the imagination in a very powerful manner, great care ought to be taken, that *children,* from the first notice they have of the existence of such beings, be taught to conceive of them as entirely under the control of God." Priestley and many of his allies were taught such views, and carefully revised them to fit the canons of reason.[8]

Eighteenth-century observers recognized a spreading materialism as a fact of social life. In his study of the Enlightenment's relation with death, John McManners cites an orthodox apologist's rueful lament of 1761: "it seems that it is no longer permissible to speak of the soul except to attack it and to confound it with the instinct of the animals." The long eighteenth-century debates on the powers that could be attributed to mere bodies implied that materialism was only too fashionable: "the very Beaux . . . Argue themselves into mere Machines," commented a worried enemy of "deism" in 1707. The experimental philosophy that sustained this materialism could be a political weapon: electricity and

7. For Priestley on ghosts, see Rutt, 1:1–8; 3:50; for Bentham on ghosts, see Bowring, 10:11–21.

8. For enlightenment, medicine, and enthusiasm, see Roy Porter, "Medicine and the Enlightenment in Eighteenth-Century England," *Bulletin of the Society for the Social History of Medicine* 25 (1979): 27–40; G. S. Rousseau, "Psychology," in *The Ferment of Knowledge,* ed. G. S. Rousseau and Roy Porter (Cambridge: Cambridge University Press, 1980), 143–210; Michael MacDonald, "Religion, Social Change and Psychological Healing in England," *Studies in Church History* 19 (1982): 101–126; Martin Fitzpatrick, "Science and Society in the Enlightenment," *Enlightenment and Dissent* 4 (1985): 83–106. For Doddridge, see Philip Doddridge, *Course of Lectures on the Principal Subjects in Pneumatology, Ethics and Divinity* (London, 1763), 552, 541. For the academies, see Nicholas Hans, *New Trends in Education in the Eighteenth Century* (London: Routledge and Kegan Paul, 1951), 54–62.

pneumatic chemistry demonstrated the range of powers that matter could display. Hence Priestley's notorious remark that "the English hierarchy (if there is anything unsound in its constitution) has equal reason to tremble even at an air pump, or an electrical machine."[9] Nor was this merely a matter of fashionable libertinism or pious philosophizing. Priestley, Bentham, and their allies saw immediate material necessity in the propaganda for rational knowledge. In 1772 the Scottish philosopher Thomas Reid wrote to Priestley's colleague, Richard Price, praising him for quelling "the present Epidemical Disease of trusting to visionary projects" with the tools of political arithmetic. Reasonable knowledge and the maturity of men of the "middling sort" could reform manners and order even as corrupt a society as the present. What Peter Burke has called "the reformation with the Reformation" mobilized considerable support among the laity. Burke points out the change in the sense of the term "superstition" during this period. A label for powerful and dangerous heresies was transferred to the impotent vagaries of the credulous vulgar. This gave polemical point to the comradely sentiments of the letter from the Derby Philosophical Society which Priestley received soon after the Birmingham mob had destroyed his house and laboratory in 1791: "the sacrilegious hands of the savages at Birmingham" were best combatted with "that philosophy, of which you may be called the father." Erasmus Darwin and his Derby colleagues counseled that "by inducing the world to think and reason," this philosophy "will silently marshall mankind against delusion, and with greater certainty overturn the empire of superstition."[10]

9. Louis-Antoine de Caraccioli, *La grandeur de l'âme* (Paris, 1761), xii, cited in John McManners, *Death and the Enlightenment* (Oxford: Oxford University Press, 1985), 159; John Witty, *The First Principles of Modern Deism Confuted* (London, 1707), v, cited in Yolton, *Thinking Matter*, 42; Joseph Priestley, *Experiments and Observations on Different Kinds of Air* (London, 1774), xiv.

10. For political arithmetic, see Thomas Reid to Richard Price, [?] 1773, *Correspondence of Richard Price*, ed. W. Bernard Peach and D. O. Thomas (Durham, N.C.: Duke University Press, 1983), 1:154; Peter Buck, "People Who Counted: Political Arithmetic in the Eighteenth Century," *Isis* 73 (1982): 28–45. For moral reformation, see R. W. Malcomson, *Popular Recreations in English Society, 1700–1850* (Cambridge: Cambridge University Press, 1973), chap. 7; Peter Burke, *Popular Culture in Early Modern Europe* (London: Maurice Temple Smith, 1978), 239–242. For Priestley and the Derby Philosophical Society, see Derby Philosophical Society to Priestley, 3 September 1791, in Rutt, 2:152; compare E. Robinson, "New Light on the Priestley Riots," *Historical Journal* 3 (1960): 73–75; French chemists to Priestley, July 1791, in R. E. Schofield, *Scientific Autobiography of Joseph Priestley* (Cambridge, Mass.: MIT Press, 1966), 257–258: "we have therefore resolved to re-establish your Cabinet, to raise again the Temple which ignorance, barbarity and superstition have dared profane."

The opponents of men such as Priestley and Darwin were swift to see through these assaults on "delusion" and "superstition." In his remarkable survey of the sinister conspiracies of the *philosophes* and their "illuminated" allies, the Edinburgh natural-philosophy professor John Robison argued in 1796 that a real danger lurked behind this "silent" campaign. In his *Proofs of a Conspiracy against all the Religions and Governments of Europe,* Robison compared the virtuous religion of Newton's celebrated General Scholium with Laplace's *Système du monde.* He cited Laplace's attack on "the dangerous maxim that it is sometimes useful to deceive men in order to insure their happiness." What were these "deceits"? "They cannot relate to astrology," Robison suggested, "this was entirely out of date." So Laplace was assaulting the doctrine of the nobility of man and his difference from beasts: materialism bred arrogance among the intellectuals and abasement among their followers.[11] Robison was one of many anti-Jacobin writers of the 1790s who made these points. "Is superstition the greatest of all possible vices?" Burke asked in 1791. No, for it was "the religion of feeble minds, and they must be tolerated in an intermixture of it, in some trifling or some enthusiastic shape or other." Burke and his admirers held that the disasters of the Revolution demonstrated three key principles of contemporary intellectual life. First, there were identifiable bands of self-styled enlightened philosophers whose sinister associations masked silent plots to subvert established order. Second, these associations promoted a materialist doctrine of mind, bolstered with a false natural philosophy, in which the status of the intellectual reformer was exaggerated and the aspirations of men reduced to the level of beasts. Last, the exaggeration of the powers of reason was no better than a revamped enthusiasm. There was nothing to choose between the radical savants and the enthusiast mob. Nor was there much difference between the wilder shores of philosophical materialism and the old doctrines of spirits, witches, and ghosts. New enlightenment was but old illumination. The enthusiastic visions of the philosophers helped this set of claims: it was not always easy to distinguish the language of the rational dissenters from that of their Methodist enemies. Priestley's Yorkshire bred both. His work on "the scriptures, Ecclesiastical History and the Theory of the Human Mind" was often couched in the metaphor of light and applied directly to

11. John Robison, *Proofs of a Conspiracy against all the Religions and Governments of Europe,* 3d ed. (London, 1798), 229–233. For Robison and the Laplacians, see J. B. Morrell, "Professors Robison and Playfair and the Theophobia Gallica: Natural Philosophy, Religion and Politics in Edinburgh, 1789–1815," *Notes and Records of the Royal Society* 26 (1971): 43–64.

radical secular change. Thus in his learned dissertation of 1782 on the scriptural foundations of unitarianism, Priestley made use of an obviously visionary language: "happy are those who contribute to diffuse the pure light of this everlasting gospel."[12]

In his own *Everlasting Gospel* of 1818 Blake drew a sharp distinction between his vision of spirituality and that of the rational unitarians: "Like dr. Priestly [sic] & Bacon & Newton—Poor Spiritual Knowledge is not worth a button!" But in the 1790s it was easy to see the connections between the proclamations of the empire of reason and the older forms of spiritual knowledge. In France and Britain astrology, mesmerism, alchemy, the Eleusinian mysteries, electrotherapy, and prophecy all became linked to the radical cause. If, as Robert Darnton has suggested, mesmerism marked the end of the Enlightenment in France, mesmerists found it possible to trace respectable natural-philosophical ancestry for their doctrines among the views on active matter developed by eighteenth-century electrical and pneumatic experimenters. But Paris physicians found it more plausible to compare Mesmer with occultists such as Paracelsus, Fludd, Greatrakes, and Bruno. Roy Porter is right to point out that the disciples of animal magnetism proffered materialist stories to explain their successes while the established academicians referred Mesmer's cures to psychosomatic possessions in order to explain them away.[13] In the 1790s, Britain witnessed a wide range of such radical

12. Edmund Burke, *Reflections on the Revolution in France* (1791; London: Dent, 1910), 155; Joseph Priestley, *Doctrine of Philosophical Necessity Illustrated* (London, 1777), xvi; Rutt, 5:4. For the anti-Jacobin reaction, see M. D. George, "Political Propaganda, 1793–1815: Gillray and Canning," *History*, n.s., 31 (1946): 66–68 (on the *Anti-Jacobin*); Norton Garfinkle, "Science and Religion in England, 1790–1800: The Critical Response to the Work of Erasmus Darwin," *Journal of the History of Ideas* 16 (1955): 276–288; Goodwin, *Friends of Liberty*, chaps. 4, 6, 10.

13. Blake, *Complete Writings*, 752; for mystical sciences and radical politics in Britain, see Clarke Garrett, *Respectable Folly: Millenarians and the French Revolution in France and Britain* (Baltimore: Johns Hopkins University Press, 1975); J. F. C. Harrison, *The Second Coming: Popular Millenarianism, 1780–1850* (London: Routledge and Kegan Paul, 1979). For mesmerism, see Robert Darnton, *Mesmerism and the End of the Enlightenment in France* (Cambridge, Mass.: Harvard University Press, 1968); Roy Porter, "Under the Influence: Mesmerism in England," *History Today* 35 (September 1985): 22–29. Mesmer connects his views with natural philosophy in "Mémoire sur ses découvertes" (1799), in *Mesmerism*, ed. George J. Bloch (Los Altos, Calif.: Kauffmann, 1980), 118–121. For English mesmerism, see Roger Cooter, "The History of Mesmerism in England," in *Mesmer und die Geschichte des Mesmerismus*, ed. Heinz Schott (Stuttgart: Franz Steiner, 1985), 152–162. For the psychosomatic explanation of mesmeric cures, see F. Azouvi, "Sens et fonction épistémologique de la critique du magnétisme animal par les Académies," *Revue de l'histoire des sciences* 29 (1976): 123–142. For Mesmer and Paracelsians, see J. J. Paulet, *L'antimagnétisme* (Paris, 1784). For the "Eleusinian mysteries," see Erasmus Darwin, *The Temple of Nature* (London,

and mystical activity. Conservatives documented groups such as the "ancient deists" at Hoxton, a center of London dissent, who combined the views of "infidel mystics" with French politics and occult sciences. The activities of the popular prophets such as Joanna Southcott and Richard Brothers were also greeted with a mixture of amusement and alarm. The work of the inspired attracted considerable support in regions such as those where dissent was strong. The events of the 1790s suggested at least three targets for conservative comment: millenarians and prophets who foresaw an imminent change in the civil and moral order; radical physicians who appealed to a materialist knowledge of the mind and the soul in order to change humanity; and rationalist metaphysicians who applied the principles of their philosophy to the reconstruction of the state. Priestley and his allies, such as Theophilus Lindsey and Richard Price, talked in explicitly millenarian terms: "I have little doubt," Priestley announced in 1798, "but that the great prophecies relating to the permanent and happy state of the world, are in the way of fulfilment." These hopes were backed by a specifically materialist account of the capacities of the human mind. As fashionable physicians and radical natural philosophers, both Thomas Beddoes and Erasmus Darwin attracted particular hostility from the conservatives. As Maureen McNeil has shown, Darwin was attacked in the same way as his ally Joseph Priestley for "constantly blending and confounding together the two distinct sciences of matter and mind." Writers in the *Anti-Jacobin* made fun of these visions. In their satire of 1798 on Darwin's *Loves of the Plants,* Canning and Frere paraphrased the radicals' view of the progress of humanity. "We have risen from a level with the *cabbages of the field* to our present comparatively intelligent and dignified state of existence, by the mere exertion of our own energies." The future prospects were ludicrously glorious and based on a risible natural philosophy: the wits claimed that the radicals hoped to raise man "to a rank in which he would be, as it were, *all* MIND; would enjoy unclouded perspicacity and perpetual vitality; feed on *oxygene,* and never die, but by *his own consent.*"[14]

1803), 13n. Compare Herbert Loventhal, *In the Shadow of the Enlightenment: Occultism and Renaissance Science in 18th Century America* (New York: New York University Press, 1976).

14. For the "ancient deists," see William Hamilton Reid, *The Rise and Dissolution of the Infidel Societies in This Metropolis* (London, 1800), 91; for prophecy, see Harrison, *The Second Coming,* 57–134; D. M. Valenze, "Prophecy and Popular Literature in Eighteenth-Century England," *Journal of Ecclesiastical History* 29 (1978): 75–92; Clarke Garrett, "Swedenborg and the Mystical Enlightenment in Late Eighteenth-Century England," *Journal of the History of Ideas* 45 (1984): 67–81. For popular dissent, see E. P. Thompson, *The Making of the English Working Class* (Harmondsworth: Penguin Books, 1968), chap. 2. For Priestley and

The apostles of reason often seemed to be tools of unreason. Bentham recognized this: in the 1770s he already accepted that "the world is persuaded, not without some colour of reason, that all reformers and system-mongers are mad. . . . I dreamt t'other night that I was a founder of a sect; of course, a personage of great sanctity and importance: it was called the sect of the Utilitarians." The language of the sects was a powerful tool for the reformers. It became a devastating weakness when attacked in the 1790s. Burke's immediate target, Richard Price, preached that "every degree of illumination which we can communicate must do the greatest good. It helps prepare the minds of men for the recovery of their rights and hasten the overthrow of priestcraft and tyranny." Their opponents identified the social habits of the reformers with their mental constitution. Their covert associations of like-minded intellectuals allegedly fostered the strategy of an insinuation of the false and dangerous beliefs of materialist metaphysics and silly natural philosophy. Thus derangement became dangerous when it seized power. In 1796 Burke picked on the geometricians and chemists whose "dispositions" made them "worse than indifferent about those feelings and habitudes which are the support of the moral world. Ambition is come upon them suddenly; they are intoxicated with it." Sometimes, as in the satires directed against Beddoes's use of gaseous medicines in Bristol in the 1790s and the "pneumatic revelries" of his friends, the "intoxication" became literal. The mental habits of these men were viewed as the cause of their threatening policy. Approaching dangerously, if characteristically, the excessive fury which he condemned, Burke said that "the heart of a thoroughbred metaphysician comes nearer to the cold malignity of a wicked spirit than the frailty and passion of man. It is like that of the Principle of Evil himself, incorporeal, pure, unmixed, dephlegmated, defecated evil." Accusations of insanity provided much of the language of the polemic on the *Reflections on the Revolution in France.* Both Burke and Robison, who was well known for his opium habit, might also be shown to be mentally disturbed. Bentham was irate that "the National Assembly of France has been charged with madness for pulling down

prophecy, see Priestley to Lindsey, 1 November 1798, in Rutt, 2:410; Jack Fruchtman, Jr., *The Apocalyptic Politics of Richard Price and Joseph Priestley* (Philadelphia: American Philosophical Society, 1983), 8–45, 81–93. For attacks on Darwin, see *Edinburgh Review* 2 (1803):449, cited in Maureen McNeil, "The Scientific Muse: The Poetry of Erasmus Darwin," in *Languages of Nature: Critical Essays on Science and Literature,* ed. Ludmilla Jordanova (London: Free Association Books, 1986), 159–203 at 172; Charles Edmonds, ed., *Poetry of the Anti-Jacobin* (London: Sampson Low, Marston, Searle and Rivington, 1890), 147 (April 1798).

establishment," and he condemned Burke's book as the "frantic exclamation" of a "mad man, than whom none perhaps was ever more mischievous."[15]

Burke was only the most effective of those who argued for the devastating effects of the connection between the associations formed by the reforming philosophers and the political havoc they had wrought. The natural philosophy of the reformers provided fruitful targets for wit: in a famous figure, Burke compared "the spirit of liberty in action" to "the wild *gas,* the fixed air": "but we ought to suspend our judgement until the first effervescence is a little subsided, till the liquor is cleared, and until we see something deeper than the agitation of a troubled and frothy surface." The most obvious—and most humorous—connection which the anti-Jacobins spotted between this natural philosophy and the politics of the Terror was the endorsement of materialism. Robison commented at some length on Priestley's use of David Hartley's theory of association and aethereal vibrations in the mind. "Dr. Priestley again deduces all intelligence from elastic undulations, and will probably think, that his own great discoveries have been the quiverings of some fiery marsh *miasma.*" From here it was but a short step to the dangerous lunacies of the intellectuals. Their overestimate of their own mental capacity was accompanied by the bestialization of humanity. "They find themselves possessed of faculties which enable them to speculate and to discover; and they find that the operation of those faculties is quite unlike the things which they contemplate by their means." The consequence was reformist arrogance and corrupted politics: "they feel a satisfaction in this distinction."[16] An insistence on the material basis of mind seemed to be leading to the creation of a new elite of intellectuals, a new breed of "saints." The resonance with the "Good Old Cause" was deliberate. The admirers of reforms also helped themselves to this hagiographic language. The connections between the English philosophers, such as the Bowood group, and their French colleagues were

15. For Bentham on the sect of utilitarians, see David Baumgardt, *Bentham and the Ethics of Today* (Princeton: Princeton University Press, 1952), appendix 1, printing Bentham MSS, University College London, 169.79. For Price, Richard Price, *Discourse on the Love of Our Country* (London, 1789), 15. For Burke's attack, Edmund Burke, *Letter to a Noble Lord* (1796), in *Burke's Politics,* ed. R. Hoffman and P. Levack (New York: Columbia University Press, 1949), 532–534. For attacks on Beddoes, see Dorothy Stansfield, *Thomas Beddoes* (Dordrecht: Reidel, 1984), chap. 7; T. H. Levere, "Dr. Thomas Beddoes: Science and Medicine in Politics and Society," *British Journal for the History of Science* 17 (1984): 187–204. For Bentham on Burke and the Revolution, see Bowring, 2:404–405; 4:338.

16. Burke, *Reflections on the Revolution,* 6; Robison, *Proofs of a Conspiracy,* 429–430.

often figured in these terms. The Girondin leader J. P. Brissot, guillotined in 1793 and later satirized as a vindictive ghost in the *Anti-Jacobin*, saw Bentham as a modern saint, one of "those rare beings, whom Heaven sometimes sends down upon earth as a consolation for woes, who, in the form of imperfect man, possess a heavenly spirit."[17]

The attack on the new "saints" was the basis of what amounted to a critique of the new social function of the intellectual. The reformers' associations were held to be the principal site of subversive philosophy and politics. Burke named these associations in the *Reflections* and then defended his decision to do so: "I intend no controversy with Dr. Price, or Lord Shelburne, or any other of their set," he claimed. But his purpose was to destroy their credentials as disinterested men of knowledge: "I mean to do my best to expose them to the hatred, ridicule and contempt of the whole world; as I always shall expose such calumniators, hypocrites, sowers of sedition and approvers of murder and all its triumphs." This was the sense given to the term "Illuminati." The Masonic conspiracies spread through Europe provided the appropriate model with which to analyze the behavior of the English reformers. "The detestable doctrines of Illuminatism have been preached among us," Robison claimed, and named both Priestley and Price as examples. Robison implied that there was a significant contrast with the proper form of natural philosophy developed in such organizations as the Royal Society of Edinburgh, of which he had been Secretary. It was argued that the materialist doctrines of the illuminated philosophers provided a model of the mind which only invited the habit of conspiracy. They had made morality a problem for subtle metaphysics, when it was really a question of public orthodoxy and private sentiment. So their revolution followed from a false natural philosophy. "They have much, but bad, metaphysics; much, but bad, geometry; much, but false, proportionate arithmetic," Burke wrote against the *philosophes*. Political subversion was the same as natural disorder. When Burke turned his gaze upon the French dissolution of the monasteries, he explicitly compared bad policy with bad cosmology: "to destroy any power growing wild from the rank productive force of the human mind, is tantamount, in the moral world, to the destruction of the apparently active properties of bodies in the material." When he explained his own horror at the deposition of the king, he pointed to the natural constitution of the mind: "we behold such disasters in the moral, as we should behold a miracle, in the physical, order of things." Any group of intellectuals which

17. Bowring, 10:192; Edmonds, *Poetry of the Anti-Jacobin*, 165–168 (April 1798).

claimed to be able to understand, reform, and manage these mental faculties was at best insanely optimistic about the capacity of metaphysics and, at worse, destructive of those natural sentiments which actually governed proper moral life.[18]

The anti-Jacobin assault repeatedly contrasted the rational technology of mental management proposed by the radicals with a proper interpretation of the established powers of the mind. The radicals were compared with wily impresarios, or with cunning magicians, or with dissolute gamblers. Burke sought an aesthetics of the state: "to make us love our country, our country ought to be lovely." The machinations of the materialists would be incompetent because they could not hope to understand or to force these aesthetic judgments. The Jacobin theater of politics was a world of illusion and crude spectacle. Their philosophical supporters were no better than wizards, making use of "poisonous weeds and wild incantations." It was scarcely surprising that deluded chemists and natural philosophers found such allies congenial. In the 1770s, Burke had contacts with Priestley's natural philosophy, but by the 1790s he viewed this work as a dangerous error. John Robison was a leader of the British resistance to the new-fangled French chemistry, but Priestley was held to be guilty of overconfidence in his mere hypotheses. Newton's aether was wrongly treated by the materialists as having the certainty of Euclid. It was easy to connect materialist natural philosophy with conjuring. The *Anti-Jacobin* imagined a pneumatic chemist whose "skin, by magical means, has acquired an indefinite power of expansion, as well as that of assimilating to itself all the *azote* of the air . . . an immense quantity which, in our present unimproved and uneconomical mode of breathing, is quite thrown away."[19] This was a well-aimed barb, for the

18. Burke to Philip Francis, 20 February 1790, *Letters of Edmund Burke,* ed. Harold Laski (Oxford: Oxford University Press, 1922), 283–284; Robison, *Proofs of a Conspiracy,* 481; Burke, *Reflections on the Revolution,* 178, 154, 78.

19. Burke, *Reflections on the Revolution,* 75, 93; Robison, *Proofs of a Conspiracy,* 484; Edmonds, *Poetry of the Anti-Jacobin,* 160. For Burke's attack on Jacobin histrionics, see P. H. Melvin, "Burke on Theatricality and Revolution," *Journal of the History of Ideas* 36 (1975): 447–468 and the interesting comments in UEA English Studies Group, "Strategies for Representing Revolution," in *1789: Reading Writing Revolution,* ed. Francis Barker et al. (Colchester: University of Essex, 1982), 81–109. For Burke and Priestley's pneumatics, see Priestley to Burke, 11 December 1782, in Schofield, *Scientific Autobiography of Priestley,* 216; for Robison and French chemistry, see J. R. R. Christie, "Joseph Black and John Robison," in *Joseph Black 1728–1799,* ed. A. D. C. Simpson (Edinburgh: Royal Scottish Museum, 1982), 47–52. For Jacobin and anti-Jacobin natural philosophy, see W. L. Scott, "Impact of the French Revolution on English Science," in *Mélanges Alexandre Koyre,* ed. R. Taton, 2 vols. (Paris: Hermann, 1964), 2:475–495.

reformers did base their authority on their understanding of the atmosphere and the economy of powers that circulated through it. The joke turned sour when these conjurers claimed to be able to reconstruct society. Their charms and spells deceived, and did not comprehend, the moral faculties. Burke argued that "on the principles of this mechanic philosophy, our institutions can never be embodied, if I may use the expression, in persons; so as to create in us love, veneration, admiration or attachment." The materialists did not know these passions and so were foolish to rationalize about them: they knew of "nothing that relates to the concerns, the actions, the passions, the interests of men." This attack applied both to the general possibility of a rationalist metaphysics of the moral order and to the intimate details of political reform. Since the state was a "body politic," a failure to understand the "true genius and character" of any natural body would lead to a failure to understand proper politics. Hence the disasters of the new French financial regime: revenue was "the sphere of every active virtue" of "all great qualities of the mind which operate in public." Mechanistic policy made civil philosophy into a branch of gambling. A principal consequence of the Revolutionary settlement had been to hand over control to the few urban intellectuals who would "understand the game." "The many must be the dupes of the few who conduct the machine of these speculations."[20]

The controversies of the 1790s used the civic humanist language of corruption and virtue and turned it back upon the radical reformers. Burke pointed out that the new intellectual regime privileged the politics of "combination and arrangement (the sole way of procuring and exerting influence)." He argued that "the deceitful dreams and visions of the equality and rights of men" would end in "an ignoble oligarchy" form of coteries of rootless men, recognizable only for their self-styled expertise in management and manipulation. The habit of association was a natural consequence of the reformers' intellectual position. Robison listed the "Corresponding - Affiliated - Provincial - Rescript - Convention - Reading Societies" as British manifestations of this habit. Those linked with politically interested patrons, such as Shelburne or the radical Whig lord and natural philosopher Charles Stanhope, and with groups and clubs of inquirers, such as the Bowood group or the

20. Burke, *Reflections on the Revolution*, 75, 178, 223, 190. Compare R. W. Kilcup, "Reason and the Basis of Morality in Burke," *Journal of the History of Philosophy* 17 (1979): 271–284.

Lunar Society, were obvious targets for this critique. The anti-Jacobins found it fitting that the Lunar Society has been destroyed by the Birmingham mob for whom Priestley's friends claimed to act as spokesmen. "Peace to such Reasoners! . . . Priestley's a Saint," chortled the *Anti-Jacobin.* The attack upon intellectual associations extended to a critique of the "enlightenment" they sought. This light was derived from the wrong use of the inquiring mind. "We see that it is a natural source of disturbance and revolution," wrote Robison. The paradox that the philosophical societies of virtuous men bred nothing but corruption was matched by the paradox that enlightenment bred disorder. "*Illumination* turns out to be worse than darkness."[21]

BOWOOD AND THE REFORMERS' DREAM

Conservatives tried to make enlightenment look like illumination. They saw the social groupings of the reforming intellectuals as the wrong kind of organization for men of knowledge. They also claimed that the true purposes of the reformers were now revealed. Controversies within the radical camp—as for example Priestley's violent attack on the infidelity of Volney's *Ruines* in 1797—were treated as signs of the incoherence of the Jacobin cause. But philosophers such as Bentham and Priestley had very specific proposals for reform. They presented the work performed since the 1770s as an ideal of the reformers' task. One such ideal was provided by the work in natural and moral philosophy which Priestley pursued with his colleagues at Bowood and elsewhere. The patronage provided by Shelburne for these philosophers was a key resource for their projects. The accounts of this relationship provided by Priestley and Bentham are extremely revealing, because in describing their relationship with their noble master they also described the function which they claimed to discharge. The idealization of this relationship is an important contrast with the harsh realities of late-eighteenth-century patronage and its vicissitudes. There is an interesting tension between the tortuous paths followed by Priestley and Bentham as they sought backing from their potential allies, and the utopian models which they presented of how this support might change society. Hence Bentham's extraordinary presentation of the contrast between himself, "an unseated, unofficed, unconnected, insulated individual," whose "blameless life" had been entirely devoted to the promotion of the Panopticon, and

21. Burke, *Reflections on the Revolution,* 190–192; Robison, *Proofs of a Conspiracy,* 479, 431; Edmonds, *Poetry of the Anti-Jacobin,* 278 (July 1798).

his enemies, such as George III: "Imagine how he hated me. . . . But for all the paupers in the country, as well as all the prisoners in the country, would have been in my hands." This tension demonstrates two important features of intellectual life at this period: First, the role of medical manager, equipped with the knowledge of pneumatic chemistry and the right principles of the philosophy of mind, provided the appropriate model for reform. Second, a complex network of political and theological aims was centered on this search for patronage and provided the reformers with their interests and goals.[22]

Bentham presented his contact with Shelburne in extraordinarily messianic terms. By the end of the 1770s, Shelburne was one of the leaders of a discredited and divided opposition to the American war and to North's Tory administration. Bentham was an impoverished legal writer, author of the important *Fragment on Government* (1776), and at this stage by no means sympathetic to the rebels' cause. His text on the law was a radical critique of the great jurist William Blackstone, whom Bentham had heard lecture on the laws of England at Oxford. Bentham proceeded to the M.A. there in 1767 and spent the intervening years working on his commentaries on Blackstone and on other essays on legal reform, including texts on prison reform and criminal punishment. His friends at Slaughter's Club and the London coffeehouses included chemists and physicians, such as George Fordyce, Jan Ingenhousz, Felice Fontana, and the Austrian F. X. Schwediauer, who were also working closely with Priestley during this period. In spring 1780 Bentham collaborated with Schwediauer on a translation of the *Usefulness of Chemistry* by the great Swedish chemist Torbern Bergman. Yet his principal labors centered on what he baptized his "Code" and his "Punishments," of which the *Fragment* was a highly condensed and preliminary extract. Bentham's remarkable memoir recalled that it was this book which prompted Shelburne to seek him out at Lincoln's Inn. "I felt as men used to feel when Angels used to visit them." In another

22. For Priestley and Volney, see Joseph Priestley, *Observations on the Increase of Infidelity* (Philadelphia, 1797) and Brian Rigby, "Volney's Rationalist Apocalypse," in Barker, *1789*, 22–37. For Bentham's presentation of himself, see Bowring, 5:160–161 and 10:212, discussed in Himmelfarb, "The Haunted House of Jeremy Bentham," 70–71. For problems of patronage, see Michael Foss, *The Age of Patronage: The Arts in England, 1660–1750* (Ithaca, N.Y.: Cornell University Press, 1971), chap. 7; John Brewer, "Commercialization in Politics," in Neil McKendrick et al., *The Birth of a Consumer Society* (London: Hutchinson, 1983), 197–262; W. A. Speck, "Politicians, Peers and Publication by Subscription, 1700–1750," in *Books and Their Readers in Eighteenth-Century England*, ed. Isabel Rivers (New York: St. Martin's, 1982), 47–68; for an excellent example of Shelburne's patronage, see Dorothy Stroud, *Capability Brown* (London: Faber and Faber, 1975), 90–92.

reverie, Bentham used explicitly apocalyptic imagery: "There came out to me a good man named Ld. S. and he said unto me, what shall I do to be saved? I yearn to save the nation. I said unto him—take up my book and follow me. . . . We had not travelled far before we saw a woman named Britannia lying by the waterside all in rags with a sleeping lion at her feet: she looked very pale, and upon inquiring we found she had an issue of blood upon her for many years. She started up fresher farther and more alive than ever; the lion wagged his tail and fawned upon us like a spaniel."[23]

Bentham's dream about Shelburne, though recollected in tranquillity, transfigured the actual relations with patronage and the proposals for reform which he offered in his juridical work. Connection and influence dominated the political strategies of the 1770s. To understand the role which the reformers made for themselves in this jungle of deference and obligation, it is necessary to describe the political programs they espoused and the model they chose for their campaigns. In a public culture that spoke the language of "candour" and abhorred "interest," patronage was always a fraught relationship. Burke seized upon these resources in his anti-Jacobin polemic against the Bowood group in the 1790s, risking the charge of hypocrisy as he did so. In 1771, Priestley was apparently barred from serving with Cook and Banks on a voyage to the South Seas by "Dr. Blackstone and his friends in the Board of longitude," allegedly on the grounds of his heretical theology and animosity against the government lawyers. Priestley wrote sarcastically that the ministry would support "a high churchman or a known atheist, tho' his reputation for philosophy or virtue should stand very low." The sarcasm implied an accurate assessment of the standards of public patronage. For example: Shelburne was struck by Bentham's apparent disinterest when he approached him in 1780, though Bentham was more prosaic: "Ld. S. puts in members," he told his brother. Another possible supporter Bentham tried was the Empress Catherine of Rus-

23. For Bentham's life in the 1770s, see Everett, *Education of Bentham,* 57–70; Mack, *Bentham,* 335–351. For Blackstone at Oxford, see Bowring, 10:45. For connections at Slaughter's, see Bowring, 10:133 and Bentham to John Lind, [?] 12 June 1776, *The Correspondence of Jeremy Bentham,* ed. T. L. S. Sprigge (London: Athlone Press, 1968), 1:328; Bentham to Samuel Bentham, 6 March 1779, ibid. 2:246–247; F. W. Gibbs, *Joseph Priestley* (London: Nelson, 1965), 94–98. For collaboration with Schwediauer, see Bertel Linder and W. A. Smeaton, "Schwediauer, Bentham and Beddoes: Translators of Bergman and Scheele," *Annals of Science* 24 (1968): 259–273. For Bentham's reveries about Shelburne, see Mack, *Bentham,* 370–372; J. H. Burns and H. L. A. Hart, eds., *Comments on the Commentaries and the Fragment on Government* (London: Athlone Press, 1977), 523–526; Norris, *Shelburne and Reform,* 141–143.

sia. Catherine had hired several British experts, including Robison, who worked at Kronstadt as mathematics professor between 1772 and 1774. One function that Bentham made his chemist friends serve was to get better contacts with Russia. He persuaded Schwediauer to translate the introduction to the Code, later to appear as *An Introduction to the Principles of Morals and Legislation.* During early 1779, Schwediauer and Priestley helped Bentham contact Shelburne through a junior treasury lord, and keen mathematician, Francis Maseres. When Bentham's brother went to St. Petersburg in August, Bentham was to pose as an expert political and technical journalist, submitting information to Shelburne for his consideration. But the crucial meeting was necessarily delayed, because Bentham felt that Shelburne should see the Code before they met, and because "my letters I was afraid had gone rather too far on the side of humility." The role play was crucial: Bentham had to present himself as the right kind of expert in order to set up the appropriate relationship with his new master.[24]

Priestley provided Bentham with an avenue—he also made his own vocation through his contacts with Bowood. The relation between Priestley's political strategy in the 1770s and his contacts with Shelburne was particularly important here. Priestley was a leader of the group of "rational dissenters" who sought the emancipation of dissent from legal disabilities. Allies included both Price and Theophilus Lindsey. Rational dissent connected the familiar civic humanist critique of the established institutions of civil and ecclesiastical corruption with a program based on the progressive unmasking of "prejudice" and the establishment of true philosophy through putative matters of fact about matter and spirit. Such matters of fact were best exemplified in the research on pneumatic chemistry which Priestley launched in Leeds just before his departure for Wiltshire. The label "rational dissent" was first coined by Priestley and his colleagues in texts such as their 1769 attack on Blackstone, an inspiration for Bentham's *Commentaries.* Bentham was impressed by the

24. For Burke and patronage, see Albert Goodwin, "The Political Genesis of Edmund Burke's *Reflections on the Revolution in France,*" *Bulletin of the John Rylands Library* 50 (1968): 336–364. For Priestley and the South Seas voyage, see Priestley to William Eden, 4 December and 10 December 1771, Priestley to Joseph Banks, 10 December 1771, in Schofield, *Scientific Autobiography of Priestley,* 95–98; David Mackay, *In the Wake of Cook: Exploration, Science and Empire, 1780–1801* (London: Croom Helm, 1985), 3–27. For Shelburne and Bentham, see Bowring, 10:225; Bentham to Samuel Bentham, 25–26 September 1775, including Priestley to Bentham, 23 August 1775, in *Correspondence of Bentham* 1:265; Bentham to Samuel Bentham, 16 May 1779, ibid. 2:257–258; Shelburne to Bentham, 27 July 1780, ibid. 2:471; Bentham to Samuel Bentham, 6 August 1780, ibid. 2:480.

"well-applied correction" which the rational dissenters had given to Blackstone's "holy zeal" for the established religion. He also judged Blackstone's publications by the standards demanded from "demonstrators" in experimental natural philosophy. Most importantly, the rational dissenters' campaigns provided the immediate context both for Priestley's initial links with the Earl, and for his subsequent formulation of a combined program of philosophical materialism, pneumatic chemistry, and political reform.[25]

Rational dissenters initially sought to speak the language of "candour" in their appeals to established power and their relationships with their patrons. Priestley told Price that "all that candour requires is that we never impute to our adversary a bad intention or a design to mislead, and also that we admit his general good understanding, though liable to be misled by unperceived biases and prejudices from the influence of which the wisest and best of men are not exempt." So this language allowed the rational dissenters to describe the way their political strategy should be structured and the way philosophical debate should be conducted. It provided a contrast with the views of the allies of the ministerial interest. An American Tory, writing in 1783 in the *Gentleman's Magazine,* helped himself to the talk of mind and body to analyze "Lord Shelburne's connection with the Dissenters." He suggested that the dissenters had been "carnalized" by Shelburne, rather than the "Peer spiritualized" by them. "Seeing more fire and spirit in Dr. Priestley's Disquisition on civil liberty," Shelburne had then offered a place at Bowood to the Doctor. In fact, it was to the "wisest and best of men," such as Shelburne, that Priestley and his allies began their appeal from 1769, following the return of John Wilkes at the Middlesex election. Shelburne's support was important in 1772, when the rational dissenters mounted an unsuccessful appeal for the extension of the Toleration Act. The defeat of this so-called Feathers Tavern Petition was immediately interpreted by Priestley and Lindsey in prophetic, if not millenarian, terms, and they used the more eschatological passages in David Hartley's *Observations on Man* to understand their own troubles: "to me everything looks like the approach of that dismal catastrophe described, I may say

25. For rational dissent, see J. G. McEvoy and J. E. McGuire, "God and Nature: Priestley's Way of Rational Dissent," *Historical Studies in Physical Science* 6 (1975): 325–404; Priestley on "those of us who are called Rational Dissenters," in Rutt, 1:349–357; Michael Watts, *The Dissenters from the Reformation to the French Revolution* (Oxford: Oxford University Press, 1978), 464–478. For Bentham on Blackstone, see Jeremy Bentham, *A Fragment on Government* (1776), ed. F. C. Montague (Oxford: Oxford University Press, 1931), 102–103n, 117n.

predicted, by Dr. Hartley in the conclusion of his essay and I shall be looking for the downfall of Church and state together." It was during this crisis that Priestley got his place at Shelburne's house and inaugurated his new set of philosophical and chemical researches.[26]

Priestley's introduction to Shelburne in 1772–1773 won him a salary increased from the £100 he earned as a minister at Leeds to £250 as Shelburne's librarian and traveling companion. It was preceded by anguished debate in London and Leeds. In September 1772, Franklin sent Price and Priestley a "moral and prudential calculus" that encouraged the move to Wiltshire. Franklin, Priestley, and Price were important members of the group of self-styled "Honest Whigs," who moved to the London Coffee House in 1772 and combined natural-philosophical and reformist political interests through this decade. Others included John Pringle, president of the Royal Society and a pneumatic physician who was an enthusiastic admirer of Priestley's chemistry. By 1773, many of Priestley's allies, including Lindsey, had left the established church and joined the rational dissenters at Essex Street Chapel in London, set up as a propaganda center for Shelburne's allies and to foment emancipation. Priestley worked actively for Shelburne's political maneuvers and gained the support of men such as the leading reformist Whig George Savile, a Yorkshire M.P. who was now acting as patron for the great natural philosopher and clergyman John Michell. Michell and Priestley had already collaborated with Savile in Leeds, both on technical projects and on joint research on the active powers of matter, the materiality of the soul, and the properties of light. During 1773–1774, Priestley led the dissenters to abandon the slogan of "candour," which involved support merely for relief from the Test, and encouraged a move to an analysis of humanity, which the whole of established civil philosophy was called in question. Catholic emancipation and support for the American cause became part of their campaigns. A reconstructed account of human nature and the sources of prejudice and opposition to "rational evidence"

26. For "candour," see Joseph Priestley, *A Free Discussion of the Doctrines of Materialism and Philosophical Necessity* (London, 1778), xxx; R. B. Barlow, *Citizenship and Conscience* (Philadelphia: University of Pennsylvania Press, 1962), 171–220. For the Tory attack, see "An Account of the Origin and Dissolution of Ld. Shelburne's Connection with the Dissenters," *Gentleman's Magazine* 53 (January 1783): 22–23. For the theory of civil liberty, see Joseph Priestley, *Essay on the First Principles of Government* (London, 1768), 10; A. H. Lincoln, *Some Political and Social Ideas of English Dissent* (Cambridge: Cambridge University Press, 1938), 160. For Priestley and Lindsey on the defeat of the petition, see Priestley to Lindsey, 23 August 1771, in Rutt, 1:146; Fruchtman, *Apocalyptic Politics of Price and Priestley*, 40.

would allow the dissenters to "cancel the obnoxious name of Christians, and ask for the common rights of humanity."[27]

Thus the conjuncture in which Priestley moved to Bowood provided him with all the resources he needed. His work in natural philosophy with Michell, Price, Franklin, Pringle, and the members of the Bath Philosophical Society, situated near his new home, provided him with important contacts. Shelburne gave him £40 a year for equipment and materials. The campaign of rational dissent provided him with an epistemology and a new and urgent need for a revised analysis of the mind. His targets included the Common Sense philosophers and the apparently irreligious skeptics in France and Scotland. The close links between Bowood and the *philosophes,* together with Priestley's journeys to Paris on Shelburne's business, confirmed his views of the important tasks of the true philosophy. This was a watershed in Priestley's philosophical and religious views. "My own sentiments are very different from what they used to be," he wrote in 1778. He dated his unitarian views in religion from the moment he went to Leeds in 1769, and he dated his "philosophical materialism" to the mid-1770s, first made public in the stream of works on matter theory and religion produced in London and Wiltshire. His productivity was extraordinary: he published a long series of works on pneumatic chemistry, a series of metaphysical texts, of which the *Disquisitions on Matter and Spirit* (1777) was the most important, and a detailed series of polemics, including amicable debates with Richard Price on materialism and determinism. All this work involved a deliberate construction of what Priestley saw as the right role the natural philosopher should serve. Pneumatics, as an account of the activity of matter and the vitality of the airs, and pneumatology, a philosophical account of the mind and the soul, were the principal concerns of this project.[28]

27. On the offer of a place at Bowood, see Franklin to Priestley, 19 September 1772 and to Price, 28 September 1772, in *Correspondence of Price* 1:138–139. For the "Honest Whigs," see V. W. Crane, "The Club of Honest Whigs: Friends of Science and Liberty," *William and Mary Quarterly,* 3d ser., 23(1966): 210–233; for work with Michell and Savile, see Norris, *Shelburne and Reform,* 100; Gibbs, *Joseph Priestley,* 91–93; Priestley to Price, 23 November 1771, in Schofield, *Scientific Autobiography of Priestley,* 93–94. For the "appeal to humanity," see Barlow, *Citizenship and Conscience,* 190, 221–271; Priestley (1773) in Rutt, 23:443–450.

28. For support by Shelburne, see Schofield, *Scientific Autobiography of Priestley,* 139–141, and for work at Bowood see Priestley to Caleb Rotheram, 31 May 1775, ibid., 146; for the change in his philosophy and theology, see Priestley to Caleb Rotheram, April 1778, in Rutt, 1:315; Joseph Priestley, *Letters to Dr Horsley* (Birmingham, 1783), iii–iv. For an analysis of Priestley's finances, see M. P. Crosland, "A Practical Perspective on Joseph

Bentham was well aware of this work: he had already read Priestley's *Essay on the First Principles of Government* (1768); in August 1767 he also received an abstract of the *History of Electricity* from his fellow attorney Richard Clark. In later life he used Priestley's edition of Hartley in his own psychological research, and he praised Priestley's attack on the Scottish philosophers. In January 1774 he began a thorough analysis of the publications on pneumatic chemistry and sent his brother copies of successive versions of the *Experiments and Observations on Different Kinds of Air*. In his "Essence of Priestley," as Bentham called it, he read the full statement of a progressive and historically sensitive account of the course of natural philosophy and the role the natural philosopher should play. The summer after he completed his "Essence," he contacted Priestley directly. The opening of Bentham's *Fragment on Government*, which he published the following year, spelled out Priestley's vision, paraphrasing the opening of the *Experiments and Observations* on pneumatics. It must have impressed Shelburne with its bold indication of the work that natural philosophy could perform:

> The age we live in is a busy age; in which knowledge is rapidly advancing towards perfection. In the natural world, in particular, every thing teems with discovery and with improvement. The most distant and recondite regions of the earth traversed and explored—the all-vivifying and subtle element of the air so recently analyzed and made known to us—are striking evidences, were all others wanting, of this pleasing truth.[29]

Just as in the case of his relationship with Shelburne, so here too Bentham provided a dreamlike account of his first encounter with Priestley's work. Much later in his life, it was important for Bentham to display his debt to the utilitarianism of rational dissent and to play down

Priestley as a Natural Philosopher," *British Journal for the History of Science* 16 (1983): 223–237.

29. Bentham, *Fragment on Government*, 93; for the use of Hartley, see Bentham, *Introduction to the Principles of Morals and Legislation*, 124n; for the praise of Priestley's attack on the Common Sense philosophy, see Alan Sell, "Priestley's Polemic against Reid," *Price-Priestley Newsletter* 3 (1979): 41–52; Bhikhu Parekh, ed., *Bentham's Political Thought* (London: Croom Helm, 1973), 152n: "Another says he has a sense . . . that pronounces what is right and wrong. This is the way that . . . the triumvirate of doctors lately slaughtered, not to say butchered, by Dr Priestly [sic] make laws of nature" (1776). For Priestley's attack on Hume, see Rutt, 4:398 and Richard H. Popkin, "Joseph Priestley's Criticisms of David Hume's Philosophy," *Journal of the History of Philosophy* 15 (1977): 437–447. For Bentham and Priestley's pneumatics, see Bentham to Richard Clark, 5 August 1767, *Correspondence of Bentham* 1:119; Bentham to Samuel Bentham, 28 January 1774, July 1775, 20 July 1774, ibid. 1:176, 186, 189; Bentham to Priestley, 1774, ibid. 1:208.

the marked division between his own views of the rights of humanity and those preached at Essex Street. Bentham recalled reading Priestley's remarkable *Essay on the First Principles of Government* in a coffeehouse in Oxford in 1768. There he read the sentiment that the "great standard" of civil society was "the good and happiness . . . of the majority of the members of any state." "At the sight of it he cried out, as it were in an inward ecstasy like Archimedes on the discovery of the fundamental principles of Hydrostatics, *Eureka*."[30] Despite Bentham's claim that he "purloined" the happiness principle from this book, he was also able to assemble a lengthy litany of key figures for his conception of the doctrines of utilitarianism. He told d'Alembert in spring 1778 that it was Helvetius who had provided him with the important hint. Debates on influence here are inevitably sterile and obviously reflect Bentham's capacity for the ingenious reconstruction of his own vocation. In the *Fragment* Bentham wrote of the English edition of Beccaria's work on penology, *On Crimes and Punishments*, which contained the phrase "the greatest happiness of the greatest number." He used just the terms he would later use to describe Shelburne. Bentham claimed that Beccaria was "received by the intelligent as an Angel from heaven would be by the faithful." Links with the *philosophes* were crucial for Bentham's development, and they were energetically pursued via Romilly and Mirabeau when he reached Bowood in the 1780s.[31] The "fundamental principles" which Bentham gained from Priestley involved a path to political power and a role model for the reformer, that of the pneumatic chemist and devotee of moral progress through technical change. Bentham shared Priestley's views on the character of the corrupt enemy and the false philosophy they peddled. In his draft preface for the Bergman translation, Bentham recalled his own Oxford career as a picture of the wrong kind of natural philosophy. Even though he heard mechanics lectures from Nathaniel Bliss, "I learnt nothing of the air I breathed in, except that the mischief it was apt to do was owing to the spitefulness

30. For Bentham's story about reading Priestley's *Essay*, see draft of 1829, Bentham MSS, University College London, 13.360, printed in Amnon Goldworth, ed., *Deontology, Together with A Table of the Springs of Action and the Article on Utilitarianism* (Oxford: Clarendon Press, 1983), 291–292, compared with Bentham, *Fragment on Government*, 34. For a very useful criticism of this story, see Margaret Canovan, "The un-Benthamite Utilitarianism of Joseph Priestley," *Journal of the History of Ideas* 45 (1984): 435–450.

31. Bentham to d'Alembert, spring 1778, *Correspondence of Bentham* 2:117; Bentham, *Fragment on Government*, 105n; Goldworth, *Deontology*, 52, citing Bentham MSS, University College Library, 158. See Harrison, *Bentham*, 113–117; Mack, *Bentham*, 105–110, 417–420; C. Blount, "Bentham, Dumont and Mirabeau," *University of Birmingham Historical Journal* 3 (1952): 153–167; Jarrett, *Begetters of Revolution*, 130–132.

of a god who when he was in an ill humour used to get a parcel of overgrown schoolboys to blow it in people's faces." He claimed that the Oxford professors held that chemistry was a science "fit only to make a man an atheist or an apothecary." The proper chemistry was precisely directed at reform of learning and cure of aerial disease. Thomas Beddoes, chemistry lecturer at Oxford from 1787 until his departure under a political cloud in 1793, argued famously that "nothing would so much contribute to the rescue of the art of medicine from its present helpless condition as the discovery of the means of regulating the atmosphere." Beddoes built this medical meteorology into his attack on the Pitt administration. So did his ally Joseph Priestley: hence, for example, his image of the pathology of the established universities. Priestley told Pitt in 1787 that they "resemble pools of stagnant water secured by dams and mounds, and offensive to the neighbourhood." Pneumatics and discovery were the key items in the collective strategy. The projector and the experimenter were the ideal types of the interests for which rational dissenters and utilitarians spoke.[32]

Bentham's contacts with Priestley, and then with Shelburne, were dominated by these new interests. Priestley had an explicit account of how experimenters should work together. In a preface to one of the volumes Bentham abstracted in spring 1774, Priestley explained that "this rapid progress of knowledge" would mark "an end to all undue and usurped authority in the business of religion as well as science." This gave a political role to the projector and the discoverer. In 1791 Priestley answered Burke with the claim that commerce and true philosophy would help to inaugurate "the social millennium."[33] Bentham worked strenuously as just such a projector of schemes in the arts and philosophy in the 1770s. He plotted an approach to the Longitude Board with whom Priestley had had such strife, suggested an improved chronometric design, investigated the rewards for discovery, and prop-

32. For Bentham on his Oxford studies, see Linder and Smeaton, "Schwediauer, Bentham and Beddoes," 268–270, printing Bentham MSS, University College London, 156.5–7; Bentham to Jeremiah Bentham, 10 March 1762, 15 March 1763, 4 April 1763, *Correspondence of Bentham* 1:60, 67, 70. For Beddoes, see Thomas Beddoes, *Observations on the Nature and Cure of Calculus, Sea Scurvy, Catarrh and Fever* (Oxford, 1792), cited in Stansfield, *Beddoes,* 147–149; Trevor H. Levere, "Dr Thomas Beddoes at Oxford: Radical Politics in 1788–1793 and the Fate of the Regius Chair in Chemistry," *Ambix* 28 (1981): 61–69. For Priestley on the universities, see Rutt, 19:128 (1787).

33. Joseph Priestley, *Experiments and Observations on Different Kinds of Air* (London, 1774), xiv; *Letters to the Right Honourable Edmund Burke* (Birmingham, 1791), 239–243. See Arnold Thackray, "Natural Knowledge in Cultural Context: The Manchester Model," *American Historical Review* 79 (1974): 672–709.

osed projects for a refrigerator to be used in times of glut, a canal through Nicaragua, and state-sponsored expeditions to the southern ocean to follow those of Cook and Banks. In 1787 Bentham took Adam Smith to task for his criticism of the projecting spirit. The Panopticon was merely the most spectacular of these schemes, energetically touted in Russia from 1785 and published in 1791. The famous manifesto which Bentham prefaced to his scheme precisely captured his account of the function of the reforming projector and the knowledge which the future guardians of the moral order would command: "morals reformed—health preserved—industry invigorated—instruction diffused—public burthens lightened—economy seated as it were upon a rock."[34]

Such knowledge depended on a revised account both of morality and of pneumatics. Bentham learned his pneumatics from Priestley, and so learned much of the rules of the experimental life. He addressed Priestley as "the Adopted father" of his chosen sciences. By the end of 1774, Bentham had sent Priestley a long essay on an improved method of making and collecting different airs, together with some important comments on chemical nomenclature. Priestley replied courteously the following month: "if you were to go to work in good earnest you would do something considerable." Many of their subsequent exchanges related to the details of chemical practice. Bentham told Priestley of new techniques for testing the virtue of air, and invented a machine, called the "Athanor," for improving Priestley's standard tests for measuring this virtue. These were highly prized techniques of pneumatic chemistry, shared, too, with other chemists such as Fontana, Schwediauer and Ingenhousz. In the following section, it will be argued that these pneumatic techniques were practical examples of what was proposed as a more general technique of medical meteorology, in which an understanding of health and disease in the atmosphere could be developed into a model of the moral economy. That analysis provides a basis, in the final sections of the paper, for the interpretation of the moral philosophy and philosophy of mind which licensed Bentham's more remarkable claims for the basis of his new science: "the science of jurisprudence," he claimed, was "as strictly and properly a science of experiment

34. For Bentham's projects, see Mack, *Bentham,* 137; "Defence of Usury" (1787), in *Jeremy Bentham's Economic Writings,* ed. W. Stark, 2 vols. (London: Royal Economic Society, 1952), 1:167–187; on the Panopticon, see Bowring, 4:39. For the Panopticon as a project, see L. J. Hume, "Bentham's Panopticon: An Administrative History," *Historical Studies* 15 (1973): 703–721 and 16 (1974): 36–54.

as any branch of natural philosophy." But this meant the natural philosophy pursued at Bowood in the 1770s.[35]

FROM PNEUMATICS TO PNEUMATOLOGY

I have argued for the importance of the relationship between Priestley's pneumatic chemistry and Bentham's legal reform. This relationship provided a knowledge which reformers could use; a description of their social function; and an account of the strategies by which reform could be achieved. This knowledge included the understanding of matter and its powers developed in the laboratories of the pneumatic chemists. Such understanding involved a new practice of rather specific policy recommendations for the better management of the social economy and the human body. The atmosphere was taken to be a major site at which principles of health and disease were produced. Under Priestley's aegis, this practice was also used to revise the picture of body. The distinction between mind and body was erased, by changing the definition of the attributes of matter. Since the mind now became just as accessible to material analysis, it also became just as accessible to management. So medical managers, using their knowledge of medical meteorology, could also be moral managers, using their knowledge of the powers of the mind. When medical management turned its attention to the discipline of minds, it produced a new story about the way interests and passions should be governed for the cause of social welfare. A revised account of pneumatology was therefore a necessary companion of the science of pneumatics. Priestley's pneumatics and Bentham's panopticism were both versions of this model of mind and body. As Foucault suggested, Bentham's Panopticon was an exercise in the economy of powers, "a marvellous machine" where the effects of power could be deployed in the setting of a laboratory: "it could be used as a machine to carry out experiments on men." Bentham explicitly considered the claim that the Panopticon made "machines under the similitude of men." It became an experimental machine for experiments upon machines. "O chemists!" Bentham exclaimed, "much have your crucibles shown us of dead matter—but our industry-house is a crucible for men!" If the Panopticon

35. Bentham to Priestley, November [?] 1774, and Priestley to Bentham, 16 December 1774, *Correspondence of Bentham* 1:209, 210–216, 225–226. For work on eudiometry, see Bentham to Samuel Bentham, 9 November 1779 and December 1779, ibid. 2:314–315, 344. For Bentham on jurisprudence as a science of experiment, see Harrison, *Bentham*, 133, citing Bentham MSS, University College London, 70A.22.

was an exercise in political anatomy and the mechanics of power, then Priestley's technology of airs provided a similar repertoire of strategies for the investigation of powers under a regime of observation, classification, and experiment. His pneumatics investigated those powers on which life depended, and modeled an economy in which these powers were distributed. The move from pneumatics to pneumatology was the key tactic in these philosophies of mind and body.[36]

The preface to Bentham's *Fragment* provides evidence of his use of Priestley's pneumatics as the mark of progress. In 1767 Priestley contrasted three forms of historiography. The first was "civil history," which had the appeal of human interest but showed the horrors of human depravity: "a man . . . cannot help being shocked with a view of the vices and miseries of mankind." The second was "natural history," which displayed wise natural order but lacked concern with "human sentiments," a necessary condition for the association of mind. Priestley argued that the history of natural philosophy was the best way of capturing human interests, through the processes of association, for the cause of progress: no history "can exhibit instances of so fine a rise and improvement in things, as we see in the progress of the human mind in philosophical investigations." Hartley's principles worked to good effect here: in Priestley's histories of electricity, optics, and pneumatics, the sympathetic reader could recapitulate the course of actual experimental advance. This was a way of showing what was wrong with Blackstone. Bentham identified the Oxford lawyer as an enemy of progress because he stood opposed to the true principles learned from the history of natural philosophy. "Correspondent to *discovery* and *improvement* in the natural world, is *reformation* in the moral." Blackstone resisted such a reformation. Yet the successes of the pneumatic chemists could and should be extended to the moral realm:

> If it be of importance and of use to us to know the principles of the element we breathe, surely it is not of much less importance nor of much less use to comprehend the principles, and endeavour at the improvement of those *laws*, by which alone we breathe it in security.[37]

The axiom of utility, the analogy between natural improvement and moral reformation, and the aim of the "security" of respiration were all

36. Foucault, *Discipline and Punish*, 202–203; Bowring, 4:63–64.

37. Joseph Priestley, *History and Present State of Electricity*, 3d ed. (London, 1775), ii-iv; Bentham, *Fragment on Government*, 93–94. For Priestley's historiography, see J. G. McEvoy, "Electricity, Knowledge and the Nature of Progress in Priestley's Thought," *British Journal for the History of Science* 12 (1979): 1–30; J. J. Hoecker, "Joseph Priestley as an Historian and the Idea of Progress," *Price-Priestley Newsletter* 3 (1979): 29–40.

aspects of the meteorological program which both Bentham and Priestley pursued. In the 1770s Priestley and his colleagues aimed to show how a benevolent aerial economy functioned and to mark the processes that governed this economy. Human beings were an integral part of this system, and their welfare was a consequence of its actions. Priestley's isolation of nitrous air in 1772 and dephlogisticated air in 1775 was part of this strategy. He described a series of processes that vitiated common air, by phlogisticating it. Such processes included "the amazing consumption of air by fires of all kinds, volcanos, &c." together with respiration and putrefaction. The air left above calces or remaining after animal respiration was revealed to be highly phlogisticated by a test comparison with nitrous air. "It is not peculiar to nitrous air to be a test of the fitness of the air for respiration. Any other process by which air is diminished and made noxious answers to the same purpose but the application of them is not so easy or elegant and the effect is not so soon perceived. In fact, it is *phlogiston* that is the test." Bad air supported neither respiration nor combustion and did not diminish in volume when shaken with nitrous air. This gave the test its key place in his pneumatics. Because Priestley applied an axiom of benevolence, he argued that the aerial economy must act to preserve the virtue of airs. So there must be processes that restored vitiated air and rendered it virtuous and respirable. "It becomes a great object of philosophical inquiry, to ascertain what change is made in the constitution of the air by flame, and to discover what provision there is in nature for remedying the injury which the atmosphere receives by this means." Evidence of restorative processes was produced in the long series of pneumatic trials Priestley made at Bowood between 1774 and 1779 using the "noble apparatus" Shelburne provided him. These processes included atmospheric purification by shaking over water and the beneficient action of green vegetable matter on air under the influence of light. Thus his isolation of dephlogisticated air and his production of evidence for photosynthesis were easily fitted into the scheme of a well-judged economy that balanced vitiation with restoration.[38]

38. Joseph Priestley, "Observations on Different Kinds of Air," *Philosophical Transactions* 62 (1772): 147–252 at 162; *Experiments and Observations on Different Kinds of Air and Other Branches of Natural Philosophy,* 3 vols. (Birmingham, 1790), 1:359. For Priestley's account of the restoration of the atmosphere, see Priestley, *Experiments and Observations on Different Kinds of Air,* 2d ed. (London, 1776), 2:91–103; J. G. McEvoy, "Joseph Priestley, Aerial Philosopher: Metaphysics and Methodology in Priestley's Chemical Thought, 1772–1781," *Ambix* 25 (1978): 1–55, 93–116, 153–175, and 26 (1979): 16–38, at 25:96–101, 158–164. For the importance of the nitrous air test, see A. J. Ihde, "Priestley and Lavoisier," in *Joseph Priestley: Scientist, Theologian and Metaphysician,* ed. L. Kieft and B. R. Willeford

These researches were closely linked with human welfare through the scheme of medical meteorology—restoration of respirable air and its variation in quality governed the physiological fate of the human and the social frame. The standard of the atmosphere was a mark of its fitness for human existence. This had initially suggested to Priestley that while atmospheric air was no doubt a compound of variously virtuous sections, nevertheless it must now be the best possible air for human respiration. "I had no idea of procuring air purer than the best common air." Yet his work of 1774–1775 did yield such an air, dephlogisticated air. It was only after eighteen months that Priestley managed to position his new "luxury" air as the ultimate in his scale of virtue, and thereby developed a set of techniques which the medical meteorologists, such as Ingenhousz and Fontana, soon baptized "eudiometry," a strategy for matching the virtues of airs to their physiological benevolence. Priestley planned a collection of airs from different sites. In 1777 he asked his friend, the Birmingham manufacturer Matthew Boulton, for "air as it is actually breathed by the different manufacturers in this kingdom." He also sampled the air left in rooms at Shelburne's house after gatherings there. "Eudiometric tours" were common. Beddoes and Price also worked on the "insalubrity" of varying airs. Fontana and his colleagues in Tuscany and Milan used eudiometry for hospital reform and proposed marsh drainage to remove the evils of "bad air." Ingenhousz was an early advocate of seaside holidays for consumptives, identifying ocean air as peculiarly virtuous for the human frame. Priestley himself wrote that the new "pure air" might be "peculiarly salutary to the lungs in certain morbid cases," and that "pure dephlogisticated air might be very useful as a medicine," even if too powerful in common measure: "a moralist may say that the air which nature has provided for us is as good as we deserve."[39]

(Lewisburg, Pa.: Bucknell University Press, 1980), 62–91; for the "aerial economy," see H. Laboucheix, "Chemistry, Materialism and Theology in the Work of Joseph Priestley," *Price-Priestley Newsletter* 1 (1977): 31–48.

39. Priestley, *Experiments and Observations on Different Kinds of Air,* 2d ed. (London, 1776), 2:40–49, 100–103; Priestley to Matthew Boulton, [?] 1777, in Schofield, *Scientific Autobiography of Priestley,* 161–162; on eudiometry, see ibid., 164–166, 174–175, and Joseph Priestley (with Richard Price), "On the Noxious Quality of the Effluvia of Putrid Marshes," *Philosophical Transactions* 64 (1774): 90–98; Felice Fontana, "Of the Airs Extracted from Different Kinds of Waters," *Philosophical Transactions* 69 (1779): 432–453; Jan Ingenhousz, "Observations sur la construction et l'usage de l'eudiomètre de M. Fontana," *Journal de physique* 26 (1785): 339–359; and P. Knoefel, "Famine and Fever in Tuscany: Eighteenth-Century Italian Concern with the Environment," *Physis* 21 (1979): 7–35 at 20–35; H. Reed, "Jan Ingenhousz: Plant Physiologist," *Chronica Botanica* 11 (1949): 285–396.

Bentham began work on eudiometry when he contacted Priestley in 1774–1775. He told Priestley that "in using nitrous air as a test of the comparative purity of the atmosphere in different places, it is of importance to be certain of its being utterly free from all previous admixture with Common air." To use such a test in this way was to declare allegiance to the principles of pneumatics. Throughout the 1770s Bentham was concerned with the development of this program: his "Athanor" was one contribution to it, anticipating eudiometers made by Cavendish and Fontana in the 1780s. He talked to Fontana about publications on the improvement of the virtue of airs and better ways of making artificial airs. He also became involved in Priestley's disputes with chemists such as Scheele, who denied that vegetation purified airs.[40] Natural philosophical understanding of the atmospheric powers was to become ever more closely linked with civil policy. John Pringle was a typical practitioner in this field. His treatises in the 1750s on hospital and jail fevers based themselves on the pneumatics of restored and corrupted airs. As Christopher Lawrence has suggested, Pringle and his reformist colleagues, including Priestley, were instrumental in the construction of a specifically aerial analysis of epidemic fevers, locating their aetiology in noxious components of the atmosphere detectable by pneumatic chemistry. Priestley defended Pringle's doctrine against Scottish critics in 1773, while successive volumes of *Experiments and Observations on Air* during the 1770s carried testimonies by physicians on the medicinal uses of airs and the aerial causation of fever. When Pringle presented Priestley with the Royal Society's Copley Medal in 1773, he placed Priestley's pneumatics in the context of the aerial system of fevers, and also linked it with the model of a benevolent economy which Priestley had begun to map: "from these discoveries, we are assured that . . . every individual plant is serviceable to mankind, if not always distinguished by some private virtue, yet making a part of the whole which cleanses and purifies our atmosphere." Storms and tempests would shake "the waters and the air together to bury in the deep those putrid and pestilential effluvia which the vegetables upon the face of the Earth have been insufficient to consume."[41] The pneumatic system pro-

40. Bentham to Priestley, November [?] 1774, and Priestley to Bentham, 16 December 1774, *Correspondence of Bentham* 1:210–216, 225–226. For work on eudiometry, see Bentham to Samuel Bentham, 9 November 1779 and December 1779, ibid. 2:314–315, 344. For Priestley's dispute with Scheele, see Priestley to Kirwan, August 1780, in Schofield, *Scientific Autobiography of Priestley,* 182–186.

41. For Pringle's work on pneumatic medicine, see D. W. Singer, "Sir John Pringle and His Circle," *Annals of Science* 6 (1948–1950): 127–180, 229–261 at 150–153 and 229–247 for work with Priestley; for the Copley address of 1773, see the reprint in Douglas

posed by Priestley and Pringle gave an account of the circulation of virtuous power in the world. It was deeply influential on the work of radical physicians in the 1790s, including both Darwin and Beddoes. It also provided an image of the perfectly managed economy in human society, where medical administration and civil hygiene, the "burial of pestilential effluvia," were equally important.[42]

Hygiene became a key principle of Bentham's vision of civil order. In his mature survey of that order, the *Constitutional Code,* the "Health Minister" was to discharge a range of eudiometric functions. What he called the "exemplificational-antimalarial function" involved the control of dangerous exhalations; other roles included registration of changes in the air and its relation to health. These were, perhaps, Hippocratic commonplaces: their management and the knowledge that sustained them were not. The utilitarian state was to be compared with the strategy of medical police fostered by the German cameralists. Where authorities such as Justi, Sonnenfels, and Frank argued during the period 1750–1780 for a centralized state bureaucracy invigilating over social and moral conduct in order to control welfare and population growth, Priestley and Bentham proffered an account of philosophical necessity and reasoned self-interest in civil society; the role of the state was as guarantor of that society, not as its despot. The progress of society was safely left in the hands of expert philosophers and medical managers whose legitimacy was derived from their understanding of the natural powers, not from their subservience to the civil powers.[43] Pneumatics

McKie, "Joseph Priestley and the Copley Medal," *Ambix* 9 (1961): 1–22. For Priestley's medical interests, see Christopher Lawrence, "Priestley in Tahiti: The Medical Interests of a Dissenting Chemist," in *Science, Medicine and Dissent: Joseph Priestley,* ed. R. G. W. Anderson and C. Lawrence (London: Wellcome Trust, 1987), 1–10; for Priestley's defense of Pringle, see Priestley, "On the Noxious Quality of the Effluvia of Putrid Marshes," 91; compare Priestley, *Experiments and Observations on Different Kinds of Air,* 2d ed. (London, 1775), vol. 1, appendix, 288–324.

42. For pneumatic medicine in the 1790s, see Stansfield, *Beddoes,* chap. 7; Ludmilla Jordanova, "Earth Science and Environmental Medicine: The Synthesis of the Late Enlightenment," in *Images of the Earth,* ed. L. J. Jordanova and Roy Porter (Chalfont St. Giles: British Society for the History of Science, 1978), 119–146. For Beddoes, see Thomas Beddoes and James Watt, *Considerations on the Medicinal Use of Factitious Airs* (Bristol, 1794), vol. 1; for Darwin, see Erasmus Darwin, *Temple of Nature,* 21n and *Zoonomia; or, The Laws of Organic Life* (London, 1796), 1:115.

43. For the work of the Health Minister, see Bowring, 9:439–445. For medical police and cameralism, see George Rosen, *From Medical Police to Social Medicine: Essays on the History of Health Care* (New York: Science History Publications, 1974), 120–141, 189–190; Michel Foucault, "The Politics of Health in the Eighteenth Century," in Gordon, *Power-Knowledge,* 166–182; Marc Raeff, *The Well-ordered Police State: Social and Institutional Change*

was an important example of this understanding. The Benthamite reforms of the 1830s testify eloquently to this fact. Edwin Chadwick was Bentham's amanuensis at the time when his master was composing the *Constitutional Code*. Chadwick's great 1842 *Report on the Sanitary Condition of the Labouring Population* was a homage to the connections between management and medical meteorology which Bentham had discussed: "bad ventilation or overcrowding, and the consequences on the moral habits" were demonstrably based on "an original cause we have high scientific authority for stating to be easily and economically controllable." As Roger Cooter has suggested, Bentham's loyal disciples among reforming physicians made the atmosphere the key site of medical management: Cooter cites the work of Southwood Smith, a convert from Calvinism to Priestley's unitarianism and the personal physician to Bentham. Southwood Smith's anticontagionism refused to speak of disease-causing miasmas and refused to define the aerial principle that might be pathogenic. In his *Treatise on Fever* (1830), he argued that disease was spread via air because "poverty in her hut . . . striving with all her might to keep out the pure air and to increase the heat, imitates Nature but too successfully." As a result, "penury and ignorance can create a mortal plague." Cooter argues that at the hands of the Benthamite anticontagionists, the air became the proper concern of expert managers and the way to moralize society. The human and the social body were engrossed by pneumatics.[44]

Bentham's campaign was to go further: the legislator could wisely extend the accomplishments of the medical manager. In the 1770s he argued that "the art of legislation is but the art of healing practised upon a large scale. It is the common endeavour of both to relieve men from

through Law in the Germanies and Russia, 1600–1800 (New Haven: Yale University Press, 1983), 119–135. For Bentham and medical reform, see Benjamin Spector, "Jeremy Bentham: His Influence upon Medical Thought and Legislation," *Bulletin of the History of Medicine* 37 (1963): 25–42.

44. Edwin Chadwick, *Report on the Sanitary Condition of the Labouring Population of Great Britain* (1842), ed. M. W. Flinn (Edinburgh: Edinburgh University Press, 1965), 29–43, 167; Thomas Southwood Smith, *Treatise on Fever* (London, 1830), 324; Roger Cooter, "Anticontagionism: History's Medical Record," in *The Problem of Medical Knowledge: Examining the Social Construction of Medicine*, ed. P. Wright and A. Treacher (Edinburgh: Edinburgh University Press, 1982), 87–108. Compare Southwood Smith, *Treatise*, 349: "Vegetable and animal matter, during the process of putrefaction, give off a principle or give origin to a new compound, which, when applied to the human body, produces the phenomena constituting fever." For Southwood Smith's career, see Mrs. C. L. Lewes, *Dr. Southwood Smith: A Retrospect* (Edinburgh: Blackwood, 1898); F. N. L. Poynter, "Thomas Southwood Smith—the Man," *Proceedings of the Royal Society of Medicine* 55 (1962): 381–392.

the miseries of life. But the physician relieves them one by one: the legislator by millions at a time." This was just the sense of Southwood Smith's parliamentary evidence in 1840: the Government must relieve the poor of "the sources of poison and disease," for otherwise "the effect is the same as if twenty or thirty thousand of them were annually taken out of their wretched homes and put to death." The accumulation of numbers and the collective origin of social pathology were essential principles of reformist medical management. Bentham insisted that "this is not a fanciful analogy": it was to be taken as a literal account of the managers' work.[45] Once again, the comparison of the body politic and the body natural was banal, but by using a specific account of how medical management worked, Bentham gave his political reform a peculiar slant. The attention to detail and the production of "docile bodies" were characteristics of this anatomical strategy. The "Code" and the "Punishments" were respectively described by Bentham as the "principles" and the "materia medica" of his political therapeutics. But, most importantly, the references to medical management pointed to the significance of a science of mind, a pneumatology. The reformer stood in urgent need of a science that would locate the "springs of action." This was the principle of utility. Bentham called it a "moral thermometer" in the hands of the expert jurist and natural philosopher. In his texts on *Legislation,* first drafted in the late 1770s, Bentham argued, with Priestley, that the progress of philosophy was opposed by prejudices, which enlightened understanding of the springs of mental and physical action would remove. The name for the branch of philosophy that investigated and extirpated such obstacles was "mental pathology." "By *pathology,* I mean the study and the knowledge of the sensations, affections, passions, and of their effects upon happiness." Thus it was a founding axiom of Bentham's reform that the link between aerial physiology, natural philosophy, and materialist epistemology be made more than a figure of speech: "Medicine, commonly so called . . . has for its basis the observations of the axioms of pathology, commonly so-called. Morals is the medicine of the soul. The science of legislation is the practical part of this medicine." Hence, "mental pathology" should provide the axioms for the science of legislation: "God forbid that any disease in the constitution of a state should be without its remedy."[46]

45. Mack, *Bentham,* 264, citing Bentham MSS, University College London, 27.13; Lewes, *Southwood Smith,* 104.

46. For "docile bodies," see Foucault, *Discipline and Punish,* 135–141. For Bentham on the medical comparison, see Bowring, 1:304–305, 367 and 2:204; Harrison, *Bentham,* 141, citing Bentham MSS, University College London, 32.6; Mack, *Bentham,* 264–266. For

Mental pathology was a foundation of reform. Bentham's successive drafts for his *Table of the Springs of Action* examined the relationship between this psychology, the philosophy of mind, and the reformer's work. This "Table" was supposed to be the analogue of an "anatomical table," which showed "the seats of physical enjoyment and sufferance and the source of physical action." Bentham proposed the same for psychology. Equipped with such a table and the utility calculus, the wise expert would show that certain actions were in citizens' interests, and the legislator would make these actions depend on these interests. In a manuscript of the 1770s, Bentham figured this relationship in heavenly terms:

> Between us two might the philosopher and the lawyer say, there is a great gulph. I have endeavoured to throw a bridge over this gulph: so that on it, as on Jacob's Ladder, if not Angels, man, however, may continually henceforth be seen ascending and descending. . . . Should I be found so happy as to succeed in bringing these celestial artizans into a more close acquaintance, what a rich and serviceable manufacture may not be hoped for from their united labours.[47]

The *Introduction to the Principles of Morals and Legislation,* completed by 1780, was Bentham's first sustained analysis of the link between these powers and his juridical and political plans. The study of mental pathology identified the sources of pleasure and pain, sensibility and will. So this reconstruction of pneumatology indicated two functions for the study of mind: understanding and control. Such an inquiry would provide a knowledge of mental powers which the reformer needed. For Bentham, "intellectual powers" were always compared to the appropriate "physical powers," and this was an identity guaranteed by the medical function of the philosophical reformer. The "science of *law*" was merely a branch of the superior "*logic* of the will." It would also locate the sources of resistance to reform derived from corruption and interest. The interests that opposed reform were just as susceptible to analysis and management as those on which reform depended.[48]

"mental pathology," see Bentham, *Introduction to the Principles of Morals and Legislation,* vii; for the cure of disease in the state, see Bentham, *Fragment on Government,* 224.

47. Bentham, *A Table of the Springs of Action,* in Goldworth, *Deontology,* 71; Mack, *Bentham,* 130, citing Bentham MSS, University College London, 27; Harrison, *Bentham,* 270–271. For a discussion of the *Table,* see Paul McReynolds, "The Motivational Psychology of Jeremy Bentham, part 1," *Journal of the History of the Behavioural Sciences* 4 (1968): 230–244.

48. For the "logic of the will," see *Introduction to the Principles of Morals and Legislation,* xiii. Compare Parekh, *Bentham's Political Thought,* 146–156, which prints Bentham MSS, University College London, 69.70–75.

The doctrine of association, developed in Hartley and edited by Priestley, satisfied these demands. The mind was materialized since matter could think. Mental principles could be translated, or, as Bentham put it, "paraphrased" as their physical correlates. Speech about the pernicious "fictions" in which the law dealt must be turned into talk of material entities. Punishments must be spelled out in physical terms, just as pain and pleasure must be read as corporeal principles. Because it used fictions, the existing condition of the legal establishment was marked by all the evils of the condition of natural philosophy before the recent advances of the pneumatic chemists. Common law was a "fictitious composition which has no known person for its author, no known assemblage of words for its substance . . . like that fancied aether, which, in default of sensible matter, fills up the measure of the universe."[49] Bentham's assault on this form of legal fiction was part of a strategy that modeled itself on the reforms of pneumatic chemists and in particular on the language they used. In 1774, as we have shown, he began corresponding with Priestley on the proper nomenclature to be used in medical and chemical philosophy. "Much more I could offer you on the same subject . . . other articles on Nomenclature." Bentham condemned Scheele for his "metaphysical" inquiry as to whether "fire be a real or fictitious entity." At the same period, he identified the close connection between the forms of chemical nomenclature and the flourishing of corrupt fantasy. "In speaking of an *pneumatic* (or say *immaterial* or *spiritual*) object, no name has ever been employed, that had not first been employed as the name of some *material* (or say *corporeal*) one. Lamentable have been the confusion and darkness produced by taking the names of *fictions* for the names of *real* entities." Priestley agreed: his pneumatics showed the proper understanding of spirits and the disasters visited upon true philosophy by assuming that material entities were really immaterial substances. Utilitarianism expelled fictions from legal discourse: pneumatic chemistry expelled them from philosophy. This great expulsion was accompanied by a revision of the principle that individuated human subjects. The belief in an immortal soul was simply the understandable consequence of the wrong state of mind: "a human soul would be a *ghost*," according to Bentham, if it were separable and

49. For Bentham on "paraphrasis" and fictions, see *Introduction to the Principles of Morals and Legislation*, xiii; for an analysis of these techniques, see Ogden, *Bentham's Theory of Fictions*, cxiii-cxxi, on Bowring, 3:177, 241; Harrison, *Bentham*, 53–74. For Bentham's comments on the connection between the disease of fiction and the immaterial principles of mind, see Bowring, 8:174; Parekh, *Bentham's Political Thought*, 48; Ogden, *Bentham's Theory of Fictions*, 18.

immaterial. "At this time of day, *custom* scarcely does, *fashion* certainly does not, command us to believe in ghosts."[50]

GHOSTS AND MACHINES

The reformers' strategies were built on the principles learned in pneumatics and mental pathology. Their roles aped those of medical managers and expert naturalists. As we have seen, this made them a vulnerable target for anti-Jacobins in the 1790s. It was alleged that the friends of the Revolution had the wrong state of mind, because they abandoned the established moral sanctions for a rationalized account of the right structure of society and of human nature. Brissot offered Priestley and Bentham seats in the National Convention: Burke said that Brissot's sanguinary addresses to the nation would allow the English "to judge of the information of those who have undertaken to guide and enlighten us."[51] Guidance and enlightenment looked occult and enthusiast because when the reformers condemned orthodox religious pneumatology as a tissue of fictions, they had nothing better than a heretical ghost story with which to replace it. This story, exemplified in schemes for social machines such as the Panopticon, seemed to destroy conventional moral sanctions and install tyranny in their place. Bentham answered possible criticisms of his "inspection house": was it advisable "to give such herculean and ineludible strength to the gripe of power?" Yes, for this was a power that could manage the mind and guarantee its happiness. What authority could this new machinery of mental powers command? Priestley's answer helped itself to the combination of pneumatics and philosophy developed in the 1770s. The theology he proposed from the 1770s was supposed to satisfy the demands of reform. Anglican and Calvinist priestcraft was challenged quite directly with the rational principles of unitarianism, a denial of the immortal soul, an empirical psychology, and the claims of reformist managers to discharge functions hitherto the proper preserve of the pulpit and the

50. For Bentham on nomenclature see Bentham to Priestley, 1774, *Correspondence of Bentham* 1:214, 216; for Scheele, see Bentham to Samuel Bentham, 9 November 1779, *Correspondence of Bentham* 2:315; for pneumatic objects, see Bowring, 8:119–120; for souls and ghosts, ibid., 195–199, and Ogden, *Bentham's Theory of Fictions*, 8–9.

51. For Bentham, Priestley, and the Convention, see J. H. Burns, "Bentham and the French Revolution," *Transactions of the Royal Historical Society*, 5th ser., 16 (1966): 95–114; Goodwin, *Friends of Liberty*, 246–257; Gibbs, *Priestley*, 152, 216. For Burke on Brissot, see "Preface to the Address of M. Brissot to his Constituents" (1794), in *Works of Edmund Burke*, 6 vols. (London: George Bell, 1891), 3:525.

bench. The Panopticon's chapel was placed inside the guard tower, where there would be no "thronging or jostling on the way to church," rather than occupying its traditionally independent site as autonomous from the system of discipline. Thus in order to complete an analysis of the social setting of the philosophy of mind and body made by reformers in the 1770s, it is necessary to provide an account of the countertheology which they developed. As Foucault suggested, the reformers replaced the established Christian soul with a new "non-corporal" element, now defined as the product of disciplines and the target at which discipline should be directed. This substitution had important implications: the new model of the soul was used to explain why error had survived and how it could be corrected. It explained this error both in individual humans and in the body politic. Reformers sought to accomplish these aims with a therapy, the philosophical history of mind. That history gave each individual a chance of redemption and immortality: redemption through the pursuit of the calculated dictates of reason, and immortality through the progress of reform.[52]

Both Bentham and Priestley lambasted established religion as superstition and false consciousness, that is, as a case of mental pathology. In a manuscript of 1773 entitled "Obstacles to Improvement," Bentham declared that "a man who after reading the scriptures can bring himself to fancy the doctrines of the Athanasian Creed" was in "that state of prepared imbecility which is necessary to a mind for the tranquil reception of one parcel of Nonsense." Priestley referred the prevalence of patent absurdities in church doctrine to political interest: rational clergymen in the established church "must every time they officiate not only profess, but in reality act upon the profession, of what they do not believe."[53] Because of the bad faith of such priests, their religion was merely an ally of corruption. Their mental state was to be contrasted with that of the enlightened philosopher. An enlightened mind was both the most important subject for natural-philosophical research and the most important resource possessed by the researcher. Thus the mind was rep-

52. Bowring, 4:47, 63. For Foucault on the "non-corporal" soul, see *Discipline and Punish,* 29. For Priestley's materialist theology, see Ira V. Brown, "The Religion of Joseph Priestley," *Pennsylvania History* 24 (1957): 85–100 and Erwin N. Hiebert, "The Integration of Revealed Religion and Scientific Materialism in the Thought of Joseph Priestley," in Kieft and Willeford, *Priestley,* 27–61. For an analysis of Bentham's anticlericalism, see James E. Crimmins, "Bentham on Religion, Atheism and the Secular Society," *Journal of the History of Ideas* 47 (1986): 95–110.

53. Bentham, "Obstacles to Improvement," in Mack, *Bentham,* 300; Priestley, "General History of the Christian Church," in Rutt, 10:538–541.

resented as a "laboratory," since it could be subjected to experimentation and observation, and as a "state," since it could be managed and reformed. In 1775 Priestley argued that mind was the result of "a certain organized system of matter," the brain, which was itself a "great laboratory and repository" for the purpose of converting phlogiston into electric fluid. Further inquiry would reveal the details of the forms of matter that acted in this way. It was demonstrated in pneumatics and optics that matter exhibited a wide range of power. "Nothing but a precise and definite knowledge of the nature of perception and thought can authorize any person to affirm whether they may not belong to an extended substance which has also the properties of attraction and repulsion." These "mental powers" were just as accessible to "observation and experiment" as were the powers of pneumatics and optics, even though "we ourselves are the subjects of the observations and experiments."[54]

These remarks implied that a materialist philosophy of mind was the guarantee of the accessibility of the mind to research. Such research, however, was itself a means of reforming the mind, purging it of false doctrine and destroying its prejudices. Priestley referred to Hartley's celebrated claim that "the greatest and noblest use of philosophical speculation is . . . the opportunity it affords of inculcating benevolent and pious sentiments upon the mind." Ultimately, this mind would be a communal property, not exemplified in any specific individual but in the enlightened state of the whole social body. Priestley's example encouraged many of his colleagues to argue that only through the understanding and transformation of mind could reform succeed. This had implications for the collective work of radical natural philosophers, lawyers, divines, and writers. In 1778 Priestley encouraged his Cumbrian friend Adam Walker to take up public natural-philosophy lectures in London. Walker interspersed his lectures with the argument that governments warped the "qualities and tendencies" of the human mind, while proper natural philosophy restored them. In the 1780s, under Priestley's influence, William Godwin abandoned Calvinism for Socinianism, experimental philosophy, and the doctrines of David Hartley. These concerns were made evident both in his political treatises and fictions of the 1790s. In his *Enquiry concerning Political Justice* (1793) Godwin based his celebrated critique of government on a psychology

54. Joseph Priestley, *Disquisitions Relating to Matter and Spirit* (London, 1777), 24–30; *Experiments and Observations on Different Kinds of Air*, 2d ed. (London, 1775), 277–279; *An Examination of Dr. Reid's Inquiry into the Human Mind on the Principles of Common Sense* (London, 1774), lvii.

that relied explicitly on the doctrine of association, while in his reflections on the work of the novelist he described his enterprise as "the analysis of the private and internal operations of the mind, employing my metaphysical dissecting knife in tracing and laying bare the involutions of motive, and recording the gradually accumulating impulses." For these men a combination of natural philosophy and the "logic of the will" was the key to moral understanding and progress. This was because the mind was no ghost but a part of the bodily machine.[55]

In 1776 Bentham attacked traditional talk of the "will" as a faculty. He ridiculed the view that "there is really any such thing as a little being that under the name of will gets into men's heads, and exercises acts of volition or any other acts. . . . it is Man that exercises those various acts, that perceives these various emotions." The following years, in his *Disquisitions concerning Matter and Spirit* and in his comments on the doctrine of philosophical necessity, Priestley agreed with this monism. Will was unitary and identified with bodily powers. Insofar as notions such as "will" or "soul" were used as the specially privileged principle of individuation in each human subject, they would lead to delusion and philosophical error. Just as the term "our country" corresponded to "a part of the world subject to that form of government by the laws of which we ourselves are bound, as distinguished from other countries," so "the idea of self" referred to a "substance, which is the seat of that particular set of sensations and ideas of which those that are then recollected make a part, as distinguished from other substances which are the seats of similar sensations and ideas." Each body was to be seen as a unified state, constituted by a single network of powers, ruled as a single polity.[56] It was for this reason that knowledge of material powers brought the right state of mind. Bentham explained that "the vast mass of mischief, of which perverted religion is the source," had a "preventive remedy" in a natural philosophy that generated "that mental strength and well-grounded confidence which renders him proof against so many

55. Priestley, *History of Electricity,* xix; compare David Hartley, *Observations on Man* (London, 1749), part 2, 245–248. For uses of these principles, see Adam Walker, *A System of Familiar Philosophy* (London, 1799), preface; William Godwin, *Caleb Williams,* ed. D. McCracken (1794; Oxford: Oxford University Press, 1970), 339; *Enquiry concerning Political Justice,* ed. Isaac Kramnick (1798; Harmondsworth: Penguin Books, 1976), 360–376. Compare Martin Fitzpatrick, "William Godwin and the Rational Dissenters," *Price-Priestley Newsletter* 3 (1979): 4–28.

56. Parekh, *Bentham's Political Thought,* 146, printing Bentham MSS, University College London, 69.70 (1776); for Priestley on the will, see Rutt, 3:451 (1777) and 25:96 (1791). For Priestley on the "self" as a state, see Priestley, *Disquisitions,* "Objections to the System of Materialism Considered: 5, from a Separate Consciousness Not Belonging to the Brain," 89–91.

groundless terrors." This was to be a natural philosophy that laid ghosts and anatomized minds. He drew an important contrast between the law of terror, spirits and fictions, and the law of utility, bodies and material interests. The former "drags men to its purpose in chains, from which . . . the captives break loose in crowds," while the latter, "transcendental legislation, leads men by silken threads round their affections and makes them its own for ever." This remark avoided all reference to a doctrine of the suffering soul—no threats of sin and redemption were present in "transcendental legislation." The Panopticon, which substituted the illuminated space for inspection for the dark confinement of the dungeon, relied on the power of these "silken threads" over subjects' minds and the knowledge of how they worked.[57]

Bentham's language of "groundless terrors" and "bungling clumsiness" in castigating existing schemes of justice referred to real features of the treatment of the condemned. Historians as different as Douglas Hay and Michel Foucault have argued for the importance of awesome spectacle and the physical presence of power at the moment of the execution of justice upon the body of the eighteenth-century criminal. Clumsy executions were loudly criticized by large and enthusiastic audiences; on the scaffold, the priest, the surgeon, and the criminal joined in a state-supported theatrical performance. Bentham and his English allies sought to emulate the influence which Beccaria's utilitarian critique of these performances had enjoyed in France. One of the more significant aspects of the ritual was the explicit connection between secular and divine judgment, for the rituals of execution were also rituals of the fate of the soul. This was what utility challenged. Michael Ignatieff cites the sermon preached by John Wesley at Bedford Assizes in 1758: Wesley contrasted "the few" who would "stand at the judgement seat this day" with the fate of all his audience. "We shall all, I that speak and you that hear, *stand at the Judgement Seat of Christ.* And we are now reserved on this earth which is not our home, in this prison of flesh and blood, perhaps many of us in chains of darkness too, till we are ordered to be brought forth."[58] While by no means blind to the force of imagination

57. Bowring, 8:13; Mack, *Bentham,* 293, printing Bentham MSS, University College London, 149.63 (1794).

58. For the eighteenth-century spectacle of punishment, see Douglas Hay, "Property, Authority and the Criminal Law," in Douglas Hay et al., *Albion's Fatal Tree: Crime and Society in Eighteenth-Century England* (Harmondsworth: Penguin Books, 1977), 17–64; Foucault, *Discipline and Punish,* 32–69. For popular protest, see E. P. Thompson, "The Moral Economy of the Eighteenth-Century Crowd," *Past and Present* 50 (1971): 76–136. For Beccaria and Brissot, see McManners, *Death and the Enlightenment,* 392–401. For Wesley, see Ignatieff, *Just Measure of Pain,* 55.

on the multitude, neither Bentham nor Priestley held that such sentiments could bind men to right action or proper morality. The sanction of damnation disappeared. This was a fundamental assault on the commonplaces of law and religion. In 1792 Thomas Beddoes argued that the experience of temporal justice generated subjects' false doctrines of divine retribution and of the torments of Hell. A better society would change the state of mind of its citizens. He agreed with Priestley that "the material world easily supplied the notion of power," while reaching the extreme conclusion that hence "visible tribunals . . . led to the idea of remunerative justice, and that with scarce an exception in another life. Thus man created God, an Heaven and an Hell." Priestley and his allies supposed that "Chains of darkness" were removed by the science of "mental pathology," not the dictates of atonement and resurrection. Priestley classed these as "corruptions" of true Christianity, and their use alongside the public spectacle of state terror and popular enthusiasm was a mark of this corruption.

> Our mode of respiting, for the sake of benefiting the souls of the Criminals, has arisen from a notion that such repentance as that of a condemned criminal may be of some avail to him with respect to his future state; a notion false and dangerous in the extreme, as it encourages the whole community to persist in evil courses, thinking that a few days, or hours, of repentance may cancel all their guilt, and prepare them for future happiness.[59]

Bentham, as usual, took a calculated view of the problematic effects of established religion on criminality. He told Dugald Steward that since Scots Calvinists paid clerics less than did English Anglicans, and since the crime rate was lower north of the border, religious work was obviously more effective in Scotland. In general, as he argued in 1780, "the dictates of religion would coincide in all cases with the dictates of utility," were men possessed of the right account of God. This account would recognize divine benevolence in the sense in which it was attributed to humans, and thus account for the "theological sanction" in mental pathology as a derivative case of utilitarian rationality. Bentham envisaged no minister of public religion in his ideal polity: the correct analysis

59. Thomas Beddoes, *Letter to a Lady on Early Instruction* (London, 1792), 16–17, cited in Stansfield, *Beddoes,* 84; Joseph Priestley, *Lectures on History and General Policy* (Birmingham, 1788), Lecture 47. For interesting remarks on Bentham's mission and law reform, see Himmelfarb, "Haunted House of Jeremy Bentham," 34–36.

of the powers of the human mind would fulfill all the functions hitherto discharged by priestcraft.[60]

Priestley shared this view. The principle of benevolence, rather than retribution, was the key to his theology. "Benevolence" was given a remarkably secular interpretation. We have seen that this principle governed his pneumatics and the model of the natural economy he made in the 1770s. The argument against retributive justice also dominated his critique of Anglican or Calvinist accounts of the soul and its fate. The doctrines of a future state and of an immortal, separable, soul were fundamental resources for the natural philosophy, the legal philosophy, and the established religions which Bentham and Priestley attacked. In his metaphysical texts composed after his abandonment of Calvinism and of Arianism, Priestley turned against the textbooks he had studied in the dissenting academies. Doddridge had introduced the pneumatology of John Locke and of the Aberdonian metaphysician Andrew Baxter into the curriculum at Northampton, and they had remained as standard authorities at Daventry. Doddridge himself had insisted upon the immateriality of the soul and denied that matter could think. Doddridge and Baxter deduced from the principle that inertial force was essential to matter the consequence that it could not possess any innate activity. Doddridge's readings of Locke and Baxter were extremely influential, and they provided Priestley with much of the target he chose in establishing philosophical materialism in the 1770s. In these texts, he turned the weapons of Hartleian associationism and pneumatic chemistry on the devotees of immaterialism. Spirits were redefined as rarer forms of matter; powers were revealed in the laboratory and in the mind; the political and theological dangers of using the immaterial soul as the principle of consciousness and of subjectivity were spelled out in considerable detail.[61]

60. For Bentham on Scottish priests, see Bentham to Dugald Steward, 27 June 1783, in Bowring, 10:129–130; on religion and utility, see Bentham, *Introduction to the Principles of Morals and Legislation,* 138–139. For the state indifference to religion, see Crimmins, "Bentham on Religion."

61. For "benevolence" in Priestley's pneumatics, see J. G. McEvoy, "Enlightenment and Dissent: Joseph Priestley and the Limits of Theoretical Reasoning," *Enlightenment and Dissent* 2 (1983): 47–67 at 49–50. For Doddridge's teaching, see Doddridge, *Course of Lectures,* 52–53, 205–209. For Doddridge and Andrew Baxter on immaterialism, see Yolton, *Thinking Matter,* 94–97, 144; P. M. Heimann and J. E. McGuire, "Newtonian Forces and Lockean Powers: Concepts of Matter in Eighteenth-Century Thought," *Historical Studies in Physical Sciences* 3 (1971): 233–306. For Doddridge and dissenting textbooks, see Isabel Rivers, "Dissenting and Methodist Books of Practical Divinity," in Rivers, *Books and Their Readers*

The critique of immaterialism involved a sensitive reformulation of the language of philosophy and a direct attack on the established authority in philosophical discipline. The reassessment of the status of matter was accompanied by a reassessment of the power exercised by Newton and his interpreters. Immaterialism made matter too base. Priestley described Baxter as "the ablest defender of the strict immaterial system" while suggesting that Baxter's metaphysics implied that it was a "pity that so mischievous a thing as he every where represents matter to be, should have been introduced at all." In Priestley's vocabulary, "matter" was to be defined as the subject of powers. He attacked Locke's timorous hesitancy before this obvious conclusion. In the *Disquisitions,* Priestley argued that it was "unaccountable in Mr. Locke" to concede that "the faculty of thinking may be a property of the body, and yet to think it more probable that this faculty inhered in a different substance, viz., an immaterial soul." Baxter himself was a well-chosen target. He was held up by Anglican apologists as the best example of the way Newtonian natural philosophy could be used against the joint dangers of deist materialism and the extreme immaterialism of the Tory philosophers such as Berkeley. Bishop Warburton described Baxter as "a great genius," whose metaphysics was unjustly neglected and "infinitely" superior to Berkeley's "miserable sophisms." Baxter's system emphasized the most committed form of voluntarism, for since matter was always and everywhere utterly inert, His subjects could see that "God hath not given the reigns of the world out of his hands, nor planted the laws by which it is governed, in brute matter."[62]

By choosing Baxter as his main enemy, Priestley could blacken court Whig naturalists, such as Samuel Clarke and Henry Pemberton, with the sins of their Scottish contemporary. They had all succumbed to the hypochondriac fear of what Priestley called "the contagion of matter." Priestley replied that matter was the source of life, not death. In the *Disquisitions* he implied that Newton's immediate circle of interpreters had betrayed their master's legacy. Their false conception of matter defined

in Eighteenth-Century England, 127–164. For Priestley's early reading, see R. E. Schofield, "Joseph Priestley: Theology, Physics and Metaphysics," *Enlightenment and Dissent* 2 (1983):69–81 at 71–72.

62. Priestley, *Disquisitions,* 8, 66, 31–32. For Warburton on Baxter and Berkeley, see A. C. Fraser, ed., *Works of George Berkeley* (Oxford: Oxford University Press, 1901), 3:400; S. C. Rome, "The Scottish Refutation of Berkeley's Immaterialism," *Philosophy and Phenomenological Reseach* 3 (1943): 313–325. For Baxter on God's power, see Andrew Baxter, *An Enquiry into the Nature of the Human Soul* (London, 1733), 45, and compare ibid., 11 on inertia and "a new theory of matter."

body as the mere object of divine will, rather than the noble seat of activity in the world. His controversies with Price in the 1770s concentrated on the propriety of Priestley's rewording of Newtonian utterances in the *Opticks.* A direct assault on Newtonian orthodoxy was a very dangerous strategy. As John Yolton has shown, controversies soon flared in the public sheets about the relative merits of Priestley's materialism and its Newtonian enemies. Contributors to *The London Review* and *The Monthly Review* during 1775 strenuously debated the mortalism and materialism they found in Priestley's new version of Hartley. Newtonian authority was satirized by Priestley's friends: "Dr. Clarke was confessedly so merely a reasoning machine, that he would almost tempt one to think that matter might think and that he himself was a living proof of it."[63] In his own succession of defenses, Priestley implied instead that with the new lessons of experimental philosophy and reformed religion it was possible to purify Newton's doctrine of its more corrupt implications, notably those about the impenetrability and passivity of bodies. From an early age, Priestley had greeted new phenomena in the laboratory with the exclamation: "Oh, had Sir Isaac Newton seen such an experiment!" Indeed, in his *Disquisitions* Priestley argued that a strict application of Newton's rules of reasoning, to which he professed "a uniform and rigorous adherence," was precisely the strategy needed to show how little ground there was to the orthodox notion of inert matter. "The principles of Newtonian philosophy were no sooner known that it was seen how few, in comparison, of the phenomena of nature, were owing to solid matter, and how much to powers." Hence Priestley's use of the "nutshell" image to describe the quantity of solid matter in the world. He treated the transmission of Newtonian natural philosophy as he did any other important and established doctrine: he contrasted the purity of an original revelation with the subsequent corruption of the creed due to the interests of its interpreters.[64]

63. Priestley, *Disquisitions,* 170–173 on Andrew Baxter, *Matho; or The Cosmotheoria Puerilis,* 2d ed., 2 vols. (London, 1745), 2:212. For a critique of Newton's interpreters, see *Disquisitions,* 112 on the "rigid immaterialists"; for remarks on the *Opticks,* see ibid., 114 and Priestley, *Free Discussion of the Doctrines of Materialism and Philosophical Necessity* (London, 1778), 8–9, 26–31, 231, 237. For assaults on Priestley and his defense, see Yolton, *Thinking Matter,* 117, which cites *The London Review of English and Foreign Literature,* November 1775, 564.

64. Timothy Priestley, *Funeral Sermon Occasioned by the Death of the Late Joseph Priestley* (London, 1805), 42–43; *Disquisitions,* 1–2, 5–7, 17. For Priestley's defense of his own version of natural philosophy against critics, see Priestley to Bretland, 7 March 1773, in Schofield, *Scientific Autobiography of Priestley,* 116–118, and Priestley to Kenrick, June 1778, in *Free discussion,* 183.

Priestley used exactly the same strategy in his analysis of the true idea of matter and the true idea of the soul. Both involved this appeal to the history of pristine truth and subsequent decay into error. Both could be restored by an appeal to the authority of experimental philosophy. It is important to emphasize the significance of this "historical method" in the philosophy of reform. We have already seen the way Bentham used Priestley's account of the history of philosophy in his own critique of Blackstone in the 1770s. Priestley's technique was useful because it showed how to establish truth against the errors of what Bentham baptized "sinister interests." The work that established the true pneumatology was coextensive with the work that analyzed the dangers of established interests. Priestley argued that "an opinion, and especially an opinion adopted by great numbers of mankind, is to be considered as any other fact in history, for it cannot be produced without an adequate cause, and is therefore a proper object of philosophical inquiry." This set up a very close connection between the philosophy of mind and the correction of error. A proper philosophy of mind would simultaneously correct these errors and explain their source. Thus this philosophy contested the orthodoxies of immaterialism by writing the history of immaterialism.[65]

The events of the 1770s show how this therapeutic historiography worked. It was during this period that Priestley broke with the dogmas of immaterialism and then reflected on his conversion experience. He told his fellow rational dissenter Caleb Rotheram that only after 1775, when he began working on an edition of Hartley to accompany his experiments at Bowood, did he recognize that the doctrine of the immaterial soul "had been imported into Christianity" and was "the foundation of the capital corruptions of our religion." The scale of this break is most marked in the comparison between Priestley's *Institutes of Natural and Revealed Religion,* composed at Daventry Academy in the 1750s and completed in early 1772, and the doctrines of the *Disquisitions,* written in Wiltshire in 1776–1777 to defend his interpretation of Hartley and Newton. In the earlier text, matter was characterized as "sluggish and inert," while God was an ominpotent and omnipresent "immaterial being or spirit." In the latter text, God was "far from being immaterial" and matter was in no way different from the dynamic conception of spirit. In the *Institutes,* the doctrine of the "sleep of the soul" as a separate

65. Rutt, 5:15 and 480; see Margaret Canovan, "The Irony of History: Priestley's Rational Theology," *Price-Priestley Newsletter* 4 (1980): 16–25. For Bentham on "sinister interests," see Harrison, *Bentham,* 200–206.

immaterial substance was stoutly defended, while by the later 1770s Priestley argued that this view was the basis of false religion.[66] Both in his *Disquisitions* and in his debates with Richard Price in 1777–1778, he then analyzed the process by which this false view of the soul had commanded such authority. Characteristically, this analysis took the form of therapeutic history. Priestley said that in its pristine form the soul was "conceived to be an aerial or an igneous substance," "what we should now call *an attenuated form of matter*." What had gone wrong? The defenders of priestcraft had realized that this original and truthful account would imply that "the soul and the body being in reality the same kind of matter must die together." So dualism was invented to keep mortalism at bay and the wrong authority in power. Both Locke and Descartes were authors of this falsehood. The Scottish philosophers of Common Sense were merely the most recent defenders of this corruption, and Bentham applauded this assault on the interests of Thomas Reid and his allies. Finally, when pneumatics, optics, and electricity demonstrated just how powerful matter could be, the resources were available for a philosophically authoritative attack on immaterialism. His experiments showed that "spirits" were indeed developed from rarer forms of matter, and so returned the pneumatology of the philosophers to its original truth.[67]

This philosophy posed as a restoration of pristine truths established through rational analysis of mind and controlled experiments on body. It carried a history of civil society and of the doctrines that society had produced. All this made the philosophers look like a new sect. Any new sect needed sacred texts, well-established authorities, and a means of proselytizing. Both Priestley and Bentham spoke the language of sectarianism. New "saints" were found, new scriptures were edited. For example, during the 1770s Priestley produced his heavily edited version of Hartley's revelation of the powers of mind. He also made a remarkable new use of the natural philosophy of the Jesuit Roger Boscovich, who had argued for a model of matter as a network of point centers of forces. Both the treatment of Hartley and that of Boscovich were controversial because many protested against the new meanings Priestley found in these texts. Just as Priestley was forced to defend his rereading of Hartley against criticisms from Price, so he was forced to defend his use of Boscovich against the comments of fellow dissenters and those of

66. Priestley to Caleb Rotheram, April 1778, in Rutt, 1:314–315; Priestley, *Institutes of Natural and Revealed Religion*, vol. 1 (London, 1772), 15–16, 156–159; *Disquisitions*, 16, 145–146; compare Priestley, *Hartley's Theory of the Human Mind* (London, 1775), xx.

67. Priestley, *Disquisitions*, 72, 170–173; *Free Discussion*, 262–268.

the author himself. Boscovich met Priestley in 1775 and they discussed shared views of the penetrability of matter and the relation of body and power. Priestley then combined his own pneumatics, the views of John Michell on the forces innate in matter, and Boscovich's doctrine that "matter consists of *powers* only, without any substance" and published them in 1777. The Jesuit was horrified. He wrote to Shelburne protesting Priestley's use of his ideas to prove materialism and mortalism. Priestley was equally angry at the danger this posed to his relationship with his patron, and told Boscovich that "I have not made *you* an accomplice" in establishing the principles of philosophical materialism. Boscovich was unconvinced by these "impieties and absurdities."[68] The life of body and the death of the soul were the most important principles which Priestley sought to establish through these editions. He made two shifts of emphasis in his interpretation of Hartley. First, he chose to emphasize Hartley's argument that "the whole man is of some *uniform composition*" rather than spelling out in detail the mechanism of vibration which Hartley used to explicate the process of thought. An ontology of pneumatic powers could do the work hitherto performed by an aether. The uniformity of body effaced the division between matter and spirit and guaranteed the truth of mortalism. Priestley told Price that powers of thought "reside in the organized body itself and therefore *must* be suspended till the time when the organization shall be restored." Mortalism was a central doctrine because it was the best way to guarantee the proper faith and the proper civic philosophy. So, secondly, Priestley swept aside Hartley's reservations about mortalism. Hartley's text argued that if body "could be endued with the most simple kinds of sensation," then it might also "arrive at all that intelligence of which the human mind is possessed." But he also pointed out that "the immateriality of the soul has little or no connexion with its immortality." Priestley disagreed. To show from pneumatics that the soul was material was to show that it was as mortal as body. This demonstration was a precondition of the proper conduct of philosophy and the proper conduct of moral life.[69]

68. For Priestley and Boscovich, see Priestley, *History and Present State of Discoveries Relating to Vision, Light and Colours* (London, 1772), 390, 393–394; *Disquisitions*, xii and 11; Priestley to Bretland, 7 March 1773, in Schofield, *Scientific Autobiography of Priestley*, 117; Priestley to Boscovich, 19 August 1778 and Boscovich to Priestley, 17 October 1778, ibid., 166–171.

69. Priestley, *Hartley's Theory*, xx; Priestley to Caleb Rotheram, 31 May 1774, in Schofield, *Scientific Autobiography of Priestley*, 146. For Hartley and mortalism, see *Free Discussion*, xvi; Hartley, *Observations on Man*, part 1, 511–512.

THE USES OF THE DEAD

Ultimately, the lessons of a philosophy of mind and body were made manifest at death. As has been argued, Hartley's system was at least as important for Priestley because of its account of life in the world to come. The combination of philosophical materialism and conjectural history implied a revised account of a future state. The rational subject would find consolation and hope in the prospects of general enlightenment rather than an individual fate. Visionary accounts of society's advance were consequences of this revised account of the progress of reason. Philosophical materialism argued that body and soul were indistinguishable in life. Orthodox pneumatology argued that the two substances became separated at death. So the materialists needed to define their own art of making a good end. For the pious, the idealized setting of the deathbed showed the superiority of secure faith over the darkness of irreligion. The existence of spirit was meant to sustain important moral sanctions. The stories told of the horrors of impious suffering, or of deathbed conversions, were important elements in the contest with materialism. Bentham was extremely critical of the force of these anecdotes: rational subjects "should be exempt from those horrors—from those pains of mind . . . infused . . . by the opium of the existence of man in a life to come." This "opium" should be replaced by a prospective account of the development of the new social and intellectual order, wisely guided by expert managers and gradually advancing toward a rational utopia. Optimism became a regulative principle for the reformer's life, and the future reputation of his philosophical sect took the place of the soul's immortality. This was a commonplace among the *philosophes.* Diderot put the point pithily: "posterity is to the philosopher what the next world is to the religious believer." Bentham echoed the sentiment at the end of his life: "my fear was—lest by dying . . . my fellow men . . . should be deprived of the happiness which it is my hope thereby to give them."[70]

70. For Hartley's millennium, see R. Marsh, "The Second Part of Hartley's System," *Journal of the History of Ideas* 20 (1959): 264–273; Fruchtman, *Apocalyptic Politics of Price and Priestley,* 16–20. For Bentham on the future see "J. B.'s Instructions for Living Happily or Not At All" (1831), in Mack, *Bentham,* 213. For enlightenment and orthodox immortalism in France, see Bernard Groethuysen, *The Bourgeois: Catholicism versus Capitalism in 18th-Century France* (London: Barrie and Rockliff, 1968), 50–77 and McManners, *Death and the Enlightenment,* 148–190; Diderot's remark is cited at p. 168. For an important treatment of the role of "posterity" in the formation of the intellectual, see Daniel Roche, "Talent, Reason and Sacrifice: The Physician during the Enlightenment," in *Medicine and Society in France,* ed. Robert Forster and Orest Ranum (Baltimore: Johns Hopkins University Press, 1980), 66–88.

This implied that accounts of the future state were important items of a politics of philosophy. By the 1790s, it was obvious that the reformers' account of death had at least two political consequences. First, despite their own criticisms of the sanctions of public executions, many reformers seemed to endorse the judicial murders of the Revolution. As early as 1790, Jacobin pamphlets published in Birmingham debated Priestley's mortalism. The following year, just days after the Birmingham riot, the cartoonist James Gillray imagined a conversation between George III, facing death on the scaffold, and Priestley, ministering to the condemned monarch. "We must all die once," Priestley is envisaged as saying; "in fact a Man ought to be glad of the opportunity of dying, if by that means he can serve his country in bringing about a glorious Revolution. As to your soul, or any thing after death, don't trouble your self about that; depend on it, the idea of a future state is all an imposition." It was held that materialism licensed murder by making men machines. During the Revolutionary decade the regicide Terror was all too easily displayed as an inevitable consequence of the philosophy espoused by writers such as Beddoes, Godwin, or Erasmus Darwin. Since these materialists banned spirits from nature, anti-Jacobins could make fun of their enemies by populating the world with vengeful ghosts. Reformers would be haunted by their victims and by the souls which they had denied.[71] The second consequence of the reformer's philosophy of mind was the emphasis placed on the confrontation between the enlightened, rational mind and the prospects of the future. When he answered Burke in 1791, Priestley ended his response with an account of a blissful future. He drew a vivid contrast between his own "pleasing dream" and the darker apocalypse prophesied by his adversary. Priestley lampooned Burke's self-appointed role as establishment's mes-

71. For Priestley's mortalism in Birmingham, see John Money, *Experience and Identity: Birmingham and the West Midlands, 1760–1800* (Manchester: Manchester University Press, 1977), 145–148; for Gillray's cartoon, see James Gillray, "The Hopes of the Party Prior to July 14th," 19 July 1791, in *The Satirical Etchings of James Gillray*, ed. Draper Hill (New York: Dover, 1976), no. 21. Compare "The Progress of Man: A Didactic Poem," in Edmonds, *Poetry of the Anti-Jacobin*, 102–110, and this satire by David Davis, printed in Gibbs, *Priestley*, 99:

Here lie at rest
In oaken chest
Together packed most nicely,
The bones and brains,
Flesh, blood and veins,
And *soul* of Dr. Priestley.

siah. "If, in these circumstances, you can save the church, as well as the state, you will deserve no less than canonization, and St. Edmund will be the greatest name in the calendar." Against the deceitful pieties of the conservatives, the reformers argued that confidence and optimism must be pursued in life and demonstrated in death. Both Bentham and Priestley provided exemplary instances of the right way to die. These instances were subsequently published as demonstrations of the right principles of philosophy and as aids to the dissemination of those principles.[72]

Both Priestley and Bentham recognized the death of Socrates as the origin of philosophy and as the proper model for their own decease. The Socratic model referred both to the sufferings of the intellectual under the burdens of persecution and to the future hope of an immortal reputation. Priestley's son sent a graphic description of his father's last days to Theophilus Lindsey with the express purpose of proving the consistency and effectiveness of the doctrines of unitarianism and philosophical materialism. The account emphasized the sustained labor of composition, publication, and experiment which Priestley continued up to the moment of his death. "He had the satisfaction of witnessing the gradual spread of his religious opinions and the fullest conviction that he should prevail over his opponents in chemistry. He looked forward with the greatest pleasure to future exertions in both these fields." His final actions included plans for improvements to his laboratory and the study of the scriptural account of the raising of Lazarus, paying specific attention to the gospel's emphasis on the empirical basis of the story: "many of the Jews which had seen the things which Jesus did, believed on him." His very last deed involved correcting the proofs of a pamphlet on the comparison between Jesus and Socrates. Here virtue was displayed as care for the future distribution of rational philosophy and the strenuous exertions of the naturalist.[73]

Bentham's death was equally exemplary. As is well known, at the age of 21 Bentham planned that "if I should chance to die of any such disease" whose study would advance "the art of Surgery or science of Physic . . . by observations to be made in the opening of my body," then

72. Priestley, *Letters to Burke,* 153–154, and Fruchtman, *Apocalyptic Politics of Price and Priestley,* 83.

73. For an annotated account of the death, see Jack Lindsay, ed., *Autobiography of Joseph Priestley* (Bath: Adams and Dart, 1970), 133–139, and Joseph Priestley, *Socrates and Jesus Compared* (Northumberland, Pa., 1803); Thomas Cooper to Benjamin Smith Barton, 6 February 1804, in Schofield, *Scientific Autobiography of Priestley,* 321.

Fordyce or some other physician or surgeon should be given the body for an anatomy, "to the intent and with the desire that Mankind may reap some small benefit in and by my decease." During the 1820s, he pursued research with the anatomists John Armstrong and Edward Grainger on processes of preservation, work that culminated in the production of Southwood Smith's "The Uses of the Dead to the Living" (1824) and Bentham's own "Auto-icon; or, Farther Uses of the Dead to the Living" in 1831. The following year Bentham confirmed his original provision for a postmortem dissection and laid down strict instructions for the preservations of his body. The body was to be displayed at future meetings of "my personal friends and other Disciples"; a codicil by Southwood Smith stated that the anatomy was to be used "to communicate curious, interesting and highly important knowledge, and secondly to show that the primitive horror at dissection originates in ignorance and is kept up by misconception and that the human body when dissected instead of being an object of disgust is as much more beautiful than any other piece of mechanism as it is more curious and wonderful." In the "Auto-icon," Bentham amplified this account of the utility of a corpse, suggesting ingenious machines that could animate "Dialogues of the Dead," notably between his own body and that of Socrates on the history of the principle of happiness.[74]

In every respect, Bentham's body was used as a means of instruction and demonstration. Southwood Smith's famous performance over the corpse of his master at Grainger's Anatomy Theatre in June 1832 and the Anatomy Act of that year were irresistible symbols of "the uses of the dead." It was reported that during the postmortem, Bentham's features were dramatically illuminated by a chance thunderstorm and "rendered almost vital by the reflection of the lightning playing over them." Disciples such as James Mill and his colleagues were there as mute witnesses.

> With the feelings which touch the heart in the contemplation of departed greatness, and in the presence of death, there mingled a sense of the power which that lifeless body seemed to be exercising in the conquest of

74. Bentham's will, 24 August 1769, *Correspondence of Bentham* 1:136; Thomas Southwood Smith, "The Uses of the Dead to the Living," *Westminster Review* 2 (1824): 59–97; C. F. A. Marmoy, "The Auto-icon of Jeremy Bentham at University College London," *Medical History* 2 (1958): 77–86; Crimmins, "Bentham on Religion," 105–108.

prejudice for the public good, thus cooperating with the triumphs of the spirit by which it had been animated.[75]

From his earliest works on law reform, Bentham had connected the well-arranged "demonstrations" of rational argument with the theatrical "demonstrations" of the public lecturers. Southwood Smith's anatomy was a demonstration in both these senses. In common with the general strategy of the reformers, it was simultaneously the act of an expert in the principles of mind and of an investigator of the principles of body. The doctrine of mind explained how education and reform would work, the doctrine of body provided what educators and reformers should know. The examination of the means by which these initial aims were transmuted under the criticisms of conservatives and the realities of patronage and power has many important implications for further inquiry into the work of reformers in the nineteenth century. It has been suggested that behind the apparent simplicities of utilitarian and unitarian activists of the 1820s and 1830s lies a complex philosophy of mind and body designed to account for extraordinary future developments in the social body. Development of society demanded relentless observation of its members' habits. The ensemble of subjects' bodily and mental habits which observers could survey would replace old models of matter and spirit. With resources drawn from the principles of utility and association, educators and civil servants such as James Mill could combine a confidence about the future with a presentation of the mind as an observable network of matters of fact. New disciplines appeared: psychology, political economy, statistics. Each of these disciplines explicitly relied on the contrast between the pathological complexities of the social order and the luminous simplicities of the mental principles on which these diseases depended and from which experts could learn the means of cure. Under the care of these experts, it was intended that the whole nation become an inspection house, a Panopticon where the mentalities of citizens would be made clearly visible to the inspectors' gaze. "If I had time to write a book," Mill claimed in 1817, "I would make the human mind as plain as the road from Charing Cross to St. Paul's." The following year, pursuing this goal of clarity, Mill finished his article on the sub-

75. For Southwood Smith's lecture and its effects, see Thomas Southwood Smith, *Lecture Delivered over the Remains of Jeremy Bentham* (London, 1831); Lewes, *Southwood Smith,* 45–47; M. J. Durey, "Bodysnatchers and Benthamites: The Implications of the Dead Body Bill for the London Schools of Anatomy, 1820–1842," *London Journal,* 1976:200–225.

ject of colonies for the *Encyclopaedia Britannica*. There he added notorious remarks on the wisdom of rational birth control as a solution to the crisis of population: "if the superstitions of the nursery were discarded, and the principle of utility kept steadily in view, a solution might not be very difficult to be found." So, for the reformers, the principles of a philosophy of mind would become principles for the management of individual bodies and of entire populations. These were projected as disciplines which, as Foucault observed, "characterized a power whose highest function was perhaps no longer to kill but to invest life through and through."[76]

76. James Mill to Francis Place, 6 December 1817, in William Thomas, *The Philosophic Radicals* (Oxford: Clarendon Press, 1979), 121; Mill, "General Remarks on the Principle of Population," in *Supplement to the Encyclopaedia Britannica* (Edinburgh, 1824). 3:261. For Mill, Bentham, and Malthus, see Patricia James, *Population Malthus: His Life and Times* (London: Routledge and Kegan Paul, 1979), 382–388. For the emergence of new disciplines of the body and of population, see Foucault, *The History of Sexuality*, vol. 1 (Harmondsworth: Penguin Books, 1981), 139; Ian Hacking, "How Should We Do the History of Statistics?" *Ideology and Consciousness* 8 (1981): 15–26; T. M. Porter, *The Rise of Statistical Thinking, 1820–1900* (Princeton: Princeton University Press, 1986).

EIGHT

The Marquis de Sade and the Discourses of Pain: Literature and Medicine at the Revolution

David B. Morris

MADAME DE MISTIVAL, *opening her eyes*—Oh Heavens! Why do you recall me from the grave's darkness? Why do you plunge me again into life's horrors?
DOLMANCÉ, *whipping her steadily*—Indeed, mother dear, it is because much conversation remains to be held.

—SADE, *Philosophy in the Bedroom*[1]

Pain is among the knottiest problems in the long, tangled history of relations between body and mind; moreover, the Marquis de Sade so thoroughly offends or resists the mentality of Anglo-American literary criticism that his works—when acknowledged at all—meet with a silence deeper and more ominous than censorship. It is therefore self-evidently quixotic to propose discussing Sade and pain together, as if to a study of the Atlantic Ocean one gratuitously added the Pacific. Nonetheless, despite its unwieldy expansiveness as a subject for inquiry, pain, like love, constitutes one of the apparently permanent experiences (chang-

This essay was supported by a grant from the Division of Research Programs of the National Endowment for the Humanities. I should especially like to thank G. S. Rousseau and James Grantham Turner for their generous assistance in its preparation and composition.

1. In *The Complete Justine, Philosophy in the Bedroom, and Other Writings*, trans. Richard Seaver and Austryn Wainhouse (New York: Grove Press, 1965), 362. When citing the Grove Press translations of Sade, I will also provide (following the page number) reference to the volume and page number of the French text, as published in the definitive edition *Œuvres complètes du Marquis de Sade*, ed. Gilbert Lély et al., 16 vols. (Paris: Cercle du Livre Précieux, 1966–1967). The French text of Dolmancé's words is revealing: "Eh! vraiment, ma petite mère, c'est que tout n'est pas dit" (3:544–545). Juliette, in the novel that bears her name, argues in favor of a philosophy that seeks to "say everything" ("tout dire" [9:586]).

ing with different cultures and times) that help to define an unwritten history of Western man, and we cannot hope to understand pain—in its fullest perplexities—without confronting the obsessive, almost unreadable pages in which Sade meditated, endlessly, on the bond uniting pain with desire. Although a complete history of pain would be fruitless and impossible, we need to consider those moments when pain emerges as something that requires an explanation, something that thrusts above the plane of merely blind or unquestioned sensation. Sade's work, however resistant or offensive, confronts us with such a moment when pain enters the zone of interpretation.

My purpose in this essay is to explore Sade's literary treatment of pain, especially as his works consume and transform the conventional vocabularies in which pain was discussed. Foremost among these vocabularies—which included theology and libertinism as well as law—was medicine. Thus my specific focus will concern Sade's transvaluations of medical knowledge. Sade did not simply appropriate a scientific vocabulary borrowed from eighteenth-century medicine and (to varying degrees) evident in the work of contemporary British and Continental writers, for whom the "life" or "nature" imitated in the novel now proved inextricable from the language of Enlightenment science.[2] Sade's transvaluations alter what they appropriate. His borrowings from scientific sources are not the most characteristic feature of his style, but they have not passed unnoticed. (In 1968 Jean Deprun published an important essay entitled "Sade et la philosophie biologique de son temps.")[3] It nevertheless needs to be emphasized that Sadean transvaluations employ biomedical language and concepts in ways that ultimately estrange them from the scientific and humanitarian labor of eighteenth-century medicine. Medicine in Sade is so thoroughly transvalued that it comes to constitute the appropriately unstable foundation for an otherwise foundationless libertine world, where reason always leads back toward the irrational, where clear and graspable truths grow indistinct and unsteady as they encounter the dark, corrosive, liberating power of desire.

2. See James Rodgers, "'Life' in the Novel: *Tristram Shandy* and Some Aspects of Eighteenth-Century Physiology," *Eighteenth-Century Life* 1 (1980): 1–20. Particularly relevant to the admixture of "medical language" in erotic or pornographic texts is G. S. Rousseau, "Nymphomania, Bienville and the Rise of Erotic Sensibility," in *Sexuality in Eighteenth-Century Britain,* ed. Paul-Gabriel Boucé (Manchester: Manchester University Press, 1982), 95–119.

3. In *Le Marquis de Sade* (Paris: Armand Colin, 1968), 189–203. This useful volume (with no editor named) collects papers from the 1966 symposium on Sade at the Centre aixois d'études et de recherches sur le dix-huitième siècle.

Pain for Sade is far more than (as we tend to consider it) a medical subject, and after Sade pain would never be quite the same.

There is a fundamental level of organic life at which pain belongs to an unthinking biochemistry of nerves and neurotransmitters that connects King Lear with Skinner's rats. Unlike pleasure, which spreads far beyond specific erogenous or tactile regions in diffuse currents of well-being, pain typically takes up residence in specific bodily parts.[4] Thus we complain of a headache or toothache or bad back, but no one announces experiencing a sudden pleasure in the thumb or foot. Our ability to locate pain in specific parts of the body is what allows pain to serve effectively as a biological defense, and we automatically pull our hand back from the fire in a reflex that occurs faster than thought. Consciousness seems necessary for us to *register* pain, in the sense that someone who is drugged or unconscious will not feel the fire's heat or the surgeon's knife. Still, few people would survive childhood if pain required accurate reasoning before we ran away or cried for help. Should we adopt a Cartesian vocabulary to describe this secret (unthinking) life of pain, we might say that it belongs to the mindless realm of *res extensa,* where whatever takes up space owes allegiance to the mechanical laws of matter. It was Descartes, in fact, who provided in his treatise on human physiology—*De l'homme,* published posthumously in 1662—an illuminating diagram for what we would now call an involuntary response to pain.

4. The localized nature of pain—as opposed to the nonlocal nature of pleasure—is discussed by Gilbert Ryle, "Pleasure," in *Dilemmas* (Cambridge: Cambridge University Press, 1954), 54–67. The best introduction to modern medical research on pain is by Ronald Melzack and Patrick D. Wall, *The Challenge of Pain* (New York: Basic Books, 1983). Several books written for general readers seek to place medical knowledge of pain in wider social and historical contexts. See, for example, Peter Fairley, *The Conquest of Pain* (1978; reprint, New York: Charles Scribner's Sons, 1980) and H. B. Gibson, *Pain and Its Conquest* (London: Peter Owen, 1982). For more philosophical and more satisfying discussions of pain and its relations to pleasure, see J. L. Cowan, *Pleasure and Pain: A Study in Philosophical Psychology* (London: Macmillan, 1968); Rem B. Edwards, *Pleasures and Pains: A Theory of Qualitative Hedonism* (Ithaca, N.Y.: Cornell University Press, 1979); and Thomas S. Szasz, M.D., *Pain and Pleasure: A Study of Bodily Feelings,* 2d ed. (New York: Basic Books, 1975). A fuller bibliographical introduction to differing modern approaches to pain is available in my essay "The Languages of Pain," in *Exploring the Concept of Mind,* ed. Richard M. Caplan (Iowa City: University of Iowa Press, 1986), 89–99. Undoubtedly the finest recent study of pain in its cultural significance—ranging from torture and nuclear war to the Old Testament, Marx, and human creativity—is Elaine Scarry's *The Body in Pain: The Making and Unmaking of the World* (New York: Oxford University Press, 1985). Scarry makes very little mention of Sade.

Descartes's diagram (see plate 16) provides an indirect but helpful introduction to the Marquis de Sade because its mechanistic assumptions provided a basis for Sade's work and have long continued to dominate Western thought. In Descartes's sketch, the nerve CC runs directly from the foot to the brain. When the fire scorches the foot, the internal response goes something like this. The "thin and mobile" filaments within the nerve cord are tugged, unequally, and thus become strained, separated, or broken. The resulting motion passes instantaneously to the brain—just as (in Descartes's mechanical analogy) by "pulling at one end of a cord, one simultaneously rings a bell which hangs at the other end."[5] All nerves for Descartes originate within the brain, and thus the tugging on nerve cord CC opens the valve or pore "d/e"—in turn releasing the so-called "animal spirits" produced and stored in the brain. These animal spirits—which Descartes described conventionally as minute, rarefied particles—descend through hollow spaces within the nerve cord and cause the muscular response that removes, say, foot from flame. At least as important as Descartes's simplified diagram is the analogy he chooses to describe the process of pain. With the delight of his age in complex machines, he compares the network of nerves, muscles, and animal spirits to an elaborate mechanical fountain, like the intricate waterworks popular in gardens and grottoes throughout the century.

What I wish to emphasize in Descartes is not the quaintness of his vocabulary—which we meet more than a century later in the novels of Sade—but the modernness of his view that pain must be understood as an event of the central nervous system, including of course the brain. In this light, Descartes's diagram might be interpreted as an episode in the larger seventeenth-century encounter with antiquity sometimes known as the battle of the ancients and the moderns. The Cartesian model of pain—although far from original—implies innovations as far-reaching as the changes that champions of the moderns attributed to the invention of gunpowder, printing, and the compass. Plato and Aristotle, for example, simply have no knowledge of the central nervous system.

5. *Treatise of Man,* translation and commentary by Thomas Steele Hall (Cambridge, Mass.: Harvard University Press, 1972), 34 ("ainsi que tirant l'un des bouts d'une corde, on fait sonner en même temps la cloche qui pend à l'autre bout"). Descartes repeats this same image in his treatise *The Passions of the Soul* (1649), where the physiology of nerves, fibers, and animal spirits is also described in detail (*The Philosophical Writings of Descartes,* trans. John Cottingham et al., 2 vols. [Cambridge: Cambridge University Press, 1985], 1:333). On the origin and development of the term "animal spirits," see Walther Riese, *A History of Neurology* (New York: MD Publications, 1959), 50–52.

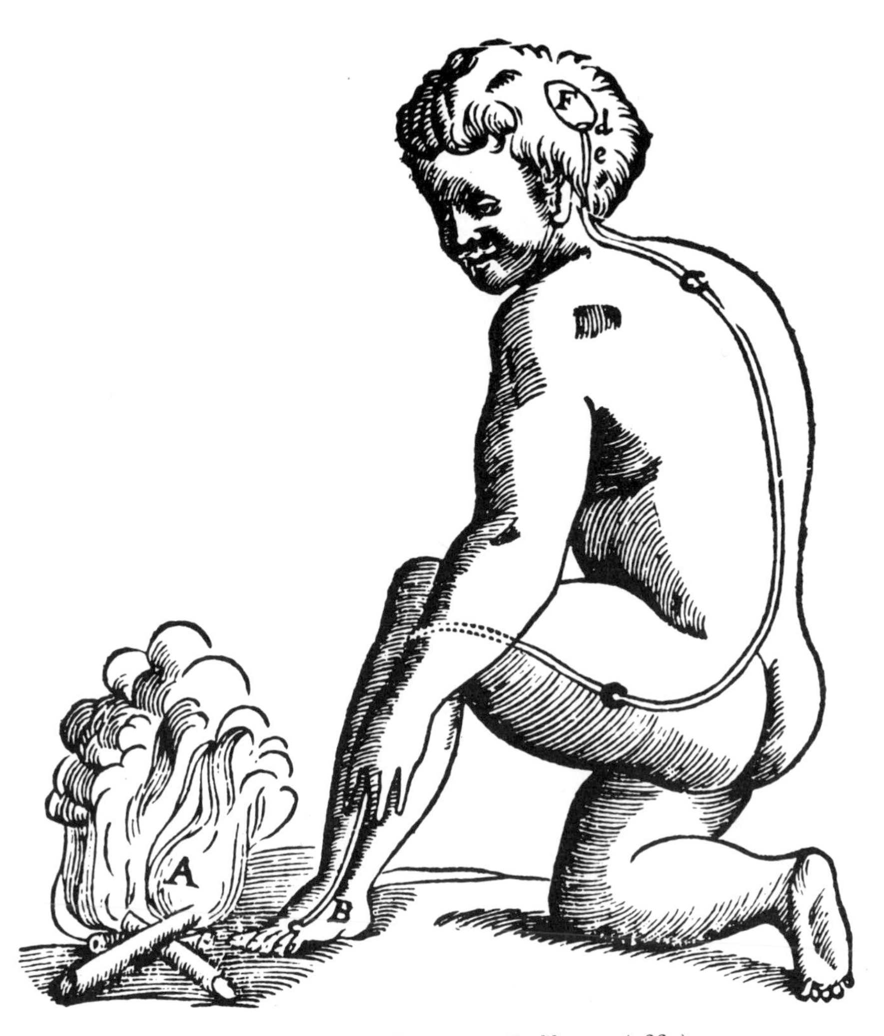

Pl. 16. From René Descartes, *De l'homme* (1662).

Indeed, Aristotle, like the biblical writers, locates thought and feeling in the heart.[6] Galen, writing in the second century A.D., established with the help of anatomical dissections a much more accurate picture of the nervous system, and in many respects Descartes's diagram is deeply indebted to Galenic physiology, which remained influential throughout the eighteenth century. Pain for Galen had a two-part explanation: in reference to nerves and in reference to organs. Nevertheless, despite its discussion of nerves, Galenic medicine mainly came to be associated with the doctrine that pain results from an imbalance of the four bodily humors. It is this Galenic physiology of organs and humoral fluids that Alexander Pope evokes in *The Rape of the Lock* when he assigns the allegorical figure of Pain its appropriate residence in the Cave of Spleen. It is significant that later in the eighteenth century "nerves" comes to replace "spleen" as the fashionable, one-word explanation of undiagnosable illness.[7] What matters most is that the Cartesian model of pain—in shifting discussion from organs and humors to the mechanics of the central nervous system—underwrites or permits a new way of thinking about man, a mode of thought that finds its most radical expression in the novels of Sade.

Sade, imprisoned for some twenty-seven years under five governments, might seem entirely isolated, remote from Cartesian physiology

6. K. D. Keele, *Anatomies of Pain* (Oxford: Blackwell Scientific Publications, 1957), 16–39. For a more detailed study concerning early theories of nerves, see Friedrich Solmsen, "Greek Philosophy and the Discovery of the Nerves," *Museum Helveticum* 18 (1961): 150–167. The best introduction to later Galenic theories of nerves and organs is two books by Rudolph E. Siegel, *Galen's System of Physiology and Medicine* (New York: S. Karger, 1968) and *Galen on Sense Perception* (New York: S. Karger, 1970). For contexts closer to Sade, see Edwin Clarke, "The Doctrine of the Hollow Nerve in the Seventeenth and Eighteenth Centuries," in *Medicine, Science, and Culture: Historical Essays in Honor of Owsei Temkin*, ed. Lloyd G. Stevenson and Robert P. Multhauf (Baltimore, Md.: Johns Hopkins University Press, 1968), 123–141; and Eric T. Carlson and Meribeth M. Simpson, "Models of the Nervous System in Eighteenth-Century Psychiatry," *Bulletin of the History of Medicine* 43 (1969): 101–115.

7. In 1786, James Adair described the popular influence of *De Morbis Nervorum* (1762), written by Robert Whytt (Professor of the Theory of Medicine at the Edinburgh Medical School, First Physician to the King of Scotland, and President of the Royal College of Physicians, Edinburgh): "Before the publication of this book, people of fashion had not the least idea that they had nerves; but a fashionable apothecary of my acquaintance, having cast his eye over the book, and having often been puzzled by the enquiries of his patients concerning the nature and causes of their complaints, derived from thence a hint, by which he cut the gordian knot—*'Madam, you are nervous'*; the solution was quite satisfactory, the term became fashionable, and spleen, vapours and hyp, were forgotten" (in R. K. French, *Robert Whytt, the Soul, and Medicine* [London: The Wellcome Institute of the History of Medicine, 1969], 166).

and from Enlightenment medicine, but medicine in fact provides one of the major discourses he puts to use in his copiously heterogeneous texts. Never has obscenity engaged such powers of erudition. Sade lost some six hundred books when the citizens of Paris liberated his recently vacated cell in the Bastille, and his reading ranged widely through the iconoclastic *philosophes* of his day, from Rousseau and Voltaire to Buffon, d'Holbach, and La Mettrie. But we need not invoke Sade's prodigious learning—or the legend of the philosopher in chains—in order to explain his knowledge of medicine. No doubt one explanation for the general commerce between fiction and physiology in Enlightenment thought involves the changed status of medicine. Like theology in the Middle Ages, medicine in the Enlightenment approached the condition of a master discourse. It is worth pausing, before we examine Sade's writing, to consider some of the ways in which medicine had changed.

In Sade's time the spectacular advances in medical knowledge—which accelerated with special vigor in late-eighteenth-century France—lent to medicine the authority of an official language and point of view that extended its influence to numerous other disciplines. French physicians ranked among the most active reformers and philosophers, whose thought penetrated far beyond medicine to questions of education, government, and law, as in the writings of Idéologue polymath Pierre-Jean-Georges Cabanis. (Sade particularly admired the work of Julien Offroy de La Mettrie, a physician-philosopher publishing in the mid-eighteenth century, whose radical views—after forcing him from France and Holland—at last found shelter at the court of Frederick the Great.) Conversely, Diderot's *Éléments de physiologie* (1774–1780) suggests how far nonphysicians felt themselves drawn to medical studies, like Samuel Johnson devouring the vast literature on diseases of the imagination. Reformers argued forcefully for a medicine that renounced "hypothetical explanations" and "imaginary systems"—associated with traditional medical teaching—in favor of scientific experiments and clinical observations.[8] Especially in pre-Revolutionary France, physicians and non-

8. Phrases in quotation cite remarks by Philippe Pinel and Pierre-François Percy in 1812 (in John E. Lesch, *Science and Medicine in France: The Emergence of Experimental Physiology, 1790–1855* [Cambridge, Mass.: Harvard University Press, 1984], 12). In addition to Lesch's lucid study of changes in French medicine about the time Sade was writing, see Erwin H. Ackerknecht, M.D., *Medicine at the Paris Hospital, 1794–1848* (Baltimore, Md.: Johns Hopkins University Press, 1967); David M. Vess, *Medical Revolution in France, 1789–1796* (Gainesville: University Presses of Florida, 1975); and *Medicine and Society in France* (selections from the *Annales,* vol. 6), ed. Robert Forster and Orest Ranum, trans. Elborg Forster and Patricia M. Ranum (Baltimore, Md.: Johns Hopkins University Press, 1980).

physicians sometimes wrote of medicine as supplying the cornerstone for an entire philosophy of man, in which improved public health would be indivisible from enlightened morality and from political reform. Medicine, in short, stands near the center of the revolution in eighteenth-century thought we call the Enlightenment (or, recently, Enlightenments). The intersection of medicine and literature in Sade's work does not simply infuse the novel with technical data or miscellaneous insights. Medicine, I claim, is foundational for Sade. It provides him with a basis for utterly reorganizing our views of man.

Sade's connection with French medicine is necessarily indirect, subordinated to his obsession with human sexual behavior, but indirect alliances sometimes prove more fruitful than direct borrowings. The indirect relation that links Sade to French medicine is at one level a powerful kinship of spirit. His entire enterprise in probing human sexuality bears resemblance to the series of events and discoveries in French medicine that Michel Foucault has termed "the birth of the clinic." This profound revision of medical thought did more than vastly extend and institutionalize the practice of clinical teaching, which in effect displaced the moribund traditions of academic medicine centered in the Paris Faculty. It signified a new emphasis on the previously subordinate arts (or, rather, trades) of pharmacy and of surgery, which were now elevated as indispensable techniques for penetrating the opaque surface of the body. (By contrast, in 1751 the Paris Faculty had required an oath from all bachelors of medicine renouncing the practice of surgery and pharmacy.) Further, it implied a new way of thinking about disease—based upon research that emphasized interior processes and conditions. "As autopsies became routine," one historian tells us, "the causes of illness came to be seen concretely in the tumors, abscesses, ulcers, inflammations, and hemorrhages located *inside* the body."[9] Monuments to this new clinical "gaze" (as Foucault calls it) are familiar to students of French medicine. They include the free instruction in clinical surgery provided by Desault in the large amphitheater he obtained at the Hôtel-Dieu; Pinel's studies of mental illness, designed to reveal correlations

For two essays—relevant to Sade—on medical views of erotic passion, see Christine Birnbaum, "La vision médicale de l'amour dans *L'Encyclopédie,*" in *Aimer en France 1760–1860,* ed. Paul Viallaneix and Jean Ehrard, 2 vols. (Clermont-Ferrand: Association des publications de la Faculté des lettres et sciences humaines de Clermont-Ferrand, 1980), 2:307–313; and Paul Hoffmann, "Le discours médical sur les passions de l'amour, de Boissier de Sauvages à Pinel," in *Aimer en France,* ed. Vaillaneix and Ehrard, 2:345–356.

9. Vess, *Medical Revolution in France,* 189, italics added.

between human passions and physiology; Bichat's systematic study of tissue, which altered medical thinking about internal organs and helped to found the science of histology. Even—however utopian it sounds—the closing of all French medical schools between 1792 and 1794, as well as the practical demands of wartime medicine in the years following the Revolution, contributed to a major change in French medicine. Paris, during Sade's long imprisonment, surpassed both Leiden and Edinburgh as the international center of new medical knowledge.

The penetrating gaze of the clinic offers more than a complex metaphor for the demystifying, unmasking tendencies of Enlightenment thought, in which Sade participated so fiercely. Clinical medicine not only brought new facts to light but also undertook a complete reorganization of the system linking the visible body to its invisible sources of illness. With the new system of relations between body and disease, between the seen and the unseen, comes as well a new system of language. As Foucault puts it: "The new medical spirit to which Bichat is no doubt the first to bear witness in an absolutely coherent way cannot be ascribed to an act of psychological and epistemological purification"—as if simply better facts or improved modes of observation were sufficient. "It is," Foucault continues, "nothing [less] than a syntactical reorganization of disease in which the limits of the visible and invisible follow a new pattern; the abyss beneath illness, which was the illness itself, has emerged into the light of language—the same light, no doubt, that illuminates the *120 Journées de Sodome* [and] *Juliette*."[10] Sade in effect renders what was previously unseen, hidden, or suppressed suddenly—if grotesquely—visible.

Foucault's emphasis on a new visibility—characterized by the emblematic "gaze" of clinical medicine—sometimes obscures his equally important discussion of nonvisual (linguistic or auditory) changes. While Sade certainly exposes to view sexual practices traditionally unseen and unrepresented, he also shares the spirit animating contemporary French medicine in his passion for organized, analytical speech. As Roland

10. *The Birth of the Clinic: An Archaeology of Medical Perception* (1963), trans. A. M. Sheridan Smith (New York: Pantheon Books, 1973), 195. Various historians of medicine and historians of science, in reviews and in footnotes, point out inaccuracies in Foucault's facts or interpretations and criticize his method of writing history, but his book remains a powerful account of well-documented changes in Enlightenment medical theory and practice. For an explanation of Foucault's approach, see Hubert L. Dreyfus and Paul Rabinow, *Michel Foucault: Beyond Structuralism and Hermeneutics* (Chicago: University of Chicago Press, 1982), 3–15.

Barthes has shown, Sadean novels employ language as a means for dividing characters, practices, even space itself into previously unsuspected categories. Sexuality finds simultaneously both a new speech and a new system, much as Sade's *120 Days of Sodom* proposes to take its structure from a sweeping fourfold reclassification of sexual passions into the simple, the complex, the criminal, and the murderous, while at the same time imparting to a generally chaotic and mute region of human experience almost a reinvented language: an organized, computational, repetitive, exhaustive speech that in some sense constitutes a wholly revised rhetoric and grammar of sexuality. (Homosexual passion instantly loses in Sade its traditional linguistic status as "that which cannot be named.") It seems incorrect to interpret Sade's unending discursiveness as merely pathological (logorrhea), the sign of obsession, imprisonment, and illness. In a spirit suggesting that literature, like science, must find a speech equivalent to its newly magnified powers of vision, Juliette explains at the end of the enormous novel that bears her name: "It is necessary for philosophy to say everything."[11]

Sade (as his critics too often forget) is not a philosopher but a novelist. That is, despite the evident philosophical ambitions of his characters, we go wrong in seeking to extract from their speech a consistent, monological doctrine we can name "Sade's philosophy." A philosophy that seeks to say everything is, in the first place, impossible. Further, in favoring the inclusiveness of rhetoric as opposed to the exclusions of traditional philosophy, Sade's novels surround his monomaniacal reasoners with a verbal context in which no one ever has the last word. (Victims must be replaced immediately—or revived—so that the discourse may go on.) Finally, in the attempt to say everything, in transgressing every bound of bourgeois decency, Sade extends language into realms where the suppressed and the unspoken border on the unspeakable. The issue is no

11. "La philosophie doit tout dire" (*L'histoire de Juliette* [1797], in *Œuvres complètes* 9:586). Austryn Wainhouse, in his Grove Press translation, renders Juliette's words as follows: "Philosophy must never shrink from speaking out." In one sense, to say "everything" implies a refusal to suppress unwelcome facts or to shrink from speaking. I suspect, however, a more radical sense appropriate to Sade's conclusion in which by saying everything philosophy approaches the scandalous possibilities of rhetoric—a rhetoric that abandons its traditional link with ethics in favor of exploring the limits of whatever can be said on any topic, such as sexuality. This "rhetorical" philosophy—in saying everything—would coincide with Sade's relentless attack on the foundations of traditional metaphysics, as well as expressing what he called "a mobility [*mobilité*] in my opinions which reflects my innermost manner of thought" (*Correspondance*, in *Œuvres complètes* 12:505). On Sadean extravagance, both verbal and nonverbal, see Marcel Hénaff, "Tout dire ou l'encyclopédie de l'excès," *Obliques* 12–13 (1977): 29–37.

longer whether obscenity will be allowed the freedom to speak its (partial) truths. Such truths remain speakable and thinkable. Sade also employs the obscene as a means for exploring man's participation in an irrationality that goes beyond speech and thought, revealing its traces in the horror that ordinarily deprives us of language. Sade, who confessed to an extreme "mobility" or irresolution in his opinions and innermost thoughts, cannot offer a coherent philosophy of the unspeakable. Rather, engaging the resources of widely different systems and modes of speech, he employs language in such a way as to emphasize the conflict and opacity that occur when normally separate discourses intersect. In place of a philosophical language for penetrating the unspeakable, he provides instead a laminated style that refuses to let us ignore and deny what we do not understand. His words force us to confront a darkness more impenetrable than the inside of the human body.

The broad parallels linking Sadean novels with a new medical speech and gaze—however seductive to students of literature and medicine—cannot of course establish patterns of direct influence. Instead, they do something equally valuable in providing a context within which more specific studies of medical and of literary relations may assume a larger significance. Historically, the understanding of pain has often fallen to the two widely diverse social practices we call literature and medicine. Nonetheless, quite often and for long periods medical and literary discourses on pain seem to occupy divided and mutually indifferent territories. In Sade's work, we encounter a moment when literature and medicine converge—under the pressure of late-eighteenth-century culture—and then, explosively, fly apart. The explosion (as Sade transvalues medical knowledge for his own purposes) is no less illuminating than the convergence. What Sade makes of pain—the meanings he both discovers and ascribes—might be said to invert or turn inside out every humanitarian impulse of Enlightenment thought, impulses especially pertinent to the progress in medical knowledge and treatment, as if Sade rigorously pursued a denial of human norms so complete that it amounts to what Georges Bataille rightly calls a quest for "the impossible and the *reverse* of life."[12]

Pain in Sade's writing is notoriously associated with its traditional opposite, pleasure. As important and far less obvious, however, is the Sadean bond that unites pain with truth. Sade is never more at home in

12. *Literature and Evil* (1957), trans. Alastair Hamilton (London: Calder and Boyars, 1973), 98.

the Enlightenment than when he joins the unmasking philosophers who sought to demystify every form of intellectual humbug, but he immediately resumes his isolated stance in equating truth (a specifically masculine version of truth) with physical pain. The libertine monk Clément argues in *Justine*: "There is no more lively sensation than that of pain; its impressions are certain and dependable, they never deceive as may those of the pleasure women perpetually feign and almost never experience."[13] An almost identical argument, with its implicit phallocentric anxieties, appears in Sade's companion novel, *Juliette*, where the arch libertine Saint-Fond declares: "I've never cared much about seeing pleasure's lineaments writ over a woman's countenance. They're too equivocal, too unsure; I prefer the signs of pain, which are more dependable by far."[14] These passages suggest that there is more to the libertine obsession with pain than an exotic, eccentric, sexual taste. Pain not only affirms (a clearly uncertain) male superiority and mastery. It also assumes the character of a sign-system that—in contrast with the slipperiness attributed to language and to appearances (no doubt to women as well)—establishes a direct, if limited, correspondence with truth. It communicates an authenticity that Sade's libertine heroes and heroines see everywhere eluding them in a world dominated by deceit, custom, equivocation, timidity, and ignorance. Here, pain for Sade has already absorbed a range of meaning that distinguishes it from merely random agonies or from meaningless sensation. Already we have entered the unstable realm of Sadean transvaluations, where familiar words and actions take on unfamiliar significance, even as libertine sexual pleasure adopts the unexpected vocabulary of screams and rage. It is a realm where medicine too cannot remain unchanged.

Medicine in fact assumes in Sade's work an appearance and function very different from what ancient or modern psychiatry might lead us to expect. Although sadism now belongs securely to the lexicon of sexual pathology, explained through theories of childhood trauma, passive-aggressive behavior, fears of impotence, repression, or a reversal of the death wish, sexuality in Sade's work is never annexed to illness, whether

13. *Justine*, trans. Seaver and Wainhouse, 606/3:206. There are three separate versions of *Justine*, which was first published in 1791. (The earliest version, entitled *Les infortunes de la vertu*, Sade composed in 1787; the vastly expanded final version, entitled *La nouvelle Justine*, was published in 1797.) Except once where indicated, I have employed the 1791 version, because it is most accessible—in several translations—to Anglo-American readers.

14. Trans. Austryn Wainhouse (New York: Grove Press, 1968), 362/8:350. The libertine hero Dolmancé asserts in *Philosophy in the Bedroom:* "pain must be preferred, for pain's telling effects cannot deceive" (252/3:436).

organic or psychological. Indeed, Sade's refusal to regard even the most abnormal or self-destructive sexual behavior as illness directly opposes the medical and political wisdom of his own day, which diagnosed his condition as "sexual dementia" and decreed that his final years be spent with the mad patients incarcerated at the Asylum of Charenton. But if Sade obstinately refuses to follow medicine in linking sexual aberration with illness, he also practices the independence of Enlightenment thought in rejecting the immemorial, church-authorized bond yoking sexuality to childbirth. As Angela Carter has observed, Sade anticipates our own era of unprecedented sexual revolution, when pleasure has abandoned its former (imperfect but inescapable) unity with biological reproduction.[15] To the libertine mind, pregnancy is intolerable, except as infants or pregnant women excite new breakthroughs in cruelty. It is common for Sade's most discriminating male libertines to renounce all contact—even visual contact—with the vagina. ("Your authentic sodomist," explains Juliette, "will always come unerect at the sight of a cunt.")[16] Male libertines not only prefer male partners. Their preference expresses a desire to affirm that sexuality must be not merely infertile but consciously sterile. Thus, in affirming a sexuality that is overwhelmingly anal, excremental, and bloody, the Sadean libertine follows a logic that leads from the denial of procreation to an embracement of death. Sexuality finds its temporary fulfillment for Sade not in childbirth but in repeated acts of destruction, with murder redefined as an unjustly suppressed form of eroticism.

The absence of expected biomedical contexts in Sade's work—the void where illness and childbirth might normally appear—provides a useful background against which his transvaluations of medical knowledge stand out as visible, crucial components of the libertine system.

15. *The Sadeian Woman and the Ideology of Pornography* (New York: Pantheon Books, 1978), introductory note. Carter takes the position that Sadean pornography serves women indirectly by its exposure of a phallocentric social structure, by its stripping away the mask of romance to reveal the sexual politics implicit in male-female relations. In her feminist reading of Sade as a critique of bourgeois, male-centered ideology, Carter shares Susan Sontag's conviction that "the pornographic imagination says something worth listening to, albeit in a degraded and often unrecognizable form" ("The Pornographic Imagination," in *Styles of Radical Will* [New York: Farrar, Straus and Giroux, 1966], 70). Other feminist critics deny pornography what Sontag calls "its peculiar access to some truth" (70–71) and regard it mainly as reflecting and promoting the oppression of women. See, for example, Laura Lederer, ed., *Take Back the Night: Women on Pornography* (New York: William Morrow, 1980), and Susan Griffin, *Pornography and Silence: Culture's Revenge against Nature* (New York: Harper and Row, 1981).

16. *Juliette,* trans. Wainhouse, 681/9:87.

"System," as a term applied to the views of Sadean libertines, does not refer to a tight, interlocking grid of clear and distinct ideas, held together by logic and constituting a coherent whole. The unsystematic libertine system depends on each individual's rigorous and total commitment to self-interest, so that reason serves a purely instrumental function in promoting the arguments of desire. Once, when fearing prosecution, Sade argued with startling lucidity—pursuing a stylistic analysis any literary critic may envy for its precision—that he could not possibly be the author of *Justine*.[17] Desire in effect performs a faultless impersonation of reason. In similarly advancing their own interests, Sade's libertines assert a wide variety of dubious (if apparently reasonable) claims, some false, self-contradictory, or in conflict with the views of other libertines. Such disparate views do not add up to a homogeneous system of logic but rather reflect a heterogeneous system of discourse, in which the need to "say everything" (which Juliette attributes to this new "philosophy") in practice authorizes saying almost anything—violating the prohibitions that bind us not only to decorum but also to reason and consistency. The force that briefly holds Sade's anarchistic libertines together is not genuine friendship or the fraternity of criminals; nor can they depend on tacit or formal codes of mutual nonaggression, which fail to survive occasions when desire, whim, or self-interest turns one libertine against another. What truly binds them together, fleetingly but repeatedly, is their need to speak endlessly about deeds and desires that would mean nothing if forbidden such verbal disclosure. (If other libertines are not present, the victim must serve the role of listener/respondent, rescuing speech from pointless monologue.) The libertine system is finally a system of speech, to which medicine makes an indispensable contribution.

The most important contribution that medicine makes to Sade's novels is in supplying what the characters invoke as a scientific physiology of pleasure and pain. Sade's physiological accounts of pain do more (as we will soon see) than merely provide an instrument for silencing or for refuting traditional moral and religious explanations. Sade initiates his transformations of medical knowledge by reversing the durable custom in medicine—evident as far back as in the ancient Hippocratic writings—that assigns pain the secondary status of a symptom. In enlarging or aggrandizing the status of pain, Sade follows the same narrative logic that permits him—while banishing midwives from a world of

17. "Note concerning My Detention," in *Justine . . . and Other Writings*, trans. Seaver and Wainhouse, 152–154/15:26–29.

marathon copulations—to sacrifice literary realism to the demands of libertine desire. Like the parricidal giant Minski in *Juliette,* whose penis (measuring eighteen inches long by sixteen in circumference) stays permanently erect, Sade's exaggerations refuse to obey the laws of normal science whenever science threatens to obscure the overriding laws of the erotic life.

Sade, quite clearly, rejects or ignores the medical tradition that regards pain as a symptom. Although its status as a symptom assures pain an important place within medicine, its importance is mainly instrumental, like the informer who tips off the police. Pain as a symptom may be forgotten or dismissed by the physician as soon as its instrumental service is over, and until very recently the history of medical interest in pain centers on the search for effective anesthetic and analgesic agents, where understanding pain is less urgent than annihilating or suspending it. Sade not only shows no interest in pain as a symptom; on the contrary, like Albrecht von Haller, whose studies of "irritability" (which he demonstrated experimentally to be a specific property of muscles causing them to contract) soon encouraged expansive ontological and theological speculations, Sade elevates pain from its secondary, instrumental status within medicine to the central position accorded basic laws of nature.

The centrality that Sade assigns to pain finds an illuminating parallel in the work of another influential late-eighteenth-century thinker, who otherwise might seem Sade's opposite. Jeremy Bentham—like Sade, born in the 1740s—brought an almost Sadean passion for reason and for enumeration to the un-Sadean goal of eradicating the irrational, both in man and in social structures. His *Principles of Morals and Legislation* (1789), while it seeks to construct a social theory rendering impossible or obsolete the abuses celebrated in Sade's dark libertine utopias, nonetheless begins from a premise that Sade would wholly accept. As Bentham declares in his first sentence: "Nature has placed mankind under the governance of two sovereign masters, *pain* and *pleasure.* It is for them alone to point out what we ought to do, as well as to determine what we shall do." This rigorous dualism of pleasure and pain, which Bentham treats as secure and indisputable, comes in Sade's work to lose its distinctness, but both Bentham and Sade start from the same point in developing their very different visions of the consequences that follow from our commitment to pleasure and pain. Pain is no longer (as in classical philosophy) subordinated to pleasure, reduced to the pedagogic office of enforcing virtuous conduct. In its centrality, pain *determines* what shall be called virtue or vice, an insight that leads Sade's libertine heroes to reject such conventional moral categories as simply a manner of speech.

Ignored as the symptom of temporary dysfunction and dismissed as the chastising pedagogue of traditional ethics, pain for Sade emerges in a new and primary role as coextensive with the truth of the body. Pain, that is, informs us truly about the state of the body. Further, this information gains immeasurable importance because the body's truth comes to define the limits of whatever Sade holds as true. It is, in effect, the sole truth in a world where every other foundation of knowledge ultimately dissolves into falsehood or uncertainty. Thus, even though Sade thoroughly alters the status of pain within medicine, medicine provides him with the knowledge indispensable for understanding the truth of the body. Sometimes this truth reflects little more than the general Enlightenment fascination with the discovery of natural facts, disentangled from theological corruptions or learned error. Medicine, for example, holds a purely positive, demystifying function in *Philosophy in the Bedroom,* where the willing ingenue Eugénie—as an introduction to her ensuing libertine education—receives a lecture in male and female anatomy, which might have come directly from a medical textbook (or indirectly from a medical textbook, through the libertine tradition in which such anatomy lectures were a recurrent narrative device). Here again Sade typically converts medicine from a healing and instructive art to an erotic practice. He seems to have understood a sense in which the penetrating gaze holds sexual as well as medical implications. As in the modern soap opera, sexuality and medicine prove inextricably entangled.

The Enlightenment emphasis upon medicine as a science—a practice grounded in experiment and in observable fact—proves fundamentally equivocal in Sade's work. Science matters to the libertine mind mainly as it permits or advances sexual practices that depend on cruelty. Thus the vivisection common to French medical experiments on animals reappears in Sade's work as a technique for generating pleasure. In *Justine* the libertine surgeon Rodin, an eminent technologist who extols "the progress of science," discovers in the probing, cutting, agonizing penetrations of (pre-anesthetic) surgery a lure that proves wholly erotic. When Rodin asserts that the science of anatomy will never reach its "ultimate state of perfection" until he has examined a child of fourteen or fifteen who has died a cruel death, experienced readers of Sade know instantly that this high-minded passion for scientific progress conceals a sexual aim and that the victim of Rodin's excited, protracted vivisection will be his own beautiful daughter.[18] Reduced to a mechanical technology for penetrating the body, medicine serves the libertine world less for relieving pain than for inflicting it. Like the ghoulish aristocrat in *Justine* who manages to achieve orgasm only by repeatedly bleeding his young wife in a vampirish simulation of phlebotomy, Sade's libertines find their ultimate erotic stimulation in blood, which is transformed from medical fact to sexual marker. The balms that miraculously restore Justine and other long-suffering victims of libertinage belong not to Enlightenment pharmacology but to primitive traditions of magic, where drugs are among the standard accoutrement of eroticism. Their Sadean purpose is simply to prepare the victim for new episodes of sexual pain.

The same process of transvaluation in Sade's work that renders medicine erotic also helps to eroticize and to medicalize pain. The most significant result of this process is not the pornographic description that it makes possible. (Sade, of course, did not invent erotic cruelty but rather refined and elaborated it within the contours of his libertine system.)[19] Placing pain within a medical context offers Sade the insuperable advantage of thereby silencing and effectively refuting other discourses traditionally concerned with human suffering. In Sade, as in American courtrooms and hospitals, medicine has a tendency to overrule or to dominate alternative systems of thought, so that priest and judge defer to the wisdom of medical testimony. Because medicine in Sade carries the authority of Enlightenment science, it breaks free from the

18. *Justine,* trans. Seaver and Wainhouse, 551–552/3:150–151. Rodin's libertine accomplice remarks concerning the human victims required by medical science: "In those hospitals where I worked as a young man I saw similar experiments by the thousand" (552/3:151).

19. On cultural and literary contexts relevant to Sadean eroticism, see Robert P. Maccubbin, ed., *Unauthorized Sexual Behavior during the Enlightenment* (Williamsburg, Va.: College of William and Mary, 1985), a special issue of the journal *Eighteenth-Century Life* (9, n.s. 3), reissued under the title *'Tis Nature's Fault: Unauthorized Sexuality during the Enlightenment* (Cambridge: Cambridge University Press, 1987); Boucé, *Sexuality in Eighteenth-Century Britain*; Ann Thomson, "L'art de jouir de La Mettrie à Sade," in *Aimer en France,* ed. Viallaneix and Ehrard, 2:315–322; and Aram Vartanian, "La Mettrie, Diderot, and Sexology in the Enlightenment," in *Essays on the Age of Enlightenment in Honor of Ira O. Wade,* ed. Jean Macary (Geneva: Librairie Droz, 1977), 347–367. (Two studies forthcoming are *Sexual Underworlds of the Enlightenment,* ed. G. S. Rousseau and Roy Porter [Manchester: Manchester University Press] and Peter Wagner's *Eros Revived: Erotica in the Age of Enlightenment* [London: Secker and Warburg].) Although now outdated, *The Romantic Agony* by Mario Praz (trans. Angus Davidson, 2d ed. [New York: Oxford University Press, 1951]) was revolutionary and influential when it first appeared. Praz, of course, has much to say about Sade.

literary heritage that portrays the doctor as a greedy quack. Indeed, Sade's libertine surgeon Rodin is an anti-quack: a wealthy man-of-science whose reasoning is formidable. In its relentless appeal to the facts of human anatomy and physiology, medicine as Sade employs it thoroughly displaces the more speculative discussions of pain that had been a traditional employment of philosophers and theologians. The Sadean libertine ultimately empties virtue and vice (or sin and innocence) of their familiar content in classical and Christian writing, where our attraction to pleasure and aversion from pain seem changeless, natural, God-given responses that provide a foundation for the ethical life. In one sense, Sade exposes the unforeseen conclusions that follow from a Benthamite reliance upon pleasure and pain as a philosophical bedrock for ethics. In another sense, all traditional foundations crumble in Sade when virtue and vice are redefined as cultural artifacts characterized by their greater or lesser powers to stimulate the nervous system. Medicine, as various Enlightenment *philosophes* had predicted, now gives direction to philosophical thought.

Theology fares even worse than philosophy at the hands of Sade's libertine medicine. The voluminous Christian meditations on human suffering might be said to take their origin from the iconography of the cross and from the prophetic words of Isaiah: "With his pain we are healed" (54:4). Pain in Augustinian theology enters the world with original sin, but Christian pain is ultimately redemptive. Christ suffers so that man might find eternal life. The body suffers in order that the soul might be saved. Sade's contemptuous and relentless assault on Christianity as "incompatible with the libertarian system" includes his parodic transvaluation of Christian attitudes toward redemptive suffering.[20] In fact, his fullest response to this pervasive Christian reading of pain is simply the plot of *Justine*. The innocent Justine's faith in God and her love of virtue are the qualities that generate each new episode of outrage and violence, as if the novel—far from reflecting picaresque randomness—were a demonstration in logic. Sade contrives Justine's imitation of Christ to establish the absence of redemptive suffering. The world that she encounters inside the church mirrors exactly the libertine cruelties that she meets everywhere else. There is no inside, no outside. Even

20. *Philosophy in the Bedroom,* trans. Seaver and Wainhouse, 301/3:483. Among numerous studies of the relation between pain and theology, see especially C. S. Lewis, *The Problem of Pain* (1940: reprint, New York: Macmillan, 1944); John Bowker, *Problems of Suffering in Religions of the World* (Cambridge: Cambridge University Press, 1970); and David Bakan, *Disease, Pain, and Sacrifice: Toward a Psychology of Suffering* (Chicago: University of Chicago Press, 1968).

when she escapes from the debauched monks at St. Mary-in-the-Wood, Justine simply encounters their doubles wherever she turns.

Sade's equivocal representation of Enlightenment medicine mirrors an ambivalence in his treatment of Christianity. It is possible that Sadean atheism—so vocal and jubilant as to undermine its own claims—expresses (as Pierre Klossowski has argued) his unacknowledged need for God.[21] It is certain that Christianity contains for Sade, as if despite itself, a hidden ground for affirmation. What Sade affirms in Christianity is not its doctrines but its historical concern with pain, from original sin, martyrdom, and self-flagellation to inquisitorial torture and the torment of the damned. The final episode of *120 Days of Sodom* thus provides a culminating image of Sade's secular transvaluation of Christianity in the horrifying erotic carnage of a pastime called "The Hell Game"—complete with impersonated demons and agonized sinners. By comparison, the parody of Christian pain in *Justine* seems oblique and almost subtle. In Sade's work, theology—like philosophy—provides only a mocking, empty, archaic language for interpreting pain, no match for the up-to-date physiology of nerve impulses and electrical fluids. As Justine suffers each new excruciating episode of sexual abuse, her suffering leads nowhere, illuminates nothing, redeems no one.

Sade's transvaluations of medical knowledge will grow clearer if we focus upon two specific passages from *Juliette* and *Justine*. The first brings us openly to a question at the heart of Sade's work. How is it, asks the libertine statesman Saint-Fond, that we arrive at pleasure through the sight of others undergoing pain and, stranger still, through suffering pain ourselves? To this central problem in Sade's fiction—which might seem so complex as to evoke cloudbanks of obscure evasions—Saint-Fond's fellow libertine Noirceuil delivers an absolutely explicit reply. Like similar demystifying exercises of Enlightenment reason, it begins by citing the error it proposes to unmask, quoted in the exact words of the Port-Royal Jansenist theologian Pierre Nicole:

> "Pain, logically defined, is nothing other than a sentiment of hostility in the soul toward the body it animates, the which it signifies through certain movements that conflict with the body's physical organization." So says Nicole, who perceived in man an ethereal substance, which he called soul, and which he differentiated from the material substance we call body. I, however, who will have none of this frivolous stuff and who consider man as something on the order of an absolutely material plant, I shall simply

21. Pierre Klossowski, *Sade mon prochain* (Paris: Seuil, 1947).

> say that pain is the consequence of a defective relationship between objects foreign to us and the organic molecules composing us; in such wise that instead of composing harmoniously with those that make up our neural fluids, as they do in the commotion of pleasure, the atoms emanating from these foreign objects strike them aslant, crookedly, sting them, repulse them, and never fuse with them. Still, though the effects are negative, they are effects nonetheless, and whether it be pleasure or pain brewing in us, you will always have a certain impact upon the neural fluids.[22]

Although Noirceuil and Nicole are both French, they speak in effect two different languages. Noirceuil's confident talk of atoms, organic molecules, and neural fluids—however garbled by the standards of twentieth-century science—represents an effort to silence theology by invoking as a superior or superseding discourse the empirical language of Enlightenment medicine. Behind their use of these two distinct languages or systems of discourse stand two utterly opposed visions of man. Nicole's theological paradigm of pain requires the concept of an eternal, immaterial soul at odds with a material, ephemeral body. By contrast, for Noirceuil pain becomes the occasion for asserting a materialism so comprehensive that it denies substantial differences separating bodies from minds or souls. As another libertine philosopher explains: "All we attribute to the soul is all simply the effect of matter."[23]

The word "soul" sounds particularly strange on the lips of Sade's atheistical libertines because they have redefined it in ways that drain off its traditional attributes. Descartes, for example, despite his innovations, essentially followed religious tradition in preserving an absolute difference between bodies (*res extensa*) and souls (*res cogitans*). For Descartes, body is material, ephemeral, mechanical, and unthinking, while soul is immaterial, immortal, conscious, and defined by its power of thought. For Sade's libertines there is no gap between body and soul. Sometimes, in fact, the soul itself simply disappears, swallowed up in matter. As Juliette's libertine instructor Delbène reports: "I am not aware of having any soul. . . . It is the body which feels, which thinks, which judges, which suffers, which enjoys." Here is a peculiarly modern solution to the mind/body problem. The problem simply dissolves into a comfortable monism. "Body and soul," Delbène continues, "they are one."[24] As in La Mettrie, the monism of body and soul in Sade's work is

22. Trans. Wainhouse, 267/8:255–256.

23. *Juliette*, trans. Wainhouse, 386/8:372.

24. *Juliette*, trans. Wainhouse, 44, 50/8:52, 59. Thinking (*cogitans*) is of course the defining function of the soul for Descartes. Delbène's assertion reflects the process by which soul came to be supplanted in eighteenth-century discussions by the mind. This transition

dynamic—not fixed or static—in the sense that different temperaments and different activities call forth a changing ratio in the relations between spirit and flesh. Still, Sade's libertines move in a world where everything—including minds or souls—is material. All belong to the same continuous moil and turmoil of molecular change.

Descartes's views on pain offer a particularly good contrast in helping to clarify the absolute materialism of Sade's libertines. For Descartes, soul alone is what gives us the ability to feel pain. Although the mechanical network of nerves (transporting the equally material animal spirits) allows the body to relay information automatically to and from the brain, Descartes emphasized that we do not *feel* pain—that is, we do not experience pain *consciously*—until the mechanical, neural impulse is communicated to the pineal gland, which he notoriously designated as the point where the material body intersects with the immaterial soul. Only when the thinking soul perceives what the mechanical responses of the nervous system tell it do we experience the feeling of pain. The evidence for this view Descartes drew in part from the puzzling phenomenon of phantom limb pain, in which amputees report painful cramps in a missing hand or arm or leg. This pain, Descartes reasoned, could not reside in the missing limb and must therefore exist in the mind or soul alone. Buttressed by traditional Christian doctrine, Descartes's argument led him to the extreme conclusion that animals feel no pain. He recognized, of course, that animals exhibit all the normal behavior *associated* with pain, for such signs belong simply to the mechanism of the body. Animals, however, because (by definition) they do not possess minds or souls, cannot in Descartes's view feel or experience pain. Pain for Descartes thus offers a privileged example for confirming the absolute dualism of soul and body. Sade in effect captures pain as his privileged counterexample for implicitly disputing Cartesian dualism and for discarding the immaterial soul as a Scholastic illusion.

Pain as it concerns nerve fibers and neural fluids—not the welfare of an immaterial soul or the effects of original sin—is the explicit subject of a second passage I wish to examine, from the novel *Justine*. Here again we can observe how medicine functions for Sade in providing a language opposed to the discourse of theology, but it is the erotic implications of his dryly technical language that deserve special attention. The passage, which appears as a note attached to a speech by Justine's libertine tempt-

from soul to mind is part of John O. Lyons's subject in *The Invention of the Self: The Hinge of Consciousness in the Eighteenth Century* (Carbondale: Southern Illinois University Press, 1978).

ress Dubois, sounds less like novelistic talk than like textbook physiology and opens with a hyperbole typical of Sade, which perhaps only an anatomist could take seriously:

> There is no part of the human body more interesting than the nerve. . . . Life and indeed the entire harmony of the body as a machine depend on the nerves. From them come sensations and pleasures, thoughts and ideas; they constitute, briefly, the center of the whole human structure. The soul is located there, that is to say the principle of life, which dies out among animals, which grows and declines in them, and is by consequence wholly material.
>
> The nerves are imagined to be tubes destined to carry the animal spirits into the organs to which they are distributed and to report back to the brain the impressions of external objects on these organs.

Let me interrupt the passage to make two brief comments. First, the word translated here (and generally in Sade) as "pain" is "*la douleur.*" "*Douleur*" retains its traditional contrast with "*peine*" (also translated as "pain"), which implies physical injury or indefinite harm with no accompanying mental or emotional anguish. It is precisely the mental and emotional suffering of their victims—which includes the victims' awareness of their victimization—that makes Sade's libertines vastly prefer *douleur* to *peine.* Second, in defining the soul as the "principle of life" Sade remains securely within the boundaries of libertine materialism. There is no real difference—merely a change in vocabulary—between Noirceuil's vision of man as an "absolutely material plant" and the view, expressed in Sade's note, that the body is a "machine" animated by a life force. (Again, La Mettrie could provide Sade with a source for *both* metaphors: each pointing toward the same restrictive range of meaning.) In other writers, the metaphorical shift from machine to plant might well reflect conceptual changes important to medical and scientific controversies of the time, measuring the distance separating an older, strictly mechanistic physiology from the newer, vitalist physiology centered in Montpellier; in Sade's hands, however, both metaphors—plant and machine—equally serve to exclude the possibility of an immaterial spirit that survives independent of the body.[25]

25. The movement from a mechanistic to a vitalist-dynamic physiology—in which the nervous system is understood not as a lifeless machine but as a point of contact (controversial, it goes without saying) between body and soul/mind—is discussed by Robert E. Schofield, *Mechanism and Materialism: British Natural Philosophy in an Age of Reason* (Princeton: Princeton University Press, 1970). On this change, see also two studies by Theodore M. Brown: "From Mechanism to Vitalism in Eighteenth-Century English Physiology," *Journal of the History of Biology* 7 (1974): 179–216, and *The Mechanical Philosophy and the*

Sade's abandonment of the Christian and Cartesian immaterial soul is unmistakable as the note continues. Whether we attribute the note to author, character, or impersonated editor, its physiological language explains that the nervous system alone provides everything necessary to account for the experience of pleasure and pain:

> An intense inflammation excites to an extraordinary degree the animal spirits that flow into the nerve tubes which, in turn, induce pleasure. If the inflammation occurs on the genitals or nearby parts, this explains the pleasures imparted by blows, stabbings, pinches or floggings. From the extreme influence of the mental on the physical comes likewise the painful or agreeable shock of the animal spirits, by reason of the mental sensation one receives. From all this it follows that with such principles and philosophy—with the total annihilation of prejudice—one can extend unbelievably (as we have said elsewhere) the sphere of one's sensations.[26]

This passage does not contain the sort of writing that immediately springs to mind when someone mentions Sade, yet it is almost as typical of Sadean narrative as scenes of sexual cruelty. Sadean eroticism establishes its difference from unreflective violence—violence unconscious of its own nature—by insisting upon the replacement of antiquated theological doctrine with up-to-date, physiological fact.

Fact, we should recognize, plays a different role in Sadean narrative from that which it plays in scientific and medical writing. Thus the reader who seeks to extract a single, self-consistent Sadean physiology will go wrong exactly in the manner of readers seeking a unified, self-consistent Sadean philosophy. Sade's characters employ—and frequently mix—elements drawn from quite different systems of physiology. Pain may be explained with reference to stinging atoms, to excited animal spirits, to stretched nerve fibers, to irritated tissue. There is some reason for feeling that Sade has brewed up a gigantic, simmering soup

"*Animal Economy*" (New York: Arno Press, 1981). For France and Europe, see Jacques Roger, *Les sciences de la vie dans la pensée française du XVIIIe siècle: La génération des animaux de Descartes à l'Encyclopédie* (Paris: Armand Colin, 1963); Thomas S. Hall, *Ideas of Life and Matter: Studies in the History of General Physiology, 600 B.C.–1900 A.D.*, 2 vols. (Chicago: University of Chicago Press, 1969); Elizabeth L. Haigh, "Vitalism, the Soul, and Sensibility: The Physiology of Théophile Bordeu," *Journal of the History of Medicine and Allied Sciences* 31 (1976): 30–41; and Sergio Moravia, "From *Homme Machine* to *Homme Sensible*: Changing Eighteenth-Century Models of Man's Image," *Journal of the History of Ideas* 39 (1978): 45–60.

26. *La nouvelle Justine; ou, Les malheurs de la vertu*, in *Œuvres complètes* 7:108–109, translation mine. G. S. Rousseau cites this passage and notes the provenance in d'Holbach (see "Nymphomania, Bienville and the Rise of Erotic Sensibility," 111–112).

of fact in which pieces borrowed from widely disparate sources—early and late—float around together in suspension. What matters to Sade is not whether his characters have access to a final truth of science (too many questions are still in doubt) but whether their facts support a demystified vision of man. The passage we have just encountered, for example, might have come nearly verbatim from the celebrated encyclopedist, philosopher, atheist, and materialist d'Holbach. The exact source of Sade's facts, however, is far less important than their implications within his vastly heterogeneous narrative texture. When we examine what "follows" from the often mixed-up facts of Sadean physiology, it will soon be clear that the now antiquated vocabulary of hollow nerve tubes and of racing animal spirits entailed serious—even deadly—consequences.

Pain belongs at the center of Sadean eroticism because, as I have suggested, it serves as a comprehensive metaphor for truth. The truth that it affirms, however, appears from the perspective of theology or of ordinary life to be simply outrage, perversion, and scandalous error. As Georges Bataille writes of Sade: "He went as far as the imagination allows: there was nothing respectable which he did not mock, nothing pure which he did not soil, nothing joyful which he did not frighten."[27] Sade's truth is in effect the negation of beliefs so basic to normal human life that we regard them as self-evidently true. The only self-evident truth in Sade's world, however, is the truth of the body, and it is pain that serves as spokesman for the body's truth. Pain for Sade is what we cannot deny, cannot evade, cannot forswear, while pleasure inevitably deceives, rhetoric beguiles, and logic unweaves its own constructions with the cunning of a false Penelope.

The truth of the body is, of course, exactly what Enlightenment medicine undertook to disclose, finding its most potent instrument and symbol in the newly routine practice of autopsy. Yet, Sade did not stop with the eroticized versions of anatomy and surgery we have seen him employ. Biomedical learning also provided crucial support for his explorations into previously unexplored areas of human sexual behavior, where the truth of the body makes itself known as desire. Pornography, of course, is an ancient and mostly superficial art dedicated to the description of sexual acts. Before Sade, however, never in the history of the novel had a writer employed the license of pornography to create such a blinding, exhaustive vision of desire freed from its normal social

27. *Literature and Evil,* trans. Hamilton, 99.

constraints. The truth of desire for Sade leads both through and beyond the description of sexual acts to a comprehensive yet flexible system in which bodies, minds, and politics are complexly interlocked. If we follow the sequence leading from body to mind to politics, we will be better prepared to understand how Sade employs pain as the ultimate figure of desire.

The body constitutes for Sade not just the indispensable locus of sexual behavior but, far more important, the force that defines and determines our sexuality. Thus Sade's work posits as a central dogma that we live out a sexual destiny imposed not by God, not by gender, not by culture, but solely by the nerves and tissues of our individual bodies. He once wrote to his wife that his outrageous manner of thought "holds with my existence" (as he put it): "with the way I am made."[28] Perhaps the best gloss on this slightly enigmatic statement is the explanation that the Count du Bressac offers Justine in discussing the libertine preference for anal sex. Here too we find physiology providing a discourse opposed to a more traditional language. The Count begins:

> Do not suppose, Thérèse [as everyone calls Justine], we are made like other men; 'tis an entirely different structure we have; and, in creating us, Heaven has ornamented the altars at which our Celadons sacrifice with that very same sensitive membrane which lines your temple of Venus; we are, in that sector, as certainly women as you are in your generative sanctuary; not one of your pleasures is unknown to us, there is not one we do not know how to enjoy, but we have in addition to them our own, and it is this delicious combination which makes us of all men on earth the most sensitive to pleasure, the best created to experience it; it is this enchanting combination which renders our tastes incorrigible, which would turn us into enthusiasts and frenetics were one to have the stupidity to punish us.[29]

The Count's delicacy as he encodes blunt sexual description in a mythological language of love perhaps explains why he is the single tormenter for whom Justine feels desire. Beneath his flowery rhetoric, however, lies the bedrock physiology to which Sade continually returns.

In Sade, physiology is destiny. What mankind calls virtue and vice (so runs the libertine argument) reflects merely the facts of biochemical fate.

28. "Ma façon de penser est le fruit de mes réflexions; elle tient à mon existence, à mon organisation. Je ne suis pas le maître de la changer" (in *Œuvres complètes* 12:409). A portion of Sade's correspondence is available in *Selected Letters,* ed. Margaret Crosland, trans. W. J. Strachan (London: Peter Owen, 1963).

29. *Justine,* trans. Seaver and Wainhouse, 512/3:111–112.

"Our constitution, our scheme, our organs, the flow of liquids, the animal spirits' energy," declares a typical Sadean libertine, "such are the physical causes which in the same hour make for the Tituses and the Neros."[30] Sodomy and pyromania in effect are hardwired in the body. This conviction, which implicitly absolves Sade's libertines from the moral censure that only adds zest to their crimes, appeals for its support to the same progressive spirit of inquiry underlying Enlightenment medicine. As the dissolute monk Clément concludes, after laborious reference to the language of fluids, fibers, blood, and animal spirits: "When the study of anatomy reaches perfection they will without any trouble be able to demonstrate the relationship of the human constitution to the [sexual] tastes which it affects."[31] Anyone foolish enough to punish a libertine will discover that it cannot be done. A taste for pain—like the monks' delight in blaspheming a God whom they believe not to exist—stands fully comprehensible for Sade as a proven truth of the libertine body, inscribed in a personal biology of nerves, tissues, and membranes.

The body in Sade's work sometimes seems entirely detached from mind, like the adjacent blocks of pornographic description and of argumentative reasoning that provide the alternating structure of his books. But the apparent separation of mind and body is always a temporary state or narrative illusion that conceals their fundamental unity. Mind, as we have seen, is not for Sade alien to the body, opposed in an irreconcilable division. In fact, we should recall Delbène's assertion to Juliette that it is the body which feels, suffers, enjoys, judges, and *thinks*. The concept of a thinking body is Sade's response to the Cartesian dualism that rigorously opposes material bodies and immaterial thoughts. Sade's libertine system, on the contrary, considers body and mind equally material, although they differ in the same degree as steam might differ from ice. Mind and body are for Sade not just equally material but also (as they were, surprisingly, for Descartes) mutually interactive. The mind relies wholly for its contents—"all sensations, knowledge and ideas" (as Sade noted in *Justine*)—upon the impulses that it receives through the nervous system. What complicates this far from original psychology—which Sade might have borrowed from various

30. *Philosophy in the Bedroom,* trans. Seaver and Wainhouse, 254/3:438.

31. *Justine,* trans. Seaver and Wainhouse, 603/3:203. On the eccentricity of libertine sexual tastes, the same speaker says: "sa singularité est le résultat de ses organes" (3:202). The studies most helpful to me in exploring the relations between Sadean eroticism and physiology are Jean Deprun's "Sade et la philosophie biologique de son temps" (see n. 3 above) and Marcel Hénaff's *Sade: L'invention du corps libertin* (Paris: Presses universitaires de France, 1978).

empiricist philosophers, including his near contemporary Condillac—is his insistence that the sensations communicated through our nerves and fibers may in turn be altered radically by our thoughts, as if mind triumphed over matter.

The triumph of mind over matter in Sade is figurative ("as if")—not literal or actual—because, as we have seen, the libertine system regards mind as material: mind cannot literally triumph over itself. In this uncompromising materialism, Sade resembles such modern thinkers as John Searle, who in *Minds, Brains and Science* (1984) dismisses the traditional mind/body problem as a false dilemma or nonproblem. (For Searle, thinking is caused by and realized in functions of the brain, much as digestion is caused by and realized in functions of the stomach. He compares the mind/body problem to a digestion/stomach problem, finding them both equally comical and futile enterprises for philosophy.) What sets Sade apart from many materialists and monists, both ancient and modern, is the enormous power that he grants to consciousness or thought in reshaping the ways in which we normally experience our bodies. Mind, that is, possesses for Sade sufficient force to overrule or to alter organic responses (such as the response to pain) usually considered natural. The experience of pain, despite its organic basis in the functioning of the nervous system, may be changed, radically, by the intervention of mind, thus altering the almost physical revulsion normal in contemplating such typical Sadean practices as incest, torture, and the consumption of excrement. In imparting to the libertine body a dynamic (almost unlimited) power of change, mind thoroughly complicates Sade's description of physiology as destiny. Our physiology—through its union with mind—includes the potential for remaking our destinies.

Pain, like pleasure, in effect expands or contracts according to the play of the libertine mind. This play of mind is especially remarkable in Sade for harmonizing or reconciling the two normally antithetical powers of reason and imagination. Reason makes its most notorious appearance in the endless Sadean dissertations justifying libertine erotic tastes. Reason indeed proves a formal requirement of libertine sexuality in Sade, regularly preceding and following each episode of debauchery with an erudite harangue, and for dedicated libertines such as Juliette this Sadean dissertation serves less as an excuse or rationale than as an aphrodisiac. Her sodomite activities with the pope on the high altar of St. Peter's do not inflame her more than the thought of hearing his private lecture on the propriety of murder. Sade is among the few major writers to explore an eroticism of reason. It is not simply that his libertines reason about sexual topics or acts. Reasoning itself—as a mode of personal power—holds erotic attractions. (Juliette: "I loved Noirceuil for his libertinage, for his mental qualities: I was not by any means captivated by his person.")[32] Reason confers attractions as palpable as any of Sade's impossibly rounded buttocks or sensual perfections. In this office reason complements rather than opposes the work of imagination. It is important to recognize that imagination, like reason, has been assigned specific responsibilities or labor in Sade's erotic economy, which depends on mind for its more obvious fleshy exchanges. In Saint-Fond's aphorism: "The imagination's fire must set the furnace of the senses alight."[33]

The power of the imagination to inflame the senses depends on the unity of mind and body basic to Sade's outlook, wherein sensuality is never merely an affair of the senses. This reciprocal interpenetration of mental and of physical states had preoccupied several innovative physicians among Sade's contemporaries, especially Cabanis and Alibert, who sought to understand the mind's power over specific bodily conditions.[34] For Sade, the reciprocity linking the realms of the "*physique*" and "*moral*" (to cite the French terms commonly employed to indicate differences between bodily and mental states) extended even to the relationship be-

32. *Juliette*, trans. Wainhouse, 159/8:157. On the aesthetics and semiotics of Sadean eroticism, see Roland Barthes, *Sade/Fourier/Loyola* (1971), trans. Richard Miller (New York: Farrar, Straus and Giroux, 1976).

33. *Juliette*, trans. Wainhouse, 341/8:329. On this subject, see Pierre Fedida, "Les exercices de l'imagination et la commotion sur la masse des nerfs: Un érotisme de tête," in Sade's *Œuvres complètes* 16:613–625. The effect of the imagination upon the body—and vice versa—was a subject of continuing medical controversy during the eighteenth century, as in discussions of how the mother's imagination might affect the fetus (see Lester S. King, M.D., *The Philosophy of Medicine: The Early Eighteenth Century* [Cambridge, Mass.: Harvard University Press, 1978], 152–181). The physiological basis of the imagination is discussed by G. S. Rousseau, "Science and the Discovery of the Imagination in Enlightened England," *Eighteenth-Century Studies* 3 (1969–1970): 108–135.

34. Cabanis develops the connections linking medicine and physiology with mind and culture in his *Rapports du physique et du moral de l'homme* (1802). For a fine discussion of Cabanis and of his ideas, see Martin S. Staum, *Cabanis: Enlightenment and Medical Philosophy in the French Revolution* (Princeton: Princeton University Press, 1980). (The *Rapports* is available in English translation, with helpful introductions by Sergio Moravia and George Mora, under the title *On the Relations between the Physical and Moral Aspects of Man*, ed. George Mora, trans. Margaret Duggan Saidi, 2 vols. [Baltimore, Md.: Johns Hopkins University Press, 1981].) A similar emphasis underlies the treatise entitled *Discours sur les rapports de la médecine avec les sciences physiques et morales* (1798) by Jean-Louis Alibert—a young colleague of Cabanis associated with the Hôpital Saint-Louis. I have been unable to determine whether Sade knew the work of Alibert or of Cabanis (whose ideas circulated via lectures in the decade preceding publication), but in any case I am not concerned here with questions of direct influence.

tween text and reader. He anticipates that the imaginative, mental stimulation of reading will excite measurable, physiological changes in the reader. (In *120 Days of Sodom* the narrator explains: "Many of the extravagances you are about to see illustrated will doubtless displease you, yes, I am well aware of it, but there are amongst them a few which will warm you to the point of costing you some fuck, and that, reader, is all we ask of you.")[35] In addition to authorizing this pornographic variant of reader-response criticism, the regulating power of imagination makes itself felt in the aesthetic arrangements inseparable from Sadean eroticism. Rarely are passions satisfied in a chaotic haste and tangle. Sexual partners and groups observe a carefully discussed choreography. Setting—like the elaborate theatrical scene specially constructed at the chateau Silling—often requires costly and ingenious preparations. Crimes are seldom merely perpetrated but rather lovingly premeditated with an artistic attention to minor details, and libertines who survive long enough frequently develop a brilliant flair for spontaneous dramatic gestures, as when Juliette (after climbing to the summit of a volcano) decides to cast a tiresome companion into the bowels of the earth and then follows this gothic performance with impromptu copulations staged imaginatively on the very brink of the gaping crater.

It is the imagination that permits Sade to approach the perfect freedom represented by libertinage: a freedom whereby nature as well as society may be overcome. Sade once defended himself by explaining that while he had imagined every possible form of sexual crime, he had not performed everything he imagined. He was a libertine but not a criminal.[36] Yet, he also composed the speech in which a libertine—distressed at the idea of crimes limited to a single lifetime—is urged to consider the "moral crime" of writing, whereby the imagination permits a writer to extend corrupting fantasies far into the future. For Sade, our imagination—both in its intensity and in its tastes—depends on our physiology (on "the peculiar organization a particular individual is endowed with"), but our physiology thereby contains the power to remake both ourselves and the world. As the dissolute monk Clément expresses Sade's dark version of Romantic idealism: "Objects have no value for us save that which our imagination imparts to them."[37] Pain, when objectified in a suffering victim, proves to be a supreme example of the imagination's power to transform *anything* into pleasure.

35. *The 120 Days of Sodom and Other Writings,* trans. Austryn Wainhouse and Richard Seaver (New York: Grove Press, 1966), 254/13:61.

36. *Correspondance,* in *Œuvres complètes* 12:276.

37. *Justine,* trans. Seaver and Wainhouse, 599/3:200.

The imagination's power to transvalue (or to drain of value) the conventional world of objects and of bodies holds implications that extend beyond individual bodies or minds to politics. Political power is implicit in the imaginative capacity to reshape the world according to our own desires, at least when Sade's libertines possess the wealth, guile, and social standing that permit them to impose their desires upon other persons. The political implications of Sadean eroticism are not farfetched or oblique, as the recent history of feminist readings of Sade makes unmistakably clear.[38] My choice here is not to focus on what might be called—somewhat metaphorically—Sade's sexual politics. The representation of women in Sade's novels, with its sources in social and economic structures as oppressive as any libertine desire, is a subject that leads far beyond the scope of this essay and that Angela Carter has discussed brilliantly at book length. Consistent with a study centering on transvaluations of medical knowledge, my focus concerns the less apparent moments when Sade takes as his subject, directly or indirectly, politics construed in its literal sense as the art or condition of government.

Sade's sexual themes are so prominent, so overwhelming, that they tend to obscure his representations of political power. Yet, he recognized a close link between sexuality and government. For example, he insisted upon a social and political significance in fiction where critics for generations have reported finding only sensationalism and debauchery. In his *Reflections on the Novel* (1800), Sade had high praise for Matthew Lewis's gothic extravaganza *The Monk,* observing that it was "the inevitable result of the revolutionary shocks which all of Europe has suffered."[39] *Philosophy in the Bedroom* places Sade's secluded libertines within a historical setting where incendiary pamphlets are distributed openly outside the palace of Equality. One such pamphlet Sade actually incorporates in his text—the famous libertine manifesto *Yet Another Effort, Frenchmen, If You Would Become Republicans,* with its guidelines for a uto-

38. For a helpful discussion of feminist approaches to Sade, see Donna Landry, "Beat Me! Beat Me! Feminist Appropriations of Sade," *Enclitic* (forthcoming). In addition to discussing the work of Simone de Beauvoir and Angela Carter, Landry rightly devotes major attention to the feminist-Lacanian studies by Jane Gallop, *Intersections: A Reading of Sade with Bataille, Blanchot, and Klossowski* (Lincoln: University of Nebraska Press, 1981) and *The Daughter's Seduction: Feminism and Psychoanalysis* (Ithaca, N.Y.: Cornell University Press, 1982).

39. *Reflections on the Novel* (1800), in *The 120 Days of Sodom and Other Writings,* trans. Wainhouse and Seaver, 109/10:15. It is in this essay that Sade defines the novel as "le tableau des moeurs séculaires" (15) and locates the novelist's subject in those revelations that occur when mankind drops the "*masque*" of public dissembling. Clearly, the "revolutionary shocks" to which Sade refers cannot be restricted to political thought and action.

pian state in which legitimate forms of personal freedom now include prostitution, incest, rape, sodomy, and murder. From his cell in the Bastille Sade was a firsthand spectator of the gathering Revolutionary shock (the authorities removed him for inciting passers-by); during his less than four years of freedom after the fall of the Bastille, he held for a time the improbable office of assessor or judge on one of the innumerable Revolutionary committees; and upon his rearrest in 1793, the house in which he was temporarily imprisoned became the location for a guillotine, where some eighteen hundred victims of the Terror were executed. For Sade, who defined the novel as "the representation of secular customs" and who spent most of his adult life imprisoned because of his unorthodox tastes and writings, it would be hard indeed to avoid observing the link between sexual practice and political power.

Politics for Sade is closely and inseparably related to what he regards as the truth of the body. "The Body Politic," as one of his libertine heroes asserts, "should be governed by the same rules that apply to the Body Physical."[40] More is at work here than the spell of analogy. Sadean politics is not just indirectly linked to the body through a physiology that includes the imagination. The body for Sade—through its nerves, fibers, and animal spirits—directly authorizes a larger, encompassing distribution of social power. "Stripping people of their liberty amuses me," explains one libertine, "I like holding captives." "Man likes to command," reports another, "to be obeyed, to surround himself with slaves compelled to satisfy him."[41] Although Sade professed to distinguish between what he called "absurd political despotism" and the "delightful despotism" of the libertine, French political life under the ancien régime finds its perfect miniaturization (as Roland Barthes has observed) in the despotic power which Sade's libertines exercise over their powerless victims. Thus in a note to *Juliette* Sade writes that one of his grasping libertine statesmen resembles "those monsters that abounded under the *ancien*

40. *Justine,* trans. Seaver and Wainhouse, 690/3:291 ("Le corps politique doit avoir sur cela les mêmes règles que le corps physique").

41. *Juliette,* trans. Wainhouse, 712/9:116; *Philosophy in the Bedroom,* trans. Seaver and Wainhouse, 317/3:500. Noirceuil instructs Juliette, in a language that reveals the connections among religious, political, and sexual despotism: "this tool is my god, let it be one unto thee, Juliette: extol it, worship it, this despotic engine, show it every reverence, it is a thing proud of its glory, insatiate, a tyrant; I'd fain make the earth bend its knee in universal homage to this prick, I'd like to see it guised in the shape of a terrific personage who would put to a death of awful torments every last living soul that thought to deny it the least of a thousand services" (185/8:180). On the development of Sade's political thought, see Jean-Pierre Faye, "Changer la mort (Sade et la politique)," *Obliques* 12–13 (1977): 47–57.

régime and personified it."[42] This sexualized, social, and absolute power authorized by the body amounts to what we might call a politics of sensibility.

Sensibility, of course, is a crucial concept in late-eighteenth-century medicine and literature, where it permitted the development of a tightly woven argument about that favorite Enlightenment object of study, human nature. This argument, so pervasive that it operated usually in abbreviated versions accepted or offered as an unspoken assumption, rested on the belief shared by Sadean libertines that our sensibility or power of feeling depends ultimately upon the refinement of our individual nervous system. The stages of this argument have been reconstructed by G. S. Rousseau in the following series: "(A) the soul is limited to the brain, (B) the brain performs the entirety of its work through the nerves, (C) the more 'exquisite' and 'delicate' one's nerves are, morphologically speaking, the greater the ensuing degree of sensibility and imagination, (D) refined people and other persons of fashion are born with more 'exquisite' anatomies, the tone and texture of their nervous systems more 'delicate' than those of the lower classes."[43] All we need in order to transform this physiological argument into a politics of sensibility is the conclusion supplied in a fascinating essay by Christopher Lawrence. Lawrence shows in a detailed study of Scottish Enlightenment thought how the argument based on physiology was employed to advance the political and social interests of an autocratic, landed minority, whose heightened capacity for exquisite feeling supposedly earned them a natural right as governors and custodians of power in a backward land.[44]

Sade—in the transvaluations he so often performed upon Enlightenment thought—effectively converted the politics of sensibility into a sexual despotism based on pain. Understood solely as a phenomenon of nerves and tissues, pain supplies the foundation for a Sadean politics in

42. *Philosophy in the Bedroom,* trans. Seaver and Wainhouse, 344/3:529; *Juliette,* trans. Wainhouse, 234/8:225. On the political and specifically antiroyalist bias of pornography written under the ancien régime, see Robert Darnton, *The Literary Underground of the Old Regime* (Cambridge, Mass.: Harvard University Press, 1982), 199–208.

43. "Nerves, Spirits, and Fibres: Towards Defining the Origins of Sensibility," *The Blue Guitar* 2 (1976): 143.

44. "The Nervous System and Society in the Scottish Enlightenment," in *Natural Order: Historical Studies of Scientific Culture,* ed. Barry Barnes and Steven Shapin (Beverly Hills, Calif.: Sage Publications, 1979), 19–40. Lawrence cites David Hume's view as representative: "The skin, pores, muscles, and nerves of a day-labourer are different from those of a man of quality: So are his sentiments, actions and manners" (*A Treatise of Human Nature,* ed. L. A. Selby-Bigge, 2d ed., rev. P. H. Nidditch [Oxford: Clarendon Press, 1978], 402).

which mastery requires that other people suffer. If the Enlightenment man of feeling—whose acute sensitivity to pain was legendary—implicitly lent support to the political suppression of persons whose sensibility was deemed less delicate, Sade's libertines argue openly that their individual powers of feeling give them an absolute right over other people. "I affirm," declares the libertine statesman Saint-Fond, "that the fundamental, profoundest, and keenest penchant in man is incontestably to enchain his fellow creatures and to tyrannize them with all his might."[45] Pain, however, plays a curious double role in this Sadean tyranny. Sade emphasizes that a taste for cruelty depends on a particularly sensitive nervous system, so that women—according to the libertine argument—are especially cruel. ("The extreme delicacy of their fibers, the prodigious sensitivity of their organs," explains a Sadean annotation, "cause them to go a great deal farther than men in this direction.")[46] At the same time, the disposition for inflicting pain also requires a paradoxical deadening of the emotions in order that cruelty might be enjoyed to the utmost. It is said of Madame Clairwil—"the most exceptional libertine of her century"—that for lack of sensibility she had no equal: "she indeed prided herself on never having shed a tear."[47]

The paradox of libertine sensibility—simultaneously hypersensitive and numb—may be traced ultimately to the Sadean monism of body and mind. It is the body's "organization"—to use Sade's favorite biological term—that ensures our leaning toward what the world calls virtue or vice. Thus, in comparing women with men, Sade repeats the familiar argument that physiology is destiny. ("Their organs are more finely constructed, their sensitivity profounder, their nerves more irascible: barbarity is not a trait of the individual of inferior sensibility.")[48] The libertine's superior sensibility, nonetheless, requires for the perfection of barbarism a complementary mental development. Sade's libertines therefore take particular care to harden their sensibilities against the normal pity or distress we are disposed to feel at the sight of human suffering. They cultivate the *apathy*—a rational indifference to feeling—

45. *Juliette,* trans. Wainhouse, 317/8:305.

46. Ibid., 797/9:201.

47. Ibid., 1042/9:440 and 274/8:262. As Clairwil explains to Juliette: "La sensibilité, ma chère, est le foyer de tous les vices, comme elle est celui de toutes les vertus" (8:266). She goes on to describe the source of individual sensibility as physiological: "Cette sensibilité, purement physique, dépend de la conformité de nos organes, de la délicatesse de nos sens, et, plus que tout, de la nature du fluide nerveux."

48. *Juliette,* trans. Wainhouse, 1058/9:456. Juliette summarizes the Sadean link between sensibility and pain in an aphorism: "la cruauté n'est elle-même qu'une des branches de la sensibilité" (9:456).

which Max Horkheimer and Theodore W. Adorno identify as a basic strain of Enlightenment thought: what Kant called "a necessary presupposition of virtue."[49]

Sadean apathy is a necessary deadening of the emotions and elevation of reason that finds its significance not as a goal or end of conduct—and certainly not as a presupposition of virtue—but as one stage in a dialectic of pain. Because Sadean libertines must deaden their feelings in order to feel more intensely, their condition bears less resemblance to a generalized, Stoic apathy (in which reason everywhere dominates passion) than to a highly selective, local anesthesia (which eliminates only a specific band or zone of feeling, while thereby heightening the sensation that remains). Specific emotions such as pity are eradicated to assure a cold detachment; reason is magnified; imagination inflames the senses. Thus Sadean libertines encourage the tendency they discover within themselves for enjoying the intensest shocks to the nervous system that accompany both their own pain and the spectacle of pain in others. A body politic governed by the same rules that apply to the libertine body will find apathy a necessary precondition of social life. Selective anesthesia is perhaps what permits every ruling elite to transform its own principles and sensibility into a license for oppression. Sade's libertine societies are unique not in their brutality but in their undeceived awareness and open enjoyment of the suffering they inflict.

The twofold libertine education of the feelings—simultaneously hardening the sensibility to pity and enlarging its relish for pain—issues finally in the murderous supremacy which Saint-Fond and his fellow libertines accept as their natural right. In the sexualized torture they inflict upon their victims, Sade's libertines reveal how pain serves so often to reify or give visible shape to the political power that, as Elaine Scarry has argued, is always implicitly or explicitly claimed by the torturer.[50] Unquestionably, the pain that Sade's work emphasizes is closely linked to social conventions of gender, so that women (represented by the pious, submissive, piteous Justine) are its normal site. Even Sade's emancipated libertine woman—as we see in Juliette—depends, like his male libertines, on a supply of victims who are usually powerless and mostly female. In Sade's work, however, the politics of sensibility does not co-

49. *Dialectic of Enlightenment* (1944), trans. John Cumming (New York: Herder and Herder, 1972), 96. Horkheimer and Adorno cite Kant's view.

50. *The Body in Pain*, 27–59. Two excellent studies that recognize the political uses and implications of pain are Helen Neal's *The Politics of Pain* (New York: McGraw-Hill, 1978) and Martin S. Pernick's *A Calculus of Suffering: Pain, Professionalism, and Anesthesia in Nineteenth-Century America* (New York: Columbia University Press, 1985).

incide exactly with a conventional sexual politics, in which males are invariably oppressors and women victims. Power in Sade is ultimately genderless, and gender sometimes grows as shifty as pain. The ultimate libertine erotic adventure—death—seems finally beyond gender, a mode of autoeroticism in which pleasure transcends distinctions of female and male. Like the brigand chief Roland, who trusts Justine to cut the rope, submissively, just when he hangs himself, the libertine mind makes use of gender in order to seek a state more archaic and indistinct, where social and biological differences between male and female dissolve in an erotic embrace of death. The victims of Sade's libertines—often mutilated past all recognition—divide simply into the dead and the about-to-die. In Sade's transvaluation of Enlightenment norms, the politics of sensibility leads logically to the androgynous or bisexual libertine witch Durand and to the final extension of undifferentiated, tyrannous power that she contemplates: genocide.

It was not tyranny, however, but revolution that provided for Sade the political metaphor best summarizing the meanings he discovered in pain. Sade settles for tyranny, we might say, because it represents a durable substitute for the transient purity of revolution. Revolution for Sade is the anarchic dream of absolute freedom realized in the moment when an established government falls and its successor has not yet come into being. In the temporary release from all law and all authority, it confronts us with a condition of utter ambiguity as the state dissolves into an elemental, inchoate, and primal disorder. "Lawful rule," as a Sadean libertine explains, "is inferior to anarchy: the greatest proof whereof is the government's obligation to plunge the State into anarchy whenever it wishes to frame a new constitution. To abrogate its former laws it is driven to establish a revolutionary regime in which there are no laws at all."[51] The revolutionary regime is by definition unstable and transitional. It soon calls forth a new state with new laws and new authority, where absolute freedom is once again merely a dream. Indeed, politics as a social practice—as the day-to-day art of government—held almost no interest for Sade compared to the intoxicating and almost purely theoretical moment of revolution when all government dissolves. It is this moment of complete freedom and utter ambiguity when ordinary structures fly apart that fascinated Sade. Like the tumultuous moment of orgasm for Sadean libertines, it provides an image of the terrifying, exhilarating vertigo that ensues when human beings live fully the consequences of their own desire. Pain, I suggest, comes to signify for Sade

51. *Juliette,* trans. Wainhouse, 733/9:137.

the vast and never wholly communicable ambiguity that he understands as implicit in the truth of desire.

Desire is an overworked topic in literary criticism of the novel, but it is also the central point to which Sade's treatment of body, mind, and politics continually returns. Within the almost limitless perimeters set by desire, what concerns me here is a quite limited, concluding issue: the relation of desire to pain. Indeed, Sadean desire seems nearly unique in selecting pain as its favored object. Sade's paradoxical argument—making pain a source of pleasure—in effect profoundly revises several powerful traditions that precede, but by no means predict, his work. In Sade, the ancient erotic topos of the lover's pain—a pain the lover half-enjoys because its poignancy and its intensity seem inseparable from love—reappears completely altered: love simply vanishes (along with religion) as a source of libertine feeling. Eros for Sade has little or nothing to do with Cupid. Similarly, Sade turns on its head the Socratic theory that desire always presupposes a painful lack or absence. (For Socrates, at least in the earlier dialogues, pain activates and accompanies desire, disappearing when desire attains its object, much as the pangs of hunger disappear after one eats.) Sadean pain not only arouses and accompanies desire but also satisfies it—or, more accurately, promises to satisfy it. Pain thus achieves a special value for Sade exactly in proportion to its capacity for *resisting* disappearance. It is something to be cherished and enjoyed and protracted: an additive that both prolongs and even replaces lesser modes of pleasure. Indeed, in its quest for permanence, Sadean desire no longer flees from absence and pain but actively courts them. It recognizes in pain the promise of an ultimate and unending and undeceiving satisfaction.

The Sadean embrace of pain is not merely a search for intense sensation. Desire, in seeking pain, seeks more than the satisfaction of carnal appetite, which is why bodies alone (gluttonously consumed) are never enough for Sade's libertines: they demand reasons and meanings as well. The two main clusters of meaning enfolded within the experience of Sadean pain should be now quite familiar. First, there is pain defined (against powerful religious and ethical traditions) strictly as an event of the central nervous system, measured through the shock that it delivers to the body and described in a biomedical language of neural fluids, animal spirits, and hollow nerve tubes. The social and sexual implications of this Sadean perspective on pain are, as I have tried to indicate, far-reaching. Second, there is the libertine insistence that pain somehow unites us with truth. Pleasure deceives, pain informs. Pleasure is always doubtful, pain provides certainty. Pain, as I have argued, is regarded as expressing the truth of the body, and the truth of the body proves coextensive with the normally suppressed, repressed, and openly denied truth of desire. It is now necessary to complicate this picture, briefly but unmercifully.

Sadean desire, which we might define as a normally unheard and unheeded voice prior to all laws and all authority, always returns to pain—as if to its source or origin. Explanations for this recurrent pattern no doubt require an awareness that pain and desire share exactly the same structure within the libertine system. Pain, as we have seen, promises absolute certainty, a bedrock for belief that cannot be questioned because it is self-evidently true, an unfeigned and unambiguous speech uttered as if involuntarily by the body, a forced confession. At the same time, this bedrock truth proves far less firm than it appears. Within the libertine body, pain swiftly and imperceptibly passes into its opposite, pleasure, in a process that is never simply or solely a reversal, as if pleasure now meant pain, and pain pleasure. Their relation is more unstable, fluid, and shifting. For Descartes, the physiological differences between pleasure and pain involve potentially measurable changes in nerve fibers. In the sensation of pleasure, the fibers are merely stretched, while pain finds them strained and torn. (Quite different organs are also involved in exciting the joy of pleasure and despondency of pain.) For Sade, the physiological differences between pleasure and pain involve potentially measurable changes in "the neural fluid particles which circulate in the hollow of our nerves." Yet the differences that for Descartes seemed absolute and binding now for Sade appear relatively ambiguous. Inscribed on the victims of libertine cruelties, the signs of pain may still look certain. Within the libertine body, however, pleasure and pain no longer hold their normative role of opposites but commingle in uncertain and changing patterns. Like desire, pain for Sade leads away from clarities.

Pain in Sade is not just the object of desire but in some sense its double. Sadean desire is thus drawn to pain as to its own mirror image. What they share fundamentally is a negative power to block satisfaction, to prevent any firm or final accommodation with meaning. Sade's libertines obsessively follow the instructions of desire but discover (in or through satiety) a perpetual dissatisfaction, lack of fulfillment, the void from which desire springs anew. "Nothing measures up to the stature of my desires," explains a voracious female libertine, whose usual debaucheries continue for twenty-four hours and reduce her genitals to what she calls "an open wound": "a hash."[52] Desire—in seeking satisfaction through pain—remains unappeasable. The monk Clément, after putting Justine through a terrifying sexual ordeal indistinguishable from torture, regrets that her vividly physical sufferings are inevitably "a very pale image of what one should really like to do."[53] Behind the breathtaking atrocities Sade's libertines perform there lies an unattainable—perhaps even unknowable—level of cruelty that always defeats them. Like pain, desire reserves to itself something that finally remains always unspoken, beyond or against language. In this sense Sade's work is a sea of horrors in which pain continually seeks and perpetually fails to drain dry the unspeakable.

Anyone who wishes to explore the assumptions underlying four decades of quite extraordinary French writing on Sade should begin with the belief that Sadean horrors represent an assault on the unspeakable. Simone de Beauvoir puts it this way: "He is trying to communicate an experience whose distinguishing characteristic is, nevertheless, a tendency to be incommunicable." Maurice Blanchot writes of Sade: "Everything which is said is clear, but seems to be at the mercy of something left unsaid"; "everything *is* expressed, is revealed, but also everything is plunged back again into the obscurity of unformulated and inexpressible thoughts." Georges Bataille comments: "The evident monotony of Sade's books is due to the decision to subordinate literature to the expression of an inexpressible event."[54] This consensus does not guarantee

52. Ibid., 709/9:114.

53. *Justine,* trans. Seaver and Wainhouse, 598/3:198.

54. Simone de Beauvoir, "Must We Burn Sade?" (1951–1952), in *The 120 Days of Sodom and Other Writings,* trans. Wainhouse and Seaver, 4; Maurice Blanchot, "Sade" [from *Lautréamont et Sade* (1949)], in *Justine,* trans. Seaver and Wainhouse, 39; Georges Bataille, *Literature and Evil,* trans. Hamilton, 94. In comparison with the brilliant French writing on Sade since the Second World War—by writers (in addition to Beauvoir, Blanchot, and Bataille) including Pierre Klossowski, Jean Paulhan, Albert Camus, Jacques Lacan, Roland Barthes, and Philippe Sollers—Anglo-American criticism of Sade seems less passionate and less adventurous, when it appears at all. When I mentioned the "silence" that has greeted Sade, I did not mean to ignore or to disparage the strong work on Sade by Lester G. Crocker, Ihab Hassan, Nancy K. Miller, R. F. Brissenden, and Joan De Jean. Still, any standard bibliography will indicate how far scholarly studies on Pope, Defoe, Molière, or Goethe (for example) vastly outnumber—almost bury—the few straggling Anglo-American entries on Sade.

Why has Sade received so much attention in France (and neglect abroad)? Most important, French intellectuals must come to terms with Sade (and with Racine) almost as a rite of passage into their national life. But Sade's work also provides unusually fertile ground for exploring connections—especially well recognized in France—among politics, sexuality, and psychoanalysis. The meditations on criminality and on self-punishment so prom-

that its claim is correct, but it both defines a basis for the modern re-valuation of Sade and helps to suggest why Sadean desire—in its endless torrent of repetitive images and words—finds in pain an appropriate vehicle for a quest characteristic of Romantic writing: the pursuit of the inexpressible. Pain in Sade draws to itself the speechless, erotic mysteries culminating and cohering in the embrace of death.

In its intrinsic contact with the inexpressible and the unspeakable, pain takes Sade far beyond the medicine of his day, when madness and unreason were still locked within the secure (if no longer absolute) classical confinement that Michel Foucault describes in *Madness and Civilization*. Foucault reads Sade as a figure of the late Enlightenment who exposes a truth that Enlightenment medicine mostly resisted. "Sadism," he writes, "is not a name finally given to a practice as old as Eros; it is a massive cultural fact which appeared precisely at the end of the eighteenth century, and which constitutes one of the greatest conversions of Western imagination: unreason transformed into delirium of the heart, madness of desire, the insane dialogue of love and death in the limitless presumption of appetite."[55] Sade, I would guess, is among the crucial, ambiguous monuments that Foucault's unfinished history of sexuality would unavoidably reconsider. In such a reconsideration, Sade should appear not as the author of a few vast, unreadable pornographic novels but as an almost impersonal force giving voice to a newly transformed discourse on the erotic life. It is not only as a sign of mastery or as a well-recognized surrogate for death—with its speechless myster-

inent in postwar French thought find a cornucopia of illustrative material in Sade, where images of "mutilation" similarly serve to suggest a radical decentering of the stable ego inherited from classical psychology (see Carolyn Dean, "Law and Sacrifice: Bataille, Lacan, and the Critique of the Subject," *Representations* 13 [1986]: 42–62). Further, recent French history has exposed the fragility of assumptions underlying Western liberal democracies, and Sade offers a full-scale assault on such assumptions. In *celebrating* cruelty, he in effect reverses the gesture basic to all Western liberal democracies, which put cruelty first in the rank of moral, social, and political offenses (see Judith Shklar, *Ordinary Vices* [Cambridge, Mass.: Harvard University Press, 1984], 7–44). Finally, in France the presence of Sade has made it easier to accept and to develop Freud's insight that "the history of human civilization shows beyond any doubt . . . an intimate connection between cruelty and the sexual instinct" (*Three Essays on the Theory of Sexuality* [1905], in *The Standard Edition of the Complete Psychological Works of Sigmund Freud,* trans. and ed. James Strachey et al., 24 vols. [London: Hogarth Press, 1953–1974], 7:159). Anglo-American resistance to Freud on this point naturally coincides with a repugnance to Sade. It also does not help Sade's reputation in England and America—where literary analysis is closely tied to academic institutions—that Sade seems almost unteachable.

55. *Madness and Civilization: A History of Insanity in the Age of Reason* (1961), trans. Richard Howard (New York: New American Library, 1965), 210.

ies and sensual affiliations—that pain served Sade. Modern clinical treatment now frequently begins with the Sadean assumption that pain is always solitary and private, full of sound but essentially inarticulate, a measure of the immense distance that separates individuals. Against cultural pieties proclaiming a human community, an almost infinite space opens between the person in pain and the comforters or tormenters who stand close by. Not even the physician or research scientist who seeks to relieve pain, tracing its shared vocabulary and redefining the biochemistry of the brain, can as yet successfully collapse the distance. Words and knowledge carry poorly across this abyss. Pain, as one modern treatment center advises its staff, is "anything that the patient says it is."[56] "Pain," wrote Emily Dickinson, "has an Element of Blank."[57] The blankness, the anythingness of pain, especially its power to summon up experience ultimately inaccessible to language, its power to engage ambiguities too slippery for even the slickest libertine reasoners: these are among the meanings with which Sade endowed the mechanical rush of animal spirits through hollow, fibrous nerves.

56. B. L. Crue et al., "Observations on the Taxonomy Problem in Pain," in *Chronic Pain: Further Observations from City of Hope National Medical Center,* ed. Benjamin L. Crue, Jr., M.D. (New York: SP Medical and Scientific Books, 1978), 20. Dr. Crue and his colleagues are writing specifically about *chronic* (as distinguished from *acute*) pain. In Sade's work, this distinction is often difficult to apply, because all pain inflicted in libertine sexuality tends toward the repetition and totalization characteristic of chronic pain. For an authoritative discussion, see John J. Bonica and C. Richard Chapman, "Biology, Pathophysiology, and Therapy of Chronic Pain," in *American Handbook of Psychiatry,* ed. Silvano Arieti, 2d ed., 8 vols. (New York: Basic Books, 1974–1986), 8:711–761. Volume 8 is edited by Philip A. Berger et al.

57. In *The Complete Poems of Emily Dickinson,* ed. Thomas H. Johnson (Boston: Little, Brown and Co., 1960), 323 (no. 650).

NINE

Mind and Body in the Clinic: Philippe Pinel, Alexander Crichton, Dominique Esquirol, and the Birth of Psychiatry

Dora B. Weiner

> . . . *so this league of mind and body, hath these two parts,* How the one discloseth the other, and how the one worketh upon the other, Discoverie, & Impression.
>
> *The former of these hath begotten two Arts. . . . The first is PHYSIOGNOMIE, which discovereth the disposition of the mind, by the Lyneaments of the bodie. The second is the EXPOSITION OF NATURALL DREAMES. . . .*
>
> *In the former of these, I note a deficience. For* Aristotle *hath verie ingeniously, and diligently handled the factures of the bodie, but not the gestures of the bodie; which are no less comprehensible by art, and of greater use, and advantage.*
>
> —SIR FRANCIS BACON, *The Two Bookes of the Proficience and Advancement of Learning* (London, 1605)

THE DOCTOR AS CLINICIAN

The vast seventeenth- and eighteenth-century literature about mind and body derives its major themes from philosophers trained in medicine. John Locke discussed sensation and reflection while David Hartley explored the association of ideas. Julien Offray de La Mettrie depicted the body as a machine and Georges Cabanis envisioned the brain as an organ that secretes thought, just as the stomach processes food. All these men were practicing physicians.[1] Materialistic philosophy motivated

1. This essay is indebted to the stimulating and apt criticism of George Rousseau, to the medical wisdom of my scholarly colleague and husband, Dr. Herbert Weiner, to the thought-provoking critique of professors Ludmilla Jordanova and Dieter Jetter, and to courteous and prompt help from Victoria L. Steele, former Head of the History and Rare Books Division, Biomedical Library, UCLA. Thanks are also due to the staffs of the Wellcome Institute Library, London, the Bibliotheek der Rijksuniversiteit, Leiden, and the Bibliothèque de la Faculté de médecine, Paris.

An earlier version of the section on Crichton was presented at the thirtieth Interna-

many medical investigators of mental functions to study the bodily substrate of human thought and emotion: from Thomas Willis to Gall and Spurzheim, they dissected and scrutinized nerves and brains. But William Harvey had taught them to conceptualize bodily functions in terms of systems: therefore they focused on circulatory, respiratory, digestive, or nervous physiology. Researchers curious to understand the relationship of mind and body concentrated on the nervous system. However, a categorical difference separates a physiologist, such as Harvey, who experimented on living animals and man, from anatomists or neurologists who work on dead animals and human corpses. It is impossible to apprehend human thought and feeling by studying the inert body and

tional Congress of the History of Medicine, Düsseldorf, West Germany, on 2 September 1986 and was published in its *Proceedings.*

Some of the outstanding general treatments in the vast literature on seventeenth-to-early-nineteenth-century "medical psychology" are the following:

For Great Britain, W. F. Bynum, Jr., "Rationales for Therapy in British Psychiatry, 1780–1835," in *Madhouses, Mad-Doctors, and Madmen: The Social History of Psychiatry in the Victorian Era,* ed. A. Scull (Philadelphia: University of Pennsylvania Press, 1981), 35–57; D. Leigh, *The Historical Development of British Psychiatry: Eighteenth and Nineteenth Centuries* (Oxford: Pergamon Press, 1961); R. Porter, "A Rage of Party: A Glorious Revolution in English Psychiatry?" *Medical History* 27 (1983): 35–50; and G. S. Rousseau, "Psychology," in *The Ferment of Knowledge: Studies in the Historiography of Eighteenth-Century Science,* ed. G. S. Rousseau and R. Porter (New York: Cambridge University Press, 1980), 143–210.

For France, the outstanding recent contribution is J. Goldstein, *Console and Classify: The French Psychiatric Profession in the Nineteenth Century* (Cambridge: Cambridge University Press, 1987). I regret that the present essay had gone to press when this book appeared so that I could not include Goldstein's insightful comments. See also P. Carrette, "Un demi-siècle d'assistance aux aliénés avant la loi de 1838," *Annales médico-psychologiques,* 151st ser., 1 (1938): 674–680, and the relevant segments of the following books: M. Laignel-Lavastine and J. Vinchon, *Les malades de l'esprit et leurs médecins, du 16ème au 19ème siècle* (Paris: Maloine, 1930); Y. Pelicier, *Histoire de la psychiatrie* (Paris: Presses Universitaires de France, 1971); J. Postel and C. Quétel, *Nouvelle histoire de la psychiatrie* (Toulouse: Privat, 1983); and C. Quétel and P. Morel, *Les fous et leurs médecines, de la Renaissance au 20ème siècle* (Paris: Hachette, 1979).

For Germany, K. Dörner, *Madmen and the Bourgeoisie: A Social History of Insanity* (Oxford: Blackwell, 1981); K. W. Ideler, *Grundriss der Seelenheilkunde,* 2 vols. (Berlin: Enslin, 1835); Th. Kirchhoff, *Grundriss einer Geschichte der deutschen Irrenpflege* (Berlin: Hirschwald, 1890); E. Kräpelin, "Hundert Jahre Psychiatrie," *Zeitschrift für die gesamte Neurologie und Psychiatrie* 38 (1918): 161–275; and G. Verwey, *Psychiatry in an Anthropological and Biomedical Context: Philosophical Presuppositions and Implications of German Psychiatry, 1820–1870* (Dordrecht: Reidel, 1984).

For Spain, D. Desmaisons, *Des asiles d'aliénés en Espagne: Recherches historiques et médicales* (Paris: Baillière, 1859), and J. E. Iborra, "La asistencia al enfermo mental en España durante la Ilustraciòn y el reinado de Fernando VII," *Cuadernos de historia de la medicina española* 5 (1966): 181–215.

brain, and therefore postmortem dissection proved unrewarding for physicians interested in mental illness. They could not ascertain how a nervous fluid might affect the mind, and where in the brain to locate thought, pain, or the emotions. They rather turned to another method favored by their eighteenth-century colleagues in anatomy and physiology, namely the intensive and systematic observation of the living patient, preferably in the clinic.

This practice was fundamental to the diagnostic method of Philippe Pinel (1745–1826), and he stands out as the eighteenth-century clinician who made the mentally ill patient his central concern. His *Traité médico-philosophique sur l'aliénation mentale ou la manie* (Medico-philosophic treatise on mental alienation or madness) became famous immediately upon publication in 1800:[2] no doubt his mythical feat during the Terror—unchaining the insane at the Salpêtrière, known in France as *le geste de Pinel*—served as publicity for the book.[3] Its true merit also found outstanding admirers, including the philosopher Georg Wilhelm Friedrich Hegel; and when Stendhal wanted to buy the *Traité* in 1806, it was sold out.[4] Pinel's was the only work on the nascent medical specialty, psychiatry, to achieve universal fame.[5] Most commentators underlined the novelty and psychologic aptness of his case histories, and indeed Pinel's first concern was neither theory, nor classification, nor clinical research, nor therapy, even though he made fundamental contributions to all of them. He believed that a doctor, and particularly a doctor concerned with mental illness, must first of all get to know his patients well. To do this, he must listen and observe.

In order to explore the subject of mental illness Pinel also read widely, and he was particularly familiar with contemporary British medical thought, having edited three volumes of a twelve-volume abridgment of

2. (Paris: Caille et Ravier, 1800). For a complete Pinel bibliography, including foreign translations of the above work, see Appendix, Biobibliographic Note 1.

3. The controversy and the demise of this myth were first discussed by G. Swain in her brilliant thesis, *Le sujet de la folie* (Toulouse: Privat, 1977). The arguments are summarized in English in D. B. Weiner, "The Origins of Psychiatry: Pinel or the Zeitgeist?" in *Zusammenhang: Festschrift für Marielene Putscher,* ed. O. Baur and O. Glandien, 2 vols. (Cologne: Wienand, 1984), 2:617–631.

4. Swain, *Le sujet,* 39 and 96–97. For Hegel's acknowledgment of Pinel's contribution, see G. W. F. Hegel, *Encyclopädie der philosophischen Wissenschaften im Grundrisse* (1830), ed. F. Nicolin and O. Poggeler (Hamburg: Meiner, 1969), 338.

5. On the comparative importance and popularity of the early books on psychiatry, see D. B. Weiner, "The Madman in the Light of Reason, Part II: Alienists, Asylums, and the Psychologic Approach," in *Handbook of the History of Psychiatry,* ed. E. R. Wallace, IV and J. Gach (New Haven: Yale University Press, forthcoming).

the *Philosophical Transactions of the Royal Society.*[6] He found plentiful confirmation for the validity of his approach in a British book that came to his attention in 1798, when his own was already written, but in time for lengthy comment in his Introduction. That book was the work of the Scottish physician Alexander Crichton (1763–1856), an author virtually unknown in the medical literature, entitled *An Inquiry into the Nature and Origins of Mental Derangement, Comprehending a Concise System of Physiology and Pathology of the Human Mind, and History of the Passions and Their Effects.*[7] Crichton's importance in the context of the present study is threefold: his book, particularly part 3, "On the Passions," confirmed Pinel's belief that his reliance on observation of the patient's feelings, as expressed in words, gestures, moods, and attitudes toward others, offered a reliable—indeed, the only reliable—path toward a diagnosis of mental illness in the living patient. Furthermore, Crichton's work alerted Pinel to German learning in medical psychology. Crichton had resided for three years in various German university towns, learned the language, and acquired a keen interest in contemporary German research and writing in anthropology, natural history, and the literature of what would become psychiatry—then called *Erfahrungsseelenkunde.* And lastly, Crichton's emphasis on the passions helped shape the thought of Pinel's favorite student and intellectual heir, Jean Dominique Esquirol (1772–1840).[8] For these combined reasons, and because Crichton's career has remained almost totally undocumented, he is discussed at length later in this essay.

The meeting of minds between Pinel and Crichton in the fall of 1798 marks a significant moment in the history of medical ideas. It is surprising, given Britain's close ties to Germany at the time, that her physicians

6. See Jacques Gibelin, ed., *Abrégé des Transactions de la Société royale de Londres,* 12 vols. (Paris: Buisson, 1789–1791). Pinel was sole editor of volumes 5–7, entitled *Chimie, anatomie et physique animale,* and *Médecine et chirurgie,* and coedited part 2 of *Matière médicale et pharmacie.*

7. (London: Cadell and Davies, 1798). There are only two scholarly studies of Crichton: H. Hopf, *Leben und Werk Alexander Crichtons (1763–1856)* (Munich: Medical Thesis, 1962) and E. M. Tansey, "The Life and Works of Sir Alexander Crichton, F.R.S. (1763–1856): A Scottish Physician to the Imperial Russian Court," *Royal Society of London: Records and Proceedings* 38 (1983–84): 241–259. For a complete Crichton bibliography, including foreign translations of the *Inquiry,* see Appendix, Biobibliographic Note 2.

8. The present essay is greatly indebted to M. Gauchet and G. Swain, *La pratique de l'esprit humain: L'institution asilaire et la révolution démocratique* (Paris: Gallimard, 1980). Marcel Gauchet is a philosopher and Gladys Swain a psychiatrist: it is her contribution that is most relevant here. She is among the rare historians who pay any attention to Crichton (pp. 347–349), and she elucidates the relationship between Pinel and Esquirol.

only discovered German writings on mental illness at the turn of the nineteenth century. The deafness of French doctors to German thought is more easily explained because, ever since the days of the "sun king," the French saw themselves as the most civilized of European nations, a model for their neighbors on the Continent. Despite the cosmopolitanism of the Enlightenment, French attention continued to focus on France and on Paris, and the dramatic unfolding of the Revolution concentrated all energies on ideas and events at home. French medical thinkers shared in this national involvement. By the turn of the century, however, this introversion gave way to new interests in foreign lands: just as Madame de Staël's *De l'Allemagne* (1811) revolutionized French attitudes toward German literature and philosophy, so active interest in German medical writings evidenced a new openness to Continental ideas in the French medical milieu. A set of translations and two journals represent significant examples of the new literature: the *Recueil des mémoires sur les établissements d'humanité,* the *Recueil périodique de littérature médicale étrangère,* and the *Bibliothèque médico-chirurgicale germanique* all began publication in the Year VII (1798–99).[9] The prominence of translations is significant: ever since German physicians and medical scientists had begun to publish in their own language instead of Latin, the French lost touch, for hardly any Frenchman knew German, and Pinel was typical of his countrymen in this respect.

That is why Crichton's work, with its emphasis on German sources, was a revelation for him. But he also shared Crichton's approach to patients as well as his diagnostic and therapeutic outlook. For Pinel as for Crichton, a reliance on personal and prolonged observation held numerous implications: it demanded a rejection of all "systems" and of almost all ancient as well as modern writers, except the few who were committed to the inductive method and proceeded as medical scientists. It called for a critical reexamination of the traditional a priori categories of mania, melancholia, dementia, and idiocy. It implied a refusal to indulge in speculation about nervous fluids and vapors circulating through the nerves, and it meant renouncing diagnosis based on

9. Under the auspices of the minister of foreign affairs, François de Neufchâteau, Adrien Cyprien Duquesnoy edited *Recueil des mémoires sur les établissements d'humanité,* 18 vols. (Paris: Agasse, An VII–XIII), which contained translations of foreign, including German, humanitarian writings. *Recueil périodique de littérature médicale étrangère,* an offshoot of *Recueil périodique de la société de médecine* under the editorship of Sédillot, jeune, began publication in the Year VII (1798–99), and *Bibliothèque médico-chirurgicale germanique; ou, Traduction des meilleurs auteurs allemands qui ont écrit sur l'art de guérir* also began in the Year VII under the editorship of Oedenkoven and Thiriart.

humoral and pneumatic theory with the consequent activist therapeutic regimen of bleeding, purging, sweating, and puking. The new approach relied on data gathered in the clinic.

Pinel developed a method of systematic observation that helped him understand his patients' minds by studying their behavior. In 1793 he had finally reached a position commensurate with his interests and talents when the government appointed him "physician of the infirmaries" at the male division of the General Hospital in Paris, Bicêtre Hospice. From this experience Pinel developed a new conceptualization of mental illness, the conviction of its curability, and the notion that distinct "species" of patients needed to be separately lodged. He incorporated that idea into his detailed prescription about "policing" the asylum, that is, managing it with firmness, but in a humane manner, with the help of attendants restricted to using psychologic treatment only. He was delighted to find his views confirmed on reading Crichton a few years later.

Specifically, Pinel watched and recorded the behavior of each of the two hundred internees at Bicêtre: their dress; their habits and demeanor; their relationships with their companions, the servants, the supervisor; their gestures and gesticulations; their moods and mood swings; their affects as expressed on their faces and in "body language"; their words—mainly their words. Pinel engaged each patient in lengthy and repeated conversations, attempting to learn his personal history, his preoccupations, even if delusional, the precipitating event of his illness. He visited each patient, often several times a day, and took careful notes over two years. His twin objectives were to assemble a detailed case history while also improving his grasp of the natural history of the disease before him. He could often document a logical progression from a man's traumatic life experience to the pathologic symptoms he was observing.

Both in the lecture room and on the hospital ward. Pinel had many opportunities to teach his views to the young generation. It is well known that he sponsored Dominique Esquirol's thesis, published in 1805 and entitled *Des passions, considérées comme causes, symptômes, et moyens curatifs de l'aliénation mentale* (On the passions, considered as causes, symptoms, and means of cure for mental alienation).[10] The resemblance of this title to that of part 3 of Crichton's book is startling, and we are not surprised to find that Esquirol mentions Crichton in one breath with the abbé de Condillac and Pinel as the main authors who molded his thought. But instead of merely acknowledging Crichton, as Pinel had done when his own book was already in press, Esquirol had time to read the Scottish

10. On Esquirol, see Appendix, Biobibliographic Note 3.

author with care before writing his own thesis. He studied Crichton's volume on the passions and his volume on the mental functions. The contrast struck him and reinforced his conviction that certain passions might be useful as a *means of cure*. Seventeen years later, when Pinel reviewed Esquirol's paper on hallucinations before the Academy of Sciences, he confirmed that Crichton's "learned research" stood at the cradle of Esquirol's formulations on this subject.[11]

Pinel and Crichton, like many philosophers, dramatists, and observers of human nature before them, analyzed the antagonism between reason and emotion, but they were not interested in this struggle per se. Rather, in observing involuntary irrational behavior, they perceived unconscious psychologic meaning. Pursuing therapeutic strategies, they wondered whether awareness of this meaning might help the patient understand his behavior, realize its harmful consequences, and therefore change his ways. Esquirol, in contrast, following Crichton's emphasis on the passions and citing his own clinical experience, argued that the therapist could use the passions to shock the patient who, as a consequence of that experience, might regain the use of his reason. Since Crichton's analysis of the passions relies so heavily on the German literature on this subject, there is no doubt that Crichton's work forms a hitherto neglected link between German and French thought.

In fact Martin Schrenk, the most percipient German historian of this era, describes two circles of intellectual influences: one reaching from Scottish moral philosophy through Kant and his *Anthropologie* to Crichton's German student days, back to Britain, via Crichton's book; the other circle originating in German learning as absorbed by Crichton, reaching French psychiatry through Pinel and Esquirol and back to Germany, where Pinel's method of observation and Esquirol's model hospital at Charenton exerted a deep and lasting influence on academic and institutional psychiatry.[12] We shall also see that Henri Ey, in his authoritative biographic sketch of Esquirol published in K. Kolle's *Grosse*

11. P. Pinel, "Rapport sur le mémoire sur les hallucinations de M. Esquirol," *Procès-verbaux des séances de l'Académie depuis la fondation jusqu'au mois d'août 1835*, Institut de France, Académie des sciences, 11 vols. (Hendaye: Observatoire d'Abbadia, 1910–), 6:196–199.

12. M. Schrenk, "Pathologie der Passionen: Zur Erinnerung an J. E. D. Esquirol, geboren 1772," *Der Nervenarzt* 44 (1973): 195–198; see also idem, *Über den Umgang mit Geisteskranken: Die Entwicklung der psychiatrischen Therapie vom "moralischen Regime" in England und Frankreich zu den "psychischen Curmethoden" in Deutschland* (New York: Springer, 1973), 50, 123–124; see also W. Leibbrand and A. Wetley, *Der Wahnsinn: Geschichte der abendländischen Psychopathologie* (Freiburg and Munich: Alber, 1961), 360.

Nervenärzte, emphasized a "similarity of human and scientific outlook" between Esquirol and the German school of "Psychiker," namely Johann Christian Heinroth (1773–1843), Karl Wilhelm Ideler (1795–1860), Johann Christian Reil (1759–1813), and Johann Gottfried Langermann (1768–1832). Ey cannot explain the origin of this resemblance: we suggest that it lies in Crichton's book.[13]

While Pinel's explicit appreciation of Crichton's book brought the British work to French attention, Pinel himself remains the crucial figure in any international overview of early psychiatry. In the past decades, he has become the subject of lively controversy owing to Michel Foucault's *Birth of the Clinic* of 1963. That controversy has served to explode the myth of Pinel the "chainbreaker," even though every textbook still depicts him as the first to free the insane from their shackles. More interestingly, it has raised the question of Pinel's unique importance among a growing group of physicians who specialized in the theory and treatment of mental illness. Pinel's awareness of German learning and its influence on Esquirol explored in this essay matter in the early history of psychiatry mainly if Pinel was indeed a pivotal figure and founder of this medical specialty. This has recently been disputed by G. Lantéri-Laura and J. Postel, who claim that Pinel was but an "eponym" for a general European development and that the French Revolution attracted the spotlight of history to Paris and enhanced Pinel's stature beyond his intrinsic merit.[14]

In order to assess his role, and the importance of that meeting of minds among Pinel, Crichton, and Esquirol, we shall present Pinel the autodidact, the learned but unemployed modern who rejected traditional systematic theories of mental illness. We will interpret his thought in the context of the French school of scientific social reform known as Ideology, of custodial and therapeutic strategies prevalent at that time, and of the contemporary literature on medical psychology. It is hoped that, viewed in this context, his original contributions to the nascent psychiatric specialty will stand out clearly. As for Crichton, his biography, particularly the German and Russian phases, and his major work remain to be analyzed. But mainly we will assess Pinel's endorsement of Crichton's book and its impact on Esquirol. He came to conceive of the asylum superintendent as the director of a therapeutic program that used the mental hospital as a tool to control the patient's body and used the pas-

13. See p. 389 below, for discussion and documentation of this argument.

14. See G. Lantéri-Laura, *Encyclopaedia Universalis* 30:750 s.v. "Psychiatrie," and J. Postel, *Genèse de la psychiatrie: Les premiers écrits de Philippe Pinel* (Paris: Le Sycomore, 1981), 45.

sions as a means of cure. To cure meant to restore the mental faculties as agents of containment and domination over the emotions. In surveying these theories and therapeutic formulations in a broader philosophic context and in historical perspective, we may be justified in interpreting Esquirol's concept of the passions as a manifestation of Romantic *Naturphilosophie,* brought by Crichton from Germany, a challenge to the rationalism of Ideology and the Enlightenment.

THE SCIENTIFIC STANCE OF MEDICAL IDEOLOGY

Pinel should be seen as an Idéologue and a disciple of Francis Bacon, John Locke, and the abbé de Condillac.[15] The Idéologues conceptualized man as the product of his environment: by changing it, they sought to improve the human condition; they were eager to apply their "science of man" to concrete social situations and to assume the role of public servants. Among physicians, the leading exponents of Ideology were P. J. G. Cabanis (1757–1808),[16] J. L. Moreau de la Sarthe (1771–1826),[17] Philippe Pinel, and Jean Antoine Chaptal (1756–1832), Bonaparte's minister of internal affairs under the Consulate, who had special power

15. The Idéologues have, after a long delay, received appropriate scholarly attention, especially from M. Regaldo and S. Moravia. See Regaldo, *Un milieu intellectuel: La décade philosophique, 1794–1807,* 5 vols. (Paris: Champion, 1976), and Moravia, *Il tramonto dell'illuminismo: Filosofia e politica nella società francese, 1770–1810* (Bari: Laterza, 1968), *La scienza dell'uomo nel settecento* (Bari: Laterza, 1970), and especially *Il pensiero degli Idéologues: Scienza e filosofía in Francia, 1780–1815* (Florence: La Nuova Italia, 1974). Among Moravia's articles, see especially "The Capture of the Invisible: For a (Pre)History of Psychology in Eighteenth-Century France," *Journal of the History of the Behavioral Sciences* 19 (1983): 370–378; "The Enlightenment and the Sciences of Man," *History of Science* 18 (1980): 246–268; "From 'homme machine' to 'homme sensible': Changing Eighteenth-Century Models of Man's Image," *Journal of the History of Ideas* 39 (1978): 45–60; "Les idéologues et l'âge des lumières," *Studies on Voltaire and the Eighteenth Century* 154 (1976): 1465–1486, and "Philosophie et médecine en France à la fin du 18ème siècle," ibid. 89 (1972): 1089–1151. On the impact of the Idéologues on medical developments, see also G. Rosen, "The Philosophy of Ideology and the Emergence of Modern Medicine in France," *Bulletin of the History of Medicine* 20 (1946): 328–339.

16. On Cabanis, see especially the recent book by M. S. Staum, *Cabanis: Enlightenment and Medical Philosophy in the French Revolution* (Princeton: Princeton University Press, 1980). See also F. Colonna d'Istria, "La logique de la médecine d'après Cabanis," *Revue de métaphysique et de morale* 24 (1917): 59–73; S. Moravia, "'Moral'–'Physique': Genesis and Evolution of a 'Rapport,'" *Enlightenment Studies in Honor of Lester Crocker,* ed. J. Bingham and V. W. Topazio (Oxford: Voltaire Foundation, 1979), 163–174; and A. Vartanian, "Cabanis and La Mettrie," *Studies on Voltaire and the Eighteenth Century* 155 (1976): 2149–2166.

17. There appears to be no secondary literature on Moreau.

to transform theory into practice.[18] At the turn of the nineteenth century, the Ideologues exerted a pervasive intellectual influence through their newspaper, the *Décade philosophique,*[19] their membership in the National Institute, the Normal and Central School faculties, and "free" associations such as the Lycée des Arts, the Philomatic and Natural History Societies, and the Society of the Observers of Man.

Pinel was no typical Ideologue, and we can use the Introduction to the *Traité* as a convenient guide to delineate his intellectual position. He shared his colleagues' materialistic view of life, and their desire to serve society: his thirty years as physician-in-chief of the Salpêtrière Hospice bear witness to that. Among Ideologue physicians Pinel stands out as a clinician: his lifelong commitment was to minister to physically and psychologically ill patients, particularly the poor. While he followed his friend Cabanis's philosophic postulates with keen attention, Pinel believed that medical truth derived from clinical experience. Despite his interest in theory, Pinel knew that, at the sickbed, philosophy is of little use. And at the sickbed Pinel was at his best—by all accounts a brilliant diagnostician.

The Introduction to Pinel's *Traité* shows that Hippocrates remained his model because observation of the patient formed the basis of the Greek physician's writings.[20] Among other ancient authors Pinel singled out several whose opinions and attitudes paralleled his own. He praised Aretaeus of Cappadocia, the Greek physician who lived in Rome in the mid-second century A.D., for dwelling on the distinctive traits of mental alienation, the predisposition to relapses, and the physical and mental excitement that madness provokes.[21] Coelius Aurelianus also found favor with Pinel: this fifth-century Algerian doctor, living in Rome, translated and commented on the writings of the great Greek physician Soranus. Pinel praised Aurelianus because he focused on the precipitat-

18. On Chaptal, see M. Peronnet, *Chaptal* (Toulouse: Privat, 1988); J. Pigeire, *La vie et l'œuvre de Chaptal, 1756–1832* (Paris: Domat-Montchrétien, 1932); a good chapter on Chaptal in J. Savant, *Les ministres de Napoléon* (Paris: Hachette, 1959); and R. Tresse, "Jean Antoine Chaptal et l'enseignement technique de 1800 à 1819," *Revue d'histoire des sciences* 10 (1957): 167–174. See also M. Crosland, *The Society of Arcueil: A View of French Science at the Time of Napoleon I* (Cambridge, Mass.: Harvard University Press, 1967).

19. *La décade philosophique, littéraire, et politique, par une Société de républicains* [later: *gens de lettres*] (Paris: An II–An IX [1794–1801]).

20. Jackie Pigeaud has explored the ancient philosophic issues that influence the relationship of physician to patient in *La maladie de l'âme: Etude sur la relation de l'âme et du corps dans la tradition médico-philosophique antique* (Paris: Les Belles Lettres, 1981).

21. Pinel, *Traité,* Introduction, ix.

ing events in mental illness, the correct assessment of symptoms, patient management, and especially

> the happy talent of choosing the appropriate tone in communicating with mental patients, an imposing gravity or a genuine empathy to earn their respect and esteem by a frank and open manner, to inspire them with both affection and fear, a skill credited to certain Moderns whose true source I indicate here.[22]

The "Moderns" whose "skill" Pinel attributed to Coelius Aurelianus were surely the Quakers at the York Retreat whose originality Pinel thus questioned.[23]

Pursuing his review of the ancients, Pinel lauded Celsus for his attention to the therapy of mental illness, and the management of patients.[24] Galen, however talented, fell victim to his own vanity, in Pinel's judgment, and to his "rare skill for timely self-advertisement." He was so busy fighting the different sects, Dogmatists, Methodists, Empiricists, and Eclectics, that he had no time or wish to study any specific doctrine in depth.[25] (The veiled allusion to the sterile squabbles of the Paris medical faculty surely struck contemporary French readers.) The fight against Galenism and iatrochemistry, according to Pinel, gave rise to "systems," and those he castigated, like a latter-day Bacon. Thus the scant selective praise from this Enlightened physician typically singles out those rare passages in ancient medical writings that indicate psychologic sensitivity and imagination and that mirror late-eighteenth-century beliefs. With a blindness typical of the Enlightenment, this Idéologue ignored Jewish and Arabic contributors to modern medicine, as well as medieval and even Renaissance writers. Pinel indiscriminately dismissed their work as "sterile language of the Schoolmen" and condemned their unscientific and indiscriminate use of drugs.[26]

Having thus disposed of the ancients and their Renaissance imitators, Pinel proclaimed his allegiance to medical science and greeted modern

22. Ibid., xi.
23. Ibid., xliv, n. 2. See below, n. 72.
24. Ibid., xii–xiv.
25. Ibid., xi.
26. Ibid., xv–xvi. This condemnation includes the work of Daniel Sennert (1572–1637), Lazare Riverius (1589–1655), and Felix Plater (1536–1614), who wrote *Praxis medica* (1602–1608), the "first modern attempt at a classification of diseases," according to Castiglioni. These included mental illness, of which he distinguished four types: *mentis imbecillitas, consternatio, alienatio,* and *defatigatio*. In addition, Pinel dismissed as irrelevant the work of Johann Heurnius (1543–1601), Gregor Horst (1578–1636), to some the "German Asklepios," and Jan Baptista van Helmont (1577–1644).

times as a breath of fresh air, a liberation. He admired van Helmont for his auto-experiment with monkshood[27] and praised Georg Ernst Stahl (1660–1734) and Herman Boerhaave (1668–1738) for their scientific teaching of medicine and chemistry—Boerhaave in particular for establishing bedside teaching in Leiden, whence his disciples spread the practice, primarily to Edinburgh, London, and Vienna. By implication, Paris lagged behind. Therefore medical psychology must now build a firm clinical base, precisely what Pinel was engaged in doing. Taking a leaf from the book of biology and citing numerous examples, he argued that medical psychology should now become comparably scientific.[28]

The Ideologues rejected the traditional belief in a soul and adopted Albrecht von Haller's concepts of sensitivity and irritability as the only bases of sensation and movement. "We feel, therefore we are," taught Cabanis, in his famous lectures on the mind/body problem at the Institut de France in 1796.[29] Feelings emanated from matter, experiments in biology assumed major importance, and therefore Pinel particularly appreciated Crichton's reports on plant and animal behavior involving hydatids, polyps, Venus's-flytrap, and the heart rate of the hamster.[30] In the same vein, Cabanis favored examples of animal behavior with implied similarities to humans. He wrote, for instance:

> Puppies and kittens smell their mothers approaching from far away. They do not confuse them with other animals of their species and of the same sex. . . . Kittens often stretch their necks to seek the nipple while their rear and thighs are still lodged in the vagina and in the womb of the mother. (Note: I have witnessed this fact myself.)[31]

27. Pinel, *Traité,* Introduction, xvii–xviii.

28. In this connection, he referred to the Genevan Théophile Bonnet (1620–1689), author of the famous *Sepulchretum anatomicum* (1679); Marcello Donatus (1538–1602), author of *De medica historia mirabili libri sex* (1568); Friedrich Hoffmann (1660–1742), the mechanist and author of *Medicina rationalis systematica,* 9 vols. (1718–1740); Johannes Nicolaas Pechlin of Leiden (1646–1706), physician to the duke of Holstein, who practiced in Stockholm; Johannes Schenk von Grafenberg (1530–1598), author of *Observationum medicarum, rararum, novarum, etc. libri duo* (1600); Gerard Van Swieten (1700–1772), the disciple of Boerhaave whom Empress Maria Theresa called to Vienna in 1745 to reform medical education and public health; and Nicolas Tulpius (1593–1674), so famous because Rembrandt painted him at the anatomy lesson, author of *Observations medicae* (1652).

29. P. J. C. Cabanis, "Rapports du physique et du moral de l'homme," in *Œuvres philosophiques,* 2 vols., ed. C. Lehec and J. Cazeneuve (Paris: Presses universitaires de France, 1956), 1:142. See also O. Temkin, "The Philosophical Background of Magendie's Physiology," *Bulletin of the History of Medicine* 20 (1946): 10–35.

30. A. Crichton, *An Inquiry into the Nature and Origin of Mental Derangement* (London: Cadell and Davies, 1798), book I, 7, 9, 23.

31. Cabanis, "Rapports," 184.

Animal experiments were not a scientific activity that Idéologue physicians pursued for its intrinsic merit, but rather a source of information to buttress their study of human behavior, emotions, and illnesses. They believed that, like a naturalist gathering knowledge in the field, the practicing physician should gather data in the clinic. The body and, through it, the mind would become the objects of scientific observation: the body would reveal the mind.[32] Pinel and Crichton agreed with Bacon that

> the Lyneaments of the bodie doe disclose the disposition and inclination of the minde in generall; but the Motions of the countenance and parts, doe not onely so, but doe further disclose the present humour and state of the mind and will. For . . . as the Tongue speaketh to the Eare, so the gesture speaketh to the Eye. And therefore a number of subtile persons, whose eyes doe dwell upon the faces and fashions of men; do well know the advantage of this observation.[33]

In agreement with Sir Francis, Pinel and Crichton saw the mental patient as a person in ill health whose body and mind were simultaneously afflicted and whose somatic and psychologic symptoms interacted. Crichton's book offered detailed and perceptive analyses of joy, grief, fear, anger, and love, their physiologic and psychologic manifestations, particularly those that a physician judged dangerous to health. Following David Hartley, Crichton underscored the material origin of motion and even of feelings, "repeated impressions on the sensory organs."[34] Along the lines of "faculty psychology," he singled out *one* feeling at a time and explored how it affected the patient's mind and body, comparable to an infected wound from which sepsis spreads, or an ailing organ that debilitates and alters body and mind. Gone is the notion that excessively aggrieved persons "lose" their minds completely, go "out of" their minds, or go *in*-sane. Gone is all moralizing or judgmental comment. Crichton presents us with scientific observations on a clinical syndrome: the madman has become a medical patient.

This view was familiar to Pinel. It agreed with the prevailing philosophy in his circle of forward-looking French physicians. It is surprising that Crichton makes no reference to Ideology, even though he spent the winter of 1785–86 in Paris, where future Ideologues discussed

32. Ibid., 195.

33. F. Bacon, *The Twoo Bookes . . . Of the Proficience and Advancement of Learning, Divine and Human* (London: Tomes, 1605), book 2, fol. 37.

34. On Hartley, see p. 368 below. Roger Smith has recently explored this question in an illuminating article, "The Background of Physiological Psychology in Natural Philosophy," *History of Science* 11 (1973): 75–123.

and planned medical and political reform—in the press, in the coffeehouses, and especially in the salons.

PINEL IN 1800

The salon of Madame Helvétius in Auteuil opened its doors to Pinel in the 1780s, on the initiative of Cabanis, the hostess's adopted son. Thus Pinel joined a circle of brilliant men and women including the marquis A. N. de Condorcet (1743–1794), later Cabanis's brother-in-law, Benjamin Franklin (1706–1790), who attempted to lure Pinel to America, and Michel Augustin Thouret (1748–1810), a prominent member of the Royal Society of Medicine and the first dean of the Revolutionary Health School of Paris. The friendship of Thouret and Cabanis, who were soon to serve as hospital commissioners of the Seine department, would finally help Pinel reach a worthwhile professional appointment. But while Cabanis, the collaborator and doctor of the comte de Mirabeau (1749–1791), was drawn into participation in public affairs, Pinel's interest remained tied to clinical medicine. Already in his forties, he had trodden a narrow and arid path, winding from adolescence as a cleric to a medical degree in Toulouse in 1773, through twenty years of autodidactic life in Montpellier and Paris. A careful study of the biographic documents reveals Pinel's early and strong bent toward clinical medicine and psychology.[35] He left Toulouse in 1773 because the training was entirely theoretical, whereas Montpellier afforded opportunities to gather clinical experience. Pinel did not register for postdoctoral courses but, in his own words,

> faithfully attended the daily medical rounds in the main hospital, . . . took written notes at the sickbed and . . . wrote case histories of the entire course of acute illnesses; that was my general plan for four years.[36]

35. See especially the following papers by the late Pierre Chabbert of Castres: "Les années d'études de Philippe Pinel: Lavaur, Toulouse, Montpellier," *Monspeliensis Hippocrates* 3 (1960): 15–23; "L'œuvre médicale de Philippe Pinel," in *Comptes-rendus du 96ème Congrès national des sociétés savantes* (Paris: Bibliothèque nationale, 1971), 153–161; "Philippe Pinel à Paris jusqu'à sa nomination à Bicêtre," in *Aktuelle Probleme aus der Geschichte der Medizin: Proceedings of the 19th International Congress of the History of Medicine* (Basel: Karger, 1966), 589–595. See also D. B. Weiner, "Health and Mental Health in the Thought of Philippe Pinel: The Emergence of Psychiatry during the French Revolution," in *Healing and History: Essays for George Rosen,* ed. Charles E. Rosenberg (New York: Science History Publication, 1979), 59–85.

36. Quoted in Chabbert, "Les années d'études," 22. On the life of medical students in Montpellier, see also C. Jones, "Montpellier, Medical Students, and the Medicalization of 18th-Century France," in *Problems and Methods in the History of Medicine,* ed. R. Porter and A. Wear (London: Croom Helm, 1987), 57–80.

Beyond this clinical work, Pinel's autobiographic statements also reveal a long-standing interest in the patients' feelings. He wrote in 1793:

> During the years when I visited hospitals for my education, . . . I often found that patients responded well to comforting words. . . . Frequently left to themselves, abandoned to dire thoughts about their fate, often isolated from their relatives and all they loved, disgusted by the crudity and harshness of the servants, often plunged into the blackest depression by the ever-present thought of a real or imagined danger, they expressed the liveliest gratitude toward those who empathized with their sufferings and tried to inspire them with confidence in their recovery. It is an excellent remedy to go to their bedside and ask how they are, express an interest in their ailments, encourage them to persevere and to believe in a prompt return to health.[37]

An early and unusual interest in the psychologic aspects of illness thus distinguished this regular visitor to the Montpellier wards.

Even though he did not register as a student, Pinel undoubtedly attended lectures, particularly those of Théophile de Bordeu (1722–1776), who influenced him decisively. Bordeu developed his own brand of vitalism and posited "secondary centers" of sensitivity outside the brain, in the precordial and epigastric region. We shall see later how useful this concept would prove to be, particularly for Esquirol, in developing strategies for psychologic therapy.[38] In 1778 Pinel walked all the way to Paris in search of a career but had to spend fifteen years earning his living as a writer, translator, and editor because the restrictive regulations of the old regime prevented him from practicing medicine. The Paris faculty did not recognize a degree from a provincial university like Toulouse, and all he could secure was a little doctoring on the sly at the *maison de santé* of the ex-carpenter Jacques Belhomme.[39] But he used the time to educate himself further.

37. D. B. Weiner, ed. and tr., *The Clinical Training of Doctors: An Essay of 1793* (Baltimore: Johns Hopkins University Press, 1980), 84.

38. On Bordeu, see E. Haigh, "Vitalism, the Soul, and Sensibility: The Physiology of Théophile de Bordeu," *Journal of the History of Medicine* 31 (1976): 30–41. On Cabanis's debt to Bordeu, see M. S. Staum, "Medical Components in Cabanis' Science of Man," *Studies in History of Biology* 1 (1978): 1–32, particularly 11 and 23–24.

39. The most informative and best-documented source on the *maison* Belhomme is R. Bénard, "Une maison de santé psychiatrique sous la révolution: La maison Belhomme," *Semaine des hôpitaux* 32 (1956): 3990–4000. See also J. Postel, "Les premières expériences psychiatriques de Pinel à la maison de santé Belhomme," *Revue canadienne de psychiatrie* 28 (1983): 571–576. Postel has also recently published a manuscript detailing Pinel's first cures: "Un manuscrit inédit de Philippe Pinel sur 'Les guérisons opérées dans le 7ème emploi de Bicêtre, en 1794,'" *Revue internationale d'histoire de la psychiatrie* 1 (1983): 79–88.

The French Revolution emancipated this provincial physician, and the essay that Pinel submitted for a prize from the Royal Society of Medicine in 1793 led to his first full-time job.[40] Arriving at Bicêtre during the Terror, Pinel found himself in the midst of some four thousand imprisoned men—criminals, petty offenders, syphilitics, pensioners, and about two hundred mental patients. In that forbidding fortress he met Jean Baptiste Pussin (1746–1811), the supervisor of the mental ward: appreciating Pussin's outstanding talent, Pinel decided to apprentice himself to that unschooled but experienced custodian of the insane. Here was the "clinic" where Pinel learned to observe mind and body. As a first move, the new physician asked the "governors" of the various sections for medical reports: one of these has recently come to light, namely the "Observations of Citizen Pussin on the Insane."[41] It provides a picture of the St. Prix ward, where order and cleanliness reigned, violent treatment of inmates was strictly banished, and humane management prevailed. The site-visitors from the National Assembly in 1790 had already recorded their surprise about this ward, remarking particularly that very few of the inmates were chained, in most instances only at night.[42] Even more than they, Pinel appreciated Pussin's ability to practice a crude classification of new arrivals according to their complexion and temperament which permitted him to house them appropriately. Here was a modest beginning of that "division into distinct species of illness" that Pinel would later practice at the Salpêtrière. He admired Pussin's strict adherence to nonviolence: even if the governor or his underlings faced attack by an inmate, they subdued the attacker without causing injury. Pussin reported that he had to dismiss numerous employees in order to assemble a nonviolent staff. He resorted to a variety of strategies to control unruly patients, including stern warnings, the manipulative use of food and privileges, and physical restraints, if necessary, making sure that these would not cause physical pain. It was Pussin, we learn from his "Observations," and not Pinel, as every textbook tells us, who first struck the chains from the insane at Bicêtre. This strict, nonviolent, nonmedical management of mental patients has been called

40. The circumstances are explained in Weiner, *The Clinical Training*, Introductory Essay.

41. "Observations du citoyen Pussin sur les fous." The manuscript is in the Archives nationales, Paris, 27 AP 8 (doc. 2). For an annotated English translation, see D. B. Weiner, "The Apprenticeship of Philippe Pinel: A New Document, 'Observations of Citizen Pussin on the Insane,'" *American Journal of Psychiatry* 136 (1979): 1128–1134.

42. C. Bloch and A. Tuetey, eds., *Procès-verbaux et rapports du comité de mendicité de la Constituante, 1790-1791* (Paris: Imprimerie nationale, 1911), 604.

"moral treatment," owing to a misleading literal translation from the French. "*Moral*" does not mean "moral" but "psychologic," and it would be helpful if English-language terminology aligned itself with the German where the terms "*psychisch*" and "*Psychiker*" were adopted in Pinel's day.[43]

It was a rare, perhaps unprecedented, role-reversal that occurred at Bicêtre in 1793–1795: the spectacle of a middle-aged doctor who had mastered Greek, Latin, and the entire medical literature apprenticing himself to an unschooled but experienced asylum superintendent. In the Introduction to the *Traité,* Pinel wrote:

> I abandoned the dogmatic tone of the doctor. With the help of frequent visits, sometimes during several hours a day, I familiarized myself with the deviations, shouts, and uncontrolled behavior of the most violent maniacs. I then talked repeatedly with the man who was most familiar with their previous state and their delirious thoughts. I took extreme care to manage his self-esteem, and asked him numerous and repeated questions on the same subject if the answers were not clear. I never objected if he said anything doubtful or improbable, but waited for a subsequent examination to enlighten or correct him. I took daily notes on the observed facts with the sole aim of having as many accurate data as possible.
>
> Such is the course I have followed for almost two years, in order *to enrich the medical theory of mental illness with all the insights that the empirical approach affords. Or rather, I strove to perfect the theory and to provide practice with the general principles that it lacked.*[44] [emphasis added]

43. The best overviews of "moral treatment" are E. T. Carlson and N. Dain, "The Psychotherapy That Was Moral Treatment," *American Journal of Psychiatry* 117 (1960): 519–524; C. Geduldig, *Die Behandlung von Geisteskranken ohne physischen Zwang* (Zürich: Medical dissertation, 1976); R. Porter, "Was There a Moral Therapy in Eighteenth-Century Psychiatry?" *Lychnos: Annual of the Swedish History of Science Society,* 1981–82:12–26; J. Postel, "Naissance et décadence du traitement moral pendant la première moitié du 19ème siècle," *L'évolution psychiatrique* 44 (1979): 588–616; and L. Sederer, "Moral Therapy and the Problem of Morale," *American Journal of Psychiatry* 134 (1977): 267–277. An interesting account, along the lines of Michel Foucault's views, is A. Scull, "Moral Treatment Reconsidered: Some Sociological Comments on an Episode in the History of British Psychiatry," in Scull, *Madness, Mad-Doctors, and Madmen,* 105–120.

44. Pinel, *Traité,* Introduction, xlviii–xlix. All references are to the first edition, unless noted otherwise. The only English version of this text is in G. Zilboorg's *History of Medical Psychology* (New York: Norton, 1941), where the translation is, in part, sheer nonsense. A passage reads: "I held repeated conversations with whatever men knew best their former condition and their delirious ideas. Extreme care is necessary to avoid all pretensions of self-esteem and many questions on the same subject if the answers are obscure. I never object if patients make equivocal or improbable remarks but postpone my questions to a later examination, for the purpose of enlightenment and correction" (340).

All his life, Pinel would acknowledge his debt to Pussin and to Madame Pussin, her husband's talented collaborator.

During the two years' apprenticeship at Bicêtre, Pinel assembled a large collection of case histories where the reader meets individuals in distress whose past and symptoms Pinel had probed in numerous encounters and conversations. Let us adduce two examples, beginning with a musician who had "fallen into madness" because of the Revolution:

> While he was convalescing, he recalled a confused memory of his favorite instrument, the violin. I urged his family to provide him with that pleasure, so useful for his total recovery. In a few days he recaptured his old skill and, for eight months, he practiced for several hours daily. Calm and reason were decidedly returning.

At that point, an agitated patient was admitted to the same ward. His presence so upset the musician that he relapsed and became permanently insane.[45] Next, we cite this intriguing case:

> One of the most famous clockmakers in Paris, beguiled by the illusion of perpetual motion that he longed to capture, set to work with indefatigable enthusiasm. . . . His loss of reason exhibited a unique trait. He believed that his head, severed on the scaffold, got mixed up with that of other victims and that the judges . . . ordered the heads restored . . . but, through some mistake, his shoulders now carried the head of an unfortunate companion.[46]

While Pinel's examples usually depicted men from Bicêtre, he learned about mentally ill and senile women upon his transfer in 1795 to the Salpêtrière Hospice as physician-in-chief. He soon missed Pussin acutely. This immense establishment, with some seven thousand elderly indigent and ailing women, was like a large village with an entrenched bureaucracy, a teeming market and huge infirmaries in disarray. Pinel secured Pussin's transfer in 1802 and obtained the appointment of assistants, Esquirol foremost among them.[47]

Pinel needed help with clinical teaching, for students crowded into his thirty-bed ward. He and Jean Nicolas Corvisart were the most famous clinicians in Paris at the time.[48] He was professor of internal med-

45. Pinel, *Traité,* 202–203.

46. Ibid., 66–67.

47. Other collaborators were A. Landré-Beauvais (1772–1840) and Charles Schwilgué (1774–1808).

48. A good overview of clinical teaching in the early nineteenth century can be gained from M. Wiriot, *L'enseignement clinique dans les hôpitaux de Paris entre 1794 et 1848* (Paris: Thèse histoire de la médecine, 1970), and from E. H. Ackerknecht, *Medicine at the Paris*

icine ("medical pathology" in the contemporary idiom) at the Paris Health School, and in 1803 he was elected to the Academy of Sciences, succeeding Georges Cuvier (1773–1838).[49] "This M. Pinel is unique," wrote a student from Strasbourg:

> he can't say two words without a hiccup and he doesn't cure his patients better than anyone else. . . . yet . . . I admit that he made a doctor of me, though I cannot say exactly how. It was at the sickbed that he taught me to recognize the main symptoms of each illness, and to relate them to the genera and species of his nosographic scheme.[50]

And François Leuret (1797–1851), the future physician-in-chief at Bicêtre, summed up the students' experience at the turn of the century in Paris: "Under Corvisart one learned quickly; with Pinel, one learned well."[51]

Pinel taught internal medicine, but with constant reference to the psychologic parameters of bodily illness. Conversely, he never failed to explain the physical substrate of mental disorders, if these were apparent in the patient. We know this from the case histories of patients seen on this teaching ward, recorded by Pinel's assistants and published as *La médecine clinique rendue plus précise et plus exacte par l'application de l'analyse; ou, Recueil et résultat d'observations sur les maladies aigües, faites à la Salpêtrière.*[52] He thus taught what we call psychosomatic medicine, whereas the teaching of psychiatry was initiated by Esquirol at the Salpêtrière in 1817.[53] Pinel also used his data for research, and with that goal in mind and with Pussin's help he reorganized the wards, particularly the mental ward. In 1802 he wrote:

> A hospital destined for sick women and as large as the Salpêtrière, opens a great career for new research on women's diseases that have always and rightly been considered as the most difficult and complicated of all.[54]

Hospital, 1794–1848 (Baltimore: Johns Hopkins University Press, 1967). See also J. C. Sournia, *La médecine révolutionnaire, 1789–1799* (Paris: Payot, 1989).

49. Cuvier became permanent secretary.

50. P. B. Bailly, *Souvenirs d'un élève des écoles de santé de Strasbourg et de Paris pendant la révolution, publiés par . . . son arrière-petit-fils* (Strasbourg: Strasbourg médical, 1924), 17–18.

51. F. Leuret, "M. Esquirol," *Gazette médicale de Paris,* 2d ser., 9 (2 Jan. 1841): 1–6. The quotation is on p. 1.

52. For this and further editions, see Appendix, Biobibliographic Note 1.

53. For a synopsis of Esquirol's course, see his "Introduction à l'étude des aliénations mentales," *Revue médicale française et étrangère* 8 (1822): 31–38.

54. Pinel, *La médecine clinique,* 1st ed. (Paris: Brosson, Gabon et Cie, 1802), Introduction, xxxiv.

Contrasting conditions at the Salpêtrière with his previous experience at Bicêtre, Pinel explained the difference in the Preface to the second edition of the *Traité* (1809):

> Several circumstances made medical treatment quite incomplete [at Bicêtre]. The mental patients had already been treated one or several times at the Hôtel-Dieu, according to the usual methods, and they were then taken to Bicêtre to bring about or reinforce their cure. This rendered my results inconclusive.[55] The use of iron chains to restrain a great number of madmen was still very much in force (*it was only abolished three years later*);[56] and how could one distinguish between the resulting exasperation and the symptoms specific to illness? The defects of the buildings, the lack of subdivisions to separate patients according to their degree of agitation or calm, frequent changes in administration, the lack of baths, and several other necessary facilities—these were many hurdles. . . . [57] [emphasis added]
>
> At the Salpêtrière I was able to resume the pursuit of my goals: the hospital administration had just transferred the treatment of all female mental patients to that hospice and this was of enormous help to me. The buildings were vast, convenient and easy to subdivide. . . . The barbarous use of iron chains was abolished, just like three years earlier at Bicêtre, and treatment then followed its regular course, according to a new method.[58]
>
> Distinguished travelers anxious to visit the Salpêtrière and witnessing the order and calm that usually prevailed there, sometimes remarked with surprise, as they examined the hospital, "But where are the madwomen?" Little did these strangers know that this was the most encouraging praise for the establishment, and that their question underlined a remarkable difference in comparison with other hospitals.[59]

By 1800, Pinel was thus well known in French academic and scientific circles, a widely read author, popular among medical students, and an innovator in hospital administration. He therefore spoke with authority when, in the Introduction to the *Traité,* he defined the context for the study of mind and body in the clinic, that is, for French medical psychology around 1800.

55. The "usual methods" were purges, vomits, venesection, and baths. Pinel was well aware of iatrogenic symptoms produced by the administration of drugs and debilitating procedures.

56. This statement provides additional proof that it was not Pinel who first removed the chains.

57. Pinel, *Traité,* 2d ed. (Paris: Brosson, 1809), Introduction, xxxi.

58. Ibid., i.

59. Ibid., 193. This passage echoes Pussin.

PINEL'S ORIGINAL CONTRIBUTIONS TO PSYCHIATRY

Between 1796 and 1798 Pinel published three papers, "Mémoire sur la manie périodique ou intermittente" (On periodic or intermittent insanity), "Recherches et observations sur le traitement moral des aliénés" (On psychologic treatment), and "Observations sur les aliénés et leur division en espèces distinctes" (On the mentally ill and their division into separate species).[60] Numerous themes call for our attention: Pinel's respect and empathy for the patient; his use of observation, including a new diagnosis; a new concept of the doctor-patient relationship; his guidelines for therapy; the subdivisions in his nosology; his call for a thoughtful administrative policy in the asylum; and the exploration of new avenues for research.

All of Pinel's writings convey the importance of each patient as a special person endowed with reason, personal feelings, and a unique tragic history where the cause of the patient's mental illness lay hidden. The physician-in-chief of the Salpêtrière knew, of course, that the Revolutionary reformers had proclaimed the right of every ailing and needy citizen—the "citizen-patient"—to health care, and he interpreted this right to include the mentally ill.[61] As a public servant who headed the largest hospital in the world, he set an example, but he knew the difficulties of dispensing psychologically sensitive care and therapy to hundreds of inmates. All around him he witnessed young physicians on Paris hospital wards who assumed an increasingly impassive attitude toward the suffering indigent—young medical scientists who favored large series of cases that yielded numerical data. Pinel realized that two contrasting kinds of psychologic therapy were emerging at the end of the eighteenth century: individual care for paying patients and collective management for the poor.

Crucial among Pinel's original contributions is the careful observation of the patient over a long time if necessary. This led him to emphasize two aspects essential to diagnosis: one is a precise record of the precipitating event that may determine the character and course of the illness,

60. P. Pinel, "Mémoire sur la manie périodique ou intermittente," *Mémoires de la Société médicale d'émulation* 1 (An V [1796–97]): 94–119; "Recherches et observations sur le traitement moral des aliénés," ibid. 2 (An VI [1797–98]): 215–255; "Observations sur les aliénés et leur division en espèces distinctes," ibid. 3 (An VII [1798–99]): 1–26.

61. This argument was presented to the French National Assembly in 1790 by the duc de La Rochefoucauld-Liancourt, chairman of the Poverty Committee. See D. B. Weiner, "Le droit de l'homme à la santé: Une belle idée devant l'assemblée constituante, 1790–1791," *Clio Medica* 5 (1970): 209–233.

the other is the physician's knowledge of the natural history of the disease afflicting the patient. Only with such knowledge can the physician accurately assess the signs and symptoms that he must interpret. It was precise observation that led Pinel to diagnose "reasoning madness" ("*folie raisonnante*"), a definition based on the concept that mental illness often involves one faculty only while the others remain unaffected. In the case of *folie raisonnante,* reason and logical thinking are intact, but the patient is captive to an insane conviction or delusion, for example that he is the prophet Mohammed. No psychiatrist could undo such madness.

Pinel's most important contribution consists of a new approach to the doctor-patient relationship. It was based on a reinterpretation of the phenomenon of periodicity in "intermittent insanity." Observers of the mentally ill had long mused about the influence of the changing seasons, the phases of the moon and sun, and biorhythms such as the patient's menstrual cycle upon morbidity. These influences of the patient's surroundings or internal milieu (to use Claude Bernard's phrase) could cause regular or irregular successive phases of morbidity and sanity. Pinel now conceptualized intermittence or periodicity anew. He focused on the periods of mental *sanity* as the moments when a skilled therapist can establish a relationship of trust with the patient. He must build this gradually, through repeated visits and conversation. By timing his interventions with care and using the patient's intact faculties, he may involve the patient in his or her own cure. Pinel thus established a new avenue toward recovery and psychologic treatment.[62] The philosopher Georg Wilhelm Friedrich Hegel praised Pinel for this innovative approach when he wrote:

> . . . true psychologic therapy holds to the point of view that madness is not an abstract loss of reason, neither of intelligence nor of will, but only a derangement, a contradiction within the remaining rationality. Similarly illness is not an abstract and total loss of health (that would mean death), but a contradiction within health. This humane, that is kindly and reasonable treatment—Pinel deserves the highest recognition for his efforts on this behalf—assumes the patient to be rational and clings to this belief and engages the patient in this manner. Similarly the physician deals with the living body, in which health is still to be found.[63]

62. This is not possible in all species of insanity. The above paragraph is indebted to G. Swain, *Le sujet de la folie,* especially section IX, and W. Riese, "Outline of a History of Psychotherapy."

63. See *Encyclopädie der philosophischen Wissenschaften,* 338. The remark appears in part I, section I: Der subjektive Geist, A. Die Anthropologie, b. Die fühlende Seele, ß. Das Selbstgefühl. Swain discovered this passage.

Hegel thus saw the dialectic process at work in the struggle of doctor and patient to wrest health from illness.

While diagnosis fascinated Pinel, therapy was never his main interest: a correct diagnosis would produce the appropriate follow-up. As an admirer of Hippocrates he believed in the "healing powers of nature": removing harmful influences and letting nature run her course was often best. He condemned the uncritical and untested use of drugs because he was wary of side effects and iatrogenic symptoms, derided the "hotchpotch" of polypharmacy, and preferred mild natural pharmacologic agents. Diet and regimen seemed aspects of therapy that physicians must supervise closely. He agreed with William Battie that "management does much more than Medicine."[64] Patients must be treated according to their individual needs, with well-designed management and therapy.

In order to administer a mental hospital successfully, the director must follow clear rules. Therefore guidelines for "policing" the asylum form an important part of the *Traité,* and Pinel outlined them in the Introduction. He advocated the dignified individualized treatment of the mentally ill citizen-patient, cleanliness, regularity in hospital routine, the banishment of violence even though firmness was of the essence. Mainly, he believed, insanity was a curable illness.

Research was always on Pinel's mind, and to that end he favored couching his nosographic distinctions in the language of the natural sciences. His division of the mentally ill into "separate species" reflects the influence of Boissier de Sauvages, Linnaeus, and Georges Louis Leclerc, comte de Buffon (1707–1788), whom Pinel undoubtedly met at the Jardin du roi in the 1780s, while studying with his assistant L. J. M. Daubenton, who became Pinel's friend. When Crichton brought the ideas of Blumenbach to Pinel's attention a few years later, they obviously fell onto well-prepared, fertile ground. The initial objective of Pinel's research was nosographic clarity. That was his first hurdle when he entered the Bicêtre mental ward in 1793, and we have a tantalizing piece of paper, 12 × 15 inches, on which he jotted down his impromptu formulations.[65] Once he subdivided and regrouped the patients, he could observe them to better advantage. He applied the "numerical method," crude statistics.[66] Conversant with skull measurements as an index of in-

64. Battie, *A Treatise on Madness* (n. 80 below), 68.

65. See R. Semelaigne, "Notes inédites de Pinel, avec un 'Tableau général des fous de Bicêtre,'" *Bulletin de la société clinique de médecine mentale* 6 (1913): 117–221. Jacques Postel has published this "Tableau" in *Genèse de la psychiatrie,* 226–229.

66. See, for example, "Résultats d'observations et construction de tables pour servir à déterminer le degré de probabilité de la guérison des aliénés," *Mémoires de la classe des sciences mathématiques et physiques,* Institut national de France, 1st ser., 8, (1807): 169–205.

telligence, he discussed them in the *Traité* but remained skeptical, and the same can be said of dissecting patient brains in order to locate the "seat" of mental illness.[67] He tried to ascertain the therapeutic value of electricity but doubted its effects,[68] and he wrote about the relationship of psychiatry and the law.[69] However, while he was open to new trends and problems, as exemplified by his attention to Crichton's book, his major involvement was a personal relationship with students such as Esquirol and with his patients, a relationship symbolized and reinforced by his residence inside the asylum walls for thirty years.

This secluded residence did not isolate Pinel from the national nor from the international medical scene. He continued to read widely, as the contents of his library indicate, and he followed the latest developments in research: we know that he hardly ever missed a meeting of the Academy of Sciences and wrote frequent reports on new experiments and books. His Introduction to the *Traité* allows us to assess his familiarity with contemporary developments in psychiatry.

THE INTERNATIONAL CONTEXT OF MEDICAL PSYCHOLOGY IN 1800

In the Introduction to the *Traité,* Pinel generalized about the important role that experienced laymen played in the management of contemporary asylums and even in the cure of mentally ill persons throughout the Western world. He singled out the *concierge* of the Amsterdam asylum,[70] Father Pouthion at Manosque in Provence,[71] and Francis Willis, Thomas Fowler, and John Haslam in England. Pinel's facts are faulty,

67. Pinel, *Traité,* section III, "Recherches anatomiques sur les vices de conformation du crâne des aliénés."

68. P. Pinel, "Recherches sur le traitement général des femmes aliénées dans un grand hospice, et résultats obtenus à la Salpêtrière après trois années d'expérience," *Le moniteur universel,* 11 Messidor, An XIII, 1158–1160.

69. P. Pinel, "Résultats d'observations pour servir de base aux rapports juridiques dans les cas d'aliénation mentale," *Mémoires de la société médicale d'émulation* 8 (1817): 675–684.

70. Pinel, *Traité,* Introduction, xliv. Pinel refers to an article by Thouin (identified as a professor of agriculture at the Museum of Natural History in Paris) entitled "Description de la *Maison des Fous* d'Amsterdam, extraite du journal manuscrit des voyages du cit. Thouin dans la Belgique et la Hollande," *Décade philosophique littéraire et politique* (Vendémiaire-Frimaire), An IV:418–424.

71. Pinel, *Traité,* Introduction, xliv. On Father Pouthion, a Brother of the Observance, see M. Mourre, *Observations sur les insensés* (Toulon: Surre fils, 1791), and M. J. Alliez, "Un précurseur de l'assistance moderne aux aliénés dans notre région, le R. P. Pouthion, de Manosque," *Bulletin de la société de psychiatrie de Marseille et du Sud-Est méditerranéen* 6 (1966–67): 36–47.

since most of the men he listed were not laymen but physicians.[72] His judgment, however, is correct: laymen can make good psychiatric nurses. He might have adduced the example of the Brothers of Charity, experts at psychiatric nursing who played a prominent role in the custody of men incarcerated in France by *lettre de cachet*, that is, by the king or the courts. In the eighteenth century the Brothers administered thirty-eight *charités* in France alone; they charged from six hundred to six thousand livres, according to the inmates' ability to pay. They provided individually programmed custody with carefully graduated privileges and even medical care, if we can believe their admirers.[73] The Brothers' practices seem not to have been widely known at the time of the French Revolution, or perhaps the anti-Catholic temper of the times minimized the Church's achievements and Pinel adopted that attitude. His acknowledgment of Father Pouthion suggests, however, that he was unaware of the Brothers of Charity's expertise, or he would have mentioned them in this context.

One should also emphasize that it was no one's unique accomplishment to strike the chains from the insane at the turn of the nineteenth century. Progressive physicians throughout Europe were replacing traditional heavy iron shackles with leather straps or canvas tunics called "straitjackets." One might cite Dr. Abraham Joly (1748–1812)[74] and Dr. Charles Gaspard de La Rive (1770–1834) of Geneva,[75] Dr. Gastaldy of

72. Most of the men whom Pinel cited did indeed have medical degrees. The Reverend Dr. Francis Willis (1718–1807), M.D. Oxon., was the chief manager of George III's mental illness in the 1780s; Thomas Fowler (?–1801), M.D. Edin., became nonresident physician at the York Retreat in 1796; and John Haslam (1764–1844), M.D. Aberdeen, served as "apothecary" at Bedlam. (Haslam did not acquire the M.D. degree until 1816.) Pinel's incomplete information stems from reports in the *Bibliothèque britannique*, published in Geneva, the chief source of news about medico-scientific activities in Great Britain available to the French while England and France were at war, that is, for twenty-three years in the late eighteenth and early nineteenth century. On the important function of the *Bibliothèque britannique* as translator and mediator of medical information, see M. A. Barblan, "La santé publique vue par les rédacteurs de la *Bibliothèque britannique*, 1796–1815," *Gesnerus* 22 (1975): 129–146, and idem, "Journalisme médical et échanges intellectuels au tournant du 18ème siècle: Le cas de la Bibliothèque britannique, 1796–1815," *Archives des sciences* (Geneva) 30 (1977): 283–398.

73. On the Brothers of Charity, see D. B. Weiner, "The Brothers of Charity and the Mentally Ill in Pre-Revolutionary France," *Social History of Medicine* 2 (1989): 321–337.

74. L. Gautier, *La médecine à Genève* (Geneva: Jullien, 1906), 346. On Switzerland, see also W. Morgenthaler, *Bernisches Irrenwesen, von den Anfängen bis zur Eröffnung des Tollhauses, 1749* (Bern: Grunau, 1915).

75. I. Benguigui, "Charles Gaspard de La Rive (1770–1834), médecin aliéniste et physicien," *Gesnerus* 42 (1985): 245–252.

Avignon,[76] and Dr. Johann Theobald Held of Prague (1770–1851).[77] There were undoubtedly many others.

In the Introduction to his *Traité,* Pinel also reviewed contemporary medical writers and academic compendia on mental illness. He dismissed the British and German books and the international journal literature in one footnote each. The books, he wrote, "assemble scattered topics, lay them out in the scholastic manner, and often produce no more than some brilliant hypothesis."[78] The journals contain "scattered data, raw material that a skillful hand must elaborate."[79] This curt rejection of British works is startling, particularly since Pinel was well informed. He cited Battie, Harper, Arnold, Pargeter, Ferriar, Perfect, Haslam, and, of course, Crichton.[80] It is true that, in the body of his *Traité,* Pinel repeatedly acknowledged indebtedness to certain of these authors, particularly John Ferriar and William Pargeter—that is, those Britishers whose books speak of their practical experience with the hospitalized mentally ill. Nevertheless, Pinel's global rejection of British writings on insanity is surprising, even after making allowance for the anti-British feelings of a patriotic Frenchman in 1800.

It can be explained as follows: as we have seen, Pinel admired the work of practitioners, whether medical or lay, whose successful management of the mentally ill led to their patients' recovery. Therefore he praised the Retreat at York and admired the work of men like William

76. J. P. Huber, J. P. Macher, and J. Alliez, "L'hospitalisation 'forcée' des insensés à Avignon au 18ème siècle," *Information psychiatrique* 56 (1980): 1257–1266.

77. Johann Theobald Held received the M.D. degree in Prague in 1797 and became physician at the Brothers of Charity's hospital in that city where he served from 1799 until 1824. In 1806, he added one section of the municipal hospital to his duties. After the battle of Leipzig in 1813, he took over a service of the Ursuline monastery, and the mental asylum of the Brothers of Charity, where he became physician-in-chief in 1822. It was there that he introduced humane treatment for the mentally ill. He was elected dean of the university five times, and *rector magnificus,* and was made an imperial councillor in 1841. He left only minor writings.

78. Pinel, *Traité,* Introduction, xxi.

79. Ibid., xlii–xliii.

80. He lists these British books on mental alienation: William Battie (1703–1776), *A Treatise on Madness* (London: Whisten and White, 1758); Andrew Harper (?–1790), *A Treatise on the Real Cause and Cure of Insanity* (London: Stalker and Walter, 1789); Thomas Arnold (1742–1816), *Observations on the Nature, Kinds, Causes, and Prevention of Insanity, Lunacy, or Madness,* 2 vols. (London: Robinson and Cadell, 1782–1786); William Pargeter (1760–1810), *Observations on Maniacal Disorders* (Reading: The author, 1792); John Ferriar (1761–1815), *Medical Histories and Reflections* (London: Cadell and Davies, 1792–1798); William Perfect (1737–1809), *Select Cases in the Different Species of Insanity, Lunacy, or Madness, with the Modes of Practice as Adopted in the Treatment of Each* (Rochester: Gillman, 1797); John Haslam (1764–1844), *Observations on Insanity* (London: Rivington, 1798).

Perfect at Malling Place, Kent, or Thomas Arnold, at Belle Grove, Leicester. But he did not extend his admiration to the theoretical writings of these British practitioners—and how right he was! Thomas Arnold, for example, indulged in the most complex nosologic subdivisions in order to accommodate his observations; he divided insanity into "ideal" and "notional"—corresponding to Locke's "sensations" and "reflections"—and then proposed four "ideal" species of insanity, namely phrenitic, incoherent, maniacal, sensitive, and nine "notional" species: delusive, whimsical, fanciful, impulsive, scheming, vain or self-important, hypochondriacal, pathetic, appetitive. As for William Battie, the cofounder of St. Luke's Hospital for Lunaticks in 1751, one wonders how he could have taught his students how the mind worked while he hewed strictly to humoral pathology and treated his patients with an exhausting regimen of "depletion and revulsion." Pinel tended to shrug his shoulders at his British colleagues' theories while admiring their practical results.

In a different context, Continental observers found it astonishing that King George III's bouts of "madness" should provide a major topic of public discussion and even Parliamentary debate. In more conventional Continental fashion, the Spaniards, for example, kept the manic-depressive illness of King Ferdinand VI a secret even though a significant forerunner in psychiatry, Dr. Andrès Piquer of Valencia (1711–1772), cared for the king and wrote a revealing "Discurso sobre la enfermedad del Rey."[81] The Spaniards considered the king's person sacred and the manuscript lay unknown in the private archives of the duke of Osuna for one hundred years.[82] In contrast with the British physicians in charge of George III, Piquer and his colleagues never manhandled or mistreated their patient nor failed in their "respect for his Royal Person." Though he "did none of the things they prescribed . . . [m]elancholics must be treated with great gentleness and kindness," wrote Piquer, "and the hotchpotch of medications belongs to quacks rather than physicians who try to know and imitate nature."[83]

81. On Piquer, see J. L. Belinchon, "La psicología medica en la filosofía moral de Piquer (1755)," in *Actas—III Congreso nacional de historia de la medicina,* Valencia, 1969 (Madrid, 1972), 2:261–266, and V. Ll. Peset, "Andrès Piquer y la psiquiatría de la Ilustración," in *Actas del XV Congreso internacional de historia de la medicina, 1956* (Madrid, 1958), 2:433–439, published as vol. 8 of *Archivo Ibero-Americano de historia de la medicina y antropología.*

82. A. Piquer, "Discurso sobre la enfermedad del Rey nuestro Señor Don Fernando VI (que Dios guarde) escrito por Don Andrés Piquer médico de camara de S. M.," in *Colección de documentos ineditos para la Historia de España,* vol. 18 (Madrid: Viuda de Calero, 1851), 156–221.

83. Piquer, "Discurso," 186.

Piquer's younger contemporary, the Savoyard physician, Dr. Joseph Daquin (1732–1815) of Chambéry, wrote a sensitive *Philosophie de la folie* in 1791, in which he advocated humane treatment.[84] Its tone reminds one of the *Confessions* that his countryman and friend Jean-Jacques Rousseau had recently published. Daquin mixed traditional and modern attitudes: a humoralist, he spoke of "hot" and "cold" brains[85] and believed in the influence of the moon on "lunatics." Yet he pursued the scientific method to establish his thesis: he regularly examined five men and five women for sixteen years and kept notes on his findings at full and new moon, "lunistice," apogee, and perigee during a total of over eight hundred visits. But he decided against publishing his journal out of discretion and respect for his patients and unfortunately for us.[86]

Across the Alps, the Florentine Vincenzo Chiarugi (1759–1820) served as physician-in-chief at the renovated Bonifazio hospital for mental and dermatologic patients and taught students at the school of practical medicine of Santa Maria Nuova. He undoubtedly collaborated in the humane *Regolamento* for Florentine hospitals that was issued under the auspices of the enlightened Grand Duke Pietro Leopoldo in 1789. Chiarugi and Pinel were, in fact, the only full-time academic "psychiatrists" of the eighteenth century. In 1793–94, that is, six years before Pinel, Chiarugi authored a two-volume work on insantiy, *Della pazzia.* Pinel dismissed this book as utterly conventional in the Introduction to the *Traité,* but the Italian's admirers nevertheless consider him the real founder of "moral management" because he insisted on humane care for demented hospital inmates.[87]

84. J. Daquin, *Philosophie de la folie* (Chambéry: Gorrin, 1791); 2d ed. (Chambéry: Cléaz, 1804).

85. Daquin, *Philosophie,* 2d ed., 53.

86. Ibid., 207–241, passim. Gladys Swain has recently discovered the tracks of a prize essay by Daquin, dated 1787, in carton D, Archives de la Société de l'Ecole de Médecine, in the archives of the Paris Academy of Medicine. Though the essay itself seems to be lost, there subsists a "Plan du journal sur les fous tenu depuis le 1er janvier 1790, et visités à chaque phase de la lune, afin d'observer si cette planète influe sur eux," dated 9 June 1801. The latest overview and update regarding Daquin is the "Presentation" of his *Philosophie de la folie* by Claude Quétel in Collection Insania (Paris: Frénésie Editions, 1987).

87. Pinel, *Traité,* Introduction, xli. The full title of Vincenzo Chiarugi's book is *Della pazzia in genere ed in specie: Trattato medico-analitico con una centuria di osservazioni,* 2 vols. (Florence: Carlieri, 1793–1794). On Chiarugi, see the Introduction to the English edition, *On Insanity and Its Classification,* ed. George Mora (Canton, Mass.: Science History Publications, 1987). Mora is undoubtedly right in attributing the provisions for the mentally ill, spelled out in the *Regolamento,* to Chiarugi, but the physician is not mentioned as author, editor, or contributor, and his collaboration can only be inferred. See also G. B. Bock,

While Pinel was highly critical of his Italian contemporary, his treatment of the German literature on psychiatry is another matter. His main reference is contained in a footnote that reads as follows:

Faucett	*uber Mélancholie*	Léipsick, 1785
Avenbrugger	*von der stillen, etc.*	1783
Greding's	*Vermischte, etc.*	1781
Zimmermann	*von D. Erfahz.*	1765
Weickard's	*Philosoph. arzt*	Léipsick, 1775

These entries indicate that Pinel did not understand what he was writing: it seems likely that he took these references from the Introduction and Appendix of Crichton's book, adding them at the last minute, as his *Traité* went to press.[88] The footnote exemplifies the damage that the decline of Latin brought to international understanding in the eighteenth century: Germans now wrote in their own language which few foreigners bothered to learn. Not to take German-language scholarship seriously was of course a typical French attitude in 1800. The French Enlightenment expected cultured Germans to speak and write in French, like the "enlightened despot," Frederick the Great.

In contrast with Frenchmen of the late Enlightenment and Revolutionary era, those classical "pagans" whose gaze remained riveted to the Roman horizon,[89] the British had strong and recent German ties. Thus

"Ancora su Vincenzo Chiarugi: Revisione bibliografica e breve analisi critica del suo pensiero," *Acta medicae historiae patavina* 18 (1971–72): 17–37; E. Coturri, "Le sostanziale innovazioni introdotte in psichiatria da Vincenzo Chiarugi," *Episteme* 6 (1972): 251–265; E. Padovani, "Pinel e il rinnovamento dell'assistenza degli alienati: I suoi percursori: I predecessori italiani: Giuseppe Daquin e Vincenzo Chiarugi," *Giornale di psichiatria e di neuropatologia* 55 (1927): 69–124; A. Scapini, *La pazzia nell'interpretazione di Vincenzo Chiarugi (1759–1820)* (Pisa: Giardini, 1966); and L. Stroppiana, "La riforma degli ospedali psichiatrici di Chiarugi nel quadro del riformismo toscano ed europeo," *Rivista di storia della medicina* 20 (1976): 168–179.

88. This garbled footnote translates into the following: [Robert?] Faucett, *Über Melancholie* (Leipzig, 1785) [I have not been able to identify this author]; Leopold Auenbrugger (1722–1809), *Von der stillen Wut oder dem Triebe zum Selbstmorde als einer wirklichen Krankheit, mit Originalbeobachtungen und Anmerkungen* (Dessau: Verlagskasse, 1783), 71 pp.; Johann Ernst Greding (1718–1775), *Medizinisch-chirurgische Schriften* (Altenburg: Richter, 1781); Johann Georg Zimmermann (1728–1795), *Von der Erfahrung in der Arzneikunst* (Zürich: Heidegger, 1763–1764); Melchior Adam Weickard (1742–1803), *Der philosophische Arzt* (Leipzig, 1775; 2 vols., Frankfurt: Andreas, 1790). The question raised by this footnote is further explored in D. B. Weiner, "Philippe Pinel, Linguist," *Gesnerus* 42 (1985): 499–509.

89. The term "pagan" is, of course, Peter Gay's key to understanding the Enlightenment.

a young Britisher like Alexander Crichton might elect to spend three years studying in Germany, something very few Frenchmen are known to have done.[90] "In the summer of [1786]," Crichton's biographers tell us, "Dr. Crichton was prevailed upon by his friend, Dr. [Robert] Pringle, to give up his original plan, and to accompany him to Stuttgart, in order that they might study the language of the country."[91] There Crichton undoubtedly made contact with the local circle of young natural scientists, for his lifelong interest in physiology and psychology took root at that time. Crichton then spent the winter in Vienna, where Maximilian Stoll had recently replaced Gerard van Swieten as the leading physician and where emperor Joseph II had just opened the *Narrenturm*; three months in Halle, where Crichton lived with the family of the distinguished anatomist Philip Friedrich Theodor Meckel; and the winter of 1787–88 in Berlin. He ended up in Göttingen in March 1788 for a stay of six months. That is where the famous Johann Friedrich Blumenbach (1752–1840) was then teaching, surrounded by an active circle of students.[92]

What did Crichton learn at Göttingen about mental illness that he eventually conveyed to Pinel and especially to Esquirol? In German lands, it would seem, interest in mental illness grew out of an entirely different conceptual framework than in Great Britain or France. German doctors traditionally learned their medicine at the universities as a coherent philosophical system, and within this system there reigned the towering figure of Immanuel Kant (1724–1804). His long essay on insanity, "Versuch über die Krankheiten des Kopfes," appeared in 1764 in five installments in *Königsberger gelehrte und politische Zeitung*. Eventually he incorporated his brilliant though abstract classification of mental

90. I can think of only two, namely the naturalist Georges Cuvier (1769–1832), who had spent his college years in Stuttgart, and the medical and forensic hygienist Charles Marc (1771–1841). There are undoubtedly others, but few indeed.

91. *Proceedings of the Geological Society* 13 (1857): lxiv.

92. These included young medical scientists whose interests and future careers paralleled Crichton's. He may have met Karl Friedrich Kielmeyer in Stuttgart, where the young physiologist studied at the famous Karlsschule, together with Georges Cuvier and Friedrich Schiller; Kielmeyer came to Göttingen in the mid 1780s. Other personal acquaintances at Göttingen may have included the medical publicist Christian Girtanner, and Heinrich Friedrich Link, whose lifelong interest in medical botany, as well as his career, resembled Crichton's closely. Common interests may have forged connections with other Göttingen students of Blumenbach's in later years, for example with the famous naturalist and explorer Alexander von Humboldt, and with Gottfried Reinhold Treviranus, the biologist. For background, see O. Temkin, "German Concepts of Ontogeny and History around 1800," *Bulletin of the History of Medicine* 24 (1950): 227–246.

disorders into his *Anthropologie*.[93] For Kant, the distinctive human trait was reason, and he stressed the power of the rational mind over the emotions. (He once wrote a thank-you letter that became a short essay, on the theme one might paraphrase as "mind over matter.")[94] Crichton adhered to this contrast of reason and the passions, and Esquirol would use it, but in a special way.

While familiar with Kant's philosophy and anthropology, of course, Blumenbach was particularly interested in the development of the individual organism. His curiosity also focused on voyages of exploration and primitive peoples all over the globe, their physical growth and living habits; he owned a famous collection of skulls. His personality and his inquisitive mind inspired a number of young explorers, and Crichton fell under his spell. Blumenbach was also a lifelong friend of Sir Joseph Banks; he visited London in 1791, and we may assume that he saw Crichton on that occasion.[95] Blumenbach coined the concept of the "*Bildungstrieb*" as in innate biologic drive in 1781. Obviously this term held broad implications for mental illness, for, if the physician could make the patient aware of pathogenic irrational drives and explain their psychologic meaning, then he could chart a path toward the patient's recovery of his health. Crichton translated Blumenbach's brief essay into English in 1792 under the title *On generation,* a poor equivalent of the German.[96] It should have read *On the Developmental Drive*. For indeed he dealt with the central problem of contemporary physiology and develop-

93. I. Kant, *Anthropologie in pragmatischer Hinsicht* (Königsberg: Nicolovius, 1798), part I, book I, sections 35–45. See also K. Kisker, "Kant's psychiatrische Systematik," *Psychiatria e neurologia* (Basel) 133 (1957): 17–28; R. Töllner, "Kant und die Evolutionstheorie," *Clio Medica* 3 (1968): 243–249; G. B. Risse, "Kant, Schelling and the Early Search of a Philosophical 'Science' of Medicine in Germany," *Journal of the History of Medicine and Allied Sciences* 27 (1972): 145–158; and N. Tsouyopoulos, "Schellings Krankheitsbegriff und die Begriffsbildung der Modernen Medizin," in *Natur und Subjektivität: Zur Auseinandersetzung mit der Naturphilosophie des jungen Schelling: Referate, Voten und Protokolle der II. Internationalen Schelling-Tagung, Zürich 1983,* ed. R. Heckmann, H. Krings, and R. W. Meyer (Stuttgart-Bad Cannstatt: Froman-Holzboog, 1985), 265–290.

94. A thank-you letter from Immanuel Kant for a book that Christoph Wilhelm Hufeland sent him is in fact a short essay entitled "Von der Macht des Gemüths durch den blossen Vorsatz seiner krankhaften Gefühle Meister zu sein." Hufeland published it in his *Journal der praktischen Arzneikunde und Wundarzneikunst* 5 (1798): 701–751, and reissued it later, with comments (Leipzig: Reclam, 1824).

95. See H. Plischke, *Johann Friedrich Blumenbach's Einfluss auf die Entdeckungsreisenden seiner Zeit* (Göttingen: Vandenhoeck und Ruprecht, 1937).

96. Blumenbach's full title is *Ueber den Bildungstrieb und das Zeugungsgeschäfte* (Göttingen: Dieterich, 1781; 2d ed., 1791), translated as *An Essay on Generation* (London: Cadell, 1792).

ment and assumed a stance that Timothy Lenoir has recently called "vital materialism."[97]

Some German attitudes toward the mind/body problem found their most famous formulations after Crichton's visit; but since he stayed in touch and received packets of books after his return to England, these writings should be mentioned here—also because they continued to attract attention in France in the early nineteenth century. Friedrich Wilhelm Joseph von Schelling (1775–1854) reminded philosophers and psychologists that man's body and mind were part of living, ever-changing Nature. Therefore Schelling's *Naturphilosophie,* first formulated in 1799, gave German medicine a vitalistic and Romantic bent.[98] Many researchers tried to resist this "spiritualistic" development, among them the great physiologist Johann Christian Reil (1759–1813), in the opinion of some, the "German Pinel."[99] He published his first important essay, "Von der Lebenskraft," as the lead article in his new *Archiv für Physiologie* in 1795. He also wrote a book on psychiatry in 1803. It was entitled *Rhapsodieen über die Anwendung der psychischen Curmethode auf Geisteszerrüttungen* (Rhapsodies on the use of the psychologic method for the cure of mental derangement) and makes for extremely difficult reading.[100] Yet Reil had many astute and profound thoughts about the mentally ill, even though psychiatry was not his specialty and he never worked in a psychiatric hospital. In contrast with the main body of his book, Reil's Preface adopted *Naturphilosophie* and exemplified the broad undercurrent of evangelical religiosity in the German attitude toward insanity and a tendency to equate insanity with sin and recovery with salvation. Reil wrote his *Rhapsodieen* of 1803 with the original intention of contributing a short piece to the journal of his friend Pastor Wagnitz. But the short essay grew to five hundred pages, which Wagnitz refused to publish.[101] Reil's Preface conveys a sense of mission that *Naturphiloso-*

97. T. Lenoir, "Kant, Blumenbach, and Vital Materialism in German Biology," *Isis* 71 (1980): 77–108.

98. See F. W. J. von Schelling, *Erster Entwurf eines Systems der Naturphilosophie* (Jena & Leipzig: Gabler, 1799).

99. On Reil, see, for example, Sir A. Lewis, "J. C. Reil: Innovator and Battler," *Journal of the History of the Behavioral Sciences* 1 (1965): 178–190, and I. Petzold, "Johann Christian Reil, Begründer der modernen Psychotherapie?" *Sudhoff's Archiv* 41 (1957): 159–179.

100. (Halle: Curt, 1803).

101. Pastor Wagnitz had recently written a stern denunciation of German workhouses and asylums, and Reil emphasized his agreement with his friend's call for reform. See Heinrich Balthasar Wagnitz, *Historische Nachrichten und Bemerkungen über die merkwürdigsten Zuchthäuser in Deutschland, nebst einem Anhang über die zweckmässigste Einrichtung der Gefängnisse und Irrenanstalten,* 2 vols. in 3 (Halle: Gebauer, 1791–1794).

phie tried to impart to humanitarians of all nations. In a similar vein, Christoph Wilhelm Hufeland's *Journal* of the 1790s called upon doctors to become medical missionaries to the poor.

In fact, an active German journal literature, not only books, discussed and publicized philosophical anthropology, natural history, religion, and their implications for mental health and mental illness. Two new journals, *Zeitschrift für empirische Psychologie* and *Magazin für Erfahrungsseelenkunde,* began publication in 1783, the latter edited by Karl Philipp Moritz (1757–1793) and Salomon Maimon (1754–1800).[102] Moritz was a friend of Goethe's and a well-published esthete, Maimon a protégé of Lessing's and Moses Mendelssohn's and a philosopher of whom Kant thought highly. And *Erfahrungsseelenkunde* was, in fact, the scientific study of psychologic experience, the very specialty that physicians like Crichton and Pinel were about to transform into psychiatry. In the *Magazin,* Crichton found what he "had not yet met with in any other publication, a number of well-authenticated cases of insane aberration of mind, narrated in a full and satisfactory manner, without a view of any system whatever."[103] Neither of the two editors was a physician. Crichton, in contrast, brought the clinical approach to the perusal of the German case histories.

He had initially embarked on writing a physiology of mind and body in health and disease—until he read John Augustus Unzer's *Erste Gründe einer Physiologie der eigentlichen thierischen Natur thierischer Körper*[104] and found that Unzer had accomplished the task. Nevertheless Crichton continued to study German thought about anthropology, physiology, and psychology, and his "esteemed friend" Blumenbach kept sending packages with German books and journals. Crichton's indebtedness to German learning is obvious from his repeated citations of a dozen contemporary German authorities. Of particular importance to Crichton was Melchior Adam Weickard's publication, *Der philosophische Arzt,* and Johann Ernst Greding's *Sämtliche medizinische Schriften.* Crichton appended eighty-five pages of Greding's *Medical Aphorisms on Melancholy and Various Other Diseases* to his *Inquiry.*[105] It was thus the German

102. *Magazin für Erfahrungsseelenkunde, als ein Lesebuch für Gelehrte und Ungelehrte, mit Unterstützung mehrerer Wahrheitsfreunde herausgegeben,* ed. C. P. Moritz and, as of vol. 8, Salomon Maimon (Berlin: Mylius, 1785–1805).

103. Crichton, *Inquiry,* Preface, v.

104. (Leipzig: Weidmanns Erben und Reich, 1771).

105. Weickard, *Der philosophische Arzt,* and idem, *Sammlung medizin-praktischer Beobachtungen und Abhandlungen* (Ulm: Stettin, 1798); Greding, *Vermischte medizinische und chirurgische Schriften* and idem, *Sämtliche medizinische Schriften,* 2 vols. (Greiz: Henning,

philosophers and physicians who attempted new formulations for the theoretical substrate of psychiatry in the early Romantic era. Crichton found their thought fascinating because of their focus on observation, on individual case histories, and on the natural history of diseases. Yet he developed his own approach.

SIR ALEXANDER CRICHTON (1763–1856): THE MAN AND HIS WORK

We can easily imagine Pinel's surprise and pleasure when he read the Introduction to Crichton's *Inquiry*. He discovered a self-assured innovator equally impatient with ancient and modern models: Crichton proposed to practice observation and follow the analytic method including, we are amazed to read, "abstracting his own mind from himself, and placing it before him as it were, so as to examine it with the freedom and with the impartiality of a natural historian."[106] (This attempt at self-analysis seems to foreshadow Sigmund Freud.)[107] Crichton discarded traditional nosologists, even Linnaeus, as "generally and justly neglected."[108] The mainstream of new knowledge, for Crichton, flowed from Germany, that "learned nation."[109] His enthusiasm for Germany

1790–1791). Greding (1718–1775), physician to the poorhouse at Waldheim in Saxony for seventeen years, recorded numerous observations and conducted over three hundred autopsies. On Greding, see N. Bondy, "Johann Ernest Greding (1718–1776): A Contribution to the History of Modern Psychiatry," *Medical History* 16 (1972): 293–296. Among the plentiful German sources mentioned by Crichton, the following were of particular importance to him: Schack Hermann Ewald, *Über das menschliche Herz: Ein Beitrag zur Charakteristik der Menschheit* (Erfurt: Schlegel, 1784); Johann Georg Heinrich Feder, *Grundlehre zur Kenntniss des menschlichen Willens und der natürlichen Gesetze des Rechtsverhaltens* (Göttingen: Dieterich, 1779); Johann Peter Frank, for his "truly elegant and learned work," *System einer vollständigen medizinischen Polizei* (Mannheim: Schwann, 1779–1827); Christoph Girtanner, *Über das Kantische Prinzip für die Naturgeschichte: Ein Versuch diese Wissenschaft philosophisch zu behandeln* (Göttingen: Vandenhoek und Ruprecht, 1796); Marcus H. Herz, *Versuch über den Schwindel* (Berlin: Voss, 1786); Johann Gottlob Krüger, *Naturlehre* (Halle: Hemmerde, 1740–1749); Georg Friedrich Meier, *Über Gemütsbewegungen* (Halle: Hemmerde, 1759); Johann Joachim Schmidt, *Behandlung der Krankheiten des Organs der Seele* (Hamburg: Hoffmann, 1797); and Friedrich Gabriel Sulzer, *Versuch über die natürliche Geschichte des Hamsters* (Göttingen and Gotha: Dieterich, 1774).

106. Crichton, *Inquiry*, Preface, x.

107. R. Hunter and I. Macalpine suggest the comparison. See *Three Hundred Years of Psychiatry, 1535–1860: A History Presented in Selected English Texts* (Hartsdale, N.Y.: Carlisle, 1982), 559.

108. Crichton, *Inquiry*, Preface, xxvii.

109. Ibid., iii.

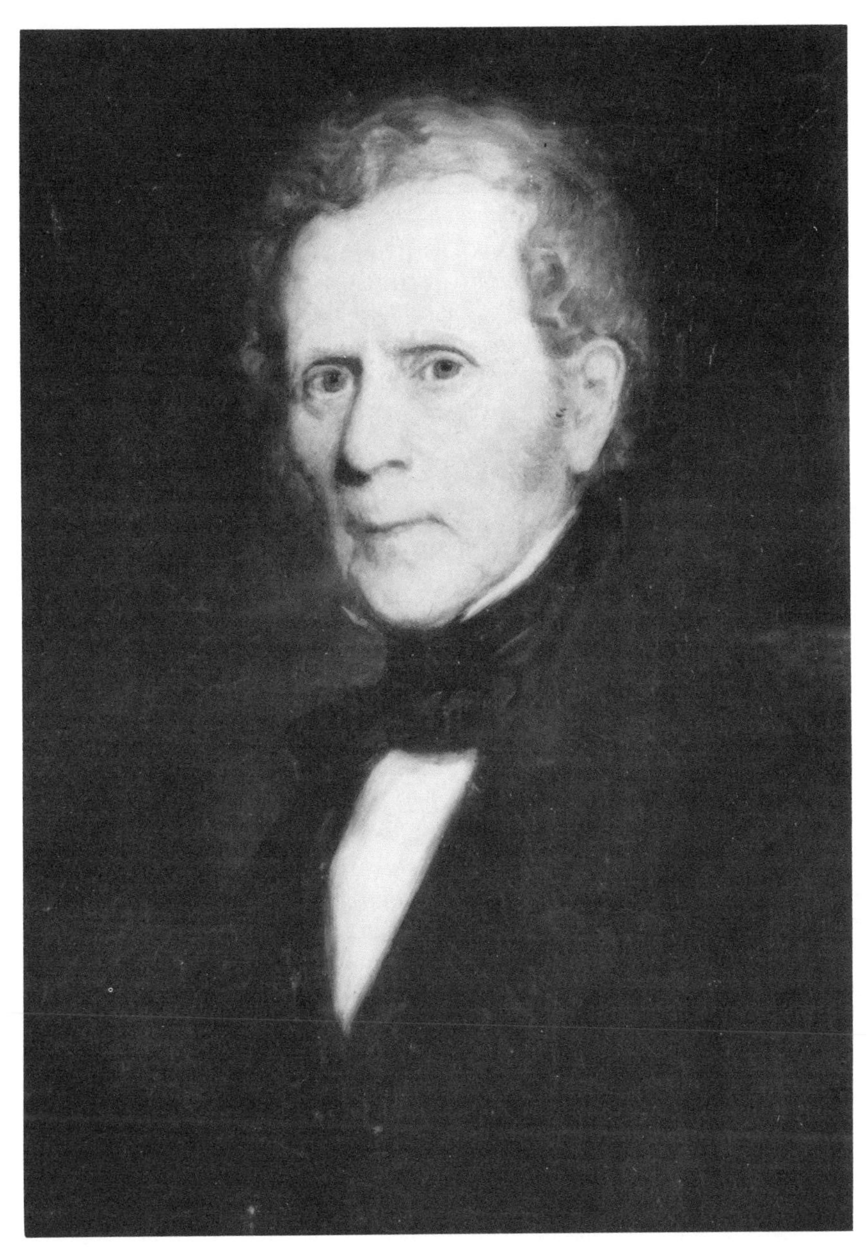

Pl. 17. Portrait of Sir Alexander Crichton attributed to C. H. Harlow (no date).

set him apart from his British medical colleagues whose travels to the Continent had long taken them to Leiden and Paris, and then to Italy and perhaps Vienna. Stuttgart, Halle, and Berlin were unusual places to visit, but Crichton did not mind taking a different track than his colleagues: he did not even mention the large group of British medical practitioners who recorded their experience with mentally ill patients in books during the last third of the eighteenth century.[110] The exception is Dr. Thomas Arnold, whose book Crichton lambastes repeatedly in his Introduction, and quite justifiably so. But Crichton spent little time on a critique of his colleagues—he was so convinced of being an innovator that he preferred to look ahead rather than backward.

He earned lavish praise from Pinel in the Introduction to the *Traité* of 1800. After heaping scorn on most contemporary writers on the subject, Pinel continued:

> I except the research of Crichton, a profound work full of new observations based on the principles of modern physiology. It focuses on the pathogenesis of mental alienation rather than on its history or therapy. I believe I should now give an exact idea of the origins, development, and effects of the human passions on the animal economy, as this author has presented them, and as they should be known, namely as the most usual cause of derangement of our psychologic functions.[111]

Pinel then proceeded to an eighteen-page paraphrase and analysis of *History of the Passions and Their Effects.* It is strange indeed that until now no one has explored the relationship of Pinel to Crichton.[112] This relationship might have blossomed had Dr. F. R. Bidault de Villiers (1775–1824) carried out his intention of publishing a translation of Crichton's book, a project revealed in a manuscript at the Wellcome Institute, London. Instead, Bidault wrote a close textual analysis and synopsis of Crichton's book but stopped short of part 3, *On the Passions,* the most novel and important section. He sent his work to his friend A. A. Royer-Collard, who eventually published it in his *Bibliothèque médicale,* but only in 1816–1817. By that time, the nascent psychiatry was turning its atten-

110. See n. 80 above.

111. Pinel, *Traité,* Introduction, xxi–xxii.

112. Swain voices the opinion that Crichton was of great importance to Pinel, but she does not pursue this insight (Gauchet and Swain, *La pratique de l'esprit,* 347–349). Goldstein argues that Pinel "sought guidance" from Crichton (*Console and Classify,* 95). Yet when Pinel read Crichton's book, his own was already being printed. I incline to argue for a meeting of minds.

tion increasingly to brains, not the mind, and thus interest in the work of Pinel and Crichton was on the wane.[113]

Who, then, was Crichton? There are only two monographic studies on Crichton in the literature,[114] and only a few historians of medical psychology acknowledge his work.[115] And yet Crichton, eventually *Sir* Alexander Crichton, born in Edinburgh in 1763, dead at the age of ninety-three at Seven Oaks, Kent, F.R.S., F.L.S., F.G.S., and a licentiate of the Royal College of Physicians, not only wrote an important early book on psychiatry but served two tsars with distinction as head of the Russian civilian medical department for fifteen years, and then lived in London for another third of a century as a respected member of his profession.[116] Crichton's education was broadly based, and his published writings are heterogeneous.[117] He had studied at the Edinburgh medical faculty with Joseph Black, Alexander Monro, *secundus,* and especially James Gregory (1753–1821), who influenced him deeply. Indeed, a comparison of the topics and opinions in Gregory's *Conspectus medicinae theoreticae* reveals striking analogies to Crichton's *Inquiry.*[118] But theory

113. See Wellcome Institute, London, MS. 1164, dossier 29, and F. T. Bidault de Villiers, "*Recherches sur la nature et le principe de l'aliénation mentale* par A. Crichton," in *Bibliothèque médicale; ou, Recueil périodique d'extraits des meilleurs ouvrages de médecine et chirurgie* 53 (1816): 30–67; 54(1816): 289–324; 55 (1817): 289–331. Bidault's essay on Crichton is not included in a collection of his *Œuvres posthumes* (Paris: Veret, 1828), whose editor comments that "M. Bidault de Villiers seems to have given up that translation and limited himself to a detailed analysis . . . published in 1816–1817" (ix).

114. See Hopf, *Leben und Werk,* and Tansey, "Life and Works;" for full citations see n. 7 above. Tansey gives a detailed account of Crichton's Scottish background and lifelong connections. She also offers some new information on his London practice and on his Continental experience.

115. The best among these are A. Boldt, *Über die Stellung und Bedeutung der "Rhapsodieen über die Anwendung der psychischen Curmethode auf Geisteszerrüttung" von Johann Christian Reil (1759–1813) in der Geschichte der Psychiatrie,* Abhandlungen zur Geschichte der Medizin und der Naturwissenschaften, Heft 12 (Berlin: Ebering, 1936), 45–51; Hunter and Macalpine, *Three Hundred Years of Psychiatry,* especially 559–564; R. Hoeldtke, "The History of Associationism and British Medical Psychology," *Medical History* 11 (1967): 46–65; Schrenk, "Pathologie der Passionen" (n. 12 above) and idem, *Über den Umgang mit Geisteskranken* (n. 12 above), 123–124.

116. Crichton was decorated by Tsar Alexander I with the order of St. Vladimir, Knight Grand Cross, second class, in 1814, and by King Frederick William III of Prussia with the Grand Cross of the Red Eagle, second class, in 1820. He was knighted by King George IV in 1821 and honored with the Grand Cross of St. Anne by Tsar Nicholas I in 1830.

117. See Appendix, Biobibliographic Note 2.

118. J. Gregory, *Conspectus medicinae theoreticae; or, A View on the Theory of Medicine*

did not predominate in Crichton's training: he served an apprenticeship with the surgeon Alexander Wood and undoubtedly also "walked the wards" of the Royal Infirmary of Edinburgh.[119] Moving to London at the age of twenty-one, he spent one year with another surgeon, William Fordyce, while also attending the hospitals. By the time he reached maturity, Crichton had absorbed three deeply influential British traditions, Baconian empiricism, Lockean Associationist psychology, and Scottish "Common Sense" philosophy. This was so obvious to Crichton that he wrote in his Introduction to the *Inquiry*; "The most useful of these authors, and their works, I shall now enumerate. . . . Those of our British Psychologists, such as Locke, Hartley, Reid, Priestley, Stewart and Kaims [*sic*] need not be mentioned."[120] And indeed Crichton incorporated these authors' ideas into his work in a casual and familiar manner.

The inductive method was basic to Crichton's approach: that is why he, like Pinel, set so much store by detailed case histories reported without reference to any preestablished "system." The absence of innate ideas and moral values—the *tabula rasa*—was another essential prerequisite for Crichton's *Inquiry*. A passage in *History of the Passions* that Pinel commented on with admiration reads:

> The passions are to be considered, in a medical point of view, as a part of our constitution, which is to be examined with the eye of a natural historian, and the spirit and impartiality of a philosopher. It is of no consequence in this work whether passions be esteemed natural or unnatural, or moral or immoral affections. They are mere phenomena, the natural causes of which are to be inquired into.[121]

Further, Crichton mentions the association of ideas as if this were a generally recognized and adopted truth: David Hartley's conclusions had by Crichton's time become obvious assumptions for the nascent psychi-

(Edinburgh: Stirling and Shade, 1823). It was first published in 1780–1782, at the very time when Crichton was a medical student in Edinburgh. A much earlier edition was translated into German as *Übersicht der theoretischen Arzneiwissenschaft,* 2 vols. (Leipzig: Fritsch, 1784–1785).

119. G. B. Risse confirms that surgeons lectured there, beginning in 1770, and their students were admitted to clinical rounds and to surgical procedures: see *Hospital Life in Enlightenment Scotland: Care and Teaching at the Royal Infirmary of Edinburgh* (Cambridge: Cambridge University Press, 1986), 266–271.

120. Crichton, *An Inquiry,* Preface, xxvii.

121. Ibid., book II, 98–99.

atric specialty.[122] For Hartley, association was a material process caused by the vibration and gravitation of particles in a fluid acting on the brain. Crichton combined this explanation with faculty psychology. According to this theory, a defective association acting on a mental faculty such as attention, will, memory, reason, or imagination will result in "derangement."[123] Crichton's ideas of faculty psychology stemmed from Dugald Stewart (1753–1828), with whom he undoubtedly studied at Edinburgh, thus absorbing the ideas of Thomas Reid (1710–1796).[124] Their "Common Sense" approach was of course more serviceable for a physician than the more famous contemporary Scottish philosophy, the skepticism of David Hume. Nor does Crichton mention the *Theory of Moral Sentiments* (1759) by another Scottish philosopher, Adam Smith (1723–1790), while a French translation of the work by the marquis de Condorcet's widow stood in Pinel's library, and he mentions it in the Introduction to his *Traité*.[125]

A Scottish education and training in surgery and medicine both in Edinburgh and London did not leave an inquisitive and ambitious young gentleman with the feeling that his preparation for a career was complete: he needed to undertake a tour of the Continent. Crichton spent four years, from 1785 to 1788, traveling abroad, and for our purposes this is the most intriguing part of his intellectual biography. One month sufficed to obtain the M.D. degree at Leiden, on 29 July, 1785, with a thesis *De vermibus intestinorum*. It is a mere eighteen pages long and—curious for a thesis in medicine—dedicated to the surgeons Alexander Wood and William Fordyce, his teachers.[126] The season 1785–

122. I have used D. Hartley, *Observations on Man, His Frame, His Duty, and His Expectations*, 4th ed., 3 vols. (London: J. Johnson, 1801). The book was first published in 1749 and translated into French by the abbé R. A. C. Sicard, *De l'homme, de ses facultés physiques et intellectuelles, de ses devoirs, et de ses espérances*, 2 vols. (Paris: Ducauroy, 1802). There is also a French version of Hartley's earlier *Various Conjectures on Perception, Motion, and Generation of Ideas*, published in 1746, translated by the abbé Jurain as *Explication physique des sens, des idées, et des mouvements tant volontaires qu'involontaires*, 2 vols. (Reims: Delaistre-Godet, 1755).

123. For a good overview, see Hoeldtke, "The History of Associationism."

124. Stewart served as professor of mathematics at Edinburgh from 1775 to 1785, and as professor of philosophy from 1785 to 1810. Reid's most influential books, popular at the time of Crichton's studies, were *Inquiry into the Human Mind on the Principles of Common Sense* (1764), *Essays on the Intellectual Powers of Man* (1785), and *Essays on the Active Powers of Man* (1788).

125. Pinel, *Traité*, Introduction, xxvii.

126. A minor indication of how blurred the boundaries between medicine and surgery had become by 1785.

DISSERTATIO MEDICA
INAUGURALIS
DE
VERMIBUS INTESTINORUM,
QUAM,
FAVENTE SUMMO NUMINE,
EX AUCTORITATE RECTORIS MAGNIFICI;
DIONYSII GODEFRIDI VAN DER KEESSEL,
J. U. D. ET JURIS CIVILIS IN ACAD. LUGD. BAT.
PROFESSORIS ORDINARII;
NEC NON
Amplissimi SENATUS ACADEMICI *Consensu*,
& *Nobilissimae* FACULTATIS MEDICAE *Decreto*,
PRO GRADU DOCTORATUS,
Summisque in MEDICINA Honoribus ac Privilegiis
rite & legitime consequendis,
Eruditorum examini submittit.
ALEXANDER CRICHTON,
BRITANNUS.
SOCIETAT. PHYSIC. CHIRURG. EDIN.
NEC NON
LYCAEI MEDICI LONDINEN. SOCIUS.
Ad diem XXIX. *Julii* MDCCLXXXV. *H. L. Q. S.*

LUGDUNI BATAVORUM,
APUD HAAK ET SOCIOS.
MDCCLXXXV.

Pl. 18. Title page of Sir Alexander Crichton's M.D. thesis, *De vermibus intestinorum* (On the worms of the intestines).

1786, spent in Paris, left no noticeable traces in Crichton's writings (nor have I found any track of his presence in France).[127] However, soon after the publication of his *Inquiry,* we find "Crickton de Londres" among the foreign associates of the official *Société de médecine de Paris,* and on 24 February 1835 he was one of 234 foreign corresponding members elected by the Paris Academy of Medicine.[128] Crichton does mention, in *Commentaries on Some Doctrines* published in 1842, that he "had the honor" of "knowing Pinel personally."[129] (That meeting must have occurred in the winter of 1785–86, when Pinel served as editor of the *Gazette de santé.* Likely places for an encounter were the Jardin du roi, where Pinel studied, the Helvétius salon, the surgeon Pierre Desault's rounds at the Hôtel-Dieu, or lectures at the Collège de France or the Sorbonne.)

Then followed Crichton's three *Wanderjahre,* spent at Stuttgart, Vienna, Halle, Berlin, and Göttingen. Late in 1788, he returned to England. On 7 May 1789 Crichton joined the Corporation of Surgeons in London but disfranchised himself after two years because, say his biographers, he "never liked the operative part of the profession." Rather, he joined the Royal College of Physicians as licentiate on 1 June 1791 and worked at a dispensary in Holborn where he gave clinical lectures "upon a plan similar to that of Göttingen University." In 1794 he was elected physician to Westminster Hospital, where he taught "The Theory and Practice of Physic," as we learn from an advertisement in the London *Times.*[130] Despite this title he actually taught a course in psychiatry since he tells us in the Preface to the *Inquiry* that he wrote the book for his students. One can indeed imagine each of the three parts as notes for a course: part 1, on the nature and origins of mental derangement; part 2, on the physiology and pathology of the human mind; part 3, on the passions and their effects. The volumes consist of five, eight, and six chapters respectively—each chapter could well have formed the subject matter for one classroom presentation. Crichton lectured at the Westminster throughout the 1790s: we can assume that he interviewed

127. Contrary to the comments of Tansey, "Life and Works," Paris was not yet "in the throes of a revolution in medical teaching," nor had the Charité Hospital been, as yet, "newly established" (243).

128. Applicants petitioned for this honor, and thus there must have been correspondence between Crichton and the academy's secretariat. That documentation lies in some of the one hundred uninventoried—and, I believe, virtually untouched—boxes stored at the Académie nationale de médecine, 16, rue Bonaparte, Paris.

129. A. Crichton, *Commentaries on some Doctrines* (London: Churchill, 1842) 180.

130. 15 April 1794, 17 September 1794, and 15 September 1797.

MEDICAL LECTURES, WESTMINSTER HOSPITAL.

THE PHYSICIANS of the Westminster Hospital, propose to read CHEMICAL LECTURES on the Cases which shall come under their care in the course of the Winter.

Dr. CRICHTON will begin his Course of Lectures on the THEORY and PRACTICE of PHYSIC, at the Hospital, on Wednesday the 1st of October, at 9 o'Clock in the Forenoon.

Dr. BRADLEY proposes to read a Course of Lectures to comprehend the most useful Parts of the Institutes of Medicine, Materia Medica, and PHARMACUTICAL CHEMISTRY, to commence the first Week in October.

A Lecture, introductory to the Chemical Courses, will be given by Dr. BRADLEY, at the Hospital, on Wednesday, October 1st, at 10 o'Clock in the Forenoon.

Mr. CARLISLE will give a general Introductory Lecture, on Saturday, October 4th, at 11 o'Clock, wherein he proposes to point out the most advantageous mode of acquring Surgical Knowledge.

Mr. LYNN and Mr. CARLISLE will afterwards continue to give such occasional Lectures on Surgery, as may be thought most useful to the Pupils; and Chemical Lectures upon every Operation, or important Case which falls under their Care.

For Particulars of the above Courses, and of attending the Practice of the Physicians, or Surgeons, apply to the Apothecary at the Hospital.

FRIENDS OF THE PEOPLE

Pl. 19. Advertisement on the front page of *The Times* (London) of 17 September 1794. The advertisement reads as follows:

MEDICAL LECTURES, WESTMINSTER HOSPITAL

THE PHYSICIANS of the Westminster Hospital, propose to read CHEMICAL LECTURES on the Cases which shall come under their care in the course of the Winter.

Dr. CRICHTON will begin his Course of Lectures on the THEORY and PRACTICE of PHYSIC, at the Hospital, on Wednesday the 1st of October, at 9 o'clock in the Forenoon.

Dr. BRADLEY proposes to read a Course of Lectures to comprehend the most useful Parts of the Institutes of Medicine, Materia Medica, and PHARMACEUTICAL CHEMISTRY, to commence the first Week in October.

A Lecture, introductory to the Chemical Courses, will be given by Dr. BRADLEY, at the Hospital, on Wednesday, October 1st, at 10 o'clock in the Forenoon.

Mr. CARLISLE will give a general introductory Lecture, on Saturday, October 4th, at 11 o'clock, wherein he proposes to point out the most advantageous mode of acquiring Surgical Knowledge.

Mr. LYNN and Mr. CARLISLE will afterwards continue to give such occasional Lectures on Surgery, as may be thought most useful to the Pupils; and Chemical Lectures upon every Operation, or important Case which falls under their Care.

For Particulars of the above Courses, and of attending the Practice of the Physicians, or Surgeons, apply to the Apothecary at the Hospital.

the mentally ill patients in front of his students—for indeed these patients were regularly admitted to his hospital in small numbers—and that he drew the students' attention to the psychologic manifestations of somatic illness.[131] Owing to his book he was asked to testify regarding the sanity of James Hadfield, the madman who attempted to assassinate King George III in 1800. The next year, Crichton became a consulting physician at the Westminster and retained that position to the end of his life.

In 1800, Crichton married and shortly thereafter was appointed physician to Adolphus Frederick, duke of Cambridge (1774–1850), the tenth child and seventh son of King George III. New family connections smoothed his path, or he may have met the young man at Göttingen, where three of the royal princes were sent for their education in 1786. Being now a courtier, he came to the attention of emissaries from the Russian tsar, who lured him to St. Petersburg in 1804. Were one to pursue research on Crichton, one would go to Edinburgh, as Tansey has done, but mainly to St. Petersburg, for Crichton spent fifteen years in the service of the tsar. In a pamphlet published in 1817, he describes himself as

> Physician-in-ordinary to their imperial majesties the Emperor and Dowager Empress of Russia; Physician-in-chief of the Civil Department of the Empire; Knight of the Order of St. Vladimir; Honorary member of the Imperial Academy of Sciences of St. Petersburg.[132]

131. The *Medical and Physical Journal* published monthly admissions figures to London Hospitals. From December 1799 to May 1800, for example, the "Diseases admitted under the care of the physicians of the Westminster" included the following cases that may well have had psychologic concomitants:

	Dec	Jan	Feb	Mch	Apr	May
amenorrhoea	3	5	4	5	4	7
asthma	2	9	2	5	1	
hypochondriasis	1		1	1		
hysteria	2		2			
dyspepsia			2			
epilepsy		2	1	2		
convulsions					2	2
palpitations						1

Medical and Physical Journal 3 (1800): 16, 112, 208, 303–304, 408–409, 505–506.

132. A. Crichton, *An Account of Some Experiments Made with the Vapour of Boiling Tar in the Cure of Pulmonary Consumption* (Edinburgh: Manners and Miller, 1817).

He published a *Pharmacopoeia pauperum* while in Russia and coedited a short-lived journal, *Russische Sammlung für Naturwissenschaft und Heilkunde.*[133] (The Leningrad Archives would undoubtedly reveal more publications.) Unfortunately the *Sammlung* contains no entries signed by Crichton, though plentiful comment by the editors collectively. This indicates much curiosity about the geology, fauna, and flora of Asiatic Russia and China, which may well reflect Crichton's avocations, and a great deal of interest in southeastern Russia, where a cholera epidemic ravaged the population. Indeed, Crichton's medals were undoubtedly rewards for his efforts in fighting this epidemic.

In connection with a subsequent typhus epidemic, Crichton established an essay prize with thoughtful guidelines. He donated a thousand rubles for the best essay on indigenous remedies, and five hundred rubles for the best description of typhus. The instructions to candidates reveal Crichton's interest in susceptibility to the disease. Candidates should take the emotions into account, and inquire

> what were the forms and characteristics of the disease among the inhabitants as the enemy came ever nearer to their homes, and later, when national enthusiasm rose to great heights, and finally, when total success rewarded the efforts of the fatherland?
>
> And how did the disease manifest itself among the enemy, first, when he was still blinded by the illusion of victory (an illusion that remained alive among prisoners), and later, when he found himself toppled from glittering heights into abject disgrace?

It might also be worth examining national differences, Crichton continues, between Europeans and Asians, with regard to typhus.

> Are there observations indicating that individuals in one nation fall ill more quickly and in larger numbers? are some more resistant to damaging influences or to contagion? or did the illness among them take on special characteristics or curious symptoms?[134]

These questions indicate an astonishing sensitivity to what we would call psychosomatic parameters of illness. Crichton's contribution of a substantial prize, and the deferential tone in which his coeditors thanked him, suggest that this personal physician to the imperial family held a well-paid and favored position at the Russian court.[135] Though eager to

133. 2 vols., ed. A. Crichton, J. Rehmann, and K. F. Burdach (Riga and Leipzig: Hartmann, 1815–1817).

134. Ibid., 2:x–xi.

135. Tansey suggests another possible motivation for the prize: Crichton had devised a new method for refining vegetable oil, together with the apothecary Konstantin Kirchoff.

come home in 1809, he did not obtain the tsar's permission until 1819, and we know little about the remaining third-of-a-century in Crichton's life. He became a respected member of the medical community, with an office in Harley Street, and was a member of the Royal, Geological, and Linnaean Societies of London. Interesting as a biographic investigation might be, we must now focus on the references, ideas, attitudes, and mainly the ideas he transmitted to Pinel and Esquirol about German anthropology, natural history, physiology, and religion, as they affected mental alienation.

THE *INQUIRY INTO THE NATURE AND ORIGIN OF MENTAL DERANGEMENT*

Crichton's *Inquiry* consists of three books on different though related subjects and a long Appendix. Book I is entitled "Inquiry into the Physical Causes of Delirium." It deals, in turn, with irritability, sensitivity, consciousness of self, pain and pleasure, and delirium. The first two sections review contemporary physiology and pay homage to Francis Glisson, Felice Fontana, and, above all, Albrecht von Haller.[136] In chapters 3 and 4, Crichton turns from physiology to psychology, from muscles to nerves, from plants and animals to man. His debt to Locke is pervasive: he argues for a categorical distinction of man from animals. In chapter 3 of the first book, Crichton discusses a complex notion for which scholars had no accurate term: they variously called it consciousness of self, self-feeling, coenesthesis, *Gemeingefühl.*[137] It combines awareness of perceptions from outside and inside the body, and of relevant mental func-

Their factory, on Aptekarskiy Island in St. Petersburg, produced 4,400 pounds of oil a day. Crichton's monetary benefits from this invention must have aroused considerable envy, and he may have decided to give away some of the money to allay these feelings. See Tansey, "Life and Works," 248, and *Dictionary of Scientific Biography,* s.v. "Kirchoff."

136. Francis Glisson (1597–1677) identified irritability as a property inherent in all living bodies. He made important contributions to knowledge of the liver and wrote the original treatise on rickets. His works include *De rachitide* (1650), *De hepate* (1654), *Tractatus de naturae substantia energetica* (1672), and *De ventriculo et intestinis* (1677). The abbé Felice Fontana (1720–1805) was a naturalist, physiologist, and forerunner of the cell theory. Albrecht von Haller (1708–1777) was one of the most productive, prestigious, and knowledgeable naturalists of the eighteenth century. He taught at Göttingen, but mainly in his native Bern, where he founded a botanical garden and an anatomic theater. He left voluminous and important writings in anatomy, physiology, and botany.

137. Crichton refers the reader to the inaugural dissertation of Christian Friedrich Hübner, *Commentatio de coenesthesi* (Halle, 1794). For a modern and critical view, see the recent article by Francis Schiller, "Coenesthesis," *Bulletin of the History of Medicine* 58 (1984): 496–515.

tions such as memory, imagination, and reason. It provides the healthy person with a consciousness of these functions and thus of him- or herself. This awareness is, of course, intact in the healthy person but impaired in the mental patient. But it is chapter 5 of book I, "On Delirium," that interests us most because Pinel translated it immediately upon its appearance in France and published his version in the new journal, the *Recueil périodique de littérature médicale étrangère.*[138] Delirium is an altered state of consciousness ("lira," in Latin, means a straight furrow) where a variety of different causes can produce similar symptoms. Alcohol, poison, strong emotions, or mental illness can all cause delirium. Crichton ascribed delirium to the action of a nervous fluid, altered in quantity and quality,[139] whereas Pinel dissented, emphasizing "vivid emotions."[140] In another note, Pinel offered a case history of his own.[141]

Pinel also added several translator's comments in which he argued with Crichton. Since these have gone virtually unnoticed in the vast Pinel literature,[142] they may be worth translating here. First, Pinel criticized the British author for basing an argument on a single case history, taken from Greding. Pinel continues:

> I have followed a quite different method when I decided to explore the same subject. For two consecutive years, I watched about two hundred mentally ill men in a hospice under my medical direction. I first divided them into separate classes, idiots or imbeciles, melancholics, maniacs; I kept exact records of the continuous or periodic manias. For the latter, I took special notes on the precipitating events of insanity, premonitory signs of periodic bouts, the variety of lesions in the understanding, the progressive series of the other symptoms, their termination, etc. and it is after this research that I published a memoir on periodic insanity.[143]

In another note, Pinel criticized Crichton for generalizing too freely about delirium and failing to classify and compare the phenomena he observed. This, of course, was Crichton's weakest point: as one of four attending physicians at an all-purpose, hundred-bed hospital, Westminster, Crichton had little occasion to observe the mentally ill. Commented Pinel:

138. P. Pinel, "Recherches sur les causes du délire, par A. Crichton," *Recueil périodique de littérature médicale étrangèere* 1 (An VII [1798–99]): 401–418, 463–478. On this journal, see p. 335 above.

139. Crichton, *Inquiry,* 168–169.

140. Pinel, "Recherches sur les causes du délire," 466 n. 1.

141. Ibid., 472.

142. The one exception is Swain and Gauchet, *La pratique de l'esprit,* 349 n. 39.

143. Pinel, "Recherches sur les causes du délire," 411 n. 1.

> It seems to me that these general considerations of delirium caused by hypochondriasis, melancholy, mania, fevers, or narcotics yield only vague knowledge since these are very different mental states, considering their accompanying symptoms, their history, and their outcome. A surer means of gaining information on this subject is to write the specific history of the different deliria, especially of maniacs, which are the least known. It is with this goal in mind that I have published my Memoir on periodic insanity [where] I traced the distinctive characteristics of maniacal delirium.[144]

In yet another instance, Pinel faulted Crichton for an imprecise differential diagnosis of delirium in drunkenness and insanity. If one pays attention to the other symptoms that characterize the two, what marked differences! exclaimed the French clinician. "Is one delirium adequately explained by the other? The author should have avoided this sort of digression and followed the analytic process. He should have written a history of maniacal delirium according to a long list of observed facts, and derived inductions from these facts only."[145]

This stern rebuke pales when compared with Pinel's most energetic editorial comment, occasioned by Crichton's mention of *mind,* as distinct from brain. Unaware of a pitfall that may topple the translator, Pinel equates the word "mind" with "*âme,*" or soul. Pinel jumps to conclusions (sensitized, no doubt, by recent French Revolutonary history, and by his own, long-rejected youth, when he wore the cassock and tonsure). Pinel lectures Crichton as follows:

> This opinion of a separate soul, as an immaterial principle, is too closely associated with theology to be introduced into medicine, in our present state of knowledge. All the more reason to exclude all the explanations the author deduces, in order to present the mechanism of delirium. Purity and severity of taste demand that the functions of the human understanding be explained only through their history. This applies to the healthy state, and to the deviations of illness in insanity. That is, one must go no further than to record the predisposition to delirium, premonitory signs, accompanying psychologic and physical symptoms, outcome, and remedies proven by an enlightened experience.[146]

Crichton would have agreed. Pinel was, in fact, being contentious, and these preliminary comments about Crichton's thoughts on delirium reveal some anxiety on his part. With his book in press, he did not relish being "scooped" by the British author. For our assessment of the two

144. Ibid., 404 n. 1.
145. Ibid., 408 n. 1.
146. Ibid., 469 n. 1.

writers it is important to underline their similar approach to a differential diagnosis of mental illness: they subjected each deranged faculty to examination through the close observation of the physiologic and behavioral pathology it produced in the patient and thus derived a diagnosis from their observation of mind and body in the clinic.

Book II of Crichton's *Inquiry* is entitled "The Natural and Morbid History of the Mental Faculties." It contains a straightforward analysis of attention, perception, memory, judgment, imagination, volition, and, surprisingly, "Genius, and the diseases to which it is most subject." Here, Crichton praises "a faithful monitor within us" that warns us "when any exertion of the mental faculties is carried too far and ought to be discontinued."[147] Pinel, in his synopsis, awards this part of Crichton's work no more than half a page.[148] This was because Pinel's attention focused on the third part of the work, namely "On the Passions, Considered as Causes of Mental Derangement, and on Their Modifications and Corporeal Effects." Here, Crichton analyzed joy, grief, fear, anger, and love, and their normal and abnormal impact on psyche and soma. He explained that emotions differ according to their cause: we may view a past action with remorse, an accident with sorrow or grief; anticipation of a future event may trigger anxiety, apprehension, or terror; an aversion may evoke anger, hatred, envy, jealousy, or shame. The effects of such emotions could be expected to vary according to a person's temperament, age, occupation, sex, and so forth.

The new contribution of our author concerns the interrelationships of emotion and physiology. In the chapter on grief, for example, Crichton sensitively probed the differences among distress, sorrow, melancholy, anguish, and despair. Then he explained major physiologic effects, for example a behavior such as sighing. When sadness slows the circulation, congestion around the heart ensues. The uneasiness caused by a sense of fullness stimulates the aggrieved person to take a deep breath followed by quick exhalation. This sigh indicates that the heart has pushed blood into the lungs where it was oxygenated and expelled.[149] Crichton favored clinical examples, even though they were rarely his own. The book has no proper ending, but peters out with an odd list of "Conclusions," a brief inventory of "Genera and Species," and the eighty-five-page Appendix of aphorisms translated from Greding's *Miscellaneous Works*.[150]

147. Crichton, *Inquiry*, book II, 26.
148. Pinel, *Traité*, Introduction, xl.
149. Crichton, *Inquiry*, book II, 175–181, passim.
150. See n. 105 above.

Pinel wanted to convey the gist and flavor of Crichton's work to his readers, and to achieve this he paraphrased Crichton's analyses of grief, fear, terror, anger, and joy. We shall quote two long examples because this earliest printed evidence of Pinel's and Crichton's perception of mind and body in the clinic represents seminal texts of early modern psychiatry. We begin with Pinel's version of Crichton's section on grief—twenty-two pages of text presented in two pages of condensed paraphrase: "Having indicated the origins of human passions," asks Crichton, "how can one conceive of their power to provoke mental alienation, without knowing the history of their effects on the animal economy?" In Pinel's version, Crichton explains:

> The consequences of great sorrow are among the most remarkable; they include a feeling of general listlessness, decline of muscular strength, loss of appetite, small pulse, tightening of the skin, pale face, cold extremities, very evident decline in the vital force of the heart and arteries, leading to an imaginary sense of fullness, a feeling of oppression and anxiety, labored and slow respiration with sighs and sobs; an exhaustion of irritability and sensitivity sometimes so complete as to entail a more or less total torpor, a comatose state, or even catalepsy.
>
> In a less extreme degree there occurs a kind of apprehension ["*ennui*"] caused by repeated impressions on the sensory organs, a reluctance to move or exercise, sometimes an acute pain in the stomach, much reduced circulation in the blood vessels of the liver and abdominal viscera. Therefrom result marasmus and a wasting state, when sadness has become habitual, that is, has turned into melancholy. The end of both is sometimes an irresistible inclination toward suicide, or a mild delirium, or a state of rage. Prior to total derangement several disturbances may occur: temporary insanity, gloomy appearance, or rather, boorish misanthropy, altered facial expressions, furtive and fierce glances, vague and confused thought, a state resembling stupor or drunkenness, and then suddenly an explosion of the most violent madness.[151]

An equally dramatic and revealing analysis is found in Crichton's differential diagnosis of terror and of anger. Here again, patient behavior alerts the experienced clinician to the possibility of serious complications. We again quote Pinel's synopsis of Crichton's text:

> . . . terror differs from fear only by its intensity and sudden onset. It has its own characteristics, namely accelerated heartbeats, spasmodic contrac-

151. Pinel, *Traité,* Introduction, xxvii–xxix. This passage represents a synopsis of Crichton's *Inquiry,* book III, 177–199.

tion of the arteries, especially near the skin, causing paleness and a sudden dilation of the large blood vessels and of the heart; a sudden arrest of respiration, as from a spasm in the muscles of the larynx; tremors of the body and legs, loss of movement in the arms that hang limp; the impression is sometimes so strong as to cause collapse with deprivation of feeling and speech.

May not such an upheaval, under certain conditions, produce the most serious harm, violent spasms, convulsions, epilepsy, catalepsy, mania, or even death? (Plater, Shenkius, Bonet, Pechlin, Donatus, Van Swieten). It can also lead to a special flux of blood toward certain body parts and dangerous hemorrhages, such as menorrhagia, hemoptysis, apoplexy.

When rapid alternations of hope and terror occur, the debilitating effect of terror can be compensated for and give rise to unheard acts of strength and courage. Terror mixed with amazement can be caused by loud thunderclaps, the spectacle of a raging fire, a dreadful precipice, a pounding cataract, a burning town. This produces specific expressions such as a fixed stare, an open mouth, pale skin, a sensation of cold in the whole body, relaxation of facial muscles, frequently an interruption in the usual trend of thought, and dizziness. . . .

How much harm anger can cause when considered from a medical point of view! It presents two remarkable varieties: a pale face and somewhat livid coloring, with a kind of weakness and trembling in the extremities, or else a red and heated face with flashing eyes and extreme muscular energy. In the latter case, the blood is pushed violently toward the body surface, producing burning heat and a strong and animated tone of voice, convulsive and irregular breathing. The return of the blood through the veins to the heart becomes difficult; it flows back to the muscles and gives them more energy and strength. Its reflux toward the head and other sensitive organs may produce more serious trouble: violent hemorrhages through the nose, ears, or lungs, intermittent or continuous fevers, delirium, or even apoplexy.

One of the strangest effects of anger acts on the secretion of bile, its quantity and quality, as attested to by the most authentic observations (Hoffmann, Tulpius, Pechlin). Hence violent colics, persistent diarrhoea, sometimes jaundice. The only favorable consequence of this passion is an occasional cure of paralysis; but what meager compensation for the innumerable harmful consequences, especially when anger is excessive: sudden exhaustion of muscular and vascular irritability, syncope, convulsions, or even sudden death.

Anger rarely results in permanent madness, even though it alters the rational faculties in such an obvious manner, or interrupts their free use for a short while. But how much a gust of anger resembles a bout of madness! Reddened eyes and face, a threatening and furious mien, harsh and offensive language. Is it surprising that anger has been called a brief madness?[152]

It is hoped that these long descriptions of grief, terror, and anger in their mental, behavioral, and bodily expressions convey the reasons why Pinel found Crichton's book so dramatically revealing. (They also exemplify Pinel's elegant style, much superior to Crichton's.) Pinel appreciated his British colleague's clinical detachment, his descriptions free from moralizing comment, and the scientific precision of his observations. He prized the ease with which Crichton moved between physiology and psychology, particularly how he deduced mental phenomena from his observation of physiologic and behavioral symptoms. One example is Crichton's analysis of paleness, which he knew to be caused by a withdrawal of blood from the capillaries but at the same time observed to have been the result of terror. Pinel was impressed by Crichton's awareness of progression in the pathogenesis of mental illness, such as the clinical signs that precede an "explosion of the most violent madness," and his differential diagnoses, as between extreme anger and madness. Many of these qualities that Pinel admired were, needless to say, the very ones he had honed in his own clinical attitude toward the mentally ill patient.

Pinel's French readers did not pay much attention to Crichton, nor was the latter's book ever translated into French. In contrast, the Germans greatly appreciated Crichton's book and translated it twice: in 1798 already, *Untersuchung über die Natur und den Ursprung der Geisteszerrüttung* attracted attention. This was three years before Pinel's *Traité* appeared in a German version. The French alienist's praise of Crichton struck the Germans as a confirmation of their own independent judgment. They were understandably pleased by the Scottish author's extensive reliance upon their scholarship in anthropology, natural history, and psychology and touched by his gratitude for the inspiration and hospitality he received from his German hosts. A second translation of Crichton's book, in 1810, contains extensive notes by Johann Christoph Hoffbauer (1766–1827), professor of law and philosophy at Halle, whose book on legal psychology Esquirol later annotated.[153] Johann

152. Pinel, *Traité,* Introduction, xxxii–xxxv, passim. This passage represents a synopsis of Crichton, *Inquiry,* book III, chapter 4, "On Fear, Its Modifications and Effects," and chapter 5, "On Anger and the Offensive Passions, and Their Effects."

153. Hoffbauer was himself an expert in the nascent psychiatry, from a philosophical and legal point of view. When he commented on Crichton's book in 1810, he had already

Christian Reil, Hoffbauer's friend and collaborator, granted Crichton, "in passing, his highest regard."[154]

Unlike the British, the Germans criticized Pinel because they found his book unoriginal and disorganized. Most of them saw nothing special in the case histories, since case studies now abounded in the German literature and they argued that humane treatment of the insane was nothing new, nor special to France. Reil derided Pinel's book as a "cock-and-bull story, prolific in some parts but sick in general conception, without principles or originality, even though his nationalistic illusions lead him to claim these."[155] At the same time, Reil borrowed from the Frenchman so copiously that Schrenk calls him a plagiarist.[156] The religiously inclined psychiatrist Johann Christian Heinroth had no patience with Pinel at all. "Pinel's descriptions are neither consistent nor complete," he commented. "First, he groups the symptoms of various illnesses under one category; then, he passes quickly over the most important manifestations. . . . Overall, he identifies himself as a typically French writer, who never explores anything, who abandons the most important topics as soon as he raises them, and thus he never treats any subject thoroughly."[157] With Crichton, in contrast, the Germans felt a deep kinship, believing themselves experts in the analysis of the passions.

The British author's book appeared at a time when Pinel was still searching for the right word to represent the misery, tension, and loneliness that he witnessed in the men and women for whom he cared. He

published two works of his own on this subject: *Untersuchungen über die Krankheiten der Seele and die verwandten Zustände*, 3 vols. (Halle: Trampen, 1802–1807), and *Die Psychologie nach ihren Hauptanwendungen auf die Rechtspflege oder die sogenannte gerichtliche Arzneiwissenschaft nach ihrem psychologischen Teile* (Halle: Schimmelpfennig, 1808; 2d ed., 1823). Hoffbauer particularly appreciated the emphasis that both Pinel and Crichton placed on the patient's mental powers. He seems to have known Pinel. His last-mentioned book was translated into French, with notes by both Esquirol and Itard, as *Médecine légale relative aux aliénés et aux sourds-muets; ou, Les lois appliquées aux désordres de l'intelligence*, trans. A. M. Chambeyron, M.D., interne de la Salpêtrière (Paris: Baillière, 1827). Esquirol's notes are rather critical in tone and emphasize his own and Pinel's clinical experience. Together with Reil, Hoffbauer coedited the influenctial, though short-lived *Beyträge zur Beförderung einer Curmethode auf psychischem Wege*, 2 vols. (Halle: Curt, 1808). It is intriguing to find, in this journal, the review of a thesis by Lenhossek, published in Pest in 1804, entitled *Untersuchungen über die Leidenschaften und Gemütsaffecten als Ursachen und Heilmittel der Krankheiten.*

154. *Rhapsodieen über die Anwendung der psychischen Curmethoden auf Geisteszerrüttungen* (Halle: Curt, 1803), 31.

155. Ibid.

156. Martin Schrenk, *Uber den Umgang mit Geisteskranken*, Introduction and passim.

157. Johann Christian Heinroth, *Lehrbuch der Störungen des Seelenlebens oder Seelenstörungen und ihre Behandlung* (Leipzig: Vogel, 1818), 117.

chose "mental alienation" to convey the separation of the patient from society (and also to create a basis for conceptualizing mental illness in terms of the law). Pinel perceived a patient who feels odd in the "normal" world, a stranger (*alienus*) in the land of sanity. A sympathetic therapist might well journey into that land of "alienation," learn the language of "in-sanity," understand the "alienated," and lead the patient back into society. Pinel's excellent Austrian translator, Dr. Michael Wagner, found a pertinent equivalent that Crichton may have appreciated, namely "*Geistesverirrung*," a term that conveys the image of a patient who has lost his way.[158] Samuel Tuke liked this term; he wrote in *The Retreat, An Institution near York*:

> I adopt this term from an opinion that the *aliéné* of the French conveys a more just idea of this disorder than those expressions which imply, in any degree, the "abolition of the thinking faculty."[159]

Rather than alienation, Crichton portrayed the antagonism between the mental faculties and the other self, the passions, that gripped body and mind. This was the core problem for the nascent psychiatric specialty that Crichton brought to France from Germany.

Strange as it may sound, Crichton may not even have known of Pinel's extraordinary praise for his book. It is likely that Crichton read the *Traité* in its guillotined English version of 1806, without the Introduction where Pinel expressed his admiration.[160] Ironically, though Pinel's Introduction of 1800 formed part of the German, Spanish, and Italian versions, the English translator substituted his own! Pinel's appreciative comments on Crichton have thus remained unknown to the English reading public, including, it would seem, Alexander Crichton. Would he not have mentioned the famous Frenchman's endorsement while reminiscing about psychiatry at the age of eighty, in 1842, when he praised "two witnesses who, for long and extensive experience in the treatment of mental derangement, and for fidelity in their narrations, have not as yet been surpassed—I mean Pinel and Esquirol"?[161] It is sig-

158. P. Pinel, *Philosophisch-medizinische Abhandlung*, trans. Michael Wagner (Vienna: Schaumburg, 1801).

159. S. Tuke, *Description of the Retreat, an Institution near York, for Insane Persons of the Society of Friends* (York: W. Alexander, 1813), 137n.

160. The English translator, Dr. D. D. Davis, substituted his own Introduction for Pinel's. While he kept, or paraphrased, numerous parts of Pinel's lengthy presentation, he shrank the section on Crichton to one colorless sentence that reads: "The psychological work of Dr. Crichton exhibits some curious facts illustrative of the morbid influence of the passions upon the functions of the intellectual faculties" (1).

161. Crichton, *Commentaries on some Doctrines*, 179.

nificant that he should mention Esquirol in the same breath with Pinel, for it is Esquirol who provides us with evidence of Crichton's impact on French psychiatric thought.

DOMINIQUE ESQUIROL: THE PASSIONS AND THEIR MASTER

In 1805 Esquirol published his medical thesis entitled *Des passions, considérées comme causes, symptômes, et moyens curatifs de l'aliénation mentale* (On the passions, considered as causes, symptoms, and means of cure for mental alienation).[162] He dedicated the essay to Pinel "in homage of my gratitude," and declared himself Pinel's disciple throughout a thesis filled with case histories, many of them his own. He derived these from the private clinic that he had established at 8, rue Buffon, across the street from the Salpêtrière, in March 1802, three and a half years before completing his thesis. This clinic began and remained under Pinel's supervision; Esquirol thus publicly committed himself to carrying out his teacher's ideas, in theory as in therapy.[163]

In his thesis, Esquirol came quickly to the point, stressing the close interrelation of psychologic and somatic phenomena and of feelings and thought:

> Few authors have studied the relationship of mental alienation to the passions. Crichton offers exact ideas on the origins and development of the passions and their effects on the organism. Professor Pinel agrees with him, regarding the passions as the most frequent cause of upset of our intellectual faculties.[164]

Having thus declared his indebtedness to these two authors, Esquirol formulated his own version of psychologic therapy. He based this on Crichton's analysis of the effect that strong emotions could exert on the mental faculties and the organism, and on Pinel's view that the therapist can intervene in order to orchestrate the struggle within the patient—strengthen the rational powers and help them master the emotions and thus promote recovery. For the formulation of his therapeutic strategy, Esquirol also drew on Bordeu's concept of "secondary centers of sen-

162. (Paris: Didot jeune, 1805).

163. The 39-page manuscript register of Esquirol's small private hospital for the years 1802–1808 has recently been acquired by the History and Special Collections Division of the Louise M. Darling Biomedical Library at UCLA. See D. B. Weiner, "Esquirol's Patient Register: The First Private Psychiatric Hospital in Paris, 1802–1808," *Bulletin of the History of Medicine* 63 (1989): 110–120.

164. Esquirol, *Des passions*, 20.

sitivity" in the epigastrium and in the precordial region. He did, in fact, revive the traditional notion of hypochondriac localization, but gave it a specific formulation. Why could not a skillful therapist, asked Esquirol, provoke a strong emotion and use it for a curative purpose? In fact, he advocated a psychologic but violent assertion of medical authority and the use of the passions as *means* of cure. To this end he proposed emotional shocks—*des secousses*—"physical or psychologic, that shake and one might say threaten the machine, and forcibly redirect it toward health."[165]

Esquirol saw two potential benefits from this shock treatment: a judicious use of certain emotions by the doctor—for example intense remorse, regret, or joy—could help the patient regain rational command over his feelings. Secondly, Esquirol argued that control over the patient is essential in the asylum, and that individually and carefully administered shock differs categorically from the indiscriminate use of "ducking" in ice-cold water, or strong cold showers on the head or abdomen that others advocated. But there is no gainsaying that awe of the director was the ruling principle in the new clinic, and Esquirol often threatened and occasionally meted out punishment: he used the straitjacket, isolation, food deprivation, and even—if rarely—cold showers. But he never permitted what he called physical violence; the patients were never beaten nor intentionally hurt. His means are mild if compared to the chamber of horrors that J. C. Reil imagined—though Reil fortunately never had occasion to carry out his ingenious strategies for stimulation, excitement, fear, horror, pain, deprivation, and slavish subjection to the asylum director.

The first step in this therapeutic process was what Esquirol called "isolation," that is, removing the patient from home and familiar surroundings, and bringing the man or woman to the clinic for treatment. "Often the first shock to the intellectual and psychologic faculties occurs in the patient's home," commented Esquirol, "among acquaintances, parents, and friends. . . . I could multiply the examples of the beneficial impact on the psychologic state of mental patients resulting from their experience in an unfamiliar establishment where care, attention, and services are tendered, in contrast with the tortures they had expected and feared that they would find there."[166] All contemporary specialists agreed on this point, whether it was the Quaker William Tuke or the Savoyard Joseph Daquin or the German physiologist Reil: therapy must take place

165. Ibid., 70.
166. Ibid., 43, 41.

in a new and neutral place far from previous emotional ties and from objects that might remind the patient of past upsetting episodes. But it was the initial encounter with the director of the clinic, Esquirol believed, that should impress if not frighten the patient. Again he had models, notably Francis Willis, the man chiefly responsible for the management of King George III's bouts of mental illness. "A great show of force and power, and a threatening demeanor and preparations designed to terrify," commented Esquirol, "can stop the patient's most obstinate and deadly designs."[167] He recounted the case history of a twenty-year-old surgeon. He told the patient upon his arrival:

> Young man, you must stay here awhile. If you want to be comfortable, behave yourself. If you act as if you had lost your reason, you will be treated as if you were mad. You must choose. See these servants? They shall do everything that you ask for, in a reasonable and sensible way. But they obey me only.[168]

He welcomed a depressed, suicidal young woman in a kindlier way. Recounts the versatile therapist:

> I seemed so frightened by her condition, I communicated such concern about the danger of her situation, that she herself asked her parents to let her stay. One must often welcome patients in a pleasant manner, with a kindly smile, with gentle concern and empathy.[169]

In either case, the patient acknowledged that the director now wielded sole authority. "In surveying the diverse circumstances where the passions can serve in the treatment of insanity," concluded the young psychiatrist, "one is surprised that most students of mental alienation have ignored their use. Some day, perhaps, with sufficient data and with precise records of successful therapy, we will be able to establish the principles of moral treatment."[170]

This hope took on new dimensions when Esquirol moved to the Salpêtrière as successor to Pussin, in 1811, and faced the challenge of adapting methods used in a small private hospital to a huge public asylum. Esquirol had been watching Pussin's authoritarian ways and he now conceptualized the establishment itself as a "therapeutic tool," using the accommodations and the routines—the food, clothing, outings, work—as so many means of commendation, enticement, reward, pun-

167. Ibid., 56.
168. Ibid., 36.
169. Ibid.
170. Ibid., 78.

ishment. In a word, Esquirol aimed to achieve the socialization of patients by regulating them, and thus helping them control themselves. This strategy was based on the belief that the fear generated in the mental patient will help dominate his passions, make him conform to social rules, and become "normal." Commented Esquirol:

> Those who know the power of habit in human psychology will not be surprised about the influence that new habits can exert on the mentally ill patient: the need to control oneself, to compromise with strangers, is a powerful aid in restoring reason. As establishment specializing in therapy for the insane offers more appropriate care, better trained servants, well-adapted accommodations.[171]

These words refer to Esquirol's private hospital, but he tried to make them true for the Salpêtrière as well, and they stayed with him as medical director of the Charenton asylum in 1826 and as chief sponsor of the Law of 1838 that still regulates internment of the mentally ill in France. Swain and Gauchet have analyzed this new relationship of powerful director to hapless inmate, and, in *Discipline and Punish,* Michel Foucault has compared this regimentation of the mental patient to other institutions that imposed uniform behavior on large groups at the beginning of the bourgeois era and of the Industrial Revolution, in the factory, the prison, or the modern hospital, which he calls a "curing machine." Klaus Dörner has amplified the theme in *Madmen and the Bourgeoisie: A Social History of Insanity.*[172] Esquirol's view of the asylum as a "therapeutic tool" can indeed be made to fit into this authoritarian and dehumanizing context. It was not until Sigmund Freud revived Pinel's concept of prolonged and private doctor-patient communication that a relationship was restored in which the patient was again encouraged to speak freely for himself.

Thus a patient-centered approach to mental illness and a focus on the passions did not predominate for long in early-nineteenth-century French psychiatry. Rather, a reductionist materialistic approach, the tradition that emphasized physical causation of mental illness, won increasing favor; it shunted the attention of clinical investigators toward the brain, even the skull, away from mind, thought, and feelings. Crucial

171. Ibid., 49. The concept of "habit" would be well worth elaborating in this context.

172. See Swain and Gauchet, *La pratique de l'esprit*; M. Foucault, *Surveiller et punir: La naissance de la prison* (Paris: Gallimard, 1975), translated into English by Alan Sheridan under the title *Discipline and Punish: The Birth of the Prison* (New York: Random House, 1978). Foucault borrowed the phrase "curing machine," out of context, from the humane masterpiece, *Mémoires sur les hôpitaux de Paris* (1788), of Jacques Tenon. On Dörner, see n. 1 above.

elements that strengthened this emphasis were the vehement attack by François Joseph Victor Broussais (1772–1834) against Pinel in *Examen de la doctrine médicale généralement adoptée* of 1816,[173] and the thesis that Antoine Laurent Jessé Bayle (1799–1858) presented in 1822, where he proved a correlation between a physical phenomenon and mental illness, namely that "arachnitis," or chronic meningitis, may be accompanied by general paralysis and a progressive and ultimately fatal dementia.[174] The primacy of the passions, in early French psychiatry, lasted only for two decades, at most.

While it lasted, Pinel and Esquirol stood at the center of French attention, but Crichton was hardly noticed in France. True, he appears in the bibliographies both men appended to their articles written for the *Dictionnaire des sciences médicales,*[175] Bidault de Villiers published a synopsis of the *Inquiry,* and several French contemporaries mentioned his name.[176] But otherwise he remained unknown, a puzzling fact, given Pinel's eighteen-page analysis in the Introduction to his *Traité* of 1800. The chief explanation is Pinel's new Introduction for the second edition of the *Traité,* published in 1809, in which he briefly refers to Crichton's book, and then discusses the various passions in pages where it is not

173. *Examen de la doctrine médicale généralement adoptée et des systèmes modernes de nosologie dans lequel on détermine par les faits et par le raisonnement leur influence sur le traitement et sur la terminaison des maladies, suivi d'un plan d'études fondé sur l'anatomie et la physiologie pour parvenir à la connaissance du siège et des symptômes des affections pathologiques et à la thérapeutique la plus rationnelle* (Paris: Moronville, 1816), amplified in *Examen des doctrines médicales et des systèmes de nosologie,* 4 vols (Paris: Delaunay, 1829–1834). On Broussais, see the magisterial chapter in Ackerknecht, *Medicine at the Paris Hospital,* and M. Valentin, *François Broussais, empereur de la médecine* (Dinard: Association des amis du musée du pays de Dinard, 1988).

174. A. L. J. Bayle, *Recherches sur l'arachnitis chronique, la gastrite . . . considérées comme causes de l'aliénation mentale* (Paris: Thèse médecine, 1822).

175. Pinel cites the *Inquiry* in the bibliography of the article "aliénation" (1812) and Crichton's *Synoptical Table of Diseases* in the article "nosographie" (1819). Esquirol cites the *Inquiry* in the articles "folie" (1816) and "délire" (1814) where he adds: "This article was translated by professor Pinel and appears in Crichton's book." He then gives the reference to the translation in the *Receuil périodique de littérature étrangère.*

176. See n. 113 above. Swain mentions two contemporaries of Pinel, both of them involved in health care for the poor, who cite Crichton: one is Dr. Jean Marc Gaspard Itard, the physician to "Victor, the wild boy of Aveyron," who refers to psychologic treatment as "the sublime art created in England by Willis and Crichton"; the other is Louis François Joseph Alhoy, for a while headmaster of the National Institute for Deaf Children, and subsequently an administrator of the National Welfare Institutions (*La pratique de l'esprit,* 348 n. 37). The reference by Itard appears at the beginning of his first report on the wild boy, recently reprinted in T. Gineste, *Victor de l'Aveyron: Dernier enfant sauvage, premier enfant fou* (Paris: Le Sycomore, 1981), 225.

177. Pinel, *Traité,* 2d ed., Introduction, xxii.

possible to distinguish his ideas from Crichton's and where the Scottish doctor does not appear as an important stimulator of Pinel's thought.[177] Also, Pinel called his new introduction "Introduction to the first edition," thus presenting his faint and brief allusion to Crichton in 1809 as if it had been written in 1800.[178]

Was it a lapse of memory to call his new Introduction the "first," or an intentional obfuscation, as some critics suggest?[179] Friends of Crichton's may well take umbrage at Pinel's elision of his eighteen-page analysis of the *Inquiry* in the Introduction to the second edition of the *Traité*. Might he have gone to the extraordinary length of calling his second Introduction the "first" in order to wipe out all memory of his early enthusiasm for Alexander Crichton, at least in the minds of French readers? Whatever the answer, Pinel's main motivation seems clear: he wished to appear as the prime analyst of the passions, and the young Esquirol echoed his thought.

There is enough internal evidence in these French physicians' writings, however, to permit the conclusion that it was Crichton who drew their attention to recent German medical research and publications. He helped introduce them to concepts such as Blumenbach's *Bildungstrieb,* Reil's *Lebenskraft,* and Schelling's *Naturphilosophie* and, more generally, to contemporary German scholarship in anthropology, natural history, and psychology, with its emphasis on developmental change, instincts, drives, and irrational forces that impel man as a biologic entity and over which he has little control.

178. Walther Riese discovered the discrepancies when he translated the Introduction of 1800 in 1969. See *The Legacy of Philippe Pinel: An Inquiry into Thought on Mental Alienation* (New York: Springer, 1969), 23–49. The two Introductions are conveniently printed side by side and provided with some editorial comment in J. Postel and P. H. Privat, "Les deux Introductions du 'Traité médico-philosophique' de P. Pinel," *Annales médico-psychologiques* 129 (1971): 14–48. The totally revised Introduction to the second edition, written in 1809, was translated by Gregory Zilboorg, who mistakenly believed it to be the first Introduction because Pinel gave it that title. See Zilboorg's *A History of Medical Psychology,* 329–341.

179. P. H. Privat, *Philippe Pinel: Son temps, son œuvre* (Paris: Thèse médecine, 1969). What must give one pause is Pinel's lack of generosity toward other colleagues: his denigration of Chiarugi, whom he dismissed in Introduction, *Traité,* xli; his failure to acknowledge Joseph Daquin's feelingful dedication of the second edition of *Philosophie de la folie* in 1804; and his covert indebtedness to Dr. James Carmichael Smythe (1741–1821) that Othmar Keel has studied and that Jacques Postel has gleefully echoed. See O. Keel, *La généalogie de l'histopathologie: Une révision déchirante: Philippe Pinel, lecteur discret de J. C. Smythe* (Paris: Vrin, 1979), and J. Postel, "Un nouveau mensonge par omission de Philippe Pinel, découvert par Othmar Keel, lecteur indiscret et perspicace," *Information psychiatrique* 57 (1981): 619–622.

In his biographic sketch of Esquirol mentioned earlier, Henri Ey points to his countryman's deep sympathy for German thought, a set of convictions whose origins puzzle Ey. He alludes to Esquirol's "probable meeting" with J. C. Heinroth in Paris and comments that "agreement in their way of thinking was so fundamental" that no actual encounter was needed because their publications express the "similarity of their human and scientific convictions."[180] An even closer link that Ey might have mentioned exists through J. C. Hoffbauer, who annotated the second German translation of Crichton's book and whose treatise on legal psychiatry Esquirol commented on in turn, in the 1827 French edition.[181] Heinroth and K. W. Ideler explored the relationship between religion, morality, and psychiatry—as did Esquirol, who also shared a fascination for the "passions" with J. C. Reil and a lifelong involvement in asylum administration with J. G. Langermann. There is not room here to explore the "meeting of minds" to which Ey alludes, however rewarding this exploration would be.

This essay is merely designed to underline the importance of Alexander Crichton, who drew the attention of Pinel and Esquirol to German scholarship in psychology and psychiatry at the turn of the nineteenth century. He thus helped open the French medical world to the influence of German thought and served as unwitting ambassador of German medical Romanticism, from Göttingen to Paris.

180. H. Ey, "J. E. D. Esquirol," in *Grosse Nervenärzte,* ed. K. Kolle, 3 vols. (Stuttgart: Thieme, 1956–1963), 2:87–97.

181. See n. 153 above.

APPENDIX: BIOBIBLIOGRAPHIC NOTES

Appended are the first complete bibliographies of the three authors' writings, omitting only Pinel's numerous pre-Revolutionary journal articles.

1. PHILIPPE PINEL

Pinel's books and papers are listed in order of appearance: Translation of William Cullen, *Institutions de médecine pratique, traduites sur la quatrième et dernière édition de l'ouvrage anglais de M. Cullen, Professeur de médecine pratique dans l'Université d'Edimbourg, etc., Premier médecin du roi pour l'Ecosse,* 2 vols. (Paris: Duplain, 1785). — Edition, with notes, of G. Baglivi, *Opera omnia medico-practica,* 2 vols. (Paris: Duplain, 1788). — Jacques Gibelin, ed., *Abrégé des Transactions de la Société royale de Londres* (Paris: Buisson, 1789–1791), 12 vols. Pinel was sole editor of volumes 5–7, entitled *Chimie, Anatomie et physique animale,* and *Médecine et chirurgie,* and coedited part 2 of *Matière médicale et pharmacie.* — *Nosographie philosophique; ou, Méthode de l'analyse appliquée à la médecine* (Paris: Brosson, 1798; 2d ed., 3 vols., 1802–1803; 3d ed., 1807; 4th ed., 1810; 5th ed., 1813; 6th ed., 1818. — *Traité médico-philosophique sur l'aliénation mentale ou la manie* (Paris: Caille et Ravier, 1800). Pinel published a second, much enlarged, edition entitled *Traité médico-philosophique sur l'aliénation mentale* (Paris: Brosson, 1809). The title page states that it is "totally revised and enlarged," and the phrase "*ou la manie*" has been dropped from the title. German translation by the Hungarian physician Michael Wagner, *Philosophisch-medizinische Abhandlung über Geistesverirrungen oder Manie* (Vienna: Schaumburg, 1801). Spanish translation by Dr. Guarnerio y Allavena, *Tratado medico-filosofico de la enagenación del alma o mania* (Madrid: Imprenta real, 1804). English translation by Dr. D. D. Davis, under the unsatisfactory title, *A Treatise on Insanity* (London: Cadell and

Davies, 1806). Italian translation by Dr. C. Vaghi as *Trattato medico-filosofico sopra l'alienazione mentale* (Lodi: Orcasi, 1830). — *La médecine clinique rendue plus précise et plus exacte par l'application de l'analyse; ou, Recueil et résultat d'observations sur les maladies aigües, faites à la Salpêtrière* (Paris: Brosson, Gabon et Cie., 1802; 2d ed., 1804; 3d ed., 1815).

Pinel's articles are listed here in chronologic order, omitting a large number of short pieces on mathematics, natural history, science, and politics contributed to the *Encyclopédie méthodique (Médecine),* to Fourcroy's journal, *La médecine éclairée par les sciences physiques,* to the *Journal de physique,* the *Journal gratuit de santé,* and critiques of published works and work-in-progress submitted to the Académie des sciences and published in its *Procès-verbaux.* On the subject of Pinel's brief articles in the *Gazette de santé,* which he edited from 1784 to 1790, see Pedro Marset Campos, "Veinte publicaciones psiquiatricas de Pinel olvidadas: Contribuciòn al estudio de los origenes del *Traité sur la manie,*" *Episteme* 6 (1972): 164–195.

"Mémoire sur cette question proposée pour sujet d'un prix par la Société de médecine: 'Déterminer quelle est la meilleure manière d'enseigner la médecine pratique dans un hôpital'" (the French text was published by G. Bollotte in *Information psychiatrique* 47 [1971]: 105–128; an English translation is to be found in D. B. Weiner, ed. and tr., *The Clinical Training of Doctors*). — "Mémoire sur la manie périodique ou intermittente," *Mémoires de la Société médicale d'émulation* 1 (An V [1796–97]): 94–119. — "Recherches et observations sur le traitement moral des aliénés," ibid. 2 (An VI [1797–98]): 215–255. — "Observations sur les aliénés et leur division en espèces distinctes," ibid. 3 (An VII [1798–99]): 1–26. — "Recherches sur les causes du délire, par A. Crichton," *Recueil périodique de littérature médicale étrangère* 1 (An VII [1798–99]): 401–418, 463–478. — "Recherches sur le traitement général des femmes aliénées dans un grand hospice, et résultats obtenus à la Salpêtrière après trois années d'expérience," *Le moniteur universel,* 11 Messidor, An XIII, 1158–1160. — "Résultats d'observations et construction de tables pour servir à déterminer le degré de probabilité de la guérison des aliénés," *Mémoires de la classe des sciences mathématiques et physiques,* Institut national de France, 1st ser., 8 (1807): 169–205. — "Résultats d'observations pour servir de base aux rapports juridiques dans les cas d'aliénation mentale," *Mémoires de la Société médicale d'émulation* 8 (1817): 675–684. — See also R. Semelaigne, "Notes inédites de Pinel, avec un 'Tableau général des fous de Bicêtre,'" *Bulletin de la Société clinique de médecine mentale* 6 (1913): 221–227. Jacques Postel has published this "Tableau" in *Genèse de la psy-*

chiatrie: Les premiers écrits de Philippe Pinel (Paris: Sycomore, 1981), 226–229.

Even though written by J. B. Pussin, the following document pertains to the above list: "Observations du citoyen Pussin sur les fous," Archives nationales, 27 AP 8 (doc. 2). For an annotated English translation, see Weiner, "The Apprenticeship of Philippe Pinel."

Pinel contributed the following articles to the famous *Dictionnaire des sciences médicales,* 60 vols. (Paris: Panckoucke, 1812–1822): "âcreté," 1 (1812): 144–146; "adynamie," 1 (1812): 161–163; "agissante (médecine)," 1 (1812): 192–198; "aigües (maladies aigües," 1 (1812): 203–205; "aliénation," 1 (1812): 311–321; "analyse (appliquée à la médecine)," 2 (1812): 19–30; "asthénie," 2 (1812): 401–406; "ataxie," 2 (1812): 419–422; "bénin" 3 (1812); 78–79; "Brownisme," 3 (1812): 320–323. "cachéxie," 3 (1812): 410–412; "chronique (maladies chroniques)," 5 (1813): 171–177; "classification (des maladies internes)," 5 (1813): 276–287; "clinique," 5 (1813): 364–371; "décomposition des maladies," 8 (1814): 169–174; "dose," 10 (1814): 151–169; "doute philosophique," 10 (1814): 239–242; "expectation (en médecine ou médecine expectante)," 14 (1815): 247–254; "expérience (en médecine considérée d'une manière générale)," 14 (1815): 267–273; "fièvre," 15 (1815): 217–240; and, together with Bricheteau, "idéologie," 23 (1818): 473–483; "médecine," 31 (1819): 380–394; "nosographie," 36 (1819): 206–265.

The definitive biography of Pinel remains to be written: the secondary literature is huge, and only a few pertinent samples will be mentioned here. The books by Pinel's descendant René Semelaigne (the grandson of Pinel's nephew) have long been regarded as authoritative: *Philippe Pinel et son œuvre au point de vue de la médecine mentale* (Paris: Imprimeries réunies, 1888); idem, *Les grands aliénistes français* (Paris: Steinheil, 1894), 15–117; and idem, *Aliénistes et philanthropes: Les Pinel et les Tuke* (Paris: Steinheil, 1912). Upon investigation it appears that Semelaigne and his family have, for over a century, been extremely protective of their famous ancestor and may well have destroyed much documentation: only a handful of letters from Pinel to his brothers survive, and all the official dossiers, at the Archives nationales, the Académie des sciences, the Académie de médecine, and the Archives de la Seine in Paris, are virtually empty. This is surprising and suggests that someone may have purged the evidence. The official eulogy at the Academy of Sciences was given by Georges Cuvier, "Eloge historique de Pinel, lu le 11 juin 1827 à l'Académie des sciences," *Mémoires,* Paris, Académie des sciences, 2d ser., 9 (1830): ccxxi–cclx, and the eulogy at the Academy of Medicine was given by Etienne Pariset, "Eloge de Philippe Pinel, lu à la séance du 28 août 1827," in *Histoire des membres de l'Académie royale de médecine,* 2 vols. in 1 (Paris: Baillière, 1845), 1:209–259. The best brief evaluations of Pinel are P. Huard and M. J. Imbault-Huard, "Philippe Pinel, idéologue, nosologiste, et psychiatre," *Gazette médicale de France* 9 (1977): 161–165; M. J. Imbault-Huart, "Pinel, nosologiste et clinicien," ibid. 12 (1978): 33–38; and J. Delay, "Philippe Pinel à la Salpêtrière," *Médecine de France* 96 (1958): 10–16. The best analyses of Pinel's thought in English are W. Riese, *The Legacy of Philippe Pinel: An Inquiry into Thought on Mental Alienation* (New York: Springer, 1969), and idem, "Philippe Pinel, His Views on Human Nature and Disease, His Medical Thought," *Journal of Nervous and Mental Disease* 114 (1951): 313–323; thoughtful shorter works in English are E. Woods and E. T. Carlson, "The Psychiatry of Philippe Pinel," *Bulletin of the History of Medicine* 35 (1961): 14–25; K. A. Grange, "Pinel and Eighteenth-Century Psychiatry," ibid. 35 (1961): 442–453. In contrast with Pinel's public professional life, his early years, until his arrival in Paris in 1778, are well documented. See W. H. Lechler, *Philippe Pinel: Seine Familie, seine Jugend- und Studienjahre 1745–1778: Roques, St. Paul-Cap-de-Joux, Lavaur, Toulouse, Montpellier, unter Verwendung zum Teil noch unveröffentlichter Documente* (Munich: The author, 1959), and especially the following papers by the late Pierre Chabbert of Castres: "Les années d'études de Philippe Pinel: Lavaur, Toulouse, Montpellier," *Monspeliensis Hippocrates* 3 (1960): 15–23; "L'œuvre médicale de Philippe Pinel," in *Comptes-rendus du 96ème Congrès national des sociétés savantes* (Paris: Bibliothèque nationale, 1971), 153–161; "Philippe Pinel à Paris jusqu'à sa nomination à Bicêtre," in *Aktuelle Probleme aus der Geschichte der Medizin: Proceedings of the 19th International Congress of the History of Medicine* (Basel: Karger, 1966), 589–595.

The most innovative recent work comes from the pen of Gladys Swain: *Le sujet de la folie: Naissance de la psychiatrie* (Toulouse: Privat, 1977). She has also coauthored a profound book on the era of Pinel: Marcel Gauchet and Gladys Swain, *La pratique de l'esprit humain: L'institution asilaire et la révolution démocratique* (Paris: Gallimard, 1980). Important is the work of Jacques Postel, a mixture of appreciation and disdain: *Genèse de la psychiatrie: Les premiers écrits de Philippe Pinel* (Paris: Le sycomore, 1981) and his articles "Les deux Introductions du *Traité médico-philosophique* de Philippe Pinel," *Annales médico-psychologiques* 129 (1971): 14–48; "Phillippe Pinel: 'Observations sur une espèce particulière de mélancholie qui conduit au suicide,'" ibid. 54 (1978): 1137–1141; "Pages d'histoire: Philippe Pinel à Bicêtre," *Psychiatrie française,* n.s., 10 (1979):

173–181; "Naissance et décadence du traitement moral pendant la première moitié du 19ème siècle," *L'évolution psychiatrique* 44 (1979): 588–616; "Philippe Pinel et le mythe fondateur de la psychiatrie," *Psychanalyse à l'université* 4 (1979): 197–244; "Un nouveau mensonge par omission de Philippe Pinel, découvert par Othmar Keel, lecteur indiscret et perspicace," *Information psychiatrique* 57 (1981): 619–622; "Pinel et Mesmer: Un rendez-vous manqué," *Magazine littéraire* 175 (1981): 25–28; "Un manuscript inédit de Philippe Pinel sur les guérisons opérées dans le 7ème emploi de Bicêtre, en 1794," *Revue internationale d'histoire de la psychiatrie* 1 (1983): 79–88; "Les premières expériences psychiatriques de Pinel à la maison de santé Belhomme," *Revue canadienne de psychiatrie* 28 (1983): 571–576.

See also D. B. Weiner, "Health and Mental Health in the Thought of Philippe Pinel: The Emergence of Psychiatry during the French Revolution" in *Healing and History: Essays for George Rosen,* ed. Charles E. Rosenberg (New York: Science History Publication, 1979), 59–85; idem, "The Apprenticeship of Philippe Pinel: A New Document, 'Observations of Citizen Pussin on the Insane,'" *American Journal of Psychiatry* 136 (1979): 1128–1134; idem, "Trois moments-clés dans la vie de Philippe Pinel," in *Comptes-rendus du 27ème Congrès international d'histoire de la médecine* (Barcelona: Acadèmia de Ciencies Mèdiques de Catalunya i Balears, 1981), 1:154–161; idem, "The Origins of Psychiatry: Pinel or the Zeitgeist?" in *Zusammenhang: Festschrift für Marielene Putscher,* eds. O. Baur and O. Glandien, 2 vols. (Cologne: Wienand, 1984), 2:617–631; idem, "Philippe Pinel, père: Deux générations en conflit," *Perspectives psychiatriques* 96 (1984): 100–103; idem, "Philippe Pinel, Linguist," *Gesnerus* 42 (1985): 499–509; idem, "The Madman in the Light of Reason, Part II: Alienists, Asylums, and the Psychologic Approach," in *Handbook of the History of Psychiatry,* eds. E. R. Wallace, IV, and J. Gach (New Haven: Yale University Press, forthcoming).

2. SIR ALEXANDER CRICHTON

Crichton's books, in chronologic order, consist of: *De vermibus intestinorum* (Leiden: Medical thesis, 1785). — A translation of J. F. Blumenbach, *Über den Bildungstrieb und das Zeugungsgeschäft* (Göttingen: Dieterich, 1791), under the title *An Essay on Generation* (London: Cadell, 1792). — *An Inquiry into the Nature and Origin of Mental Derangement, Comprehending a Concise System of the Physiology and Pathology of the Human Mind, and a History of the Passions and their Effects* (London: Cadell and Davies, 1798). German translation (Leipzig, 1798; 2d ed., Leipzig, 1810, with notes and additions by Johann Christoph Hoffbauer). Dutch translation by L. Bicker (Rotterdam and Leiden, 1801, 2d ed., 1804). The library of the Wellcome Institute for the History of Medicine in London owns a 62-page manuscript synopsis of Crichton's book in French, by Dr. F. R. Bidault de Villiers (1775–1824). He undertook this for his friend A. A. Royer-Collard, the medical director of Charenton hospice, Esquirol's predecessor. This translation is not included in Bidault's *Recueil des œuvres posthumes* (Paris: Veret, 1828), but he published a synopsis in *Bibliothèque médicale* 53 (1816): 30–67; 54 (1816): 289–324; 55 (1817): 289–331. — *A synoptical Table of Diseases, exhibiting their Arrangement in Classes, Orders, Genera, and Species, designed for the Use of Students* (London: n.p., 1805). — *Russische Sammlung für Naturwissenschaft und Heilkunde*, eds. Drs. A. Crichton, J. Rehmann, and K. F. Burdach, 2 vols. (Riga and Leipzig: Hartmann, 1815–1817). — *Pharmacopoeia pauperum* (St. Petersburg: n.p., 1807). — *An Account of Some Experiments Made with the Vapour of Boiling Tar in the Cure of Pulmonary Consumption* (Edinburgh: Manners and Miller, 1817), 62 pp. French translation (St. Petersburg, 1817). German translation (Braunschweig, 1819). — *Practical Observations on the Treatment and Cure of Several Varieties of Pulmonary Consumption, and on the Effects of the Vapour of Boiling Tar in that Disease* (London: Lloyd, 1823), 228 pp. Crichton dedicated this enlarged version to the Dowager Empress of all the Russias, in recognition of "the great confidence which was placed in me during my long residence at the court of Russia by His Majesty the Emperor and Your Imperial Majesty, and your august Family." — *Commentaries on some Doctrines of a dangerous Tendency in Medicine, and on the general Principles of safe Practice* (London: Churchill, 1842).

In addition to these books, Crichton wrote the following papers: "Some Observations on the Medicinal Effects of the *lichen islandicus* and *Arnica montana*," *London Medical Journal* 10 (1789): 229–241. — "A Case of Oedema fugax and a Case of an hitherto undescribed Cause of Jaundice," *Medical Physical Journal* 6 (1802): 25–31. — "The Means by which Vitality is Supplied to the Living System," read to the Royal Society on 17 March 1814 (Crichton was still in Russia), *London Medical, Surgical, and Pharmacological Repertory* 1 (1814): 439. — "On the Climate of the Antediluvian World, and its Independence of Solar Influence; and on the Formation of Granite," *Annals of Philosophy* 9 (1825): 97–108, 207–217. This essay is cast in the shape of a letter to the editor and is sent from "Harley Street, Cavendish Square." — Crichton read three short papers to the Geological Society, namely: "On the Taunus and other

Mountains of Nassau, in Explanation of Specimens presented to the Geological Society of London," *Geological Society Transactions* 2 (1826): 265–272. This was the year when Crichton put his collection of minerals up for sale. — "On the Geological Structure of the Crimea," *Geological Society Proceedings* 1 (1832): 342–343. — "An Account of Fossil Vegetables Found in the Sandstone which underlies the Lowest Bed of the Carboniferous Limestone near Ballisadiere, in the County of Sligo, Ireland," ibid. 11 (1838): 394–395. Tansey tells us that Crichton's interest in Ireland stemmed from some lands inherited by his wife. See also his *Reflections on the Policy of Making an Ample and Independent Provision for the Roman Catholic Clergy of Ireland* (*London*: Ridgeway, 1834).

There are only two scholarly studies of Crichton: H. Hopf, *Leben und Werk Alexander Crichtons (1763–1856)* (Munich: Medical thesis, 1962), and E. M. Tansey, "The Life and Works of Sir Alexander Crichton, F.R.S. (1763–1856): A Scottish Physician to the Imperial Russian Court," *Royal Society of London: Records and Proceedings* 38 (1983): 241–259. A number of scholars devote passages of varying lengths to an analysis of Crichton's contribution to the prehistory of psychiatry, namely: A. Boldt, *Über die Stellung und Bedeutung der "Rhapsodieen über die Anwendung der psychischen Curmethode auf Geisteszerrüttung" von Johann Christian Reil (1759–1813) in der Geschichte der Psychiatrie,* Abhandlungen zur Geschichte der Medizin und der Naturwissenschaften, Heft 12 (Berlin: Ebering, 1936), 45–51; Hunter and Macalpine, *Three Hundred Years of Psychiatry,* especially 559–564; R. Hoeldtke, "The History of Associationism and British Medical Psychology," *Medical History* 11 (1967): 46–65; M. Schrenk, "Pathologie der Passionen: Zur Erinnerung an J. E. D. Esquirol, geboren 1772," *Nervenarzt* 44 (1973): 195–198; and idem, *Über den Umgang mit Geisteskranken,* 123–124.

There is a substantial entry in A. Hirsch et al., *Biographisches Lexikon der hervorragenden Arzte aller Zeiten und Völker,* s.v. "Crichton," and a full obituary in *Proceedings of the Geological Society of London* 13 (1857): lxiv–lxvi, most of which is copied by the authors of the obituaries in *Proceedings of the Royal Society of London* 3 (1856): 269–272; W. Munk, *The Roll of the Royal College of Physicians of London,* 2d ed. (London: The College, 1878), vol. 2 (*1701–1800*), 416–418, and *Dictionary of National Biography,* vol. 5 (1908), s.v. "Crichton." D. Leigh, in *The Historical Development of British Psychiatry* (Oxford: Pergamon, 1961), devotes almost all his attention to Crichton's nosology (44–47, 161), which is heavily indebted to Cullen, as we would expect. See also N. H. Schuster, "English Doctors in Russia in the Early Nineteenth Century," *Proceedings of the Royal Society of Medicine* 61 (1968): 185–190, and John Appleby, "British Doctors in Russia, 1657–1807" (Ph.D. thesis, University of London, 1979), 243, 341, 357, 364: these passages deal with seeds obtained for Kew Gardens from Russia. One passage reads: "In 1818, Sir Joseph Banks informed the Royal Botanic Garden at Kew that he had received a parcel of seeds on 18 August from Dr. Alexander Crichton of St. Petersburg. He believed them to be Siberian, but was uncertain as he had not received an accompanying letter" (364). A cursory treatment of Crichton is found in Ekbert Faas, *Retreat into the Mind: Victorian Poetry and the Rise of Psychiatry* (Princeton: Princeton University Press, 1988), 36, 52–53, 58–59, 61, 100.

3. JEAN ETIENNE DOMINIQUE ESQUIROL

Esquirol's entire œuvre consists of essays: twelve of these, first written for the *Dictionnaire des sciences médicales,* constitute his major book, *Des maladies mentales* of 1838, some are new definitions from the point of view of psychiatry or the law (for example "illusion," "hallucination," "homicidal monomania"), some are of a political and administrative nature (for example "maisons d'aliénés"), some were read to the Académie royale de médecine, of which he was a member, some to the Académie des sciences, to which he did not belong. Sometimes there only subsist synopses in contemporary journals of papers that no longer exist. Esquirol's papers are here listed in the order of their appearance in each journal, to indicate the growth and change of his interests.

Esquirol published almost exclusively in the following journals: *Annales d'hygiène publique et de médecine légale,* 1829–1923 (henceforth *AHP*), *Archives générales de médecine,* 1823–1914 (henceforth *AGM*), *Bibliothèque médicale; ou, Recueil périodique d'extraits des meilleurs ouvrages de médecine et de chirurgie,* 1803–1822 (henceforth *BMRP*), *Journal général de médecine, de chirurgie et de pharmacie; ou, Receuil périodique de la Société de médecine de Paris,* 1796–1830 (henceforth *JGM*), *Revue médicale française et étrangère,* 1820–1880 (henceforth *RMFE*).

The *AHP* contain the following articles by Esquirol: "Rapport statistique sur la maison royale de Charenton pendant les années 1826, 1827, et 1828," 1 (1829): 100–151; "Sur deux homicides commis par un homme atteint de monomanie avec hallucinations," 2 (1829): 392–405; "Monomanie érotique méconnue par des personnes étrangères à l'observation des aliénés," 3 (1830): 198–220 (with Marc, Ferrus, and Leuret); "Sur la statistique des aliénés et sur le rapport du nombre des aliénés à la population: Analyse de la statistique des aliénés de la Norvège," 4

(1830): 332–359; "Consultation médico-légale: Sur l'état mental d'un testateur, jugé d'après les actes de ses dernières volontés," 5 (1831): 370–385; "Consultation médico-légale: Sur la validité du testament d'un homme atteint d'hémiplégie, avec affaiblissement de l'intelligence," 7 (1832): 203–207; "Question médico-légale: Sur l'isolement des aliénés," 9 (1833): 131–191; "Mémoire historique et statistique sur la maison royale de Charenton," 13 (1835): 5–192; "Consultation médico-légale sur l'état mental de Pierre Rivière," 15 (1836): 202–205 (with Orfila, Marc, Pariset, Rostan, Mitivié, and Leuret); "Consultation sur un cas de suspicion de folie, chez une femme inculpée de vol," 20 (1838): 435–460; "Observations médico-légales sur la monomanie homicide," 23 (1840): 204–215; "Rapport sur un cas de bigamie," 24 (1840): 402–406 (with F. L. Leuret); "Monomanie homicide: Rapport sur l'état mental du nommé B," 24 (1840): 350–359.

In *Annuaire médico-chirurgical des hôpitaux* (Paris: Crochard, 1819), Esquirol published "Mémoire sur la folie à la suite des couches," 600–632 (see also abstract of this paper in *BMRP* 60 [1818]: 390–392.

The *AGM* contain the following articles by Esquirol: "Remarques sur les signes donnés par les auteurs comme propres à faire connaître si le corps d'une personne, trouvé pendu, l'a été après la mort ou pendant qu'elle vivait encore," 1 (1823): 1–13 (see similar article in *JGM*); "Note sur le mode de traitement employé à l'hôpital des aliénés de Moscou par le Dr. Kibaltiez," 3 (1823): 374–377; "Tumeur considérable développée dans l'intérieur du crâne," 3 (1823): 594–597; "Note sur l'institution des aliénés à St. Pétersbourg 4 (1824): 143–145; abstract, "Existe-t-il de nos jours un plus grand nombre de fous qu'il n'en existait il y a quarante ans?" 6 (1824): 290–293; abstract, "Etranglement interne de l'intestin grêle," 7 (1825): 461; "Altérations du système cérébro-spinal," report on essays submitted for a prize offered by the Académie de médecine, public meeting 5 November, 9 (1825): 598; "Note statistique sur la maison des insensés de Matti à Aversa, dans le royaume de Naples," 12 (1826): 195–202; abstract, "Des illusions chez les aliénés," 30 (1832): 275–277.

The *BMRP* contains the following articles by Esquirol: "Notice sur M. Nysten," 1818, *61*: 248–250, "Sur les déplacements du colon transverse dans l'aliénation mentale," 1818, *60*: 392–396, *61*: 388–389.

The *JGM* contains the following articles by Esquirol: "Observations sur l'application du traitement moral à la manie, par M. Esquirol, médecin d'une maison de traitement d'aliénés, située vis-à-vis la Salpêtrière," 17 (7th year) (Thermidor, An XI [August 1803]): 281–294; "Observations pour servir à l'histoire du traitement de la manie; par M. Esquirol, médecin de la maison de traitement des aliénés, vis-à-vis la Salpêtrière,

No. 8," 19 (An XII [February 1804]): 129–147; review of *Traité de matière médicale* by C. J. A. Schwilgué, 2d ed., ed. P. H. Nysten, 37 (1810): 106–109; "Sur les terminaisons critiques de la manie," 50 (1814): 3–85; "Observations sur l'aliénation mentale à la suite de couches," *62* (1818): 148–164; "De l'aliénation mentale à la suite des couches, pendant et après l'allaitement: Lu à la Société de médecine le 17 mars 1818," 62 (1818): 337–340; "Ouverture de corps d'aliénés qui présentent le colon transverse dans une direction perpendiculaire, et son extrémité splénique descendue derrière le pubis," 62 (1818): 341–358; 63 (1818): 176–184; "Obervation de fracture d'une vertèbre dorsale, suite d'une chute sur les lombes," 64 (1818): 80 (from a case report in *Bibliothèque médicale*); "Fragment d'os introduit dans les bronches, sans aucun symptôme de suffocation," 64 (1818): 235–236 (a case report); "Epanchement sanguin entre la face interne de la dure-mère et la face externe de l'arachnoïde correspondante," 64 (1818): 243–244 (an unsigned case report attributed to Esquirol); "Apoplexie suivie de paralysie et de démence, par épanchement considérable de sang entre la dure-mère et l'arachnoïde," 64 (1818): 350–352 (fatal outcome of previous case); "Observations d'hallucinations," 66 (1819): 289–305; "Extrait du rapport de MM. Esquirol et Chantourelle sur l'observation précédente," 81 (1822): 168–174 (refers to a "paralysie à l'extrémité supérieure droite, guérie par l'emploi de la noix vomique," same vol., p. 160); "Remarques sur les signes donnés par les auteurs de médecine légale, comme propres à faire connaître si le corps d'une personne trouvée pendue l'a été après la mort ou pendant qu'elle vivait encore," 83 (1823): 103–107 (see similar article in *AGM*).

The *RMFE* contains the following articles by Esquirol: "Introduction à l'étude des aliénations mentales," 8 (1828): 31–38; "De l'influence de l'épilepsie sur les fonctions du cerveau et par conséquent sur l'intelligence," 9 (1822): 5–10 (read to the Académie de médecine); "Notice sur le village de Geel," 7 (1822): 137–155 (read to the Académie de médecine on 22 January 1822.)

The *Dictionnaire des sciences médicales,* 60 vols. (Paris: Panckoucke, 1812–1822) contains the following articles by Esquirol: "délire," 8 (1814): 251–259; "démence," 8 (1814): 280–294; "démonomanie," 8 (1814): 294–318; "érotomanie," 13 (1815); 186–192; "folie," 16 (1816): 151–240; "hallucinations," 20 (1817): 64–71 (read to the Académie des sciences, 31 March 1817; reported on by commission headed by Philippe Pinel on 16 June 1817: *Comptes-rendus et rapports,* Institut de France, Académie des sciences, 6:196–199, MS in archives, Académie des sciences); "idiotisme," 23 (1818): 507–524; "manie," 30 (1818): 437–472;

"maisons d'aliénés," 30 (1818): 47–95 (Italian translation by S. Riva, *Delle case dei pazzi* [Parma: Ducale, 1927]); "mélancholie," 32 (1819): 147–181; "monomanie," 34 (1819): 114–125; "suicide," 53 (1821): 213–283.

In addition to these articles, Esquirol published the following monographs, several of which were translated into German or English: *Des passions, considérées comme causes, symptômes, et moyens curatifs de l'aliénation mentale* (Paris: Didot jeune, 1805). — *Des établissements des aliénés en France et des moyens d'améliorer le sort de ces infortunés: Mémoire présenté à S. E. le ministre de l'intérieur en septembre 1818* (Paris: Huzard, 1819). — *Note médico-légale sur la monomanie homicide* (Paris: Baillière, 1827). German translation, *Esquirol's Beobachtungen über Mord-Monomanie, mit Zusätzen von Mathias Joseph Bluff* (Nuremberg: Stein, 1831). — *Des illusions chez les aliénés: Question médico-légale sur l'isolement des aliénés* (Paris: Crochard, 1832). English translation by William Liddell, *Observations on the Illusions of the Insane and on the Medico-Legal Questions of their Confinement* (London: Renshaw and Rush, 1833). — Esquirol's major work is *Des maladies mentales considérées sous les rapports médical, hygiénique et médico-légal,* 2 vols. (Paris: Baillière, 1838). English translation by E. K. Hunt, *Mental Maladies: A Treatise on Insanity* (Philadelphia: Lea and Blanchard, 1845). German translation by K. Ch. Hille, *Allgemeine und spezielle Pathologie und Therapie der Seelenstörungen, nebst einem Anhange Kritischer und Erläuternder Zusätze von J. C. A. Heinroth* (Leipzig: Hartmann, 1827) (this collection appeared before *Des maladies mentales* but groups many of the same articles that Esquirol originally wrote for the *Dictionnaire des sciences médicales* and which constitute his own book of 1838). German translation of Esquirol's text of 1838 by W. Bernhard, *Die Geisteskrankheiten in Beziehung zur Medizin und Staatsarzneikunde vollständig dargestellt* (Berlin: Voss, 1838). German translation by E. H. Ackerknecht (Bern: Huber, 1968). Italian translation by L. Calvetti, *Dell'alienazione mentale; o, Della pazzia in genere ed in specie,* 2 vols. (Milan: Rusconi, 1827–1829). Spanish translation by R. de Monasterio y Correa, *Tratado completo de las enagenaciones mentales,* 2d rev. ed. by P. Mata (Madrid: León de Pablo Villaverde, 1858). — *Examen du projet de loi sur les aliénés* (Paris: Baillière, 1838).

Further, Esquirol annotated the French translations of two important foreign works: W. C. Ellis, *Traité de l'aliénation mentale; ou, De la nature, des causes, des symptômes et du traitement de la folie, comprenant des observations sur les établissements des aliénés, ouvrage traduit de l'anglais par Th. Archambault avec des notes et une introduction historique et statistique; enrichi de notes par M. Esquirol* (Paris: Rouvier, 1840); and J. C. Hoffbauer, *Médecine légale relative aux aliénés et aux sourds-muets; ou, Les lois appliquées aux dé-*

sordres de l'intelligence, avec notes par MM. Esquirol et Itard (Paris: Baillière, 1827). Several of his medicolegal consultations appear in C. C. H. Marc, *De la folie considérée dans les rapports avec les questions médico-judiciaires,* 2 vols. (Paris: Baillière, 1840). He took a prominent part in elaborating the law of 1838 that still regulates the hospitalization and treatment of the mentally ill in France: see *Examen du projet de loi sur les aliénés* (Paris: Baillière, 1838).

While Esquirol figures in every history of psychiatry, the monographic literature is modest. See especially L. Danner, *Etude sur Esquirol: Son influence sur la marche de la pathologie mentale* (Paris: Thèse médecine, 1858); H. Ey, "J. E. D. Esquirol," in *Grosse Nervenärzte,* ed. K. Kolle, 3 vols. (Stuttgart: Thieme, 1956–1963), 2:87–97; M. Dumas, *Etienne Esquirol: Sa famille, ses origines, ses années de formation* (Toulouse: Thèse médecine, 1971); G. Legée, "Evolution de l'étude clinique, sociale et juridique de l'aliénation mentale sous l'impulsion de Jean Etienne Dominique Esquirol, médecin aliéniste d'origine toulousaine," in *Compte-rendus du 96ème Congrès national des sociétés savantes,* Toulouse, 1971, Sciences, 1:63–81; F. Leuret, "M. Esquirol," *Gazette médicale de Paris,* 2d ser., 9 (2 January 1841): 1–6; G. Mora, "On the Bicentenary of the Birth of Esquirol, the First Complete Psychiatrist," *American Journal of Psychiatry* 129 (1972): 74–79; E. Pariset, "Eloge de J. E. D. Esquirol, lu dans la séance publique annuelle du 17 décembre 1844," *Histoire des membres de l'Académie de médecine,* 2 vols. (Paris; Baillière, 1845), 2:425–482; R. Semelaigne, "Esquirol," in *Les grands aliénistes français* (Paris: Steinheil, 1894).

PART FOUR

The Jewish Question

TEN

Medicine, Racism, Anti-Semitism: A Dimension of Enlightenment Culture

Richard H. Popkin

As Europe expanded through the Voyages of Discovery and colonized the Americas, Africa, Asia, and Polynesia, the problem of explaining the varieties of human beings became a focal point. For the most part, explanations for why people differed in skin color, hair, and eyes were offered within a framework based on the Bible. In similar fashion, religious differences were accounted for in terms of the vicissitudes of the human race since the collapse of the Tower of Babel. These differences are twofold: (1) physical, relating to bodily characteristics, and (2) mental or spiritual, relating to the workings of the mind.

As explorers, historians, and geographers studied these varying populations, they became acutely aware of the range of human characteristics. People sought explanations for why we differed so, and various theories were offered about the nature of the human race. A consideration of these theories, particularly as they apply to the physical and mental properties of Jews and Negroes as victims of racism, will be the focus of our attention. I will trace the road from scripturally based color-racism and anti-Semitism to secular versions, with a view toward science rather than revelation. And some may be surprised at the malignant role played by well-known heroes of the Enlightenment, and the benevolent role played by various unenlightened types as well.

According to Scripture, after the Flood, because Ham and Canaan saw Noah naked and drunk and did nothing to cover him, they were cursed. Noah awoke from his drunkennness, we are told, realized what his younger son, Ham, had done to him, "and he said, Cursed *be* Canaan, a servant or servants shall he be unto his brethren." Many interpreters in the seventeenth century offered the view that Noah's curse on Ham and Canaan caused both them and all their descendants to be dark, and servile.

Developments in both the crushing of the Spanish and Portuguese Jews and the exploration by enslavement of the Africans introduced further biological content to explain Jewish and African differences. In fifteenth-century Spain and Portugal, an attempt was made to eliminate religious differences after the reconquest by forcibly converting Jews and Moslems to Christianity. This act produced the only major case of Jewish converts who retained their differences and remained identifiable as Jews. They were labeled "New Christians" and "Marranos" (a slang term for pig), who, though baptized as Christians, were still, in some significant sense, Jewish, and a threat to Christianity. The notorious Spanish Inquisition was introduced to ferret out the Judaizers among the New Christians. This converted group was given a biological definition: someone was a New Christian if he or she had a New Christian or Jewish ancestor in the last five generations. People were Old Christians if they could produce evidence of *limpieza de sangre,* purity of blood.[1] Somehow, the biological feature of Jewishness became extremely hard to eradicate by usual Christian means of conversion and baptism. Hence, well into the eighteenth century, the Portuguese were keeping records of who was half New Christian, one-quarter, one-eighth, one-sixteenth, and, beyond that, "part" New Christian or Jewish. And, still, the Inquisition insisted that biological Jewishness contained the seeds of spiritual Jewishness that were dangerous to Christianity. Authorities made little progress in defending or delineating the biological features of Jewishness, except in terms of genealogy. The Spanish and Portuguese Inquisitions had lists of behavioral manifestations of Judaizing, which included any form of Jewish religious practice, especially not eating pork, not working on Saturday, wearing clean clothing and lighting candles on Friday night, fasting on Yom Kippur, and celebrating the Passover meal. Owning Hebrew books was also a sign of Judaizing, unless one had special permission. However, none of the above would indicate a biological basis of Jewishness. Almost all inquisitional cases are about behavioral practice and genealogy and beliefs.

A further complicating factor is that in some special cases, known

1. Concerning the New Christians and Marranos, see H. Charles Lea, *History of the Inquisition in Spain,* 4 vols. (New York, 1907); I. S. Revah, "Les Marranes," *Revue des études juives* 118 (1959/60): 29–77; Cecil Roth, *A History of the Marranos* (Philadelphia: Jewish Publication Society of America, 1907); and A. A. Sicroff, *Les controverses des status de pureté de sang en Espagne du XVe au XXIIIe siècle* (Paris: Didier, 1960).

D. Joh. Christoph. Wagenseils

Benachrichtigungen

Wegen einiger

die Judenschafft angehenden

wichtigen Sachen

Erster Theil/

worinnen

I. Die Hoffnung der Erlösung
Israelis oder klarer Beweiß der grossen/
und wie es scheinet / allgemach herannahenden Ju-
den-Bekehrung/sammt unvorgreifflichen Gedancken/wie solche
nechst Verleihung Göttlicher Hülffe/
zu befördern.

II. Wiederlegung der Unwarheit
daß die Juden zu ihrer Bedürffniß
Christen-Blut haben müs-
sen.

III. Anzeigung/wie leicht es dahin
zu bringen/ daß die Juden forthin
abstehen müssen/ die Christen mit
Wuchern und Schinden zu
plagen.

Leipzig/

bey Johann Heinichens Wittwe.

1705.

Pl. 20. Title page of Johann Christoph Wagenseil's *Benachrichtigungen wegen einiger die Judenschafft angehenden wichtigen Sachen, Erster Theil . . . I. Die Hoffnung der Erlösung Israelis . . .* (Leipzig, 1705).

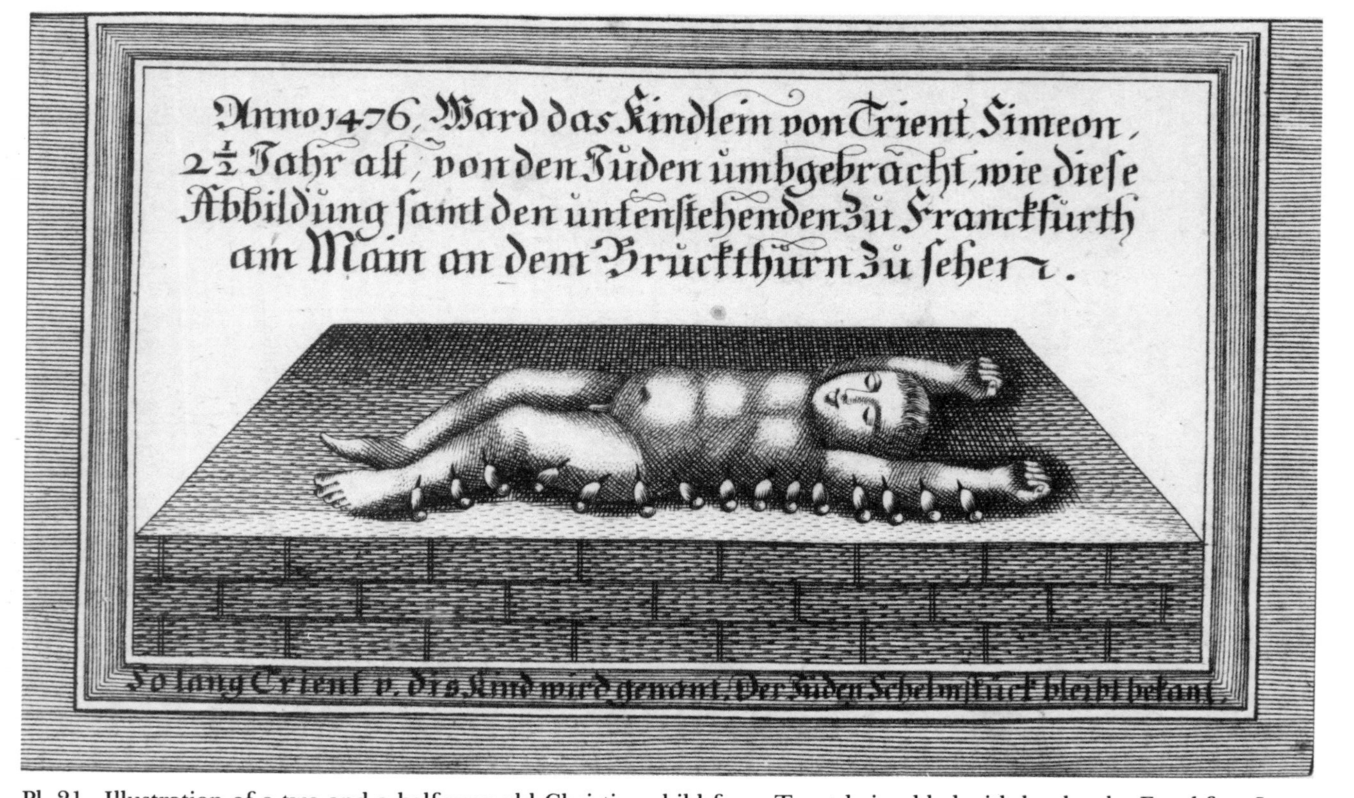

Pl. 21. Illustration of a two-and-a-half-year-old Christian child from Trent being bled with leeches by Frankfurt Jews, from Johann Christoph Wagenseil's *Die Hoffnung der Erlösung Israelis* (see plate 20).

New Christians were made honorary Old Christians, or their New Christian character was ignored because of their importance in the Christian world. For example, the family of Pablo de Santa Maria, bishop of Burgos, who had been Solomon Halevi, rabbi of Burgos, were declared honorary Old Christians. The Santa Maria family claimed to be descended from the family of Mary, the mother of Jesus, and thus, though Jewish, were traceable to the first family of Christianity.

Santa Teresa of Avila was known to be the daughter of a New Christian who had been found to be secretly Judaizing. Diego Laynez, the second general of the Jesuit order, was known as the Pope's Jew. During his lifetime several of his relatives were punished for secretly practicing Judaism.

This religious and political manipulation indicated that genealogical facts could be ignored when desirable. Cervantes proposed a solution when he had Don Quixote announce he had no ancestors, hence no genealogy.[2] In the case of color discrimination, as blacks became part of the economic world of the whites, people discoursed "upon the Grand Division of mankind into *Blacks* and *Whites*." In one of the most popular and little-used sources (by present-day scholars), *Letters Writ by a Turkish Spy at Paris,* which appeared in over thirty English editions between 1692 and 1803,[3] the spy told the president of the college of science at Fez that

2. A work of the time, the *Myth of Spanish Nobility,* tried to show that all Spanish noble families, including that of Ferdinand of Aragon and Torquemada, had Jewish blood.

3. *The Letters Writ by a Turkish Spy,* or *L'espion turc* (after its first printing), is a most important source of what was being discussed, or taken seriously, from about 1684 to 1800, among the literary public. The work is hardly used by present-day scholars, but was widely published during the Enlightenment. The first two volumes appeared in French (though written in Italian). The next six appeared in English (also an additional one, attributed to Daniel Defoe) and were translated into French, German, Dutch, and even Russian (an edition encouraged by Catherine the Great). There were at least thirty-one English editions, six French, six German, six Dutch, one Italian, and one Russian edition. The work established a genre for discussions critical of, or touching questions about, European ideas; namely having an outsider, the Turkish Spy, make dangerous and/or heretical points. *The Persian Letters,* the *Chinese Letters,* the *Jewish Letters,* the *Cabbalistic Letters,* are all sequels to the *Turkish Spy*'s technique. I believe this untapped source will be very important in assessing questions that were being discussed, and answers that were being considered. In some other articles, I am dealing with some specific cases, the view in the *Turkish Spy* of the pre-Adamite theory, the attempt to reform Judaism in the *Turkish Spy,* the *Turkish Spy* as a source about the Messianic movement of Sabbatai Zevi. For information about the *Turkish Spy* and its many editions and possible authors, see Giovanni P. Marana, *Letters Writ by a Turkish Spy,* selected and edited by Arthur J. Weitzman (London: Routledge and Kegan Paul, 1970), Introduction, vii–xix, 232–233; and C. J. Betts, *Early Deism in France* (The Hague: Nijhoff, 1984), chap. 7.

he had met an eminent physician recently and that together they had inquired

> into the Causes of the Differences of Colour; whether it proceeded from the Various Heat and Influence of the Sun, or from the Divers Qualities of the Climates wherein they live; or finally, from some Specifick Properties in themselves, in the Natural Frame and Constitution of their Bodies. He was of Opinion, that if *Adam* was *White*, all his Children must be so too; if *Black*, all his Posterity must be of the same Colour. Therefore, by Consequence, either the *Blacks* or the Whites are not the Descendants of *Adam*.[4]

These alternatives covered just about all of the possibilities considered during the eighteenth century.

During the latter part of the seventeenth century, a critique developed against biblical explanation of human phenomena. The work of Isaac La Peyrère, Baruch de Spinoza, Richard Simon, the author of the *Letters Writ by a Turkish Spy in Paris*, and the early English deists among others, questioned whether we had an accurate text of the Bible and whether the Bible as we know it is an accurate account of human history. La Peyrère's *Men before Adam* raised the possibility that there were non-Adamic origins of most inhabitants of the earth. The evidence he offered from ancient history and newly discovered cultures, together with his biblical criticism, led to the rise of an intellectual group who sought to explain human differences in natural terms.[5] Spinoza's naturalism, as well as the impact of the Italian Renaissance naturalists, produced attempts to explain the varieties of mankind apart from the Scriptures (and to explain the Scriptures as one small episode in human history). The dominant explanations were in terms of either multiple origins of man (polygenesis) or environmental and cultural influences on an initially common human stock.

La Peyrère's theory that there were men before Adam was offered for scientific and religious reasons to justify a peculiar view about the imminent culmination of Jewish and world history in which everyone, Adamite (that is, Jew), and pre-Adamite (that is, gentile), and post-Adamite would be saved.[6] While theologians ranted against the work,

4. [G. P. Marana], *The Eight Volumes of Letters Writ by a Turkish Spy, Who Liv'd Five and Forty Years, Undiscover'd at Paris* (London, 1723), 8:264. This is usually listed as the eighth edition. The text is almost the same in all editions.

5. On La Peyrère and his influence, see R. H. Popkin, *Isaac La Peyrère: His Life, His Works, and His Influence* (Leiden: E. J. Brill, 1987).

6. Cf. R. H. Popkin, "The Marrano Theology of Isaac La Peyrère," *Studi internazionali di filosofia* 5 (1973): 97–126; and *Isaac La Peyrère*, chap. 3.

and theological authorities had the work burned and banned (and Spinoza and the author of the *Turkish Spy* offered more evidence for the view),[7] some more practical people saw a wonderful application of the theory in the question of human differences. Planters in the Virginia colonies by the 1680s were using "the pre-Adamite whimsey" to justify black slavery.[8] The blacks were of separate and different origin and did not have the intellectual or spiritual properties of whites. Hence, feeling was they should not be Christianized, since they lacked the requisite mental or religious capacities. Further, the physical differences between blacks and whites showed the separate origins of each group. Therefore, an intensive study began to locate and explicate the major differences (and so a branch of physical anthropology was born). Biologists, medical practitioners, explorers, among others, offered their findings concerning the differences, and then began seeking causal explanations either in the original characteristics of different racial stocks or in the transformations that had occurred owing to climate, temperature, diet, and so forth. The explanations almost always started from one of two assumptions, either that blacks began with and have continued to have fundamental defects that make them intellectually and spiritually inferior to whites, or that blacks have developed fundamental defects that make them presently inferior to whites. The different implications of these two assumptions are enormous in terms of whether the so-called "defects" are remediable or not. Before going into further details, let us first examine the secular versions of why Jews are different from Christian Europeans.

Until the Spanish Inquisition introduced biological criteria to answer "Who is a Jew?" or "Who is a New Christian?" the prevailing Christian view was that people were Jews by choice. They willfully and stubbornly accepted certain views and practices, and hopefully could be brought to choose other views and practices, namely those of Christianity. Among seventeenth-century millenarians, the conversion of the Jews was a most

7. In the *Tractatus Theologico-Politicus* Spinoza kept pointing up internal evidence in the Bible that indicated mankind existed before Adam. The *Turkish Spy* actually offered a more complete list of reasons for taking pre-Adamism seriously than any other work of the time. In fact it offered material about oriental theories of the origins of the world that did not become part of the general European discussions until at least fifty years after its original publication. Some of these data also appear in Charles Gildon's letter to Dr. R. B., in Charles Blount, *The Oracles of Reason* (London, 1693), 177–183, but does not seem to have been picked up at the time.

8. See the criticism of this view in Morgan Godwyn, *The Negro's and Indians Advocate, Suing for Their Admission into the Church; or, A Persuasive to the Instructing and Baptizing of the Negro's and Indians in Our Plantations* (London, 1680), Preface and chap. 1.

critical matter, since it would be the penultimate event before the Second Coming of Jesus and the Commencement of His Thousand-Year Reign on Earth. Millenarians thought that great efforts should be made to prepare for the Conversion but that God alone could and would bring about the great event.[9] When the event occurred, the converted Jews would be spiritually and biologically identical with everyone else. They might even be better spiritually because so much divine effort was invested in their case.[10]

By the end of the seventeenth century, those who no longer saw the Jews as a special group in providential history who would be united with everyone else began to see them as an odd cultural group that was identifiably different from others in Europe by dress, hairstyle, occupation, eating habits, cultural activities, and so forth. For many, these differences could be eradicated by an individual's deciding to join the Christians. There is considerable testimony about Jews who individually decided to convert, who then became accepted members of the society around them, and whose descendants became indistinguishable from the other members of the society.[11] In fact, several prominent noblemen and women in Europe have been startled by genealogical inquiries that show that they are descendants of Jewish converts.[12]

9. This was the view of Isaac La Peyrère, of Joseph Mede of Cambridge, and of the leading millenarian, John Dury, among others. La Peyrère devoted a good part of his *Du Rappel des Juifs* ([Paris?], 1643) to advice on how to make Jews ready for conversion; Mede offered the theory that dominated English millennial thinking, that the conversion would occur by miracle as it did in the case of St. Paul. Dury worked on many conversion projects such as establishing a college of Jewish studies in London, publishing editions of Jewish classics like the *Mishna,* readmitting the Jews to England, but all of these were seen as only preparatory. On this, see my article "Jewish-Christian Relations in Holland and England," in *Jewish-Christian Relations in the Seventeenth Century,* ed. S. Van den Berg and E. van der Wall (The Hague: Nijhoff, 1987).

10. La Peyrère suggested this in his *Du Rappel des Juifs.*

11. In England, the converts often wrote an account of what led them to see the light. The authors of these, like Moses Marcus in the early eighteenth century, became regular members of society and often advisers on religious matters, or Hebrew teachers. Their descendants merged into the general population both in Europe and in America.

12. There is an interesting case in the unpublished Cazac papers at the Institut Catholique de Toulouse, when a local archivist, writing on Montaigne's cousin, Francisco Sanches, asked a French nobleman, the Marquis de Saporta, if the family had any papers of their illustrious ancestor, the Chancellor of the University of Montpellier in the sixteenth century, who was a New Christian. The twentieth-century nobleman tried desperately to avoid accepting his heritage until it was pointed out to him that his title came from his Jewish ancestors who were ennobled in the sixteenth century. The twentieth-century marquis suggested that he and the archivist could keep this secret, since it was not germane

Other observers of the situations saw the Jews as bearers of spiritual deficiencies that could not be overcome. The fact that Jews had accepted the superstitious views of their rabbis for centuries could be an incurable trait rather than one that could be overcome by education and assimilation. Hence, two views developed similar to those about why blacks are black, regarding the Jews. One thought that the difference between Jews and non-Jews was the outmoded adherence on the part of Jews to certain practices and views and that Jews could change this by altering their activities and beliefs. The other view was that there was a basic characteristic that made Jews Jews, and that this was a spiritual feature, a spiritual disease, which could not be changed.[13] The first view supported public contests, such as the one just before the French Revolution, for the best answer to the question, "How to make the Jews happy and useful in France?" The second view led to secular anti-Semitism, and in our century to the Holocaust.

One might expect that once scriptural explanations were dropped

to the archivist's planned book. The correspondence ends with the archivist sending the marquis the call number of the book in the Bibliothèque Nationale in Paris from which he drew his information.

13. The view of a special unchangeable characteristic that made Jews different appears in the work of many French Enlightened writers. See the quotations offered in Arthur Hertzberg, *The French Enlightenment and the Jews* (New York: Schocken Books, 1968), chap. 9; Leon Poliakov, *Histoire de l'antsémitisme de Voltaire à Wagner* (Paris: Calman-Levy, 1968), livre I, chap. 2; and Pierre Pluchon, *Nègres et Juifs au XVIIIe siècle* (Paris: Tallandier, 1984); deuxième partie, "Les lumières et les Juifs," 64–81.

The notion that Judaism is a disease appears in remarks of Voltaire where he indicated Judaism had infected Western culture with oriental ideas. At one point he said, "They are, all of them, born with raging fanaticism in their hearts, just as the Bretons and the Germans are with blond hair. I would not be the least bit surprised if these people would not some day become deadly to the human race" (Voltaire, *Œuvres complètes,* 52 vols., ed. Louis Moland [Paris: Garnier frères, 1877–1885], 28:439–440).

This theme was taken up in nineteenth-century Germany: see George L. Mosse, *Toward the final Solution: The History of European Racism* (Madison: University of Wisconsin Press, 1985), part II, "Infected Christianity." The Nazi theorist, Alfred Rosenberg, cited the Jew, Otto Weiniger, from his *Sex and Character* as saying Judaism is like an invisible, cohesive web of slime fungus, existing since time and immemorial all over the world. "From all of this it follows that Judaism is part of the organism of mankind just as, let us say, certain bacteria are part of man's body." The bacteria have to be kept under control. Cf. George L. Mosse, *Nazi Culture* (New York: Schocken Books, 1966), 76–77. Mosse quotes a Nazi judge as saying in 1938, "The Jew is not a human being. He is an appearance of putrescence. Just as the fusion—fungus cannot permeate wood until it is rotting, so the Jew was able to creep into the German people to bring on disaster, only after the German nation, weakened by the loss of blood in the Thirty Years War, had began to rot from within" (ibid., 336–337). And, of course, Joseph Goebbels referred to Judaism as a bacillus.

by intellectual leaders and replaced by the "scientific" ones of the Enlightenment, solely factual considerations would enter into explaining why various groups differ. But, alas, much more was, and still is, involved in accounting for human differences, including what roles various groups should play in social, political, cultural, and economic activities.

In the matter of black Africans, there was considerable research. On one side, scientific data were sought to show the inferiority of blacks, justifying their enslavement and exploitation. The growing group of abolitionists, on the other side, tried to show that blacks, at least potentially, are not inferior intellectually or culturally. The physical differences could be described and explained in anthropological and biomedical terms, but final evaluation seemed dependent upon what one wished to prove.

Starting with skin color, various explanations were offered such as the effect of climate and sunshine. G. S. Rousseau, in the paper he delivered before the American Society for Eighteenth-Century Studies Conference on racism held in Los Angeles in 1973, examined the views of Claude Nicolas Le Cat, an influential French physician from Rouen (1700–1768), who believed there was a substance in the organic system, ethiops, that made blacks black, and the lack of much of it made whites white.[14] In the earlier-mentioned *Turkish Spy,* there is a discussion of a medical dissection of a dead Negro. "Between the outward and inward skin of the corps was found a kind of Vascular Plexus spread over the whole Body like a Web or Net, which was fill'd with a Juice as Black as Ink." This web or net, not found in white people, accounted for the skin color, and purported to show that blacks and whites had different origins. The Turkish Spy, who accepted the pre-Adamite theory, used this dissection as further evidence for his antibiblical views.[15] In another argument, an elaborated theory of climate, diet, and way of life was developed by the great biologist, Count Buffon, 1707–1788, to explain differences in skin color. (Buffon claimed that all babies are born white,

14. On this, see G. S. Rousseau, "Le Cat and the Physiology of Negroes," in *Studies in Eighteenth-Century Culture,* vol. 3, *Racism in the Eighteenth Century,* ed. Harold E. Pagliaro (Cleveland: Press of Case Western Reserve University, 1973), 369–386.

15. Marana, *Turkish Spy* 8:265. See the discussion of the Turkish Spy's pre-Adamism in Popkin, *Isaac La Peyrère,* chap. 9; and "A Late-Seventeenth-Century Gentile Attempt to Convert the Jews to Reformed Judaism," in S. Almog et al., *Israel and the Nations: Essays Presented in Honor of Shmuel Ettinger* (Jerusalem: Historical Society of Israel and Zalman Shazar Center, 1987), xxv–xlvii.

and then some soon, within eight days, became black for environmental reasons.)[16]

Aside from the question of what is scientifically the case, the discussions during the eighteenth century involved two other matters: (1) was the condition, skin color, permanent? and (2) was this condition organically related to black intellectual and cultural inferiority? Similar issues developed concerning variation of European and African hair, that is, what physiologically causes the differences; is the difference permanent; and, is it related to the crucial matter of supposed black cultural and mental inferiority? The mere fact of the difference could be trivial, as between varieties of eye color or hair color, or it could be part of a systematic set of differences to prove that blacks were not of the same race, or even species as whites. And, there are even some attempts to find medical and biological similarities between blacks and monkeys as part of the quest for a major, even monumental, difference theory between whites and blacks. Various doctors who traveled to different parts of the world reported on physiological differences. John Atkins, an English naval surgeon, concluded that whites and blacks were different in some basic physical features.[17] Unlike Le Cat, Atkins did not try to determine the exact physiology of the differences. We are told that Baron de Lahotan, voyaging to America, had a dispute with a Portuguese doctor who had been in Angola, Brazil, and Goa about what factors accounted for differences amongst peoples. The Portuguese doctor insisted the native Americans, the Asians, and Africans each had to have different fathers. Baron de Lahotan offered both scriptural evidence and a theory that air and climate could account for the color differences.[18] There was also a doctor, John Mitchell, who offered a counter-theory to the view that mankind began as white, and because of climate and so forth, some people became dark and even black. Mitchell claimed the original state of people was closer to that of Indians and Negroes than to that of

16. Georges Louis Leclerc, Comte de Buffon, *Natural History, General and Particular,* trans. William Smellie, 2d ed., sec. 9, "Of the Varieties of the Human Species." On this, see R. H. Popkin, "The Philosophical Bases of Modern Racism," in *The High Road to Pyrrhonism,* ed. R. A. Watson and James E. Force (San Diego: Austin Hill Press, 1980), 86–87.

17. John Atkins, Surgeon, *The Navy-Surgeon; or, A Practical System of Surgery* (London, 1734), Appendix on observations about conditions on the Coast of Guiney, pp. 23–24. Atkins concluded, "From the Whole, I imagine that White and Black must have descended of different Protoplasts; and that there is no other way of accounting for it."

18. Lom d'Arce, *Nouveaux voyages de M. de Baron de Lahontan dans l'Amérique septentrionale* (The Hauge, 1703), letter dated Nantes, 10 mai 1693, 249–253.

Europeans.[19] The great biological classifier, Linnaeus (1707–1778), in his description, implied much about the significance of the differences. He stated that the Europeans were "fair, sanguine, brawny. Hair yellow, brown, flowing; eyes blue, gentle, acute, inventive. Covered with close garments. Governed by laws." In contrast, the African was "black, phlegmatic, relaxed. Hair black, frizzled; skin silky, nose flat; lips tumid; crafty, indolent, negligent. Anoints himself with grease. Governed by caprice." Linnaeus included physical differences as well as cultural, social, and intellectual ones, stated beneficially for Europeans and disparagingly for Africans.[20]

The eminent Scottish philosopher David Hume, neither biologist, medical student, nor anthropologist, stated the extreme interpretation of the differences as they presented themselves in the cultural achievements of both groups. In his essay "Of National Characters," Hume added the following in a note:

> I am apt to suspect the negroes and in general all other species of men (for there are four or five different kinds) to be naturally inferior to the whites. There never was a civilized nation of any other complexion than white, nor even any individual eminent either in action or speculation. No ingenious manufactures amongst them, no arts, no sciences. On the other hand, the most rude and barbarous of the whites, such as the ancient GERMANS, the present TARTARS, have still something eminent about them, in their valour, form of government, or some other particular. *Such a uniform and constant differences could not happen in so many countries and ages, if nature had not made an original distinction betwixt these breeds of men* [my emphasis]. Not to mention our colonies, there are Negroe slaves dispersed all over Europe, of which none ever discovered any symptoms of ingenuity, tho' low people, without education, will start up amonst us, and distinguish themselves in every profession. In JAMAICA indeed they talk of one negroe as a man of parts and learning; but 'tis likely he is admired for very slender accomplishments like a parrot, who speaks a few words plainly.[21]

As I have argued elsewhere, Hume's empirical theory of knowledge does not commit him logically to any particular view on this subject. The view he offered was presented as an empirical generalization and an

19. John Mitchell, "An Essay upon the Causes of the Different Colours of People in Different Climates," *Royal Society of London Philosophical Transactions* 43 (1744–45): 146.

20. Linnaeus (Karl von Linne), *A General System of Nature through the Three Grand Kingdoms of Animals, Vegetables and Minerals* (London: Lackington, Allen, 1806), I, section "Mammalia. Order F. Primates."

21. David Hume, "Of National Characters," in *The Philosophical Works of David Hume*, ed. T. H. Green and T. H. Grose (London: Longmans, Green and Co., 1882), 3:252n.

explanation of it.[22] However, Hume ignored all the evidence contrary to his theory, some of which will be considered shortly. There was plenty of empirical evidence to counter Hume's generalization. Hume's Scottish opponent James Beattie spent dozens of pages showing the factual falsity of Hume's views and their malevolent influence.[23] Hume discussed Beattie's whole critique by calling him "a silly—bigotted" fellow.[24] So, to my mind, Hume must be recognized as personally very prejudiced, unwilling to use his philosophical standards on this subject, and unimpressed by the fact that defenders of slavery were quoting him, and saying "as the learned philosopher David Hume has proved." The fact was, his thoughts were just a bundle of perceptions that had nothing to do with skin color. Hume's philosophy may have been racially neutral, but Hume the philosopher was not.

Hume was quoted approvingly over the next half-century by defenders of slavery in the Americas,[25] but he offered no account of the original physical difference that caused the enormous cultural and intellectual difference between whites and blacks. Skin pigmentation did not seem to indicate any cause, except that dark pigmentation was usually interpreted as a degenerative effect from the original white complexion of the entire human race. The first American edition of the *Encyclopaedia Britannica* described the many bad characteristics of Africans and offered as an explanation only that the Negroes "are an awful example of the corruption of man when left to himself."[26]

In the early nineteenth century, an American medical doctor, Samuel Morton of Philadelphia, in his *Crania Americana,* claimed to have discovered the cause of Negro inferiority in the lower cranial capacity of blacks. Morton had the largest skull collection in the world. He stuffed up the orifices of his skulls, filled them with pepper seed, and reported that the Caucasian skulls held the most pepper seed, the blacks the least, with Asiatics and American Indians in between.[27] (The eminent biologist

22. R. H. Popkin, "Hume's Racism," *The Philosophical Forum* 9 (1977–78): 211–218.

23. See James Beattie, *Essays on the Origin and Immutability of Truth,* 2d ed. (Edinburgh, 1776), 310 ff.

24. Hume, "Advertisement," which appears in all editions of Hume's work after Beattie's attack (which first appeared in 1770). This dismissal of Beattie as a bigot first appears in Hume's *Letters,* ed. J. Y. T. Greig (Oxford: Oxford University Press, 1932), 2:301.

25. Cf. Popkin, "Hume's Racism," 221–222.

26. *Encyclopaedia Britannica,* 3d ed. (Philadelphia, 1798), s.v. "Negro."

27. See Samuel G. Morton, *Crania Americana; or, A Comparative View of the Skulls of Various Aboriginal Nations of North and South America; to Which Is Prefixed and Essay on the Varieties of the Human Species* (Philadelphia and London, 1839), and *Crania Aegyptiana; or, Observations on Egyptian Ethnography, Derived from Anatomy, History and Monuments* (Philadelphia, 1844).

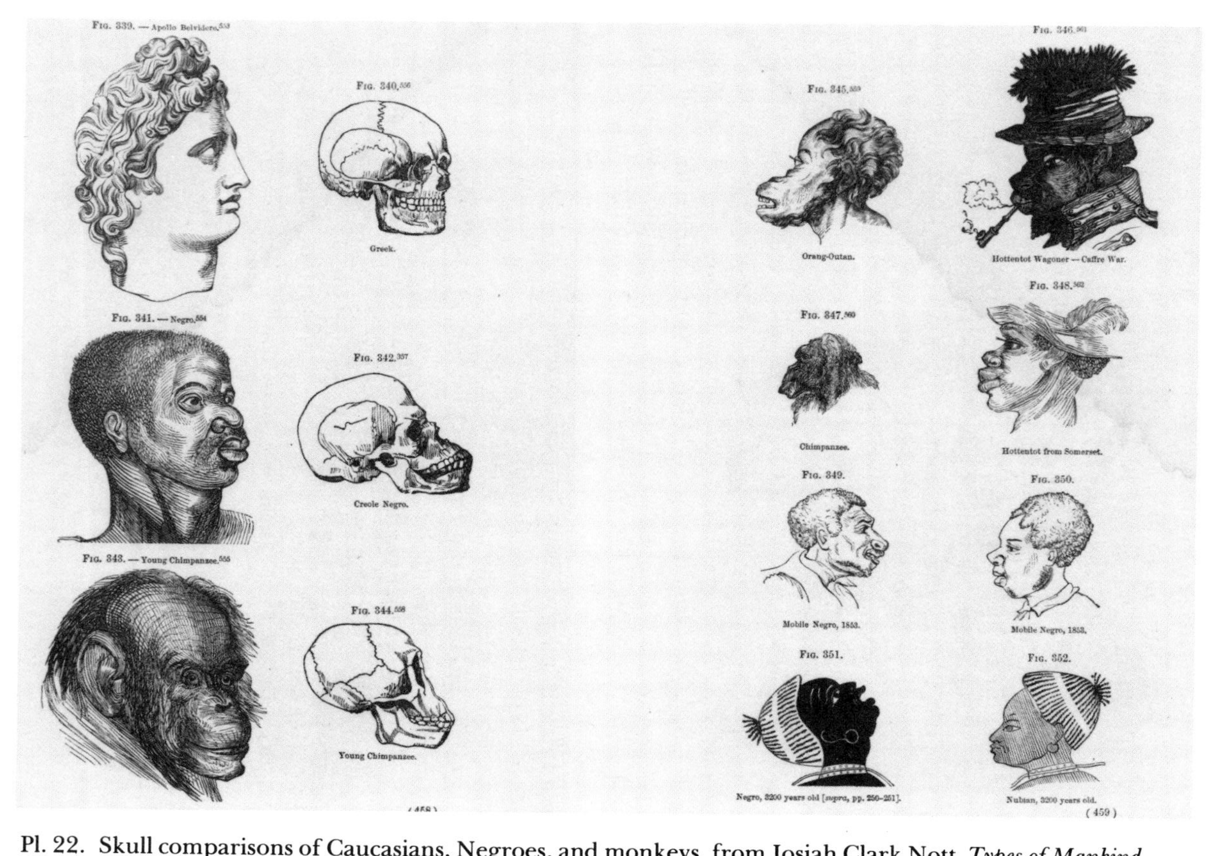

Pl. 22. Skull comparisons of Caucasians, Negroes, and monkeys, from Josiah Clark Nott, *Types of Mankind* (Philadelphia, 1854), a memorial volume for Dr. Samuel Morton.

Steven Jay Gould, who has written extensively on the history of biological theories, examined Morton's researches and concluded that Morton reported only those cases which allowed him to "fudge" his data by leaving out some results and using uneven measurement techniques that allowed more pepper seed to fill some skulls than others.[28] Morton's work was followed with a study by an Italian, Filippo Manetta, in his *La razza negra nel suo stato selvaggio*. Manetta's work was not translated, but it was extensively quoted and explained in an article entitled "Negro" in the *Encyclopaedia Britannica*. Manetta claimed that the cranial sutures of Negroes close much earlier than in other races: "to this premature ossification of the skull, preventing all further development of the brain, many pathologists have attributed the inherent inferiority of the blacks, an inferiority which is even more marked than their physical differences." Manetta's theory was that white and black children are born with equal intelligence but that at puberty, when the brain sutures close, all further intellectual development in blacks ceases.[29] The famous eleventh edition of the *Britannica* recorded Manetta's theory and added that evidence was lacking to settle the matter, but "the arrest or even deterioration in mental development is no doubt very largely due to the fact that after puberty sexual matters take the first place in the negro's life and thought."[30] And so, second to skin color, intellectual inferiority became another crucial difference. Physiological features, such as alleged smaller skull capacity or sealing of the brain sutures, became the accepted causes of black insufficiency. This account was finally removed in the present, fifteenth, edition of the *Encyclopaedia Britannica*.[31] The major issue then became whether biological or environmental factors could alter the situation or whether it was a fixed condition.

Hume, Dr. Morton, and a host of others held to a polygenetic theory about human origins, and maintained that the state of affairs was unchangeable. Still, the abolitionists and advocates of human equality

On Morton, see William Stanton, *The Leopard's Spots* (Chicago and London: University of Chicago Press, 1960); and R. H. Popkin, "Pre-Adamism in Nineteenth-Century American Thought: 'Speculative Biology' and Racism," *Philosophia* 8 (1978): 219–221.

28. Stephen Jay Gould, "Morton's Ranking of Races by Cranial Capacity: Unconscious Manipulation of Data May Be a Scientific Norm," *Science* 200 (1978): 503–509.

29. See "Negro" by Prof. A. H. Keane (of University College, London), *Encyclopaedia Britannica*, 9th ed. (New York, 1884), 17: 317.

30. "Negro" by Thomas Athol Joyce, *Encyclopaedia Britannica*, 11th ed., 19:344.

31. The present, fifteenth, edition, gives a neutral account of how Negroes differ from other races, followed by a section on "Negro, American," listing Negroes from the eighteenth century to the present who have made a significant contribution to American life.

insisted on the possibility of change in the intellectual achievements of blacks. Buffon, the leading biologist of the period; Blumenbach, the eighteenth-century "founder of modern anthropology," and various theologians and progressive-minded philosophers insisted that change was possible through environmental alterations such as moving people to healthier climates, through changing their diets, and through social engineering in terms of education, life-style, and so forth. They also believed that the best evidence of their remedial theory was the fact that black intellectuals and creative artists already existed, and presumably many, many more would come into being if environmental, biological, and social change took place.[32] There is an amazing literature in the eighteenth century, arguing against Hume, and later Thomas Jefferson, who made similar claims of black inferiority. Jefferson once ended his discussion saying,

> I advance it, therefore, as a suspicion only, that the blacks, whether originally a distinct race, or made distinct by time and circumstances, are inferior to the whites in the endowment both of mind and body.

Jefferson gave as a possible reason, black color:

> Whether the black of the negro resides in the reticular membrane between the skin and scarfskin, or in the scarfskin itself; whether it proceeds from the color of the blood, the color of the bile, or from that of some other secretion, the difference is fixed in nature, and is as real as if its seat and cause were better known to us. And is this difference of no importance? Is it not the foundation of a greater or less share of beauty in the two races?[33]

But as Henry Lewis Gates has shown, most of the cases that failed were the result of deliberate manipulation.[34] In a more positive vein, Gates

32. Johann F. Blumenbach, *On the Natural Varieties of Mankind,* trans. Thomas Bendyshe (New York: Bergman Publishers, 1969), 305–312; and Henri Grégoire, *De la littérature des nègres* (Paris, 1808), chaps. 5–8. See also Popkin, "Philosophical Bases of Modern Racism," 86–89.

33. See Winthrop D. Jordan, *White over Black* (Chapel Hill: University of North Carolina Press, 1968), "Jefferson: The Assertion of Negro Inferiority," pp. 435–440; and Thomas Jefferson, *Notes on the State of Virginia* (1782), in *The Writings of Thomas Jefferson,* ed. Paul Leicester Ford (New York and London, 1894), 3:244–250 (the first of the quoted passages appears on p. 250, the second on p. 244).

34. In a personal meeting with Professor Gates in 1981, he shared with me his dissertation done at Cambridge on black writers and artists in the eighteenth century. A revised version has been published as Henry L. Gates, *The Signifying Monkey: A Theory of Afro-American Literary Criticism* (Oxford: Oxford University Press, 1988).

tells how the Duke of Brunswick raised some black children with his own at Wolfenbüttel in Lower Saxony. One of these blacks (A. W. Amo) became *Professor* Amo of the University of Halle.[35] Also, the Governor of Jamaica raised a black boy, named Francis Williams, and sent him to Cambridge. Afterward, Williams returned to Jamaica, took charge of a school, and wrote Latin poetry. Williams was the same man Hume insulted by saying he was like a parrot who spoke a few words plainly.[36] The most famous case was Phillis Wheatley, a young West African woman settled in Boston who wrote poetry in English. She was considered such a sensation that public poetry sessions were held, where she sat surrounded by witnesses and wrote her verse. In fact, General George Washington sat in a special session. Eventually, Wheatley was taken on tour in England and was exhibited hither and yon as a black creative artist and intellectual, a living disproof of the racist views of Hume and Jefferson that the "defects" of blacks were irremediable.[37] Jefferson dismissed her case, saying her poetry was mediocre, and besides, she was a mulatto.[38] Hume said not a word about any of these cases and never revised his statement on the matter.

The racists of the eighteenth century contended that the dark complexion of the Africans was an irremediable defect that was part of a fundamental, unchangeable set of defects that made blacks inferior to whites. The human body, they maintained, limited or determined what mental development was possible. The body fixed the space the brain could occupy, and presumably brain size related to mental capacity. Dr. Morton's theory or Dr. Manetta's contended that bodily conditions, smaller cranial capacity, or early closed cranial suture accounted for lesser black mental ability. The actual scientific reasons for these differences were of less concern than the overall conclusion they pointed to, that blacks were of a different species than whites. Some form of polygenetic theory would explain how the difference began and continued, and this in turn justified keeping the blacks in an inferior status indefinitely.

35. On Amo, see K. A. Britwum, s.v. "Amo, A. W.," in *Dictionary of African Biography* 1:196–197. He is also discussed in Grégoire's *Littérature des nègres*, 198–202.

36. On Williams's career, see Grégoire, *Littérature des nègres*, 236–245. One of Williams's Latin odes is published there. Williams and his rection to Hume's remark is discussed at length in Gates's dissertation.

37. Phillis Wheatley is discussed in Grégoire, *Littérature des nègres*, 260–272, and at length in Gates's dissertation.

38. See Jefferson's *Notes from Virginia*, 246. "Religion, indeed, has produced a Phyllis Whately [*sic*]; but it could not produce a poet. The compositions published under her name are below the dignity of criticism."

PHILLIS WHEATLEY, NEGRO SERVANT to Mr. JOHN WHEATLEY, of BOSTON.
Published according to Act of Parliament, Sept. 1st 1773 by Archd. Bell,
Bookseller No. 8 near the Saracens Head Aldgate.

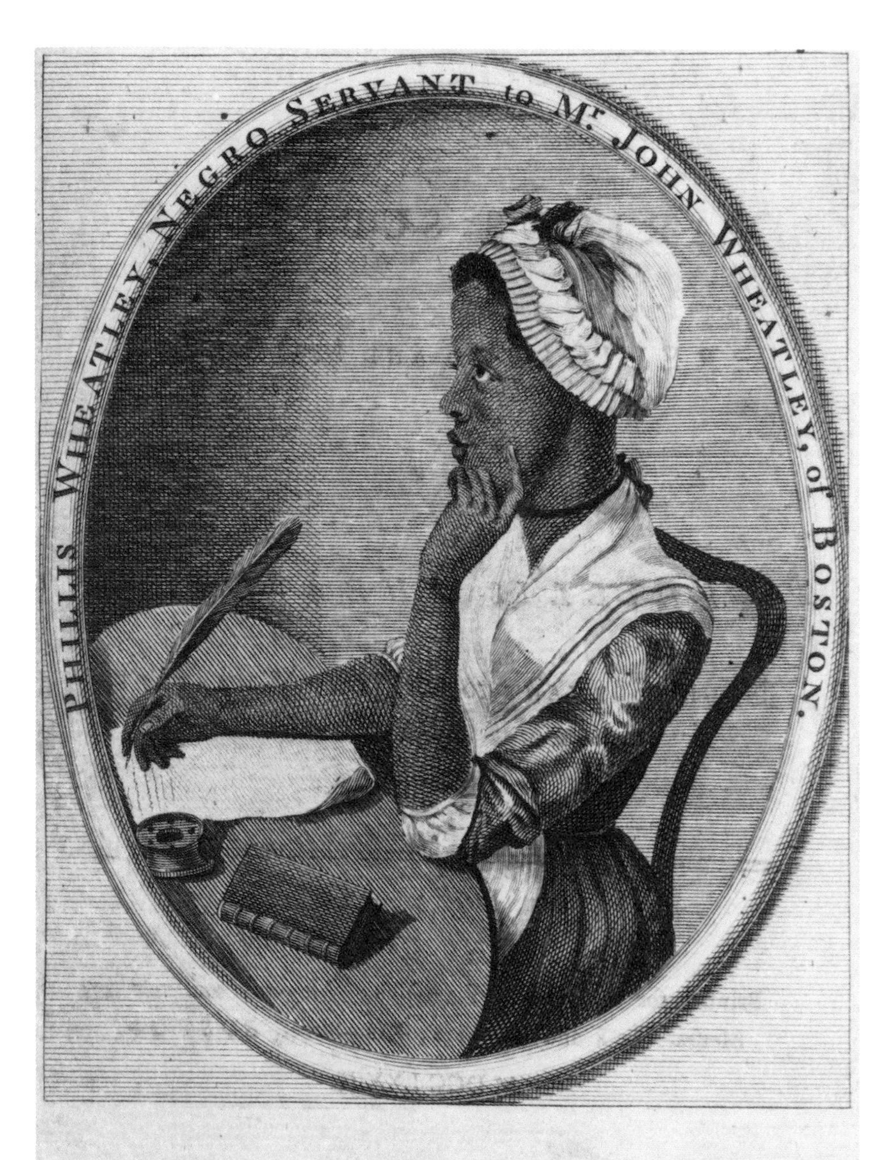

Pl. 23. Portrait of Phillis Wheatley on the title page of the 1773 London edition of her poems.

Those opposing this conclusion denied that the physical differences implied different species. Mostly, they contended that the differences in blacks from whites were degenerative, but reparable with time, effort, and good will. The emergence on the scene of black intellectuals and creative artists, usually engineered by careful nurturing, showed proof that the intellectual faculties could be awakened and restored. Such able scientists as Count Buffon believed the physical differences could be overcome in ten generations by moving blacks to a geographical band extending from northern France to the Caucasus Mountains, feeding them a good French diet, and giving them an Enlightenment education.[39] Even the most ardent abolitionists conceded that at the present time almost all blacks were in poor physical condition, and as a result were intellectually limited. The polygenetic racists, in opposition, insisted that the poor physical condition (except for ability to do hard labor under appalling conditions) was simply a sign of permanent mental inferiority. The body was the carrier of the difference, and it limited the mind, as in the theory of cranial capacity of Dr. Morton or the theory of early suture closing of Dr. Manetta. The remedialists saw the bodily differences as causing mental inferiority and believed that improving the physical conditions would improve mental abilities and that black Platos, Homers, and Pindars would soon evolve. The argument, of course, is ongoing as to whether the apparent differences in intellectual abilities between different races are due to distinct somatic conditions that are basically unalterable or to environmental conditions both inside and outside the individuals in question: one has moved from the scientific inquiries of Dr. Le Cat, Count Buffon, and Professor Stanhope Smith, Professor of Moral Philosophy at Princeton, to investigations about IQs and genetic factors that may be related to mental development.

Turning from color racism, which was secularized in the Enlightenment by justifying it on the basis of somatic distinctions between races, and the effects these were presumed to have, to the secularization of anti-Semitism, one first has to recognize that different factors and interests were involved. Color racism justified black slavery and colonialism. The Jews, especially those of western Europe where modern secular anti-Semitism developed, were neither slaves nor possessors of any territory to be colonized. In fact, from Shylock's speech onward,

39. Buffon, *Natural History*, vol. 3, sec. 9, pp. 57–207. On p. 207, Buffon said that the present unfortunate situation could be changed and improved if the causes that generated them—climate, food, mode of living, epidemic diseases, and the mixture of dissimilar individuals—ceased to operate.

about how much Jews were like everyone else, there was a recognition that physically Jews were like Europeans or Caucasians except for possibly a different smell, a slightly different coloring, a slightly different nasal configuration. A converted Jew outside of Iberia was an accepted and acceptable member of his society. The alleged Jewish smell disappeared, whether by Divine Providence, or by accepting general European washing practices. Jews became just swarthy people, of Levantine or Iberian extraction; facial characteristics were no longer matters of significance. La Peyrère, presumably himself a convert, or a child of converts, had said the darkish color would change in the course of conversion by divine action.[40] And the other physical features like the Semitic nose were overlooked.

There were many prominent converts all over Europe during the sixteenth, seventeenth, and eighteenth centuries, and except in Spain and Portugal, they were accepted as coequal members of society. Michel de l'Hôpital, Chancellor of France under Catherine de Medici, was a convert. So was Antoinette Lopes, mother of Michel de Montaigne. Nostradamus, the notorious French court astrologer, was the grandson of two rabbis, both of whom converted. There were professors in England, Tremellius in France, Philippe d'Aquin and Paulus Ricci in Rome, and many others who had personally converted. Bayle's *Dictionary* contains many biographies of university professors, political advisers, Hebrew and Arabic scholars who converted. And Bayle considered the evidence about whether Jean Bodin among others was of Jewish origin.

There was a steady trickle of converts during the Renaissance period through the Enlightenment. Whether they converted from conviction or for advantage, they were almost always accepted in their new roles. One became Harvard's Hebrew professor, another an advisor to an Anglican bishop, others court bankers and advisers. By the end of the eighteenth century, Moses Mendelssohn's children became converts, and one, Dorothea Schlegel, became a prominent intellectual and salon hostess. As Hannah Arendt has shown, in the secular early nineteenth century the converts began to find their situation strained and, for some, even

40. La Peyrère, *Du Rappel des Juifs,* 8: "Les Juifs en ce temps la n'auront plus cette couleur noire et bazanée qu'ils ont contractée en leur Exil. . . . Ils changeront de visage dans ce Rappel, et la blancheur de leur teint aura le même éclat, dit le Psaume qu'ont les ailes et la gorge d'un pigeon extrêmement blanc."

Malcolm X, having read about Spinoza when he was in jail, concluded from the fact that he was described as dark and swarthy, that Spinoza was black. "Spinoza impressed me for a while when I found out he was black. A black Spanish Jew" (*Autobiography of Malcolm X* [New York: Grove Press, 1966], 180).

untenable. Without acceptance into the Jewish community they felt they no longer had roots. Rahel Varnhagen, a nineteenth-century salon hostess and the heroine of Arendt's work, even committed suicide.[41] Others went on to become leading figures in the missionary movements, and one became the first Anglican bishop of Jerusalem.[42]

If converts were easily acknowledged except in the Inquisition world, what was the real difference between a Jew and a non-Jew? Even Old Christian Spaniards and Portuguese believed that the essential and important difference was mental or spiritual. They could describe this in terms of malign beliefs condemned by God. But for an eighteenth-century secular humanist, what difference should Jewish beliefs have made? Jews, however, could be and were classified as superstitious, unreasonable, and unenlightened by Bayle, by various English deists, and by many *philosophes*.[43] And it was accepted that living according to these unfortunate beliefs could lead to some physical disabilities because of dietary restrictions, the conditions of ghetto life, and the imposed poverty, enforced by the nasty Christian ancien régime. For people who saw what was later to be called "the Jewish question," all one needed to do to resolve or dissolve the problem was to enlighten Jews so that they became just ordinary rational Europeans. There was no shortage of evidence that Jews had the intellectual equipment to participate in European civilization. From Philo Judaeus and Flavius Josephus to Moses Maimonides to Leon de Modena, to Menasseh ben Israel to Isaac de Pinto and Moses Mendelssohn, there were a stream of significant figures who played an important role in the history of European ideas, their Jewishness notwithstanding.[44] The roles of de Pinto and Mendelssohn

41. Hannah Arendt, *Rahel Varnhagen: Lebengeschichte einer deutschen Jüdin aus der Romantik* (Munich, 1962).

42. The leading missionary for the London Society for Promoting Christianity amongst the Jews was Joseph Wolf, a convert. The leading figure in the American Society for Ameliorating the Condition of the Jews was Joseph Frey, a convert who gave thirty thousand sermons in America. The first Anglican Bishop of Jerusalem was Michael Solomon Alexander, 1799–1843, chosen because he could speak to Jesus on His Return in his native tongue.

43. The *philosophes* will be discussed shortly. Regarding the views of the English deists about the Jews, see S. Ettinger, "Jews and Judaism as Seen by the English Deists of the Eighteenth Century" (in Hebrew), *Zion* 29 (1964): 182–207. For Bayle's view, see his many articles on Old Testament characters in the *Dictionnaire historique et critique*. See also Hertzberg, *French Enlightenment*, chap. 3.

44. The theme was developed at length in such works as Jacques Basnage, *L'histoire et la religion des Juifs, depuis Jésus-Christ jusqu'à présent, pour servir de supplément et le continuation à l'histoire de Joseph* (Rotterdam: R. Leers, 1706–1707, and later editions); Henri

TRAITÉ
DE LA
CIRCULATION
ET DU
CRÉDIT.

Contenant une *Analyse raisonnée des Fonds d'Angleterre*, & de ce qu'on appelle Commerce ou Jeu d'Actions; un Examen critique de plusieurs Traités sur les Impôts, les Finances, l'Agriculture, la Population, le Commerce &c. précédé de l'Extrait, d'un Ouvrage intitulé *Bilan général & raisonné de l'Angleterre depuis* 1600 *jusqu'en* 1761; & suivi d'une *Lettre sur la Jalousie da Commerce*, où l'on prouve que l'intérêt dés Puissances commerçantes ne se croise point, &c. avec un Tableau de ce qu'on appelle *Commerce*, ou plutôt *Jeu d'Actions*, en Hollande.

*Par l'Auteur de l'*ESSAI SUR LE LUXE, *& de la* LETTRE SUR LE JEU DES CARTES, *qu'on a ajoutés à la fin.*

A AMSTERDAM,

Chez MARC MICHEL REY.

MDCCLXXI.

Pl. 24. Title page of Isaac de Pinto's *Traité de la circulation et du crédit* (Amsterdam, 1771).

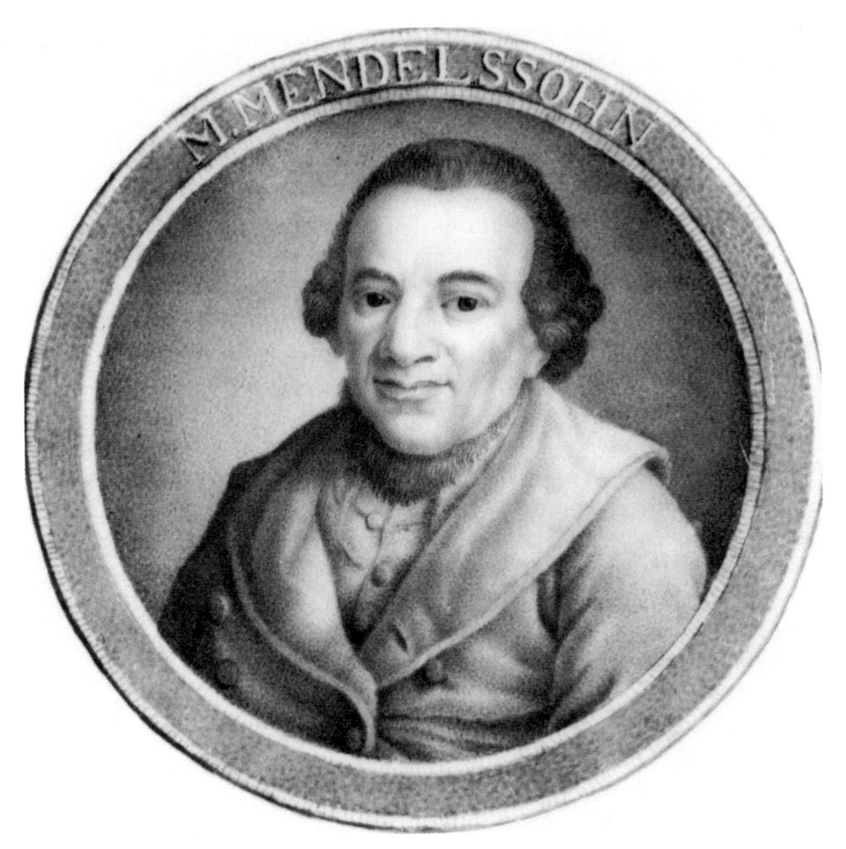

Pl. 25. Portrait of Moses Mendelssohn, from an urn in the Stadtsmuseum of Braunschweig, Lower Saxony.

in eighteenth-century Enlightenment discussions was of the highest significance. De Pinto was one of the first modern economists, a friend of Hume and Diderot, and a protagonist of Voltaire, while being the leader of the Amsterdam Synagogue.[45] Mendelssohn, the Jewish Socrates, was

Grégoire, *Essai sur la régénération morale et politique des Juifs* (Metz, 1789), and Honoré Gabriel Riquetti, Marquis de Mirabeau, *Sur Moses Mendelssohn, sur la réforme politique des Juifs* (London, 1787).

45. On de Pinto, see R. H. Popkin, "Hume and Isaac de Pinto," *Texas Studies in Literature and Language* 12 (1970): 417–430; and "Hume and Isaac de Pinto, II: Five New Letters," in *Hume and the Enlightenment: Essays Presented to Ernest Campbell Mossner*, ed. William B. Todd (Edinburgh: The University Press, 1974), 99–127, 428–429. In the first essay, I discuss de Pinto's role in the history of economic theory, from his refutation of Hume's

a friend of Lessing's, the sponsor of Kant, perhaps the leading figure of the German Enlightenment, while remaining an orthodox Jew.[46]

In both cases, irreligious or deist friends of Christian origin still indicated that there was some difference between de Pinto and Mendelssohn and other Europeans. Hume was more philo-Semitic than most of his contemporaries, and defended the Jews in his *History of England,*[47] giving a quite anti-Christian explanation of their mistreatment and expulsion from England in the Middle Ages. Hume was very friendly with de Pinto and worked hard to get him a pension from the East Indian Company. He dined with de Pinto and discussed politics and economics with him. But in writing about him, and for him, Hume felt he had to make the point that he was a good man, "tho" a Jew.[48] This may have been because the people Hume was dealing with, government leaders and India Company officials, were too conscious of de Pinto's Jewishness and not sufficiently aware of his goodness. De Pinto had other important backers, such as Lord Clive and the Duke of Bedford, who could just recommend him without qualification.[49] Lessing promoted Mendelssohn in all sorts of ways, but would not take him to, or propose him to, his lodge of the Freemasons because he was a Jew.[50] But what could this mean for Hume or Lessing? Lessing wrote *Nathan the Wise* expounding that Jews were like everybody else, a work that helped emancipate the German Jews. But like Hume, Lessing could still sense some difference that remained even in the most enlightened Jews. However, when the Swiss physiologist, Lavater, wrote Mendelssohn saying that if he was so ra-

essay on the national debt, to the discussion of de Pinto's views in Adam Smith, Dugald Stewart, Karl Marx, Werner Sombart, and others. Marx called de Pinto "the Pindar of the Amsterdam Bourse" (note in *Das Kapital,* vol. 1, pt. 2, chap. 4, p. 165, in *Marx-Engels Werke,* vol. 23 [Berlin, 1962]).

Sombart said that de Pinto was the first person to see clearly "dass die Entwicklung des modern Kreditsystems von der Vermehrung des Edelmetalle abhangig ist" (*Der Modern Kapitalismus,* III, *Das Wirtshaftsleben in Zeitalter des Hochkapitalismus* [Berlin, 1955], 191).

46. For some background on Mendelssohn's career, see Alexander Altmann, *Moses Mendelsson: A Biographical Study* (University: University of Alabama Press, 1973).

47. See the selections from David Hume's *History of England* on the Jews in medieval England in David F. Norton and Richard H. Popkin, *David Hume, Philosophical Historian* (Indianapolis: Bobbs Merrill, 1965), 119–126.

48. Letter to Thomas Rous, 28 August 1767, published in Popkin, "Hume and Isaac de Pinto, II," 104.

49. On this see the account in Popkin, "Hume and Isaac de Pinto, II."

50. Jacob Katz, *Jews and Freemasons in Europe* (Cambridge: Harvard University Press, 1970), 25. Altmann, *Moses Mendelssohn,* 311, commenting on Lessing's discussions about Freemasonry with Mendelssohn, said "Mendelssohn had never made an effort to enter the order as many Jews of the next generation would do with varying success."

tional, he had to become a Christian, Lessing, along with Herder and others, answered that there was no need for Mendelssohn to convert.[51] Mendelssohn kept out of the argument until his final work *Jerusalem* (written in 1786), where he defended Judaism and claimed he and his Enlightenment friends shared a common rational religion, and that he and other Jews had in addition a set of revealed laws they had to keep. Thus, for Mendelssohn, Jews, rationally, were or could be like everybody else, but religiously they were different. So, in Mendelssohn's own view, and in the view of his Enlightenment friends, some distinction remained. They could discuss Plato and Spinoza and human freedom, but Mendelssohn kept a kosher house.[52]

The enlightened Jews of Holland also insisted on some difference when the French Revolutionary armies conquered Holland and established the Batavian Confederacy. The French tried to enforce the new French law making Jews citizens. Both the Jewish leaders and the Dutch Calvinists joined in insisting they did not want Jews to be turned into Dutchmen. The Jews maintained they enjoyed Dutch hospitality, and enjoyed their status as legal residents, but they did not want to be Dutch, because they expected to go to their own home when the Messiah finally arrived. The orthodox Calvinists insisted the future of all mankind depended on Jews remaining separate. Only then could they play out their role in Divine History leading to the millennium.[53]

At the beginning of the Enlightenment, Dr. Isaac Orobio de Castro, one-time royal physician in Spain, later professor in the medical school at the University of Toulouse, and finally eminent physician in Holland (where he treated Queen Sophie of Prussia), wrote against Spinoza and publicly debated Philip van Limborch in the presence of Doctor John Locke on the truth of the Christian religion. Neither Locke nor van Limborch doubted the intellectual ability of Orobio, and they saw his spiritual blindness as some kind of Jewish flaw.[54] Jacques Basnage, the

51. On the Lavater affair, see Altmann, *Moses Mendelssohn,* chap. 3.

52. On Mendelssohn's *Jerusalem,* see Altmann, *Moses Mendelssohn,* 514–552.

53. See the texts of the debate in Holland, published by S. E. Bloemgarten, "De Amsterdamse Joden gedurende de eerste jaren van de Bataafse Republick (1795–1798)," I, II, III, *Studia Rosenthaliana* 1, no. 1 (1967): 66–96; 1, no. 2 (1967): 45–70; 2, no. 1 (1968): 42–65.

54. On Orobio de Castro, see Yosef Kaplan's *Isaac Orobio de Castro, and His Circle* (in Hebrew; summary in English) (Jerusalem: Magnes Press, 1982). The work was published by Oxford University Press in an English translation in 1990.

Locke and Limborch discussed Orobio at length in their correspondence. See letters 958, 959, 963, and 964 in *The Correspondence of John Locke,* ed. E. S. De Beer, vol. 3 (Oxford: Oxford University Press, 1978).

Prevenciones Divinas contra la
Jdolatria de las Gentes
PRUEVASE
QUE TODO QUANTO SE HAVIA
DE INVENTAR EN EL CRISTIA
NISMO; SELO PREVINO DIOS
A JSRAEL EN LOS CINCO
LIBROS DELA LEY: PARA
QUE ADVERTIDO NO PUDIESSE
CAER EN TALES ERRORES
POR
El Doctor Ishac Orobio
de Castro.
Copiado en AMSTERDAM
Por Abraham Machorro
Año 1704.
Empeçado en 1.º Junio
y acabado en 1.º Otubre
Año 1704.

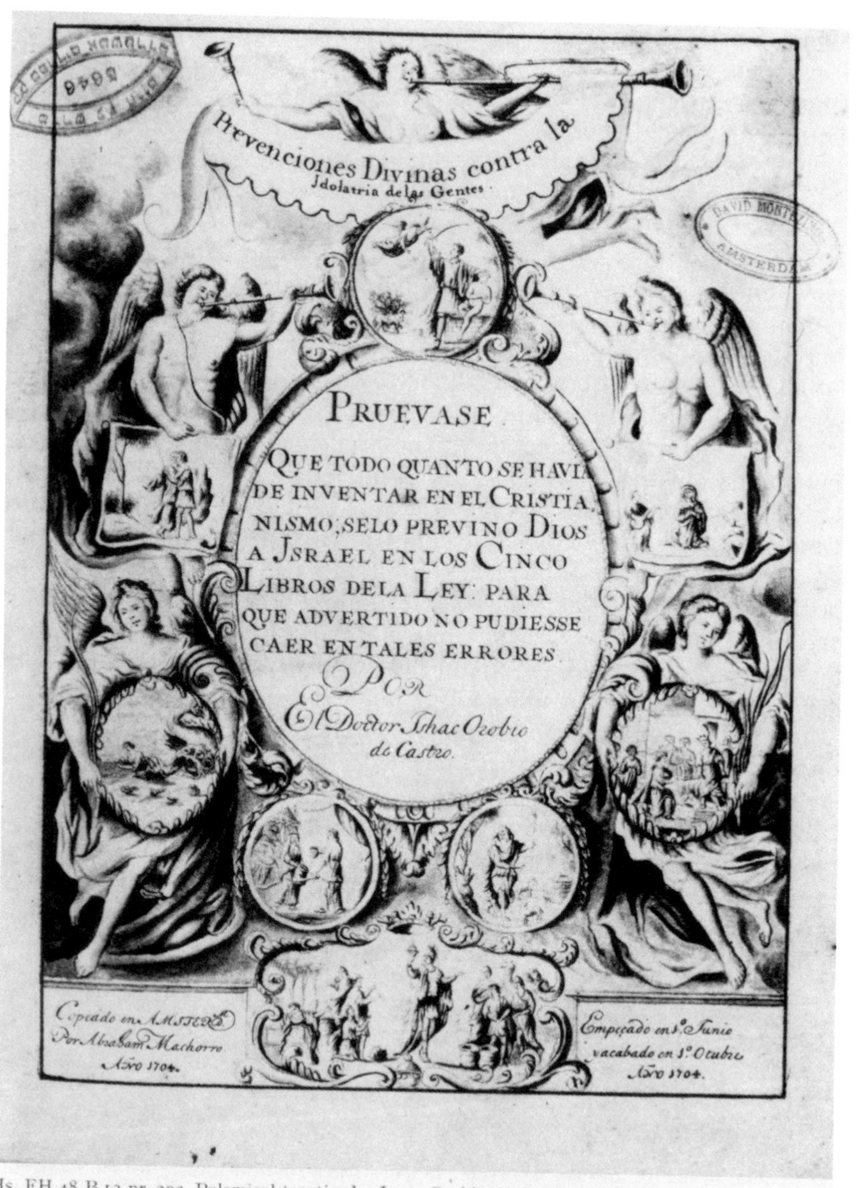

Ms. EH 48 B 13 nr. 202, Polemical treatise by Isaac Orobio de Castro, copied by Abraham Machorro
Amsterdam, 1704. Titlep.

Pl. 26. Scenes from the life of Dr. Orobio de Castro, including his having been a royal physician in Spain and professor of medicine at Toulouse.

Huguenot scholar already mentioned, who wrote the first history of the Jews since Josephus, was very concerned with the failure of the debates between Jews and Christians to bring about Jewish conversions. Basnage, following a project outlined by Menasseh ben Israel, to show how Jewish history after the Fall of the Temple was Providential up to the present, put together a vast body of information and material into a huge history showing God active in both chastising the Jews for their spiritual blindness, and protecting them because of their ultimate role in the imminently forthcoming millennium. Basnage saw the debates as hardening Jewish resistance for intellectual reasons—the Jews knew the theological material better, and they were clever arguers. Therefore, at the conclusion of his work, he urged Christians not to carry on any more debates, but rather to leave it to God to change the mental and spiritual attitude of the Jews.[55]

All of this indicates that the difference felt or sensed by eighteenth-century thinkers between Europeans and Jews centered on a mental or spiritual factor rather than a physical one. An exception should be noted. Spinoza mentioned the possibility that all of the generations of circumcising Jewish males may have made them too effeminate to play any further role in history. He states:

> The sign of circumcision is, as I think, so important, that I could persuade myself that it alone would preserve the [Jewish] nation for ever. Nay, I would go so far as to believe that if the foundations of their religion have not emasculated their [the Jews'] minds they may even, if occasion offers, so changeable are human affairs, raise up their empire afresh, and that God may a second time elect them.[56]

An attempt to delineate the difference started appearing in the writings of the English deists and the French *philosophes*. Their anti-Christianity should, and often did, remove the Christian anti-Semitic prejudices from their perspective. But only a few therefore became philo-Semites (like John Toland or Montesquieu).[57] Others began stress-

55. Cf. Basnage, *Histoire des Juifs*. An English translation appeared in 1708. Basnage's work is an all-important source for seeing the place of the Jews in the Christian world circa 1700. The work is just beginning to be taken seriously as a significant contribution.

56. Benedictus de Spinoza, *Tractatus Theologico-Politicus*, ed. R. H. M. Elwes (New York: Dover Press, 1951), chap. 3, p. 56. This text has been seized upon over and over again to show that Spinoza was a proto-Zionist, or that he still harbored Jewish leanings long after his excommunication.

57. See John Toland, *Nazarenus: A Jewish and Gentile and Mahometan Christianity* (London, 1718), and the citations from Montesquieu's writings given in Hertzberg, *French Enlightenment*, 273 ff.

ing the nasty ancient Jewish views and activities that spawned the great menace of the last millennium and a half, Christianity. Judaism was the foul root on which Christianity grew. Old Testament morality was really immorality when seen from an enlightened perspective. All sorts of mind-boggling and mind-limiting activities introduced from Moses to New Testament times infected Christianity and made it so bad. And Judaism retained those primitive customs and practices of ancient times, which enlightened theorists believed might reinfect Christianity and the Christian world.[58]

For some, a program of enlightened activity could change Jews into reasonable Europeans. The Royal Society of Metz, where the largest number of Jews in France lived, announced a prize essay contest in 1785 on the question, "How to make the Jews happy and useful in France?" The question reflected the problems of the Jews in the area, many of whom were very poor and engaged in marginal or dishonest economic activities.[59] The abbé Henri Grégoire, a priest from a heavily Jewish area in Alsace, wrote one of the prize-winning essays, entitled *Essai sur la régénération physique, morale et politique des Juifs.*[60] Grégoire saw the Ashkenazi Jews of his time as impoverished, unhealthy, immoral and antisocial, all owing to the baleful effects of anti-Semitism and in no wise to Jewish body or mind. The Sephardic French Jews he considered somewhat more enlightened. He envisaged, and during the Revolution and the Napoleonic period fought for, equal civil rights for Jews, which he believed would lead to their becoming physically, morally, and socially like the rest of French population.[61] And Grégoire, one of the greatest millenarians of the time, hoped this meant that Jews and the

58. Many of the nastiest texts are gathered together in Pierre Pluchon, *Nègres et Juifs au XVIIIe siècle: Le racisme au siècle des lumières* (Paris: Tallandier, 1984), "Les lumières et les juifs," pp. 64–82. See also Poliakov, *Histoire de l'antisémitisme,* livre I, chap. 2, "La France des lumières," pp. 87–160.

59. On the background of the essay contest, see Hertzberg, *French Enlightenment,* 328 ff., and Poliakov, *Histoire de l'antisémitisme,* 167–173.

60. These were two other winners of the prize, a Protestant, Adolphe Thiery, and a Jew, Zalkind-Hourwitz. All the essays have been republished by Editions d'Histoire Social in Paris in a series entitled *La Révolution française et l'emancipation des Juifs.* Grégoire's also appeared in English, and it is this that influenced discussions and policies in France during the Revolution of 1787–1831. On Grégoire's role, see Ruth Necheles, *Abbé Grégoire: The Odyssey of an Egalitarian* (Westport, Conn.: Greenwood Press, 1971), and R. H. Popkin, "La Peyrère, the Abbé Grégoire and the Jewish Question in the Eighteenth Century," *Studies in Eighteenth-Century Culture* 4 (1975): 209–222.

61. Grégoire, *Essai,* passim.

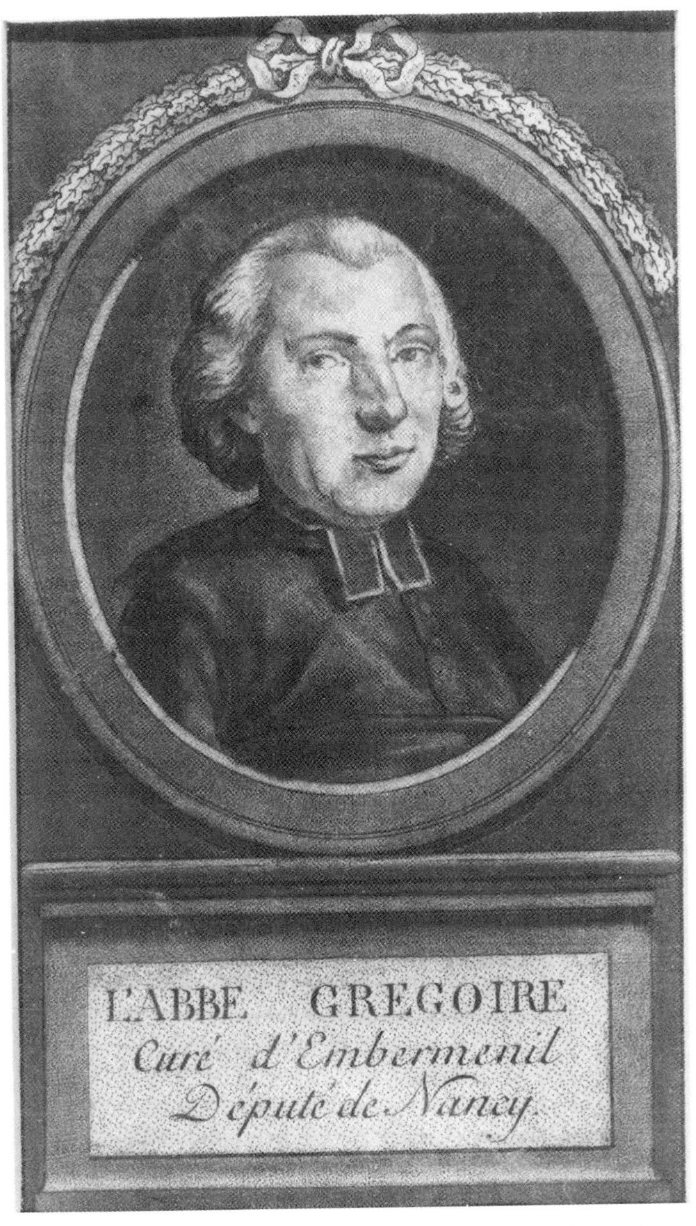

Pl. 27. Portrait of the abbé Henri Grégoire (18th cent.).

rest of the French population would become true Christians, ready for the millennium.[62]

Grégoire represented one side, the one that saw the Jews as the victims of centuries of unjustified religious and political anti-Semitism. If this persecution were abolished, and the Jews were given an Enlightenment education, he believed they would flourish. Intellectually they would produce dozens, hundreds, thousands of Mendelssohns and de Pintos. The Jew would be regenerated by the Revolution that would spread Enlightenment to the four corners of the world.[63]

As Grégoire found out, when he started his campaign for Jewish civil equality in 1787 and introduced a bill to establish it in 1789, he was opposed by radical intellectuals quoting Voltaire, Diderot, d'Holbach, and other Encyclopedists and *philosophes*.[64] Voltaire, Diderot, and d'Holbach were all quite virulent anti-Christians who in the course of their literary careers made a range of observations about the Jews. Since the publication of Arthur Hertzberg's book *The French Enlightenment and the Jews* (1968), many studies have tried to explain the context of these authors' remarks and to contend they were not really anti-Semites.[65] Among others, Voltaire said many different things, some of which became, whether intended or not, the basis of secular anti-Semitism and of the Aryan mythology. Diderot's early writings on the Jews in the *Encyclopédie* became a stock source for secular anti-Semites. Diderot apparently changed his opinion when he met actual Jews, like de Pinto, when Diderot went to Holland and visited him. D'Holbach was certainly more anti-Christian than anti-Semitic, but his *L'esprit du judaïsme* has become a classic that is still published by anti-Semitic groups in the Ukraine. Modern interpreters have ranged from seeing these remarks on Judaism by the Enlightenment greats as just typical views of their time, to claiming they are a minor part of their anti-Christian polemics, to saying these are occasional not central views, to the other extreme of seeing them as extreme and uncalled-for anti-Semitism. A recent French study by Pierre Pluchon, *Nègres et Juifs au XVIIIe siècle,* argues that even

62. Grégoire's millenarianism dominated his fight for equality of blacks and Jews, and his contributions to the fight for freedom of all sorts of groups. He died while working for Greek freedom in 1831. In his *Histoire des sectes réligieuses,* Grégoire, in his section on Jews, makes clear his hopes for the millennial union of Jews and Christians. See tome III, livre V, chaps. 1–3 (Paris, 1828).

63. See Grégoire, *Essai sur la régénération physique, morale et politique des Juifs,* chaps. 25–27.

64. See Hertzberg, *French Enlightenment,* chap. 10, "The Revolution."

65. See, for instance, Hugh Trevor-Roper's review of Hertzberg's book in *The New York Review of Books,* 22 August 1968, 11.

the philo-Semitism of the abbé Grégoire is really anti-Semitic and that the views of Voltaire, Diderot, and d'Holbach are equally inflammatory.[66] Leon Schwartz, however, has shown that, at least in Diderot's case, he changed his mind after meeting Jews and seeing their situation, and became mildly philo-Semitic.[67]

The gist of the theory offered by these great figures of the French Enlightenment was that Judaism was and is an eastern or oriental view and practice, and contained elements that were antithetical to an enlightened European point of view. In contrast, in the widely circulated *Letters Writ by a Turkish Spy,* the chief protagonist sought to convince the sultan's Jewish agent in Vienna to adopt a rational Judaism, shorn of its peculiar practices, which would be essentially a moral view based on the universal ethical elements in prerabbinical Judaism.[68] I have argued elsewhere that this is an early attempt to convert European Jews to reformed Judaism.[69]

Voltaire and Diderot often characterized Judaism as fundamentally alien to a civilized European view. Voltaire was challenged by de Pinto, who insisted that at least the Spanish and Portuguese Jews, living in Holland, France, and England, were civilized Europeans.[70] (De Pinto had been the secretary of the Dutch Academy of Sciences and gave two unpublished lectures that contain no Jewish elements but only Enlightenment scientific and deist views.)[71] Voltaire brushed aside de Pinto's arguments, and advised him, if he were so intelligent, to become a *philosophe*. De Pinto's contention that he was a *philosophe* and a Jew made no sense to Voltaire.[72] Judaism ancient and modern was and is antithetical to a life of reason. Judaism ancient and modern is Asiatic,

66. Pluchon, *Nègres et Juifs,* 64–90. See also Poliakov's evaluation of these eighteenth-century figures in *Histoire de l'antisémitisme,* livre I, chap. 2.

67. The evolution of Diderot's views on Judaism and his shift from an Enlightenment anti-Semite to a genuine universalist humanist is very well traced and examined in Leon Schwartz, *Diderot and the Jews* (Rutherford, N.J.: Fairleigh Dickinson University Press, 1981). See also my review of Schwartz's book in *Eighteenth-Century Studies* 18 (1984): 115–118.

68. See, for instance, Marana, *Letters Writ by a Turkish Spy,* vol. 4, letter V, pp. 251–259; vol. 5, letter III, pp. 70–71, and letter XX, p. 203.

69. Popkin, "A Late-Seventeenth-Century Gentile Attempt" (n. 15 above).

70. Isaac de Pinto, *Apologie pour la nation juive; ou, Réflexions critiques sur le premier chapitre du VIIe tome des œuvres de M. de Voltaire au sujet des Juifs* (Paris, 1762).

71. These are in the collection of manuscripts of the Ets Haim Library of Amsterdam, now in Jerusalem. I intend to edit these in the not-too-distant future.

72. Voltaire's main discussions of this theme appear in his *Essai sur les mœurs et l'esprit des nations* (1769), in the articles on the Old Testament in the *Dictionnaire philosophique* (1764), and in the appendixes to later editions of the *Dictionnaire.*

uninfluenced by either the good rational forces of the Hellenic or the Aryan Indian world.[73]

The rendition of this theme in Diderot and Voltaire usually allowed or suggested that this basic drawback of Judaism could be overcome by individual Jews if they broke with their traditions and communities. Voltaire's viewpoint, however, especially in *Essai sur les mœurs,* was that Europeans could be enlightened and liberated from their Christian past but that Jews are of a different biological stock, which yields their religion and character. It is unlikely that a Jew can overcome or escape his or her innate character. Even if Jews were cured of their religion, their inborn features would remain, and they would be a threat to themselves and to the Europeans with whom they lived. They infected Europe long ago with Christianity, and their natural incurable Jewishness could repeat itself. And so, at least the suggestion was made that Jews be removed from Europe so that their spiritual contagion could be stopped. At least once, Voltaire claimed that Jews were hopeless in the movement to reform humanity.[74]

D'Holbach's *L'esprit de judaïsme* went a bit further. The author, in his virulent anti-Christian campaign, had published part of Orobio de Castro's polemic against Christianity under the title *Israël vengé*. He had also published a version of *Les trois imposteurs, Moses Jesus et Mohammed,* an antireligious work circulated in the early eighteenth century containing material from Hobbes and Spinoza, among others. During the same period he wrote his notorious anti-Jewish work in which he claimed that Europe, where arts, sciences, and philosophy flourished in Greece and Rome, was then taken over by the false dream invented by imposters like Moses to deceive the Jews. Europe has to break with the unbearable yoke of religious institutions and practices to regain its intellectual force. "Leave to the stupid Hebrews, to the frenzied imbeciles, and to the cowardly and degraded Asiatics these superstitions which are as vile as they are mad; they were not meant for the inhabitants of your climate."[75]

73. See Voltaire's response in his letter of 21 juillet 1762, letter 9791, Voltaire's *Correspondence,* ed. Theodore Besterman, vol. 49 (Geneva, 1959), 131–132. The abbé Guénée defended the Jewish side in his *Lettres de quelques juifs portugais et allemands à M. Voltaire* (Paris, 1769) (*portugais, allemands et polonais* takes the place of *portugais et allemands* beginning with the 4th ed., 1776). Voltaire answered in *Un chrétien contre six juifs,* in *Œuvres* 29:558.

74. This theme runs through the *Essai sur les mœurs* in Voltaire's evaluation of Judaism. Hertzberg, *French Enlightenment,* 286–299 shows how Voltaire was taken by his contemporaries as advocating anti-Semitism.

75. On d'Holbach, see Pierre Naville, *Paul Thiry d'Holbach* (Paris, 1943). The quotation is from d'Holbach's *L'esprit du judaïsme* (London, 1770), 200–201.

The *esprit* of Judaism was thus something foreign to Europe, which had taken over and now must be overthrown. The Jews were the carriers of the *esprit* and as such were not capable of being true Europeans.[76]

Voltaire, Diderot, and d'Holbach found a basis for discerning a difference between Jews and Europeans: the difference was spiritual, and pretty much incurable. *And* the Jewish spirit had infected Europe, causing the Dark Ages, and was still a constant threat to the European point of view. In discerning the difference as one related to mind rather than body, these heroes of the French Enlightenment started the pattern of modern secular anti-Semitism. What was different and wrong with Jews was not their role in the Christian world picture but their role as evil influences who infected Europe with Christianity. This *esprit* was part of the Jew's oriental nature, which did not belong in Western society and was in danger of reinfecting Europe. This analysis blossomed in the twentieth century in the view of Hitler and Goebbels that Judaism is a bacillus that can always infect the Aryan world and can only be stopped by being eradicated.

The study of language and national identity led to a further stage in the saga of the secularization of racism in the Enlightenment, and the theory developed that Jews should be excluded from the new European nation states because their language was foreign to Europe, as was their mental outlook. It was claimed that Jews in Europe retained the social, cultural, and intellectual outlook found in the Jews of the Middle East and Asia.

The history of the discovery of the "source" of European languages is curious. In the seventeenth century, one impetus to such research was the quest for the language of Adam, the language Adam spoke and in which he named everything according to its nature. The Adamic language would therefore contain universal knowledge. All sorts of candidates were explored from the obvious Hebrew to the less obvious ones like Dutch, Swedish, and Chinese. The ancient languages of India entered into this only tangentially.[77] The *Letters Writ by a Turkish Spy* publicized the news that ancient Sanskrit writings contained a historical

76. The Scientific Academy of the Ukranian Socialist Soviet Republic keeps reissuing d'Holbach's work as if it were news to the present world.

This claim that Jews did not belong in Europe does not seem to have been part of the English opposition to enfranchising Jews there. In the 1753 opposition to Jewish citizenship, economic issues and Christian prejudice seem to have been paramount.

77. For a discussion of the search for the Adamic language, see David S. Katz, *Philo-Semitism and the Readmission of the Jews to England, 1603–1655* (Oxford: Oxford University Press, 1982), chap. 2.

cosmology long predating biblical events.[78] The first English publication by Nathaniel Brassey Halhed, a century later, translated from the Persian, pointed out the conflict of the Judeo-Christian scriptures and the Indian ones, and resolved it only as an act of faith.[79] Sir William Jones's inquiries into Sanskrit were partly motivated by an interest in showing that the Indian chronological claims were not historically accurate. Jones became the first European Sanskrit expert and reassured European Christians by telling them that the Indian chronology pre-Adam was mythological and that the rest was easily reconcilable with the Bible.[80] In an aside, Jones observed that it might be the case that all European languages from Latin and Greek onward were derivations from Sanskrit but that Semitic languages were not.[81]

Jones's view quickly became the Indo-European language theory of early-nineteenth-century German scholars. Fredrich Schlegel proclaimed that European languages and cultures derived from an ancient Indo-European language that came from the language of the Indian Aryans, namely Sanskrit.[82] Schlegel coincidentally was married to Moses Mendelssohn's daughter, Dorothea, who had converted to European *enlightened* Christianity.

It took little effort to show some of the implications of the Indo-European language theory. Joined with Herder's theory that each culture expresses its unique "idea," its mind, in its language and literature, European cultures expressed human mental outlooks in the host of languages derivative from Indo-European. Hebrew was not an Indo-European language. Hence it expressed an idea, a mind, and a culture foreign to Europe. European culture developed from Indo-European Hellenic roots and not from Hebraic ones. The culmination of this line

78. For example, see Marana, *Letters Writ by a Turkish Spy*, vol. 8, letter 12, pp. 253–258. Some of the same data appear in Charles Gildon's letter in Charles Blount's *Oracles of Reason* (1693), 182.

79. Nathaniel Brassey Halhed, *A Code of Gentoo Laws, or Ordinations of the Pundits, from a Persian Translation, made from the Original, written in the Shanscrit Language* (London, 1776), xxxviii-xxxix and xliii-xliv.

80. On Jones's life, career, and influence, see the article on him in the *Dictionary of National Biography*. His contribution to the discussion appears in his essays, "On the Gods of Greece, Italy, and India," "On the Chronology of the Hindus," and "A Supplement to the Essay on India Chronology," in *The Works of Sir William Jones* (London, 1807), vols. 3 and 4.

81. In a private letter dated 27 September 1787, Jones wrote, "You would be astonished at the resemblance between that language [Sanskrit] and both Greek and Latin," in *Memoirs of Sir William Jones*, ed. Lord Teignmouth (London, 1807), 2:128.

82. Friedrich Schlegel, "Über die Sprache und Weisheit der Inder," in *Sämmtliche Werke*, vol. 7 (Vienna, 1846).

of speculation was that the Jew by nature, by language, by culture, and by mentality is not and cannot be a European.[83] This reasoning resulted in the German saying, "A Jew can read German. A Jew can write German. But a Jew cannot think German."[84] No matter how much Heine tried, German nationalist anti-Semites said he would be writing Jewish verse, not German verse, and Felix Mendelssohn, the grandson of Moses Mendelssohn, would be writing Jewish music and not German music (according to Richard Wagner).[85] The story from then on is the development of national cultural theories that made Jews outsiders in the countries where they resided, and permanent outsiders. Hilaire Belloc stated in 1922 "that the continued presence of the Jewish nation intermixed with other nations alien to it presents a permanent problem of the gravest character: that the wholly different culture, tradition, race, and religion of Europe make Europe a permanent antagonist to Israel" and therefore the Jews had to be removed from Europe.[86] Herzl's realization that the Dreyfus case showed that Jews would never be accepted as Europeans, but would be accepted as members of a Jewish state, spurred the secular Zionist movement as the way of dealing with the new secular anti-Semitism that was taking over Western Europe.

Another dimension to this story is that of the opponents of the new secular racism. It is interesting that the United States was the first Western country to eliminate religious requirements for citizenship. Once the First Amendment to the Constitution was ratified, Jews then residing in the United States were citizens thereof. Slowly the magnitude of this development became apparent as Jewish communities were accepted as coequal with other religious groups and as Jews became full participants in the civic world. The fact that there was no established church or religion allowed the United States to have a quite different history with regard to religious racism than any European country. A year before

83. For the development of this theory, see Mosse, *Toward the Final Solution,* chap. 3, and Leon Poliakov, *Le mythe aryen* (Paris, 1971), part I, chap. 5, "Allemagne: La langue et la race," pp. 85–122.

84. This seems to be the racist result of putting together the views of Herder, Fichte, and Schlegel. See the discussion in Mosse, *Toward the Final Solution,* chaps. 3, 7, and 8; and Poliakov, livre I, chap. 3, and livre III, pp. 393–403.

85. Richard Wagner, "Das Judentum in der Musik," in *Gesammelte Schriften und Dichtungen,* vol. 5 (Leipzig, 1907), 66–85. On Wagner's views, see Mosse, *Towards a Final Solution,* 101–105, and Poliakov, *Histoire de l'antisémitisme,* "Le cas de Richard Wagner," pp. 440–467, especially 448–451.

86. Hilaire Belloc, *The Jews* (London: Constable and Co., 1922), published before Hitler's *Mein Kampf,* began by stating that the Jews had to be removed from Europe. The quotation is from p. 3.

the adoption of the United States Constitution, Moses Mendelssohn read something in a European newspaper that suggested the new American nation was considering having an established religion. He added a note at the end of his defense of Judaism, *Jerusalem,* expressing his fears about what might happen in the United States, and that this new country might not become a beacon light unto other nations.[87] As we know, his fears were groundless, and the United States began its nationhood as a secular state.

The first Jew to become a naturalized U.S. citizen was David de Cohen Nassy (1747–1806), a medical doctor from Surinam, who came to the United States in 1792. He published a book on epidemic diseases prevalent in Philadelphia in 1793 and became the first Jewish member of the American Philosophical Society.[88] In 1798, he published *Lettre politico-theologico-morale sur les Juifs*. The title is suggestive, of course, of Spinoza's work, whose importance for the enlightenment world had been spelled out by Mendelssohn. Nassy explored the significance of the kind of freedom that existed in America compared with the Revolutionary anarchy in France. He foresaw the possibilities America held out to the persecuted groups in Europe, and the cultural flowering that could occur in the United States as compared with Europe. In his analysis of anti-Semitism, he saw that its evil effects would disappear in America because of the legal equality of American citizens. "All men, then, must be equal in their rights, equal in their privileges: their birth, cults, wealth, and ranks do not determine at all their inequality."[89]

The denial of this equality represents a disease (called a "prejudice" by Nassy) affecting Europe but from which America was immune because "of that wise and enlightened philosophy which makes no distinction among men, except that which is demanded by virtue, useful talents and good *mores*."[90] Nassy saw Europe as becoming infected with the new disease or prejudice of secular racism while the United States was safe because it had eliminated religious distinctions in its laws. There is no indication of where Nassy stood on the slavery question. Others who

87. Moses Mendelsson's *Jerusalem* has the following note on the next to last page. "Leider, horen wir auch schon den Congress in Amerika das alte lied anstimmen, und von einer *herrschenden Religion* sprechen" (*Gesammelte Schriften,* vol. 8, *Schrifter zum Judentum,* ed. Alexander Altmann [Stuttgart, 1983], 203).

88. On Nassy, see Jose Faur, "David Nassy: On Prejudice and Related Matters," in *Neveh Ya'akov: Jubilee Volume Presented to Dr. Jaap Meyer,* ed. Lea Dasberg and Jonathan N. Cohen, (Assen, 1982), 87–116.

89. Quoted ibid., 89.

90. Quoted ibid., 100.

could see the menace of secular racism, and view America as a bastion against it, were some of the millenarian leaders of the American and French revolutions who saw this more thoroughly. They objected to the blacks being condemned because of their physical features and the Jews because of their mental or spiritual ones and claimed that these developments were hindering preparations for the millennium.

Elias Boudinot, the president of the Continental Congress during the end of the American Revolution (who signed the Treaty of Paris making the United States a nation) and the first director of the U.S. Mint, saw the American and French revolutions as the historical enactment of the prophecies in the books of *Daniel* and *Revelation.* He insisted as part of the preparation for the Second Advent and the millennium that there must be equality for blacks, Indians, Jews, and even women—all must be equal citizens of the premillennial American state.[91] The abbé Grégoire, a major figure in the French Revolution, fought for the equality of Jews, Protestants, and blacks, and died, like Byron, while campaigning for Greek independence, all as part of the preparation for the millennium.[92] Charles Crawford, an Englishman who took part in the American Revolution, was an important defender of equal rights for Jews, blacks, and American Indians. He left America when the deists like Jefferson took over, and joined with the London Society for Promoting Christianity among the Jews. He almost persuaded Czar Alexander I to emancipate the Russian Jews. These humane activities were all part of his millenarian plan.[93]

One of the grounds for opposing the new secular racism was the millenarian expectation that *everyone* would and should be equal physically and mentally in the world to come. The religious role in fighting secular racism has not, I think, been given its due. There was also a secular answer to secular racism that began to emerge at the end of the eighteenth century in the cultural relativism of the von Humboldt

91. On Boudinot, see R. H. Popkin, "The Age of Reason versus the Age of Revelation: Two Critics of Tom Paine, David Levi, and Elias Boudinot," in J. A. Leo Lemay, *Deism, Masonry and the Enlightenment: Essays Honoring Alfred Owen Aldridge* (Newark, Del.: University of Delaware Press, 1987), 158–170. Boudinot's defense of women's rights appears in his address to the Society of the Cincinnati, Princeton, 23 September 1783, printed in *The Life, Public Service, Addresses and Letters of Elias Boudinot,* ed. J. J. Boudinot (New York: Da Capo Press, 1971), 374.

92. On Grégoire's career, see Necheles, *Abbé Grégoire.*

93. Charles Crawford, *Three Letters to the Hebrew Nation* (London, 1817), appendix on Czar Alexander I's support of the philo-Semitic activities of the London Society, and his acts toward Jewish emancipation in 1815–1817. All of this came to a sudden end, and official Russian policy became very anti-Semitic during the rest of the nineteenth century.

brothers and in Herder's views. They stressed the denial of standards for evaluating cultural differences and the insistence that each culture be allowed to develop its own potentialities.[94]

Neither the millenarian nor the cultural relativist response to the new secular racism was able to stem its advance until it became a monstrous force dominating the events all over the globe in the nineteenth and twentieth centuries. As Disraeli said, race is the motor of history. By now, I think we have to look back and realize that the same currents that liberated us from the dominance of absolutism and religious authority in the Enlightenment also, unfortunately, spawned a new and more virulent explanation of why people differ and what should be done about it. Now, after all of the havoc wreaked in the last two hundred years, I think we have to look for some ideologies that can heal the wounds of secular racism and bring about the genuine brotherhood of man. And, perhaps, by looking at those who saw the menace of the new racial ideologies in the eighteenth century, we can find some guidance for making a more humane world.

94. See Popkin, "Philosophical Bases" (n. 16 above), 99–102.

PART FIVE

Suggestions for Further Reading

Suggestions for Further Reading

Note: The works listed below are often cited in the individual chapters and form something of a checklist of important works about the diverse aspects of the mind/body relation discussed above. The list is selective and intended to direct the reader to significant sites for these topics. As such, it will inevitably appear random to the reader who browses through it looking for tight principles for inclusion and consideration. But the subject of mind and body in our period of the Enlightenment was not restricted to any *one* set of discourses or critiques, and the reader should be prepared for the embodiment of this topic in a very wide number of discourses ranging throughout printed literature in many languages on both sides of the ocean. If this array confounds readers and students, we are altogether sympathetic. Yet it must be remembered that one of the aims of this book has been to demonstrate how widespread throughout culture was the concern with the mind/body relation. This may be small consolation for readings extending from the poetic and artistic to the technically scientific and medical. The fact of this diversity in many languages and countries remains. (GSR)

Ackerknecht, Erwin H., M.D. *Medicine at the Paris Hospital, 1794–1848.* Baltimore: Johns Hopkins University Press, 1967.

Addison, Joseph. *The Spectator.* 5 vols. Edited by Donald F. Bond. Oxford: Clarendon Press, 1965.

Altschule, Mark D. "Ideas about Anxiety Held by Eighteenth-Century British Medical Writers." Chapter 1 of his *Roots of Modern Psychiatry: Essays in the History of Psychiatry.* New York and London: Greene and Stratton, 1957.

Anscombe, G. E. M. *Ethics, Religion, and Politics: Collected Philosophical Papers.* Vol. 3. Minneapolis: University of Minnesota Press, 1981.

———. *Intention.* Oxford: B. Blackwell, 1957; 2d ed., Ithaca, N.Y.: Cornell University Press, 1963.

Ardal, Pall. *Passions and Value in Hume's Treatise.* Edinburgh: Edinburgh University Press, 1966.

Armstrong, John. "The Art of Preserving Health." In *Poetical Works of John Armstrong.* Edinburgh: Chalmers, 1847.

Arnold. T. *Observations of the Nature, Kinds, Causes, and Prevention of Insanity, Lunacy, or Madness.* 2 vols. London: Robinson and Cadell, 1782–1786.

Astruc, J. *Traité des maladies des femmes.* 5 vols. Paris: Cuvelier, 1761–1765.

Auenbrugger, L. *Von der stillen Wuth oder dem Triebe zum Selbstmorde als einer wirklichen Krankheit, mit Originalbeobachtungen und Anmerkungen.* Dessau: Verlagskasse, 1783.

Bakan, David. *Disease, Pain, and Sacrifice: Toward a Psychology of Suffering.* Chicago: University of Chicago Press, 1968.

Bakhtin, M. *Rabelais and His World.* Translated by H. Iswolsky. Cambridge, Mass.: Harvard University Press, 1968.

Barckhuysen, Otto. *Dissertatio Medica Inauguralis sistens Considerationem Terroris Pathologico-Therapeuticam.* Leiden: Conrad Wishoff, 1738.

Barker, Francis. *The Tremulous Private Body.* New York: Methuen, 1984.

———, ed. *1789: Reading Writing Revolution.* Colchester: University of Essex, 1982.

Barthes, Roland. *Sade/Fourier/Loyola.* Translated by Richard Miller. New York: Farrar, Straus and Giroux, 1976.

Bataille, Georges. *Literature and Evil.* Translated by Alastair Hamilton. London: Calder and Boyars, 1973. Original French edition published 1957.

Bateson, Gregory. "Pathologies of Epistemology." In *Steps to an Ecology of Mind,* edited by Gregory Bateson, 493–495. San Francisco: Chandler, 1972.

Battie, W. *A Treatise on Madness.* London: Whisten and White, 1758.

Beauvoir, Simone de. *Faut-il brûler Sade*— 1951–1952. Reprint, Paris: Gallimard, 1972.

Benthall, J. *The Body Electric.* London, 1976.

Bentham, Jeremy. *Panopticon; or, The Inspection-House.* In *The Works of Jeremy Bentham,* edited by John Bowring, vol. 4. Edinburgh, 1838–1848. Originally published 1791.

———. *Comments on the Commentaries and A Fragment on Government.* Edited by J. H. Burns and H. L. A. Hart. London: Athlone Press, 1977.

———. *Deontology, together with A Table of the Springs of Action and the Article on Utilitarianism.* Edited by Amnon Goldworth. Oxford: Clarendon Press, 1983.

Blackmore, Sir Richard. *A Treatise of the Spleen and Vapours.* London: Pemberton, 1725.

Blanchot, Maurice. *Lautréamont et Sade.* Paris: Minuit, 1949.

Blumenbach, J. F. *Über den Bildungstrieb und das Zeugungsgeschäft.* Göttingen: Dieterich, 1781; 2d ed., 1791, translated by Alexander Crichton under the title *An Essay on Generation* (London: Cadell, 1792).

Bond, John. *An Essay on the Incubus, or Night Mare.* London: Wilson and Durham, 1753.

Booth, Wayne. "Did Sterne Complete *Tristram Shandy*?" *Modern Philology* 48 (1951): 172–183.

Boswell, James. *Boswell's Column, Being His Seventy Contributions to the London Magazine under the Pseudonymn the Hypochondriack from 1777 to 1783.* Introduction and notes by Margery Bailey. London: Kimber, 1951.

Bottomley, F. *Attitudes to the Body in Western Christendom.* London: Lepus Books, 1979.

Bowker, John. *Problems of Suffering in Religions of the World.* Cambridge: Cambridge University Press, 1970.

Braudy, Leo. "*Fanny Hill* and Materialism." *Eighteenth-Century Studies* 4 (1970): 21–40.

Brissenden, R. F. "'Trusting to Almighty God': Another Look at the Composition of Tristram Shandy." In *The Winged Skull: Papers from the Laurence Sterne Bicentenary Conference,* edited by Arthur H. Cash and John M. Stedmond, 258–268. Kent, Ohio: Kent State University Press, 1971.

———. *Virtue in Distress: Studies in the Novel of Sentiment from Richardson to Sade.* London and New York: Macmillan, 1974.

Broad, C. D. *The Mind and Its Place in Nature.* London: Routledge and Kegan Paul, 1925.

Brodie, Benjamin Collins. *Mind and Matter.* New York: G. P. Putnam, 1857.

Brooks, Peter. *Reading for the Plot: Design and Intention in Narrative.* New York: Alfred Knopf, 1984.

Brown, N. O. *Life against Death.* London: Routledge and Kegan Paul, 1959.

Brown, Theodore M. "From Mechanism to Vitalism in Eighteenth-Century English Physiology." *Journal of the History of Biology* 7 (1974): 179–216.

———. *The Mechanical Philosophy and the "Animal Oeconomy."* New York: Arno Press, 1981.

Browne, Richard. *Medicina Musica; or, A Mechanical Essay on the Effects of Singing, Musick, and Dancing, on Human Bodies.* London, 1729.

Bucher, Heini W. *Tissot und sein Traité des nerfs: Ein Beitrag zur Medizingeschichte der schweizerischen Aufklärung.* Zürcher medizingeschichtliche Abhandlungen, Neue Reihe, no. 1. Zurich: Juris-Verlag, 1958.

Butler, Joseph. *The Works of Joseph Butler.* Edited by W. E. Gladstone. Oxford: Clarendon Press, 1896.

Cabanis, Pierre-Jean-Georges. *On the Relations between the Physical and Moral Aspects of Man.* Edited by George Mora. Translated by Margaret Duggan Saidi. 2 vols. Baltimore: Johns Hopkins University Press, 1981.

Caplan, Richard, ed. *Exploring the Concept of Mind.* Iowa City: University of Iowa Press, 1986.

Carlson, Eric T., and Meribeth M. Simpson. "Models of the Nervous System in Eighteenth-Century Psychiatry." *Bulletin of the History of Medicine* 43 (1969): 101–115.

Carter, Angela. *The Sadeian Woman and the Ideology of Pornography*. New York: Pantheon Books, 1978.
Carter, Richard B. *Descartes' Medical Philosophy: The Organic Solution to the Mind-Body Problem*. Baltimore: Johns Hopkins University Press, 1983.
Cash, Arthur. *Laurence Sterne: The Early and Middle Years*. London: Methuen, 1975.
Cheyne, George. *An Essay of Health and Long Life*. London, 1724.
———. *The English Malady: or, A Treatise of Nervous Diseases of All Kinds*. London: Strahan and Leake, 1733.
———. *Essay on Regimen*. London, 1740.
———. *The Natural Method of Curing the Diseases of the Body, and the Disorders of the Mind Depending on the Body*. In 3 parts. London, 1742.
———. *The Letters of Doctor George Cheyne to Samuel Richardson (1733–1743)*. Edited by Charles F. Mullett. Columbia, Mo., 1943.
Chiarugi, V. *Della pazzia in genere ed in specie: Trattato medico-analitico con una centuria di osservazioni*. 2 vols. Florence: Carlieri, 1793–1794.
Churchland, Patricia S. *Neurophilosophy: Toward a Unified Science of the Mind/Brain*. Cambridge, Mass.: MIT Press, 1986.
Clark, William. *Dissertatio Medica Inauguralis de Viribus Animi Pathematum in corpus humanum*. Leiden: Johannes Verbeek, 1727.
Clarke, Edwin. "The Doctrine of the Hollow Nerve in the Seventeenth and Eighteenth Centuries." In *Medicine, Science, and Culture: Historical Essays in Honor of Owsei Temkin*, edited by Lloyd G. Stevenson and Robert P. Multhauf, 123–141. Baltimore: Johns Hopkins University Press, 1968.
Clarke, Samuel. *A Discourse Concerning the Unchangeable Obligations of Natural Religion and . . . the Christian Revelation*. London, 1706. Published in 1711 as the second part of the author's *A Discourse Concerning the Being and Attributes of God*.
———. *The Works of Samuel Clarke*. London, 1738. Reprint, New York: Garland Publications, 1978.
Cleland, John. *Memoirs of a Woman of Pleasure*. Edited by Peter Sabor. Oxford: Oxford University Press, 1985.
Cogan, Thomas. *Specimen Medicum Inaugurale de Animi Pathematum vi et modo agendi in inducendis vel curandis morbis*. Leiden: Th. Haak, 1767.
Colman, John. *Locke's Moral Philosophy*. Edinburgh: Edinburgh University Press, 1983.
Cox, J. M. *Practical Observations on Insanity*. London: Baldwin and Murray, 1806.
Crichton, A. *An Inquiry into the Nature and Origin of Mental Derangement: Comprehending a Concise System of the Physiology and Pathology of the Human Mind. And a History of the Passions and their Effects*. London: Cadell and Davies, 1798.
Crimmins, James E. "Bentham on Religion, Atheism and the Secular Society." *Journal of the History of Ideas* 47 (1986): 95–110.
Crocker, Lester G. *An Age of Crisis: Man and World in Eighteenth Century French Thought*. Baltimore: Johns Hopkins University Press, 1959.

———. *Nature and Culture: Ethical Thought in the French Enlightenment.* Baltimore: Johns Hopkins Univeristy Press, 1963.
Cross, Wilbur. *The Life and Times of Laurence Sterne.* New Haven: Yale University Press, 1925.
Crue, B. L., et al. "Observations on the Taxonomy Problem in Pain." In *Chronic Pain: Further Observations from City of Hope National Medical Center,* edited by Benjamin L. Crue, Jr., M.D. New York: SP Medical and Scientific Books, 1978.
Daquin, J. *Philosophie de la folie.* Chambery: Gorrin, 1791; 2d ed., Chambery: Cleaz, 1804.
Darnton, Robert. *Mesmerism and the End of the Enlightenment in France.* Cambridge, Mass.: Harvard University Press, 1968.
———. *The Literary Underground of the Old Regime.* Cambridge: Harvard University Press, 1982.
Darwin, Erasmus. *Zoonomia; or, The Laws of Organic Life,* Parts I–III. 2 vols. London: J. Johnson, 1796.
Dean, Carolyn. "Law and Sacrifice: Bataille, Lacan, and the Critique of the Subject." *Representations* 13 (1986): 42–62.
DeJean, Joan. *Literary Fortifications: Rousseau, Laclos, Sade.* Princeton: Princeton University Press, 1984.
DePorte, Michael. *Nightmares and Hobbyhorses: Swift, Sterne, and Augustan Ideas of Madness.* San Marino, Calif.: Huntington Library, 1974.
Deprun, Jean. "Sade et la philosophie biologique de son temps." In *Le Marquis de Sade,* edited anonymously, 189–203. Paris: Armand Colin, 1968.
Descartes, René. *Treatise of Man.* Translated by Thomas Steele Hall. Cambridge, Mass.: Harvard University Press, 1972.
Deutsch, F. *On the Mysterious Leap from the Mind to the Body.* New York: International University Press, 1959.
Dictionnaire des sciences médicales. 60 vols. Paris: Panckoucke, 1812–1822.
Diderot, D., ed. *Encyclopédie; ou, Dictionnaire raisonné des sciences, des arts, et des métiers,* s.v. "Vapeurs." Lausanne and Berne: Chez les sociétés typographiques, 1782.
Diethelm, Oskar. *Medical Dissertations of Psychiatric Interest Printed before 1750.* New York: Karger, 1971.
Duden, Barbara. *Body History: Methodological Reflections upon Reading the Diaries of an Early Eighteenth-Century German Country Doctor.* Stuttgart: Klett-Cotta, 1987.
Dussinger, John A. *The Discourse of the Mind in Eighteenth-Century Fiction.* The Hague: Mouton, 1974.
———. "The Sensorium and the World of *A Sentimental Journey.*" *Ariel* 13 (1982): 3–16.
Eaves, T. C. Duncan, and Ben D. Kimpel. *Samuel Richardson: A Biography.* Oxford: Clarendon Press, 1971.
Eccles, John. *The Neurophysiological Basis of Mind.* Oxford: Clarendon Press, 1953.

Elias, Norbert. *The Civilizing Process.* 2 vols. New York: Urizen Books, 1978–1982.

Esquirol, J. E. D. *Des maladies mentales considerées sous les rapports médical, hygiénique et médico-légal.* 2 vols. Paris: Baillière, 1838.

———. *Des établissements des aliénés en France et des moyens d'améliorer le sort de ces infortunés: Mémoire présenté à son Excellence le ministère de l'intérieur en septembre 1818.* Paris: Huzard, 1819.

Essick, Robert N. "How Blake's Body Means." In *Unnam'd Forms: Blake and Textuality,* edited by Nelson Hilton and Thomas A. Vogler. Berkeley, Los Angeles, London: University of California Press, 1986.

Ewald, S. H. *Über das menschliche Herz: Ein Beitrag zur Charakteristik der Menschheit.* Erfurt: Schlegel, 1784.

Faas, Ekbert. *Retreat into the Mind: Victorian Poetry and the Rise of Psychiatry.* Princeton: Princeton University Press, 1988.

Faye, Jean-Pierre. "Changer la mort (Sade et la politique)." *Obliques* 12–13 (1977): 47–57.

Feder, J. G. H. *Grundlehre zur Kenntniss des menschlichen Willens und der natürlichen Gesetze des Rechtsverhaltens.* Göttingen: Dieterich, 1779.

Fedida, Pierre. "Les exercises de l'imagination et la commotion sur la masse des nerfs: Un érotisme de tête." In *Œuvres complètes du Marquis de Sade* 16:613–625. Paris: Au cercle du livre précieux, 1967.

Ferriar, J. *Medical Histories and Reflections.* London: Cadell and Davies, 1792–1798.

———. *Medical Histories and Reflections.* 3 vols. London: Cadell and Davies, 1795. Reprint, London: Tavistock Publications, 1970.

Figlio, Karl M. "The Metaphor of Organization: An Historiographical Perspective on the Bio-medical Sciences of the Early Nineteenth Century." *History of Sciences* 14 (1976): 17–53.

Flew, Antony, ed. *Body, Mind, and Death.* New York: Macmillan, 1974.

Forster, Robert, and Orest Ranum, eds. *Medicine and Society in France.* Translated by Elborg Forster and Patricia M. Ranum. Baltimore: Johns Hopkins University Press, 1980.

Foucault, Michel. *Madness and Civilization: A History of Insanity in the Age of Reason.* Translated by Richard Howard. New York: New American Library, 1965. Original French edition published 1961.

———. *The Order of Things: An Archaeology of the Human Sciences.* London: Tavistock Publications, 1970. Original French edition published 1966.

———. *The Birth of the Clinic: An Archaeology of Medical Perception.* Translated by Sheridan Smith. New York: Pantheon Books; London: Tavistock Publications, 1973. Original French edition published 1963.

———. *Discipline and Punish: The Birth of the Prison.* Translated by A. Sheridan. Harmondsworth: Penguin Books, 1979. Original French edition published 1975 under the title *Surveillir et punir: Naissance de la prison.*

———. *The History of Sexuality.* Translated by Robert Hurley. 3 vols. New York: Pantheon Books, 1978–1986. Original French edition published 1976–1984.

———. *Power-Knowledge: Selected Interviews and Other Writings 1972–1977.* Edited by Colin Gordon. New York: Pantheon Books, 1980.

Fox, Christopher, ed. *Psychology and Literature in the Eighteenth Century.* Illustrations by Michael DePorte. New York: AMS Press, 1987.

French, R. K. *Robert Whytt: The Soul and Medicine.* London: Wellcome Institute of the History of Medicine, 1969.

Freud, Sigmund. "Three Essays on the Theory of Sexuality." In *The Standard Edition of the Complete Psychological Works of Sigmund Freud,* translated and edited by James Strachey et al., 7:123–246. London: Hogarth Press, 1953–1974. These essays originally published 1905.

Fuller, Francis. *Medicina Gymnastica; or, A Treatise Concerning the Power of Exercise, with Respect to the Animal Oeconomy; and the Great Necessity of it in the Cure of Several Distempers.* London, 1705.

Gallagher, Catherine, and Thomas Lacqueur, eds. *The Making of the Modern Body.* Berkeley, Los Angeles, London: University of California Press, 1987.

Gallis, Francis. *Disputatio Medica Inauguralis de Anxietate.* Harderwijk: Johannes Mooyen, 1739.

Gallop, Jane. *Intersections: A Reading of Sade with Bataille, Blanchot, and Klossowski.* Lincoln: University of Nebraska Press, 1981.

Gardiner, Patrick. "Hume's Theory of the Passions." In *David Hume: A Symposium,* edited by D. F. Pears. London: Macmillan, 1963.

Garrett, Clarke. *Respectable Folly: Millenarians and the French Revolution in France and Britain.* Baltimore: Johns Hopkins University Press, 1975.

Gesenius, Wilhelm. *Medicinisch-moralische Pathematologie; oder, Versuch über die Leidenschaften und ihren Einfluss auf die Geschäfte des körperlichen Lebens.* Erfurt, 1786.

Gilman, Sander L. *Jewish Self-Hatred: Anti-Semitism and the Hidden Language of the Jews.* Baltimore and London: Johns Hopkins University Press, 1986.

Γνωθι σαυτον [Gnōthi sauton], oder Magazin zur Erfahrungsseelenkunde, als ein Lesebuch für Gelehrte und Ungelehrte, mit Unterstützung mehrerer Wahrheitsfreunde. 10 vols. Edited by C. P. Moritz and, as of vol. 9, S. Maimon. Berlin: Mylius, 1783–1793.

Goldstein, Rebecca. *The Mind-Body Problem: A Novel.* New York: Random House, 1983.

Griffin, Susan. *Pornography and Silence: Culture's Revenge against Nature.* New York: Harper and Row, 1981.

Gruman, Gerald J. *A History of Ideas about the Prolongation of Life: The Evolution of Prolongevity Hypotheses.* Transactions of the American Philosophical Society, n.s., vol. 56, pt. 9. Philadelphia, 1966.

Guislain, Joseph. *Traité sur l'aliénation mentale et sur les hospices des aliénés.* Amsterdam, 1826.

Hagstrum, Jean H. *Sex and Sensibility: Ideal and Erotic Love from Milton to Mozart.* Chicago: University of Chicago Press, 1980.

———. *The Romantic Body: Love and Sexuality in Keats, Wordworth, and Blake.* Knoxville: University of Tennessee Press, 1985.

Hallaran, W. S. *An Enquiry into the Causes Producing the Extra-ordinary Addition to the Number of Insane.* Cork: Edwards and Savage, 1810.
Haller, Albrecht von. *On the Sensible and Irritable Parts of Animals.* London, 1755.
Harper, Andrew. *A Treatise on the Real Cause and Cure of Insanity.* London: Stalker and Waltes, 1789.
Harrison, J. F. C. *The Second Coming: Popular Millenarianism 1780–1850.* London: Routledge and Kegan Paul, 1979.
Hartley, D. *Observations of Man, His Frame, His Duty, and His Expectations.* 4th ed. 3 vols. London: J. Johnson, 1801. First published 1749. Translated into French by the abbé R. A. C. Sicard under the title *De l'homme, de ses facultés physiques et intellectuelles, de ses devoirs, et de ses espérances,* 2 vols. (Paris: Ducauroy, 1802).
Haslam, J. *Observations on Insanity.* London: Rivington, 1798.
———. *Observations on Madness and Melancholy.* 2d ed. London: Callow, 1809.
Hassan, Ihab. "Sade: Prisoner of Consciousness." *TriQuarterly* 15 (1969): 23–24.
Haygarth, John. *Of the Imagination, as a Cause and as a Cure of Disorders of the Body.* Bath: Cadell and Davies, 1800.
Heimann, P. M., and McGuire, J. E. "Newtonian Forces and Lockean Powers: Concepts of Matter in Eighteenth-Century Thought." *Historical Studies in Physical Science* 3 (1971): 233–306.
Heinroth, J. C. *Lehrbuch der Störungen des Seelenlebens; oder, Seelenstörungen und ihre Behandlung.* Leipzig: Vogel, 1818.
Henaff, Marcel. *Sade: L'invention du corps libertin.* Paris: Presses universitaires de France, 1978.
———. "Tout dire ou l'encyclopédie de l'excès." *Obliques* 12–13 (1977): 29–37.
Herz, M. H. *Versuch über den Schwindel.* Berlin: Voss, 1786.
Hill, John. *Hypochondriasis: A Practical Treatise on the Nature and Cure of that Disorder, Commonly Called the Hyp and the Hypo.* London, 1766. Reprint, Los Angeles: William Andrews Clark Memorial Library, University of California, 1969, as no. 135 of the Publications of the Augustan Reprint Society. Introduction to reprint by G. S. Rousseau.
Himmelfarb, Gertrude. "The Haunted House of Jermy Bentham." In *Victorian Minds,* 32–81. New York: Alfred Knopf, 1968.
Hobbes, Thomas. *Leviathan.* Edited with Introduction by Michael Oakeshott. Oxford: B. Blackwell, 1960. Originally published 1651.
———. *The Moral and Political Works of Thomas Hobbes of Malmesbury.* London, 1750.
Hoffbauer, J. C. *Untersuchungen über die Krankheiten der Seele und die verwandten Zustände.* 3 vols. Halle: Trampen, 1802–1807.
———. *Die Psychologie nach ihren Hauptanwendungen auf die Rechtspflege oder die sogenannte gerichtliche Arzneiwissenschaft nach ihrem psychologischen Teile.* Halle: Schimmelpfennig, 1801; 2d ed., 1823.
Hoffmann, Paul. "Le discours médical sur les passions de l'amour, de Bossier de Sauvages à Pinel." In *Aimer en France, 1760–1860,* edited by Paul Viallaneix

and Jean Ehrard, 2:345–356. Clermont-Ferrand: Association des publications de la Faculté des lettres et sciences humaines de Clermont-Ferrand, 1980.

Horkheimer, Max, and Theodore Adorno. *Dialectic of Enlightenment.* Translated by John Cumming. New York: Herder and Herder, 1972. Original German edition published 1944.

Huisinga, Matthaeus. *Dissertatio Medica Inauguralis sistens Incubi causas praecipuas.* Leiden: Gerard Poortvliet, 1734.

Hume, David. *An Enquiry concerning the Principles of Morals.* In *Enquiries concerning Human Understanding and concerning the Principles of Morals,* edited with introduction and analytical index by L. A. Selby-Bigge, 3d rev. ed., edited by P. H. Nidditch. Oxford: Clarendon Press, 1975. Originally published 1751.

———. *A Treatise of Human Nature.* Edited with introduction and analytical index by L. A. Selby-Bigge. 3d rev. ed. Edited by P. H. Nidditch. Oxford: Clarendon Press, 1978. Originally published 1739–1740.

Hunter, Richard, and Ida Macalpine. *Three Hundred Years of Psychiatry 1535–1800.* London: Oxford University Press, 1963.

Hutcheson, Francis. *An Inquiry concerning Beauty, Order, Harmony, Design.* Edited with introduction and notes by Peter Kivy. The Hague: Martinus Nijhoff, 1973. Originally published 1725. This is the first of two treatises that together constitute *An Inquiry into the Original of Our Ideas of Beauty and Virtue.*

Ignatieff, Michael. *A Just Measure of Pain: The Penitentiary in the Industrial Revolution 1750–1850.* London: Macmillan, 1978.

Imbroscio, C. "Recherches et réflexions de la médecine française du dix-huitième siècle sur des phénomènes psychosomatiques." *Studies on Voltaire and the Eighteenth Century* 190 (1980): 494–502.

Jobe, T. H. "Medical Theories of Melancholia in the Seventeenth and Early Eighteenth Centuries." *Clio Medica* 19 (1976): 217–231.

Johnson, Mark. *The Body in the Mind: The Bodily Basis of Meaning, Imagination, and Reason.* Chicago: University of Chicago Press, 1987.

Jordanova, Ludmilla, ed. *Languages of Nature: Critical Essays on Science and Literature.* London: Free Association Books, 1986.

Kant, I. "Von der Macht des Gemuths durch den blossen Vorsatz seiner krankhaften Gefühle Meister zu sein." In Hufeland's *Journal der praktischen Arzneikunde und Wundarzneikunst* 5 (1798): 701–751. Reissued later, with comments (Leipzig: Reclam, 1824).

Kearns, Michael. *Metaphors of Mind in Fiction and Psychology.* Lexington: University Press of Kentucky, 1987.

Keele, K. D. *Anatomies of Pain.* Oxford; Blackwell Scientific Publications, 1957.

Kerby-Miller, C., ed. *Memoirs of the Extraordinary Life, Works and Discoveries of Martinus Scriblerus.* New York: Russell and Russell, 1966.

Kermode, Frank. *The Sense of an Ending.* Oxford: Oxford Univesity Press, 1966.

Kieft, L., and B. R. Willeford, eds. *Joseph Priestley: Scientist, Theologian and Metaphysician.* Lewisburg, Pa.: Bucknell University Press, 1980.

Kiellman, T. Z. *Dissertatio Medica Inauguralis de Incubo.* Leiden: Van der Aa, 1739.

King, L. "Mirror of Eighteenth-Century Medicine." *Bulletin of the History of Medicine* 48 (1974): 517–539.

———. *The Medical World of the Eighteenth Century.* Chicago: University of Chicago Press, 1958.

———. *The Philosophy of Medicine: The Early Eighteenth Century.* Cambridge, Mass.: Harvard University Press, 1978.

King, Peter, Seventh Baron. *The Life and Letters of John Locke, Together with Extracts from His Journals and Commonplace Books.* London: H. Colburn, 1829.

Kirchovius, Paulus. *Dissertatio Medical Inauguralis de Mentis et Animae Humanae consensu et dissensu.* Leiden: Conrad Wishoff, 1725.

Klossowski, Pierre, *Sade mon prochain.* Paris: Seuil, 1947

Kossmann, E. F. *Nieuwe Bijdragen tot de Geschiedenis van het Nederlandsche Tooneel in de 17e en 18e eeuw.* The Hague: Martinus Nijhoff, 1915.

Kraus, Pamela. "Locke's Negative Hedonism," *Locke Newsletter* 15 (1984): 43–63.

Kydd, Rachel. *Reason and Conduct in Hume's Treatise.* Oxford: Oxford University Press, 1946.

Lacan, Jacques, "Kant avec Sade." *Critique* 19 (1963): 291–313.

Laehr, Heinrich. *Die Literatur der Psychiatrie, Neurologie und Psychologie von 1459–1799.* Berlin: Reimer, 1900.

Lain Entralgo, Pedro. *Mind and Body: Psychosomatic Pathology—a Short History of the Evolution of Medical Thought.* London: Harvill Press, 1955.

Laird, John. *Hume's Philosophy of Human Nature.* London: Methuen, 1932.

La Mettrie, Julien Offray de. *L'Homme Machine: A Study in the Origins of an Idea.* Edited by Aram Vartanian. Princeton: Princeton University Press, 1960.

Lamprecht, Sterling P. *The Moral and Political Philosophy of John Locke.* New York: Columbia University Press, 1918.

Lawrence, Christopher. "The Nervous System and Society in the Scottish Enlightenment." In *Natural Order: Historical Studies of Scientific Culture,* edited by Barry Barnes and Steven Shapin, 19–40. Beverly Hills, Calif.: Sage Publications, 1979.

Lederer, Laura, ed. *Take Back the Night: Women on Pornography.* New York: William Morrow, 1980.

Lenhossek, H. *Untersuchungen über die Leidenschaften und Gemutsaffecten als Ursachen und Heilmittel der Krankheiten.* Thesis in Medicine, Pest, 1804.

Lesch, John E. *Science and Medicine in France: The Emergence of Experimental Physiology, 1790–1855.* Cambridge, Mass.: Harvard University Press, 1984.

Leventhal, Herbert. *In the Shadow of the Enlightenment: Occultism and Renaissance Science in Eighteenth Century America.* New York: New York University Press, 1976.

Lewis, C. S. *The Problem of Pain.* 1940. Reprint, New York: Macmillan, 1944.

Locke, John. *The Educational Writings of John Locke.* Introduction and notes by James L. Axtell. Cambridge: Cambridge University Press, 1968.

———. *Two Tracts on Government.* Edited with introduction, notes and translation

by Philip Abrams. Cambridge: Cambridge University Press, 1967.
———. *The Correspondence of John Locke*. Edited by E. S. De Beer. Oxford: Clarendon Press, 1976–.
———. *An Essay concerning Human Understanding*. Edited by P. H. Nidditch. Oxford: Clarendon Press, 1979. Originally published 1690.
———. *Essay on the Law of Nature*. Latin text, with translation, introduction and notes by W. von Leyden, together with transcription of Locke's shorthand in his journal for 1676. Oxford: Clarendon Press, 1954.
Long, Philip. *A Summary Catalogue of the Lovelace Collection of the Papers of John Locke in the Bodleian Library*. Oxford: Oxford University Press, 1959.
López Piñero, J. M. *Historical Origins of the Concept of Neurosis*. Translated by D. Berrios. Cambridge: Cambridge University Press, 1983.
Mabbot, John David. *John Locke*. London: Macmillan, 1973.
Maccubbin, Robert P., ed. *Unauthorized Sexual Behavior during the Enlightenment*. Special issue of *Eighteenth-Century Life* (9, n.s. 3 [1986]). Reissued as *'Tis Nature's Fault: Unauthorized Sexuality during the Enlightenment* (Cambridge: Cambridge University Press, 1988).
MacDonald, Michael. *Mystical Bedlam: Madness, Anxiety and Healing in Seventeenth-Century England*. Cambridge: Cambridge University Press, 1981.
Mack, Mary. *Jeremy Bentham: An Odyssey of Ideas, 1748–1792*. London: Heinemann, 1962.
MacKenzie, James. *The History of Health and the Art of Preserving It*. Edinburgh, 1758.
Mackie, John L. *Hume's Moral Theory*. London: Routlege and Kegan Paul, 1980.
MacLean, Kenneth. *John Locke and English Literature of the Eighteenth Century*. New Haven: Yale University Press; London: H. Milford, 1936.
Mandeville, Bernard, M.D. *A Treatise of the Hypochondriack and Hysterick Diseases in Three Dialogues*. 3d ed. London, 1730 (1st ed., 1711).
Marées, Christiaan H. de. *Disputatio Medica Inauguralis de Animi Perturbationum in corpus potentia*. Göttingen: Dieterich, 1775.
Matson, W. I. "Why Isn't the Mind-Body Problem Ancient?" In *Mind, Matter, and Method*, edited by P. K. Feyerabend and G. Maxwell. Minneapolis: University of Minnesota Press, 1966.
Maudsley, Henry. *Body and Mind*. London: Macmillan, 1870.
McDowell, John. "Are Moral Requirements Hypothetical Imperatives?" *Proceedings of the Aristotelian Society Supplementary Volume* 52 (1978): 13–30.
———. "Virtue and Reason." *The Monist* 62 (1979): 331–350.
McEvoy, J. G., and J. E. McGuire. "God and Nature: Priestley's Way of Rational Dissent." *Historical Studies in Physical Science* 6 (1975): 325–404.
McManners, John. *Death and the Enlightenment*. Oxford: Oxford University Press, 1981.
Meier, G. F. *Über Gemutsbewegungen*. Halle: Hemmerde, 1759.
Melzack, Ronald, and Patrick D. Wall. *The Challenge of Pain*. New York: Basic Books, 1983.

Miller, Jonathan. *The Body in Question.* New York: Random House, 1978.
Miller, Nancy K. "*Juliette* and the Posterity of Prosperity." *L'esprit créateur* 15 (1975): 413–424.
———. "*Justine*; or, The Vicious Circle." In *Studies in Eighteenth-Century Culture,* vol. 5, edited by Ronald C. Rosbottom, 215–228. Madison: University of Wisconsin Press, 1976.
Monje, J. J. *Specimen Medicum Inaugurale de Animi Pathematibus eorumque effectibus; nec non salutari eorundem in morbis efficacia.* Leiden: Ar. and J. Houkoop and Andr. Koster, 1785.
Montagu, Ashley. *Man's Most Dangerous Myth: The Fallacy of Race.* 5th ed. New York: Oxford Univesity Press, 1974.
Moore, C. A. "The English Malady." In *Backgrounds of English Literature, 1700–1760.* Minneapolis: University of Minnesota Press, 1953.
Moore, George. *The Use of the Body in Relation to the Mind.* London: Longman, 1847.
Moore, George Edward. *Principia Ethica.* Cambridge: Cambridge University Press, 1903.
Moravia, Sergio. "From *Homme Machine* to *Homme Sensible*: Changing Eighteenth-Century Models of Man's Image," *Journal of the History of Ideas* 39 (1978): 45–60.
Morris, Colin. *The Discovery of the Individual, 1050–1200.* New York: Harper and Row, 1972.
Morris, David B. "The Languages of Pain." In *Exploring the Concept of Mind,* edited by Richard M. Caplan, 89–99. Iowa City: University of Iowa Press, 1986.
Mullan, John. "Hypochondria and Hysteria: Sensibility and the Physicians." *The Eighteenth Century: Theory and Interpretation* 25, no. 2 (1984): 141–177.
Muratori, L. A. *Ueber die Einbildungskraft des Menschen, mit vielen Zusätzen herausgegeben.* Edited by Georg Hermann Richters. Leipzig, 1785. Originally published in Italian in 1734.
Myers, C. S. *The Absurdity of Any Mind-Body Relation.* Oxford and London, 1932.
Nagel, Thomas. *The View from Nowhere.* New York: Oxford University Press, 1986.
Neal, Helen. *The Politics of Pain.* New York: McGraw-Hill, 1978.
New, Melvyn. "'The Grease of God': The Form of Eighteenth-Century Fiction." *PMLA* 91, no. 2 (1976): 235–243.
O'Brien, Gordon W. "The Genius and the Mortal Instruments: Mind and Body and the Romantic Imagination," *Minnesota Review* 6 (1966): 316–352.
Odegard, Douglas. "Locke and Mind-Body Dualism." *Philosophy* 45 (1970): 87–105.
Onians, R. B. *The Origins of European Thought about the Body, the Mind, the Soul, the World, Time, and Fate.* Cambridge: Cambridge University Press, 1951.
Ouwens, Wilhelmus. *Dissertatio Medica Inauguralis de Horrore.* Leiden: Johannes Hasebroek, 1737.
Pargeter, W. *Observations on Maniacal Disorders.* Reading: For the author, 1792.

Pemberton, Thomas. *Dissertatio Medica Inauguralis de Metu.* Leiden: S. and J. Luchtmans, 1777.
Perfect, W. *Select Cases in the Different Species of Insanity, Lunacy, or Madness, with the Modes of Practice as adopted in the Treatment of each.* Rochester: Gillman, 1797.
Pernick, Martin S. *A Calculus of Suffering: Pain, Professionalism, and Anesthesia in Nineteenth-Century America.* New York: Columbia University Press, 1985.
Pinel, P. "Mémoire sur la manie périodique ou intermittente." *Mémoires de la Société médicale d'émulation* 1 (An V [1796–97]): 94–119.
———. "Recherches et observations sur le traitement moral des aliénés." Ibid. 2 (An VI [1797–98]): 215–255.
———. "Observations sur les aliénés et leur division en espèces distinctes." Ibid. 3 (An VII [1798–99]): 1–26.
———. *Nosographie philosophique; ou, Méthode de l'analyse appliquée à la médecine.* Paris: Brosson, 1798; 2d ed., 3 vols., 1802–1803; 3d ed., 1807; 4th ed., 1810; 5th ed., 1913; 6th ed., 1818.
———. *Traité médico-philosophique sur l'aliénation mentale ou la manie.* Paris: Caille et Ravier, 1800.
———. *La médecine clinique rendue plus exacte par l'application de l'analyse; ou, Recueil et résultat d'observations sur les maladies aiguës, faites à la Salpetriere.* Paris: Brosson, Gabon et Cie, 1802.
———. *Lettres de Pinel.* Edited by C. Pinel. Paris: Masson, 1859.
Piquer, A. "Discurso sobre la enfermedad de el Rey nuestro Señor Don Fernando VI (que Dios guarde) escrito por Don Andres Piquer, medico de camara de S.M." In *Coleccion de documentos ineditos para la historia de España* 18:156–221. Madrid: Viuda de Calero, 1851.
Pomme, P. *Traité des affections vaporeuses des deux sexes.* Lyon: Duplain, 1762.
Porter, Roy. "Against the Spleen." In *Laurence Sterne: Riddles and Mysteries,* edited by V. G. Myer, 84–98. London: Vision; Totowa, N.J.: Barnes and Noble, 1984.
Price, Richard. *A Review of the Principal Questions in Morals.* Edited by D. Daiches Raphael. Oxford: Clarendon Press, 1948. Orignally published 1758.
Priestley, Joseph. *Scientific autobiography.* Edited by R. E. Schofield. Cambridge, Mass.: MIT Press, 1966.
———. *An examination of Dr. Reid's "Inquiry into the human mind on the principles of common sense," Dr. Beattie's "Essay on the Nature and Immutability of Truth" and Dr. Oswald's "Appeal to Common Sense in Behalf of Religion."* London: J. Johnson, 1774.
———. *Hartley's Theory of the Human Mind on the Principle of the Association of Ideas.* London: J. Johnson, 1775.
———. *Disquisitions relating to matter and spirit.* London: J. Johnson, 1777.
———. *A free discussion of the doctrines of materialism and philosophical necessity.* London: J. Johnson and T. Cadell, 1778.
Purcell, John. *A treatise of Vapours; or, Hysterick Fits.* London: E. Place, 1707.
Pussin, J. B. "Observations du citoyen Pussin sur les fous." Archives nationales,

27 AP 8 (doc. 2). For an annotated English translation, see D. B. Weiner, "The Apprenticeship of Philippe Pinel: A New Document, 'Observations of Citizen Pussin on the Insane,'" *American Journal of Psychiatry* 136 (1979): 1128–1134.

Putnam, Hilary. "How Old Is the Mind?" In *Exploring the Concept of Mind,* edited by Richard Caplan. Iowa City: University of Iowa Press, 1986.

Ramazini, Bern. *A Treatise on the Disease of Tradesmen, to which they are subject by their particular Callings.* Translated and edited by Dr. James. London, 1740.

Raphael, D. Daiches, ed. *British Moralists 1650–1800.* Oxford: Clarendon Press, 1969.

Rather, L. J. "G. E. Stahl's Psychological Physiology." *Bulletin for the History of Medicine* 35 (1961): 37–49.

———. *Mind and Body in Eighteenth-Century Medicine.* London: Wellcome Historical Medical Library, 1965.

———. "The 'Six Things Non-Natural': A Note on the Origins and Fate of a Doctrine and a Phrase." *Clio Medica* 3 (1968): 337–347.

Raulin, J. *Traité des affections vaporeuses des deux sexes.* Paris: Herissant, 1758.

Reich, J. J. *Disputatio Medica Inauguralis de Passionibus Animi Corpus Humanum Varie Alterantibus.* Halle: Typ. C. Salfeldii, 1695.,

Reil, J. C. *Rhapsodieen über die Anwendung der psychischen Curmethode auf Geisteszerruttungen.* Halle: Curt, 1803.

Reil, J. C., and J. C. Hoffbauer, eds. *Beyträge zur Beförderung einer Curmethode auf psychischem Wege.* 2 vols. Halle: Curt, 1808.

Reiser, Stanley. *Medicine and the Reign of Technology.* Cambridge and New York: Cambridge University Press, 1978.

Richardson, Samuel. *The Correspondence of Samuel Richardson.* Edited by Anna Laetitia Barbauld. London: R. Phillips, 1804.

Riese, Walther. *A History of Neurology.* New York: MD Publications, 1959.

Riffaterre, Michael. "Sade, or Text as Fantasy." *Diacritics* 2 (1972): 2–9.

Rivers, Isabel, ed. *Books and Their Readers in Eighteenth-Century England.* New York: St. Martin's Press, 1982.

Robinson, Nicholas. *A New Method of Treating Consumptions: Wherein all the Decays Incident to Human Bodies, are Mechanically Accounted for.* London: 1727.

———. *A New System of the Spleen.* London: Bettesworth, 1729.

Rodgers, James. "'Life' in the Novel: *Tristram Shandy* and Some Aspects of Eighteenth-Century Physiology." *Eighteenth-Century Life* 1 (1980): 1–20.

Roger, Jacques. *Les sciences de la vie dans la pensée française du XVIIIe siècle: La génération des animaux de Descartes à l'Encyclopédie.* Paris: Armand Colin, 1963.

Rohde, Erwin. *Psyche: The Cult of Souls and Belief in Immortality among the Greeks.* Translated by W. B. Hills. London and New York, 1925.

Rosen, George. "Emotion and Sensibility in Ages of Anxiety: A Comparative Historical Review." *American Journal of Psychiatry* 6, no. 124 (1967): 771–783.

———. *From Medical Police to Social Medicine: Essays on the History of Health Care.* New York: Science History Publications, 1974.

Rousseau, G. S. "Science and the Discovery of the Imagination in Enlightened England." *Eighteenth-Century Studies* 3 (1969–70): 108–135.

———. "Nerves, Spirits and Fibres: Towards Defining the Origins of Sensibility." In *Studies in the Eighteenth Century, III,* edited by R. F. Brissenden and J. C. Eade. Toronto and Buffalo: University of Toronto Press, 1976. Reprinted in *The Blue Guitar* (Messina) 2 (1976): 125–153.

———. "Science and Literature: The State of the Field." *Isis* 69 (1978): 583–591.

———. "Psychology." In *The Ferment of Knowledge,* edited by G. S. Rousseau and Roy Porter, 143–210. Cambridge: Cambridge University Press, 1980.

———. "Literature and Medicine: The State of the Field." *Isis* 72 (1981): 406–424.

———. "Nymphomania, Bienville and the Rise of Erotic Sensibility." In *Sexuality in Eighteenth-Century Britain,* edited by Paul-Gabriel Boucé, 95–120. Manchester: Manchester University Press, 1982.

———. "Smollett and the Eighteenth-Century Sulphur Controversy." In *Tobias Smollett: Essays of Two Decades,* 144–157. Edinburgh, 1982.

———. "Mysticism and Millenarianism: 'Immortal Dr. Cheyne.'" In *Hermeticism in the Renaissance,* edited by Allen Debus, 192–230. Washington, D.C.: The Folger Shakespeare Library, 1988.

Rousseau, G. S., and Roy Porter, eds. *The Ferment of Knowledge: Studies in the Historiography of Eighteenth-Century Science.* Cambridge: Cambridge University Press, 1980.

———, eds. *Sexual Underworlds of the Enlightenment.* Manchester: Manchester University Press, 1986.

———, eds. *Exoticism in the Enlightenment.* Manchester: Manchester University Press, 1990.

Ryle, Gilbert. *Dilemmas.* Cambridge: Cambridge University Press, 1954.

Sade, Marquis de. *Juliette.* Translated by Austryn Wainhouse. 6 vols. in 1. New York: Grove Press, 1968.

———. *Œuvres complètes du Marquis de Sade.* 16 vols. Paris: Au cercle du livre précieux, 1966–1967.

———. *The 120 Days of Sodom and Other Writings.* Translated by Austryn Wainhouse and Richard Seaver. New York: Grove Press, 1966.

———. *The Complete Justine, Philosophy in the Bedroom, and Other Writings.* Translated by Richard Seaver and Austryn Wainhouse. New York: Grove Press, 1965.

Scarry, Elaine, *The Body in Pain: The Making and Unmaking of the World.* New York: Oxford University Press, 1985.

Schmidt, J. J. *Behandlung der Krankheiten des Organs der Seele.* Hamburg: Hoffmann, 1797.

Schofield, Robert E. *Mechanism and Materialism: British Natural Philosophy in an Age of Reason.* Princeton: Princeton University Press, 1970.

Schouten, Dirk. *Dissertatio Medicina Inauguralis de Anxietate.* Leiden: Johannes Luzac, 1742.

Selby-Bigge, L. A., ed. *British Moralists: Being Selections from Writers Principally of the Eighteenth Century*. Oxford: Clarendon Press, 1897. Reprint, New York: Dover, 1965.

Sena, John. "Smollett's Persona and the Melancholic Traveler." *Eighteenth-Century Studies* 1 (1968): 353–369.

Shaftesbury, Third Earl of (Anthony Ashley Cooper). *Characteristics of Men, Manners, Opinions, Times*. Edited with introduction and notes by John M. Robertson. Indianapolis: Bobbs-Merrill, 1964. Originally published 1711.

Shklar, Judith. *Ordinary Vices*. Cambridge: Harvard University Press, 1984.

Shorter, E. *A History of Women's Bodies*. Harmondsworth: Penguin, 1983.

Shortland, M. "Barthes, Lavater and the Visible Body." *Economy and Society* 14 (1985): 273–312.

Siegel, Rudolph E. *Galen's System of Physiology and Medicine*. New York: S. Karger, 1968.

Simon, Bennett. *Mind and Madness in Ancient Greece*. Ithaca, N.Y.: Cornell University Press, 1978.

Smith, Peter, and O. R. Jones. *The Philosophy of Mind: An Introduction*. Cambridge: Cambridge University Press, 1982.

Smith, Roger. "The Background of Physiological Psychology in Natural Philosophy." *History of Science* 2 (1973): 75–123.

Smollett, Tobias. *The Expedition of Humphry Clinker*. Edited by Lewis M. Knapp. London, 1966. Originally published 1771.

———. *The Letters of Tobias Smollett*. Edited by Lewis M. Knapp. Oxford, 1970.

———. *The Adventures of Roderick Random*. Edited by P. G. Boucé. Oxford, 1979. Originally published 1748.

———. *Travels through France and Italy*. Edited by Frank Felsenstein. Oxford, 1981. Originally published 1766.

Smyth, James Carmichael. *An Account of the Effects of Swinging, Employed as a Remedy in the Pulmonary Consumption and Hectic Fever*. London, 1787.

Snell, Bruno. *The Discovery of the Mind*. Oxford: Oxford Univeristy Press, 1953.

Sollers, Philippe. "Sade dans le texte." In *L'écriture et l'expérience des limites*. Paris: Seuil, 1968.

Solmsen, Friedrich. "Greek Philosophy and the Discovery of the Nerves." *Museum Helveticum* 18 (1961): 150–167.

Sontag, Susan. "The Pornographic Imagination." In *Styles of Radical Will*. New York: Farrar, Straus and Giroux, 1966.

———. *Illness as Metaphor*. London: Allen Lane, 1979.

Spillane, J. *The Doctrine of the Nerves*. London: Oxford University Press, 1981.

Staum, Martin S. *Cabanis: Enlightenment and Medical Philosophy in the French Revolution*. Princeton: Princeton University Press, 1980.

Stead, C. K. *The Death of the Body*. London: Collins, 1986.

Sterne, Laurence. *The Life and Opinions of Tristram Shandy Gentleman*. Edited by Melvyn New and Joan New. Gainesville: University of Florida Press, 1978–1984.

———. *The Letters of Laurence Sterne*. Edited by Lewis Perry Curtis. Oxford, 1965.

———. *A Sentimental Journey through France and Italy by Mr. Yorick*. Edited by

Gardner Stout. Berkelely and Los Angeles: University of California Press, 1967.

Stevenson, Charles L. *Ethics and Language*. New Haven: Yale University Press, 1945.

Stevenson, Lloyd G., and Robert P. Multhauf, eds. *Essays in Honor of Owsei Temkin*. Baltimore: Johns Hopkins University Press, 1968.

Stroud, Barry. *Hume*. The Arguments of the Philosophers. London: Routledge and Kegan Paul, 1977.

Thomas, Keith. *Religion and the Decline of Magic*. Harmondsworth: Penguin, 1973.

Thomson, Ann. "L'art de jouir de La Mettrie à Sade." In *Aimer en France 1760–1860*, edited by Paul Viallaneix and Jean Ehrard, 2:315–322. Clermont-Ferrand: Association des publications de la Faculté des lettres et sciences humaines de Clermont-Ferrand, 1980.

Thomson, David. *Wild Excursions: The Life and Fiction of Laurence Sterne*. New York, 1972.

Trotter, T. *An Essay, Medical, Philosophical and Chemical on Drunkenness*. London: Longman, 1804.

Tryon, Thomas. *A Treatise of Dreams and Visions*. London, 1695.

Tuke, S. *Description of the Retreat, an Institution near York, for Insane Persons of the Society of Friends*. York: W. Alexander, 1813.

Turner, B. S. *The Body and Society: Explorations in Social Theory*. Oxford: Blackwell, 1984.

Tuveson, E. *The Imagination as a Means of Grace*. Berkeley and Los Angeles: University of California Press, 1960.

Van Sant, Ann. *Entrapment and Display: A Study of Eighteenth-Century Sentimentality*. New York: Columbia University Press, 1990.

Veith, I. *Hysteria: The History of a Disease*. Chicago: University of Chicago Press, 1965.

Vess, David M. *Medical Revolution in France, 1789–1796*. Gainesville: University Presses of Florida, 1975.

Viallaneix, Paul, and Jean Ehrard, eds. *Aimer en France, 1760–1860: Actes du colloque international de Clermont-Ferrand*. Clermont-Ferrand: Association des publications de la Faculté des lettres et sciences humaines, 1980.

Voyer, Isaac. *Dissertatio Medica Inauguralis de Anxietate*. Leiden: Henricus Mostert, 1769.

Wagner, Peter. *Eros Revived: Erotica in the Age of Enlightenment*. London: Secker and Warburg, 1989.

Wagnitz, H. B. *Historische Nachrichten und Bemerkungen über die merkwürdigsten Zuchthäuser in Deutschland, nebst einem Anhang über die zweckmässigste Einrichtung der Gefängnisse und Irrenanstalten*. 3 vols. Halle: Gebauer, 1791–1794.

Weickard, M. A. *Der philosophische Arzt*. Leipzig, 1775. 2 vols., Frankfurt: Andres, 1790.

Wesley, John. *Primitive Physick, or, An Easy and Natural Method of Curing Most Diseases*. London, 1747.

Whytt, R. *Observations on the Nature, Causes, and Cure of those Disorders which have been called Nervous, Hypochondriac, or Hysteric, to which are prefixed some Remarks on the Sympathy of the Nerves.* Edinburgh: Becket and Du Hondt, 1765.

Wigner, E. P. "Remarks on the Mind-Body Question." In *The Scientist Speculates: An Anthology of Partly Baked Ideas,* edited by I. J. Good, 284–302. New York: Basic Books, 1962.

Wilson, M. D. "Body and Mind from the Cartesian Point of View." In *Body and Mind: Past, Present and Future,* edited by R. W. Rieber. New York, 1980.

Wittgenstein, Ludwig. *Philosophical Investigations.* Translated by G. E. M. Anscombe. London: Macmillan, 1953; 3d. rev. ed., 1967.

Wolf, Fred Alan. *The Body Quantum: The Physics of the Human Body.* London: Heinemann, 1987.

Wolfe, Richard J. "The Hang-up of Franz Kotzwara and Its Relationship to Sexual Quackery in Late 18th-Century London." *Studies on Voltaire and the Eighteenth Century* 228 (1984): 47–66.

Wollaston, William. *The Religion of Nature Delineated.* Introduction by Stanley Tweyman. Delmar, N.Y.: Scholars' Facsimiles and Reprints, 1974. Originally published 1724.

Woolf, Virginia. "On Being Ill." In *Collected Essays* 4:193–203. London: Chatto and Windus, 1966.

Wright, Peter, and Andrew Treacher, eds. *The Problem of Medical Knowledge: Examining the Social Construction of Medicine.* Edinburgh: Edinburgh University Press, 1982.

Yolton, John. *John Locke and the Way of Ideas.* Oxford: Clarendon Press, 1956.

———. *Thinking Matter: Materialism in Eighteenth-Century Britain.* Oxford: Blackwell; Minneapolis: University of Minnesota Press, 1983.

Zwager, H. H. *Nederland en de Verlichting.* Haarlem: Fibula–Van Dishoeck, 1980.

INDEX

Note: This index contains materials found in the main text only, not in the footnotes.

Designer:	U.C. Press Staff
Compositor:	Prestige Typography
Text:	10/12 Baskerville
Display:	Baskerville
Printer:	Braun-Brumfield, Inc.
Binder:	Braun-Brumfield, Inc.